DIAGNOSTIC PATHOLOGY

PLACENTA

AMIRSYS®

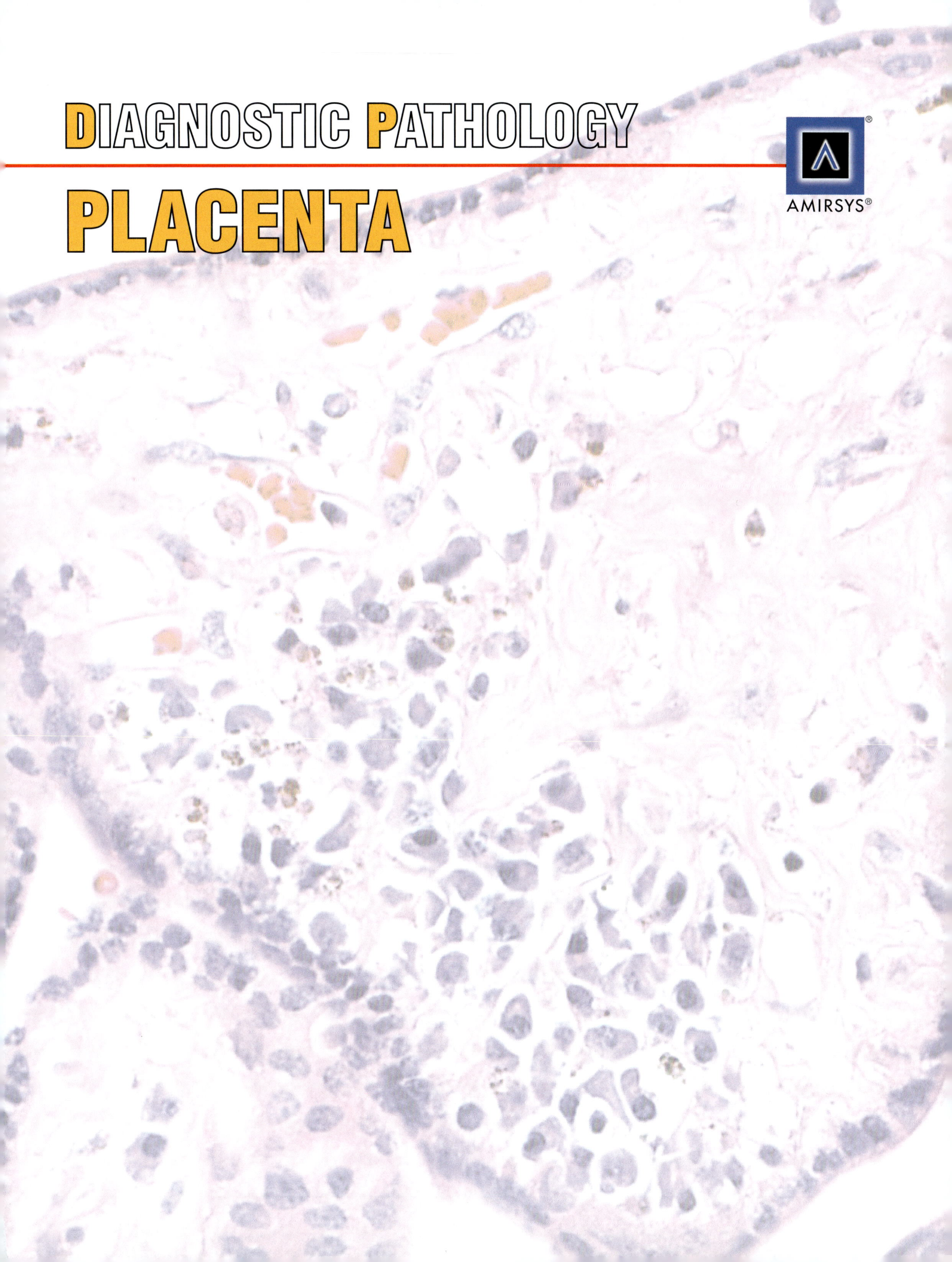

DIAGNOSTIC PATHOLOGY

PLACENTA

Amy Heerema-McKenney, MD
Contract Staff Physician
Cleveland Clinic Institute of Pathology and Laboratory Medicine
Cleveland, Ohio

Edwina J. Popek, DO
Professor of Pathology and Pediatrics
Baylor College of Medicine
Texas Children's Hospital Pavilion for Women
Houston, Texas

Monique E. De Paepe, MD, MSc
Professor of Pathology and Laboratory Medicine
Women and Infants Hospital
Alpert Medical School of Brown University
Providence, Rhode Island

Linda M. Ernst, MD, MHS
Associate Professor of Pathology
Northwestern University
Feinberg School of Medicine
Chicago, Illinois

Bahig M. Shehata, MD
Professor of Pathology and Pediatrics
Emory University School of Medicine
Pediatric Pathologist
Children's Healthcare of Atlanta
Atlanta, Georgia

Eileen Margaret McKay, MD
Assistant Professor of Clinical Pathology and Laboratory Medicine
Perelman School of Medicine
University of Pennsylvania
The Children's Hospital of Philadelphia
Philadelphia, Pennsylvania

Karen Marie Chisholm, MD, PhD
Pathology Fellow
Stanford University School of Medicine
Stanford, California

Philip J. Katzman, MD
Associate Professor of Pathology and Laboratory Medicine
University of Rochester Medical Center
Rochester, New York

Rebecca L. Linn, MD
Pathology Resident
Northwestern University
Feinberg School of Medicine
Chicago, Illinois

Jason A. Jarzembowski, MD, PhD
Program Director, Perinatal Pathology
Children's Hospital of Wisconsin
Associate Professor of Pathology
Medical College of Wisconsin
Milwaukee, Wisconsin

Caitlin Cundiff, BS
Research Scientist
Emory University School of Medicine
Atlanta, Georgia

Jessica Labib, BA
Medical Student
Emory University School of Medicine
Atlanta, Georgia

ELSEVIER

1600 John F. Kennedy Blvd.
Ste 1800
Philadelphia, PA 19103-2899

DIAGNOSTIC PATHOLOGY: PLACENTA

ISBN: 978-1-937242-22-0

Publisher Cataloging-in-Publication Data

Diagnostic pathology : placenta / [edited by] Amy Heerema-McKenney, Edwina J. Popek, and Monique E. De Paepe.
pages ; cm
Placenta
Includes bibliographical references and index.
ISBN 978-1-937242-22-0 (hardback)
1. Placenta--Diseases--Atlases. 2. Pathology--Atlases. I. HeeremaMcKenney, Amy. II. Popek, Edwina J. III. De Paepe, Monique E. IV. Title: Placenta.
[DNLM: 1. Placenta--pathology--Atlases. WQ 17]
RG591.D515 2014
618.34--dc23

International Standard Book Number: 978-1-937242-22-0

Cover Designer: Tom M. Olson, BA

Printed in Canada by Friesens, Altona, Manitoba, Canada

Last digit is the print number: 9 8 7 6 5 4 3 2 1

For Jesse, with deepest gratitude for your support in all of my endeavors.
AHM

In memory of my parents, Edward and Erna Popek, who saw that, despite multiple degrees and years of specialty training, I really was just like them: a teacher.
EJP

The placenta is the pregnancy's black box, the seat of secrets to a new life. Here is to the mothers whose placentas have contributed to our understanding of these secrets, and to the children they have nurtured.

To Valérie, Charlotte, and Sophie, for the love, the laughter, and the inspiration. And for their admirable effort to try and comprehend their mother's fascination with this intriguing organ.

And to François. Naturally.
MDP

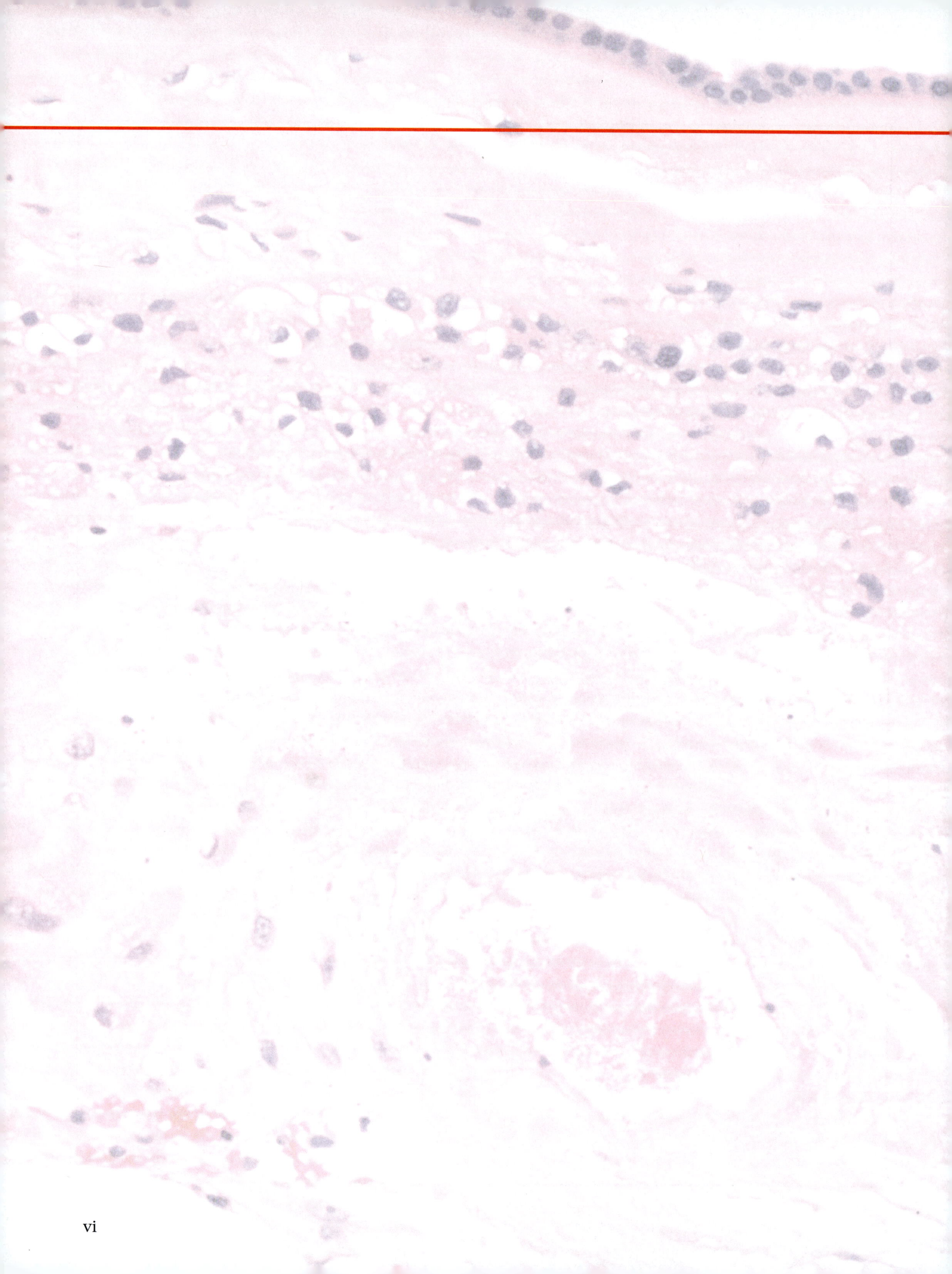

PREFACE

One of the more perplexing phenomena in the field of pathology is what could be termed the "placenta paradox": the placenta is the most accessible human organ, yet, at the same time, it is also the most poorly understood. Attributable, in part, to the rather cursory attention devoted to the placenta in most training programs and to its ever-looming medicolegal ramifications, examination of the placenta often presents an intimidating task for the general surgical pathologist. The placenta probably does not deserve its enigmatic reputation. Many of the inflammatory, immune-mediated, or vascular processes seen in the placenta have analogies in other organ systems, such as the lung, liver, or kidney. And, as in these other organs, the placental pathologies have more or less constant — and increasingly better understood — clinical (fetal and/or maternal) correlates.

Diagnostic Pathology: Placenta aims to be a practical and highly accessible complement to the existing excellent but somewhat more encyclopedic classic placental pathology literature. To this end, it uses the easy-to-access bullet format popularized by the Amirsys surgical pathology, histology, and radiology textbooks. The first section provides a systematic overview of the various placental compartments, each presented with their respective normal gross and microscopic appearance, as well as their major pathological findings. The second section addresses the most important placental pathology constellations and their typical clinical correlates. In the third section, we focus on prevalent pregnancy complications, such as preeclampsia, intrauterine growth restriction, and multiple gestations, and describe the placental findings commonly associated with these clinical scenarios.

While the focus of the text is on the placenta, we include key correlates in the gross and microscopic examination of the fetus where essential. Also, the pathology of the postpartum hysterectomy is included, as disorders of placental implantation are increasingly encountered on the surgical pathology bench. Finally, the last section provides essential reference tables as well as proposed templates that may be useful for gross and microscopic placental description.

It is our hope that this text will enhance the readers' understanding of the placenta and, ultimately, their appreciation of the critical role it plays as the unique interface between mother and fetus. We hope we may have contributed to the demystification of the placenta. Enjoy the book.

Amy Heerema-McKenney, MD
Contract Staff Physician
Cleveland Clinic Institute of Pathology and Laboratory Medicine
Cleveland, Ohio

Edwina J. Popek, DO
Professor of Pathology and Pediatrics
Baylor College of Medicine
Texas Children's Hospital Pavilion for Women
Houston, Texas

Monique E. De Paepe, MD, MSc
Professor of Pathology and Laboratory Medicine
Women and Infants Hospital
Alpert Medical School of Brown University
Providence, Rhode Island

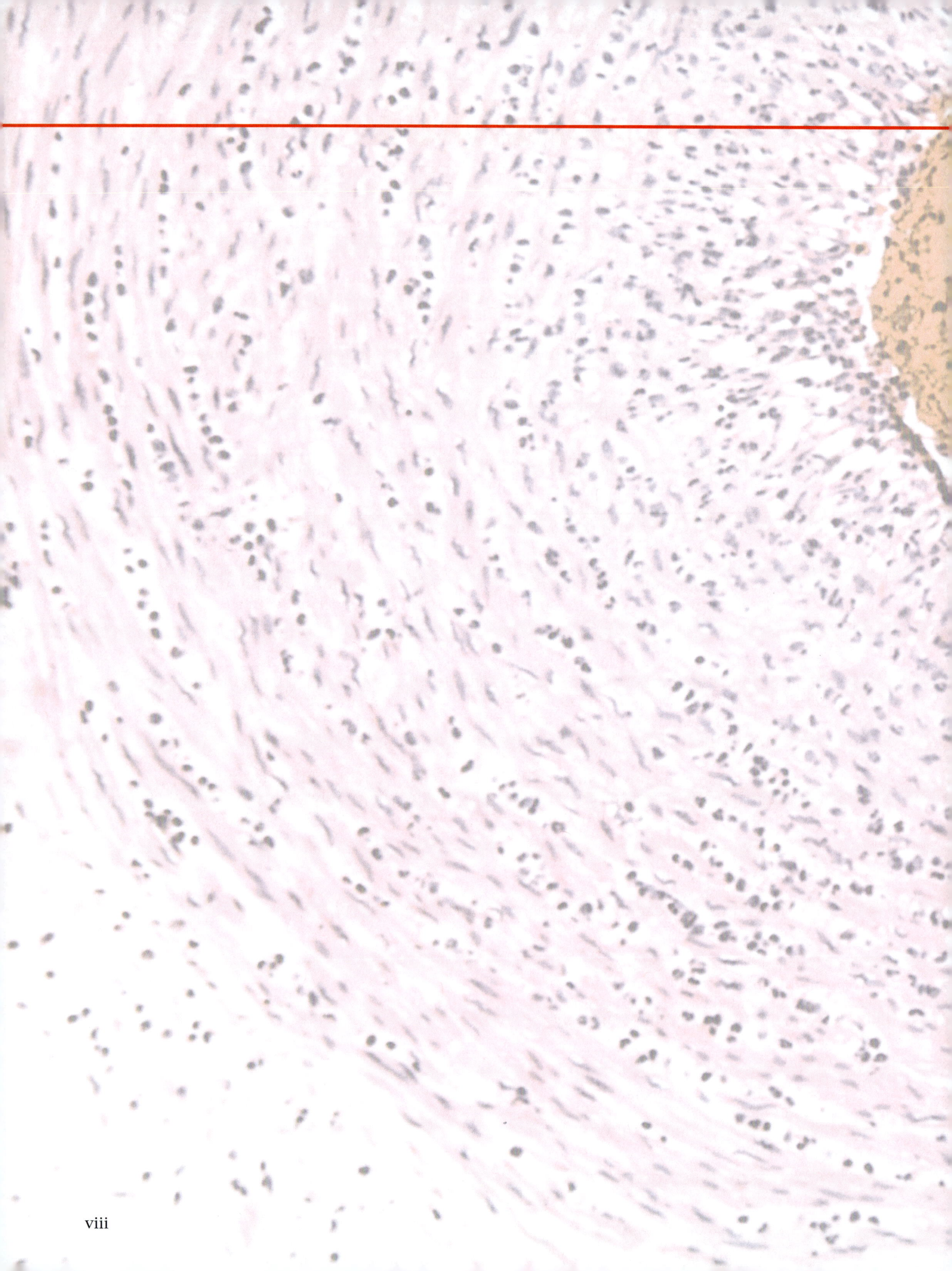

ACKNOWLEDGMENTS

Editors

Dave L. Chance, MA, ELS
Arthur G. Gelsinger, MA
Angela M. Green Terry, BA
Sarah J. Connor, BA
Tricia L. Cannon, BA
Jason D. Cronin, BA

Image Editors

Jeffrey J. Marmorstone, BS
Lisa A. M. Steadman, BS

Medical Editor

Jesse K. McKenney, MD

Illustrations

Laura C. Sesto, MA
Lane R. Bennion, MS
Richard Coombs, MS

Art Direction and Design

Laura C. Sesto, MA
Tom M. Olson, BA

Lead Editor

Rebecca L. Hutchinson, BA

Production Leads

Katherine L. Riser, MA
Rebecca L. Hutchinson, BA

AMIRSYS®
Names you know. Content you trust.®

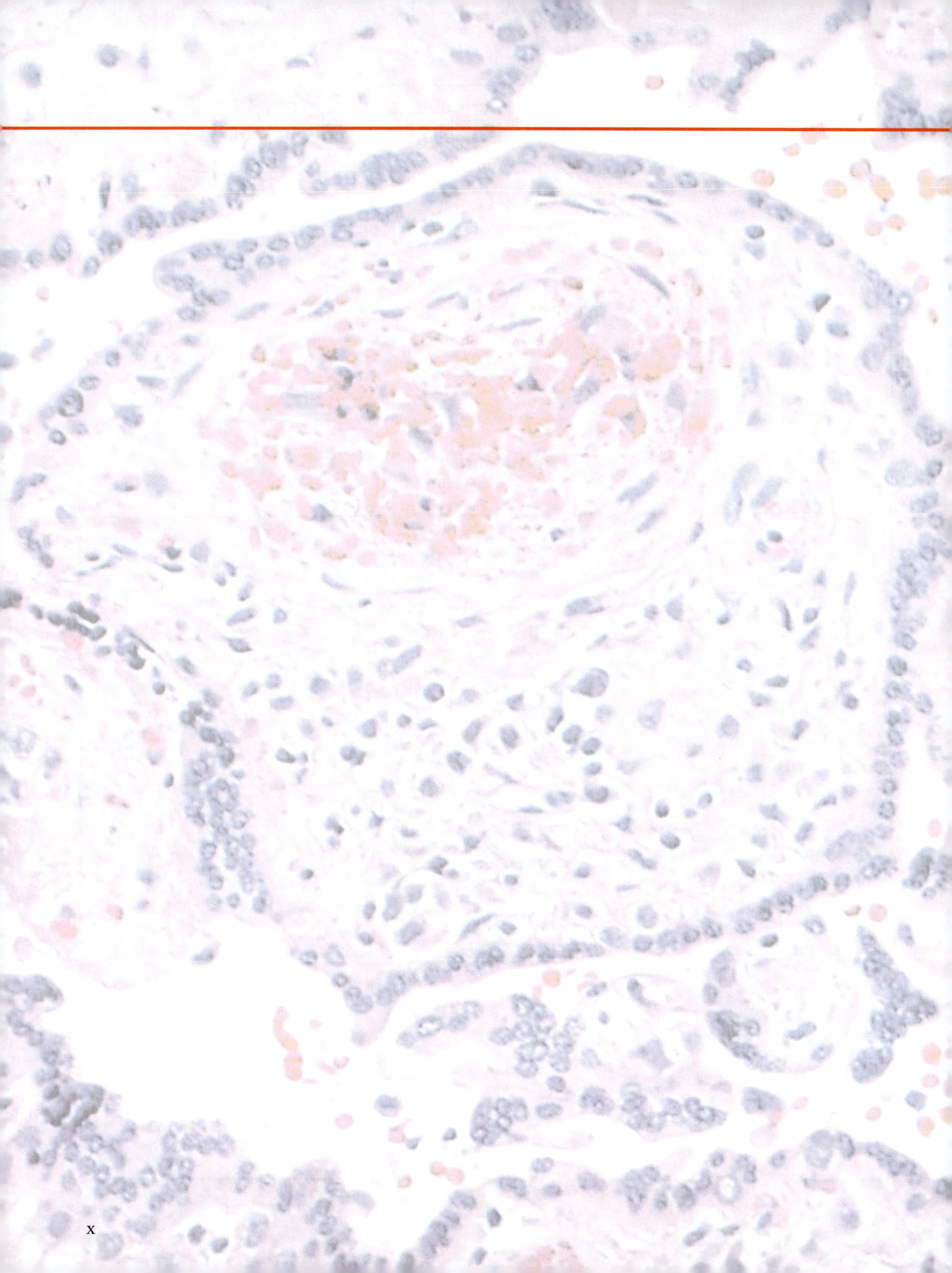

SECTIONS

TABLE OF CONTENTS

PART I
Overview of Gross and Microscopic Changes

SECTION 1
Umbilical Cord

SECTION 2
Extraplacental Membranes

SECTION 3
Chorionic Plate

SECTION 4
Stem Villi

SECTION 5
Chorionic Villi

SECTION 6
Decidua

PART II
Placental Diagnoses

SECTION 1
Meconium

SECTION 10 Placental Mesenchymal Dysplasia

PART III Placental Evaluation in Special Circumstances

SECTION 1 Gestational Diabetes

SECTION 2 Preeclampsia and Uteroplacental Malperfusion

SECTION 3 Fetal-Maternal Hemorrhage

SECTION 4 Intrauterine Growth Restriction

SECTION 5 Prematurity

SECTION 6 Abnormal Placental Implantation

SECTION 7 Intrauterine Fetal Demise

SECTION 8 Multiple Gestations

SECTION 9
The Postpartum Hysterectomy

PART IV
Appendix

SECTION 1
Reference Charts for Placental Evaluation

SECTION 2
Sample Templates for Placental Evaluation

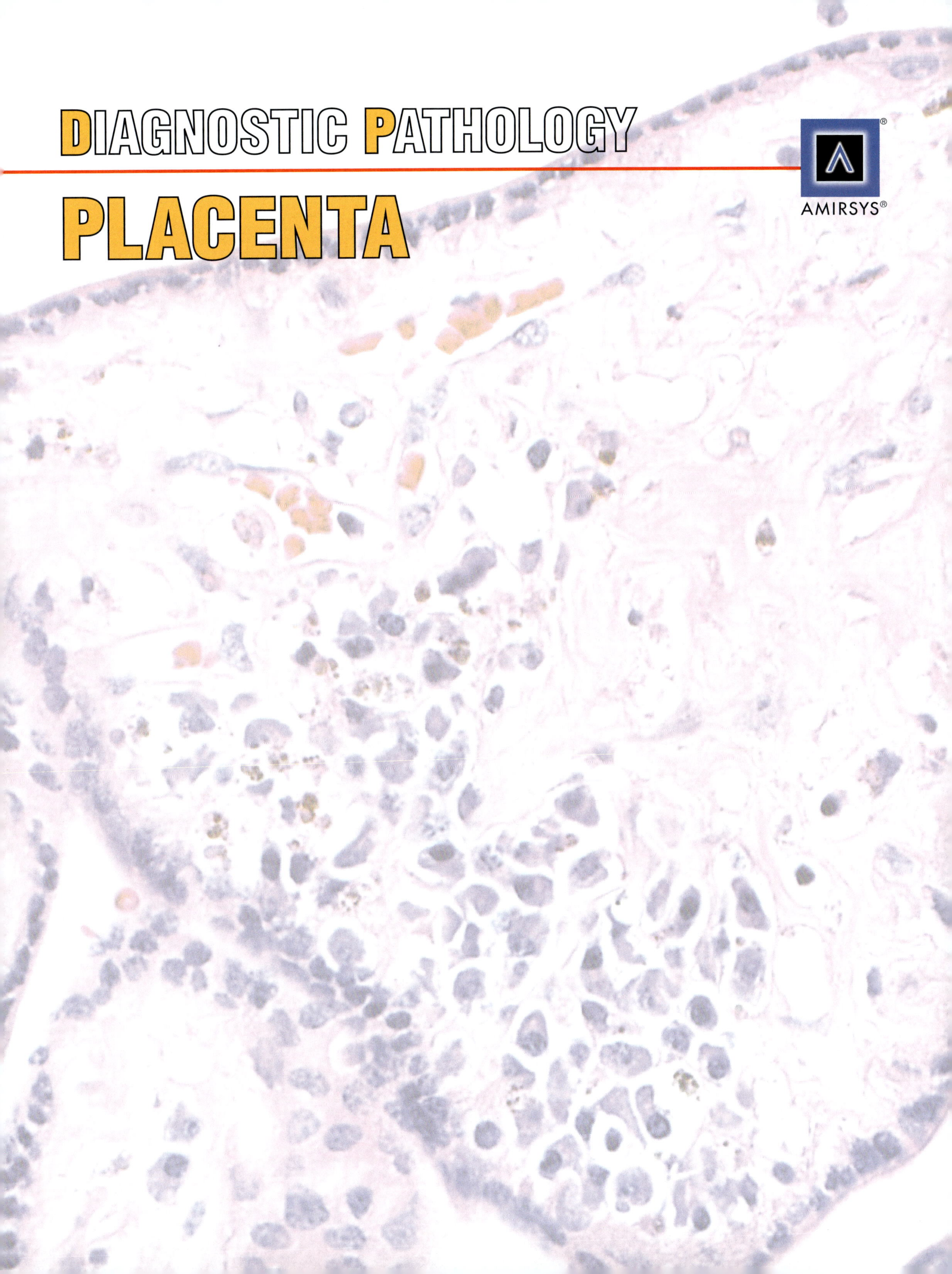

DIAGNOSTIC PATHOLOGY

PLACENTA

AMIRSYS®

Umbilical Cord

GROSS EVALUATION AND NORMAL HISTOLOGY OF UMBILICAL CORD

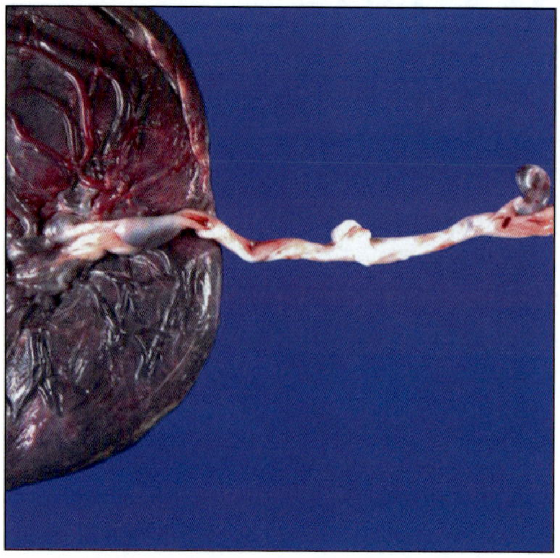

The umbilical vessels may have varicosities, commonly called "false knots." They usually arise from the vein. These have little clinical significance, although, rarely, varicosities may contain thrombi.

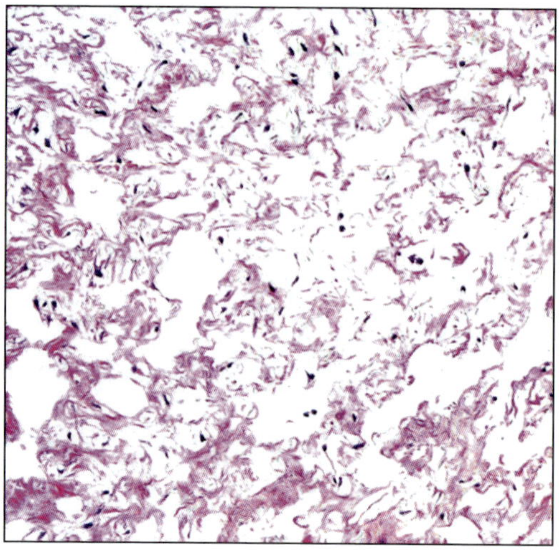

Wharton jelly is rich in extracellular matrix. It provides structural support, resisting kinking and compression. Cells include myofibroblasts near vessels, macrophages, and mast cells. The cord has no lymphatics or nerves.

TERMINOLOGY

Synonyms

- Omphalomesenteric duct and vitelline duct

GROSS EVALUATION

Gross Inspection of Cord

- One of the most important aspects of placental examination
- Abnormalities associated with fetal morbidity and mortality
  - Tight knots
  - Umbilical cord prolapse through cervix
  - Vasa previa with velamentous cords
  - Abnormal cord length
  - Abnormal cord coiling
  - Torsion/stricture
    - ± overcoiling
  - Hematoma/hemorrhage
  - Thrombosis
    - Umbilical artery &/or umbilical vein
  - Tumors
    - Hemangioma
    - Teratoma vs. acardiac twin
  - Cord entanglement about the fetal body (nuchal cord, limb/body entanglement)
    - See compressed &/or macerated regions of cord
  - Cord entanglement between monoamniotic twins
- Every exam should document the following
  - Color (note changes such as green or brown meconium staining or localized red to brown maceration)
  - Total length
  - Diameter
  - Coiling
  - Type of insertion, distance from insertion to edge of placental disc
  - Presence of amniotic web
    - Abnormal extension of amnion from cord to chorionic plate tethers cord, limiting mobility
  - Presence of knots, strictures, surface lesions
    - Small white plaques on surface of cord suggest peripheral funisitis due to *Candida* infection
  - Number of vessels on cut section and lesions of vessels, such as thrombi or concentric opacities
- Document abnormalities, such as tight knots, strictures, areas of compression, or maceration, with a gross photograph

Umbilical Cord Length

- Reference values for cord length are established and should be used in evaluation
- Cords that are very long are associated with multiple pathologies
  - Fetal heart failure due to increased work of moving blood through long umbilical cord (high output failure)
  - Increased risk of cord wrapping around neck, body, or limbs, with potential effects on circulation through affected body part as well as through cord
  - Associated with increased fetal activity and male gender
- Cords that are too short may be associated with restricted fetal movement, premature separation of placenta, and tearing during delivery
  - Length of cord received in pathology is usually < true total length, as segments may be sent from delivery room for blood gas analysis, cord blood banking, cultures, etc.

Umbilical Cord Diameter

- Reference values for cord diameter are established and should be used in evaluation
- Thick cords may be due to edema or effects of maternal diabetes

- Thin cords may reflect fetal growth restriction or effects of uteroplacental malperfusion of placenta, as in preeclampsia
- Focal swellings of cord can occur, usually near fetal end

Umbilical Cord Coiling

- Helical coiling of cord is normal and protects vasculature from compression
  - Average number of coils per 10 cm of length is recorded as cord coil index
  - Normal coiling ranges 1-3 twists per 10 cm of length
- Most cords (75%) coil counterclockwise as viewed from fetus
- Overcoiled cords may be associated with increased vascular resistance to blood flow through cord and increased afterload on fetal heart
  - Overcoiled cords may have constrictions and focally diminished Wharton jelly, further compromising flow
  - Placenta may show fetal thrombotic vasculopathy, evincing poor fetal blood flow
- Undercoiled cords may be more susceptible to kinking and acute obstruction of fetal blood flow

Umbilical Cord Insertion

- Insertion is defined as point where cord branches and its vessels are no longer covered with Wharton jelly
- "Normal" umbilical cord insertion
  - Insertion in center of disc or off center but within central 2/3 of disc (paracentral or eccentric insertion)
- Marginal umbilical cord insertion
  - Insertion within 1 cm of disc edge
  - Less efficient for perfusion of placenta
- Velamentous umbilical cord insertion
  - Insertion in membranes of placenta
  - Vessels coursing through membranes to disc are at risk for compression or injury
    - No protection from compression by Wharton jelly
    - Can tear if near site of membrane rupture
  - Less efficient for perfusion of placenta
  - Gross examination should include measuring length of longest intramembranous vessel
- Furcate umbilical cord insertion
  - Umbilical vessels branch before cord inserts
    - No protection by Wharton jelly along branched segments
    - Increased risk of compression, tearing, thrombi

HISTOLOGIC COMPONENTS

Amniotic Epithelium

- Low cuboidal epithelium
- May become squamous, especially near term and near cord insertion site
- Tightly adherent to underlying connective tissue, unlike amnion of membranes

Umbilical Arteries

- Typically paired (singular in 1-2% of infants)
- Derived from allantoic vessels accompanying allantoic duct
- Originate from internal iliac arteries in fetus
- Bring deoxygenated blood from fetal circulation to placenta
- Muscular arteries without a well-developed elastic lamina, elastic fibers present in smooth muscle
  - Vascular smooth muscle is arranged in helical bundles
- Anastomose within 2-3 cm of insertion of cord onto placental disc (Hyrtl anastomosis)
  - Equalizes pressure and ensures supply of blood throughout placenta if 1 umbilical artery is thrombosed
  - Various patterns of anastomosis, including fusion, or ≥ 1 communicating branch
- Single umbilical artery
  - More common in whites, 1% at term
  - May see atrophic remnant of 2nd umbilical artery
  - More frequent in twins, usually in smaller twin when growth is discrepant
  - 20% have additional malformations with significant morbidity and mortality
    - Abnormal karyotype and multiple malformations are more common when left umbilical artery is missing
  - Placenta may show velamentous cord insertion, circumvallation, and magistral distribution of chorionic plate vasculature
- Discordant size (difference of 0.1 cm in diameter)
  - Similar associations as single umbilical artery

Umbilical Vein

- Paired in early gestation, singular with regression of right umbilical vein by 2nd month
  - Persistence of right umbilical vein is a cause of true supernumerary vessels
    - Discern true supernumerary vessel from excessive coiling with additional sections
    - Present in < 1% of cords
- Brings oxygenated blood from placenta to fetal hepatic vein
- Derived from allantoic vessels accompanying allantoic duct
- Muscular vessel with well-developed internal elastic lamina

Wharton Jelly

- Mucoid substance protecting umbilical vessels from compression
- Rich in hyaluronic acid and chondroitin sulfate
- Scattered myofibroblast-like cells
- Scattered heparin producing mast cells
- Derived from extraembryonic mesoderm
- Liquefies under pressure
- No lymphatics or nerves are present in umbilical cord

Vestigial Remnants

- Omphalomesenteric duct remnant
  - Usually present at periphery of cord
  - Lined by various endodermal epithelia, typically intestinal type (gastric or hepatic, rarely pancreatic)
  - Commonly has smooth muscle coat

GROSS EVALUATION AND NORMAL HISTOLOGY OF UMBILICAL CORD

  - May be cystic, associated with other anomalies of omphalomesenteric duct such as Meckel diverticulum
- Vitelline vessel remnants
  - May accompany the omphalomesentic duct remnant
  - Lined by simple endothelium
  - Variable number of channels
  - May be called cord hemangioma, although not of clinical significance
- Allantoic duct remnant
  - Located between paired umbilical arteries
  - Lined by urothelium, with occasional mucin-producing cells
  - Rarely with accompanying smooth muscle
  - May contain urine if urachus (median umbilical ligament) is patent

ARTIFACTS, MIMICS, AND IATROGENIC LESIONS

Gross Artifacts

- Lesions due to clamping of cord
  - Imprint of clamp visible with careful inspection
  - Can cause hemorrhage and discoloration of cord
  - Changes should not be confused with thrombi or hemorrhages that occur before delivery
- Avulsion of cord with delivery of placenta
  - Not relevant to infant health
  - Communicate with obstetric team if in doubt as to timing of avulsion
    - True avulsion in utero is exceedingly rare and catastrophic

Microscopic Artifacts

- Inclusion "cyst" of amnion
  - Usually not a true cyst but an artifact due to tangential sectioning through spiral of cord
- Loss of 2nd umbilical artery due to incomplete sectioning of cord
- > 3 vessels on section due to excessive coiling or redoubling of vessels

Iatrogenic Lesions

- Cord hemorrhage
  - Presents with bloody amniotic fluid and fetal bradycardia
  - Rare complication of forceps delivery
  - Rare complication of cordocentesis
- Cord hematoma
  - Most cases are spontaneous and not iatrogenic
  - Blood extravasates into Wharton jelly
    - May be associated with vascular ectasia or thinning of umbilical vein media
  - Complication of cordocentesis
  - Rare complication of amniocentesis
  - Small fresh hemorrhages may be due to torsion with delivery or cord blood sampling after delivery

FINAL DIAGNOSIS REPORTING

Gross Umbilical Cord Features

- Abnormalities of vessel number (e.g., single umbilical artery)
- Excessively (> 2 standard deviations) long cord length, excessively short cord length (verified by clinician)
- Excessive over- or undercoiling
- Excessively thick or thin cord diameters
- Abnormal cord insertion (velamentous, marginal, furcate)
- Presence of thrombi, tight knots, strictures, focal edema, significant segmental compression or maceration (with length of involved area)

SELECTED REFERENCES

1. Jessop FA et al: Umbilical cord coiling: clinical outcomes in an unselected population and systematic review. Virchows Arch. 464(1):105-12, 2014
2. Ernst LM et al: Gross patterns of umbilical cord coiling: correlations with placental histology and stillbirth. Placenta. 34(7):583-8, 2013
3. Proctor LK et al: Umbilical cord diameter percentile curves and their correlation to birth weight and placental pathology. Placenta. 34(1):62-6, 2013
4. Balkawade NU et al: Study of Length of Umbilical Cord and Fetal Outcome: A Study of 1,000 Deliveries. J Obstet Gynaecol India. 62(5):520-525, 2012
5. Tantbirojn P et al: Gross abnormalities of the umbilical cord: related placental histology and clinical significance. Placenta. 30(12):1083-8, 2009
6. Asabe K et al: Iatrogenic ileal perforation: an accidental clamping of a hernia into the umbilical cord and a review of the published work. J Obstet Gynaecol Res. 34(4 Pt 2):619-22, 2008
7. de Laat MW et al: The umbilical coiling index, a review of the literature. J Matern Fetal Neonatal Med. 17(2):93-100, 2005
8. Machin GA et al: Abnormal umbilical cord coiling is associated with adverse perinatal outcomes. Pediatr Dev Pathol. 3(5):462-71, 2000
9. Naeye RL: Umbilical cord length: clinical significance. J Pediatr. 107(2):278-81, 1985
10. Itskovitz J et al: Intrauterine rupture of the umbilical cord during delivery. Eur J Obstet Gynecol Reprod Biol. 10(1):35-40, 1980

Umbilical Cord Diameter (cm)

Gestational Age (Completed Weeks)	10th Percentile	50th Percentile	90th Percentile	N	Mean	Standard Deviation
18	0.36	0.46	0.61	4	0.53	0.08
19	0.43	0.54	0.68	10	0.51	0.12
20	0.50	0.60	0.73	8	0.72	0.30
21	0.56	0.67	0.79	9	0.61	0.14
22	0.62	0.72	0.84	17	0.69	0.09
23	0.67	0.78	0.88	14	0.75	0.20
24	0.72	0.83	0.93	18	0.84	0.13
25	0.77	0.87	0.97	9	0.86	0.12
26	0.80	0.91	1.01	9	0.93	0.13
27	0.83	0.94	1.05	7	0.93	0.09
28	0.85	0.97	1.09	4	1.04	0.06
29	0.87	1.00	1.12	9	0.92	0.16
30	0.88	1.02	1.15	16	1.04	0.18
31	0.88	1.03	1.18	13	1.06	0.16
32	0.88	1.05	1.20	10	1.04	0.14
33	0.88	1.05	1.22	16	1.06	0.20
34	0.87	1.06	1.23	23	1.03	0.24
35	0.86	1.06	1.24	17	0.97	0.13
36	0.85	1.05	1.25	33	1.03	0.17
37	0.84	1.05	1.24	40	1.02	0.14
38	0.83	1.03	1.23	54	1.04	0.18
39	0.82	1.02	1.22	58	1.01	0.15
40	0.81	1.00	1.19	59	1.04	0.14
41	0.80	0.98	1.16	40	1.05	0.17

Umbilical cord diameter (UCD) percentiles and mean and standard deviation of the cohort (N = 497). UCD was calculated using the formula: UCD = 2 x √(weight/π x length). The substitution of weight in place of volume was used after showing that umbilical cord volume was similar to weight (p < 0.001; r = 0.997; y = 1.071x - 0.644). Proctor LK et al: Umbilical cord diameter percentile curves and their correlation to birth weight and placental pathology. Placenta. 34(1):62-6, 2013.

Umbilical Cord Length at Various Gestational Ages

Gestational Age (Weeks)	N	Umbilical Cord Length (cm)
20-21	16	32.4 ± 8.6
22-23	27	36.4 ± 9.0
24-25	38	40.1 ± 10.1
26-27	59	42.5 ± 11.3
28-29	80	45.0 ± 9.7
30-31	113	47.6 ± 11.3
32-33	337	50.2 ± 12.1
34-35	857	52.5 ± 11.2
36-37	3,153	55.6 ± 12.6
38-39	10,083	57.4 ± 12.6
40-41	13,841	59.6 ± 12.6
42-43	4,797	60.3 ± 12.7
44-45	1,450	60.4 ± 12.7
46-47	492	60.5 ± 13.0

Data represent mean ± 1 standard deviation. Naeye RL: Umbilical cord length: clinical significance. J Pediatr. 107(2):278-81, 1985.

GROSS EVALUATION AND NORMAL HISTOLOGY OF UMBILICAL CORD

Gross Features

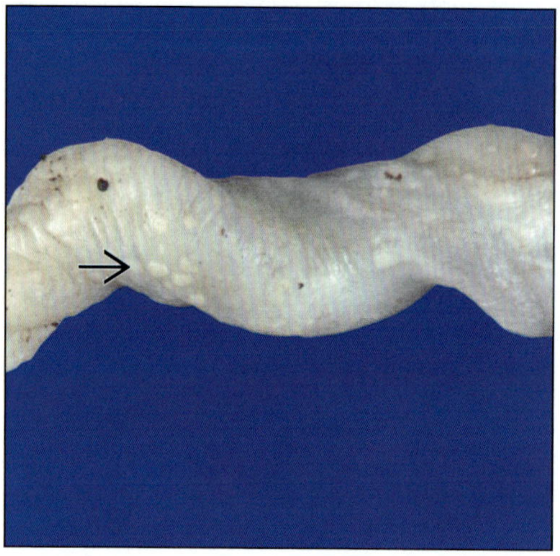

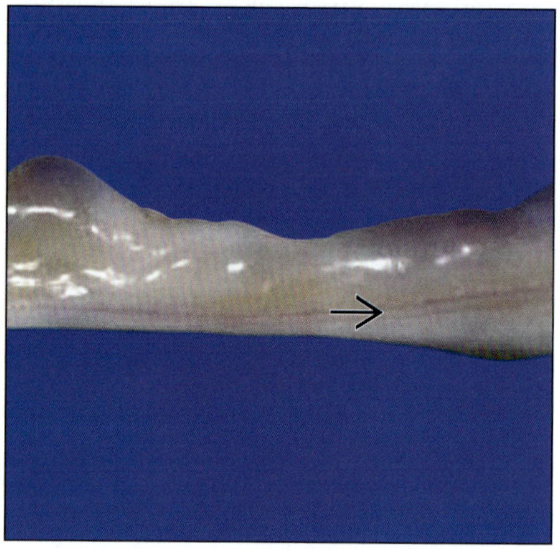

(Left) *Gross exam includes close inspection of the surface. The small white plaques* → *on the cord surface are foci of peripheral funisitis. The lesion is nearly pathognomonic for candidal infection of the amniotic fluid.* ***(Right)*** *Vitelline vessels* → *may be visible on gross inspection. They are a remnant vasculature that accompanied the omphalomesenteric duct in early development.*

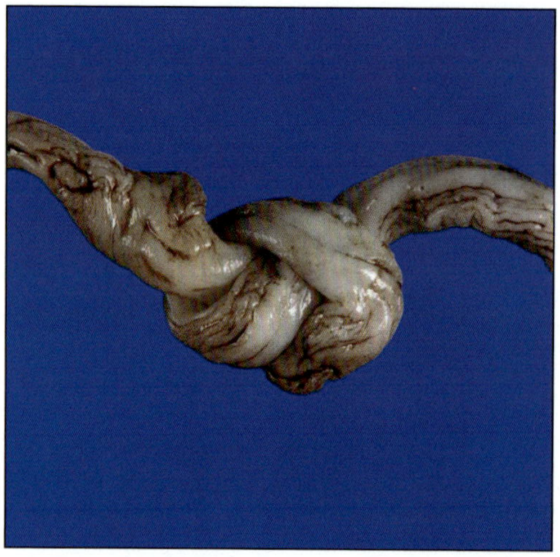

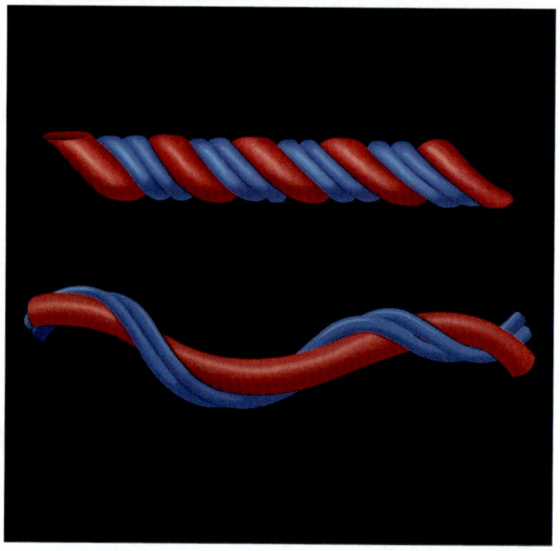

(Left) *True knots can be loose or tight. The lack of congestion on either side of this knot indicates that it is not a tight knot and may have had little clinical significance.* ***(Right)*** *Cord coiling refers to the frequency of the umbilical arteries (blue) coiling around the umbilical vein (red). Normal coiling ranges from 1-3 coils per 10 cm length of cord. Both overcoiling (top) and undercoiling (bottom) have been associated with adverse outcome in some studies.*

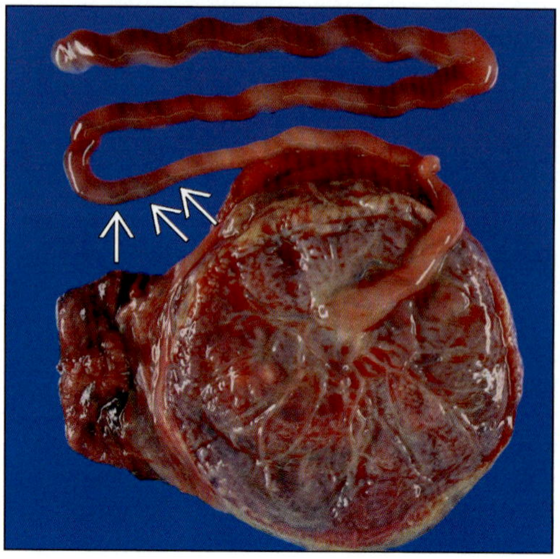

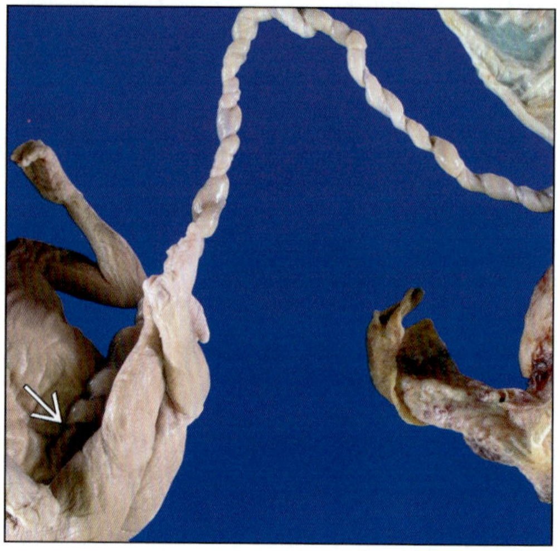

(Left) *This excessively long and hypercoiled cord led to 2nd-trimester fetal demise. Mathematical modeling suggests that excessive coiling increases resistance to blood flow. Excessive length and hypercoiling increase the work required for placental perfusion. Careful inspection of vessels* → *is needed to appreciate the coiling.* ***(Right)*** *Gross image shows a case of 2nd-trimester demise with an excessively long, hypercoiled cord. Strictures* → *are commonly seen at the cord insertion site, as in this case.*

GROSS EVALUATION AND NORMAL HISTOLOGY OF UMBILICAL CORD

Gross Features

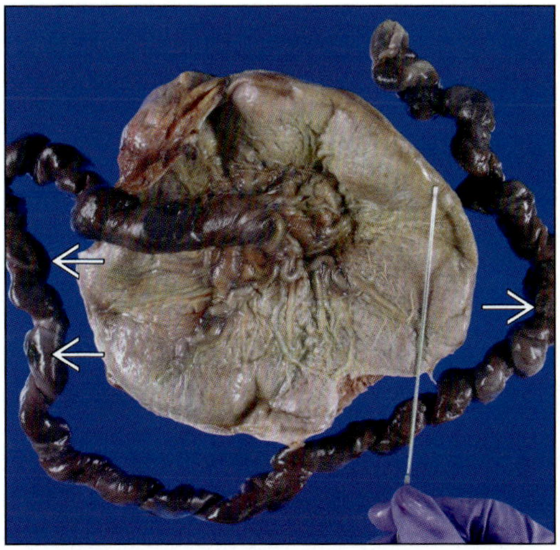

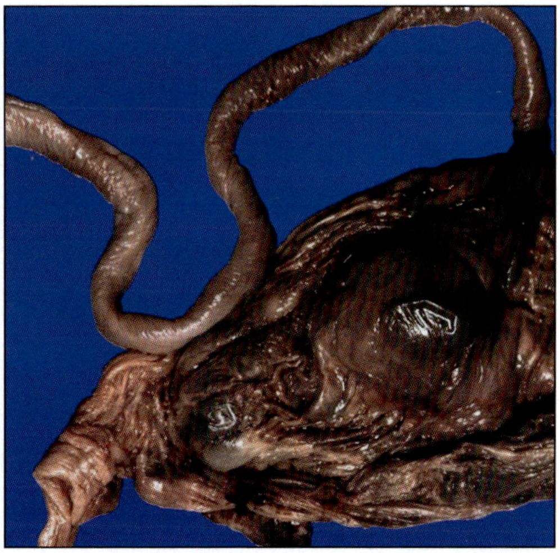

(Left) *Multiple mechanisms of cord compromise are present in this case of fetal demise. There was a tight nuchal cord, explaining the marked congestion. The cord is hypercoiled, excessively long, and shows ulcers* → *of meconium-associated vascular necrosis.* ***(Right)*** *Gross image shows a severely undercoiled cord in this case of fetal demise. Cord accidents are a significant cause of fetal death. Correlative findings, such as thrombi in the cord and placenta, help discern the cause of death.*

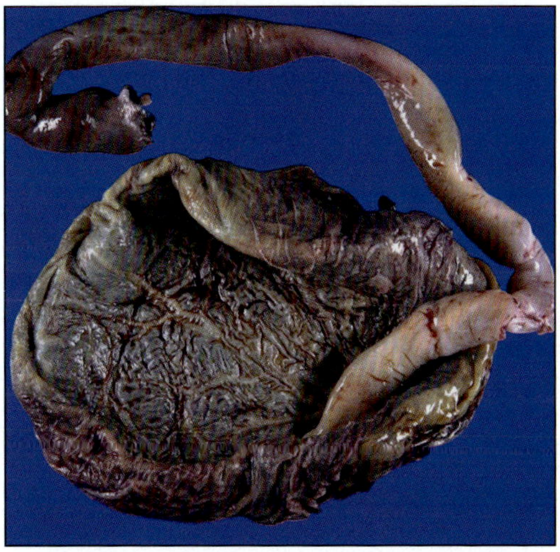

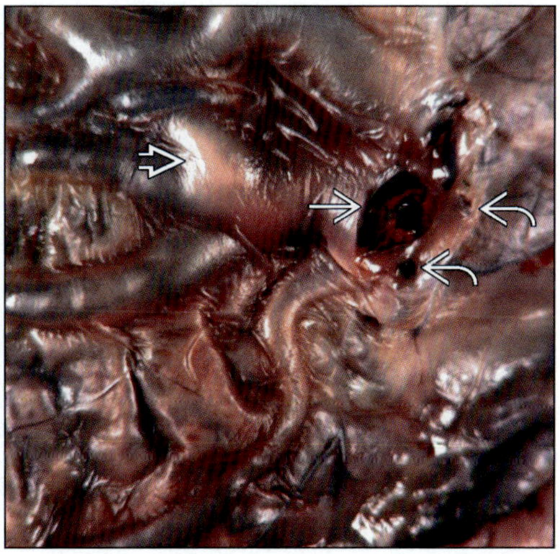

(Left) *This undercoiled cord is from a case of severe, chronic meconium staining and in utero fetal demise. Undercoiled cords are more susceptible to acute occlusion from kinking.* ***(Right)*** *Gross image shows a thrombus* → *of the umbilical vein near the cord insertion. Note the smaller diameter of the 2 umbilical arteries* ↷*. The white discoloration* ⇨ *of the proximal chorionic plate vein indicates extension of the thrombus.*

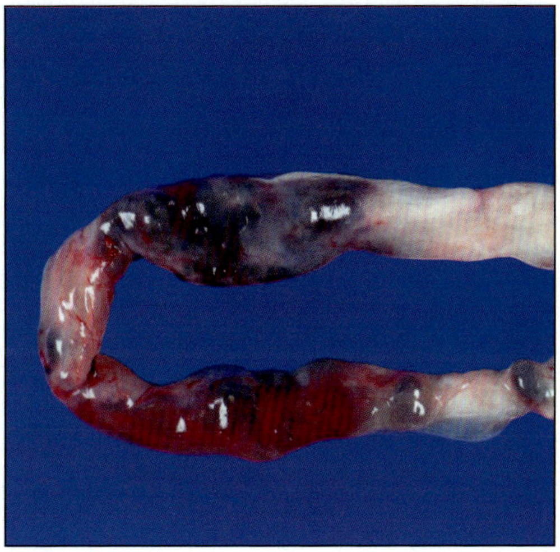

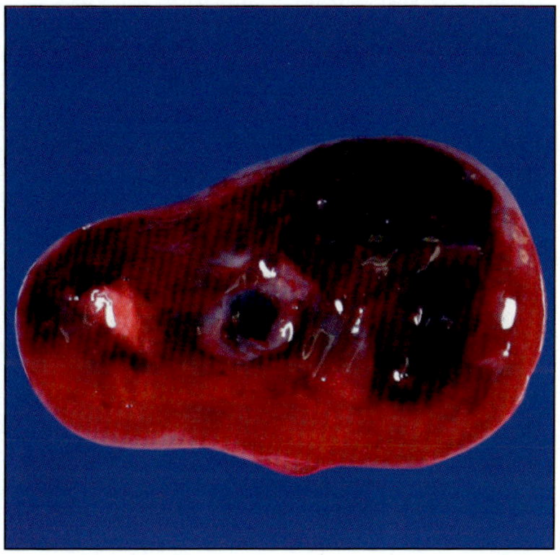

(Left) *Hemorrhage within the cord substance may be spontaneous, iatrogenic, or an artifact of delivery. The cord should be carefully inspected for clamp marks near the lesion.* ***(Right)*** *While the amount of blood that the fetus can lose in a cord hematoma is limited, the pressure may occlude flow through the remaining intact vessels.*

GROSS EVALUATION AND NORMAL HISTOLOGY OF UMBILICAL CORD

Graphic and Gross Features

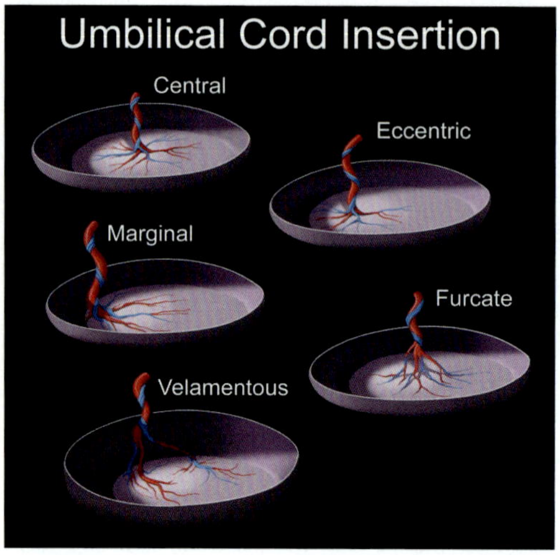

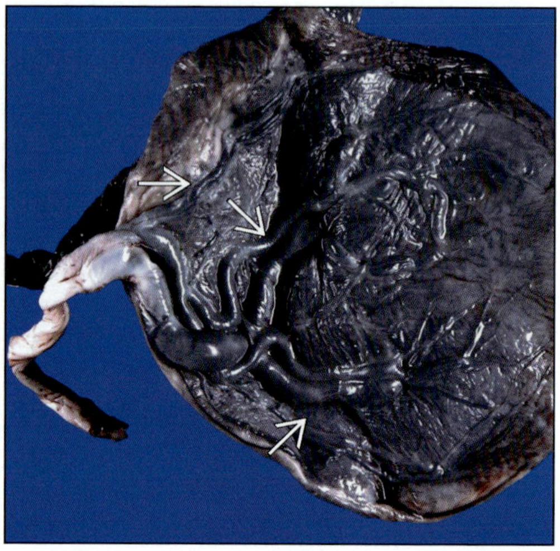

(Left) *Central and eccentric cord insertions are most common. Marginal, velamentous, and furcate are more often associated with pathology. Velamentous and furcate cords leave vessels vulnerable to injury. Marginal insertion may be less efficient for perfusion.* ***(Right)*** *Cords that insert at the margin, or within 1 cm of the margin, are deemed marginal. Marginal cord insertion is associated with magistral chorionic plate vasculature. There are few artery/vein pairs ➡, which show little decrease in diameter or branching.*

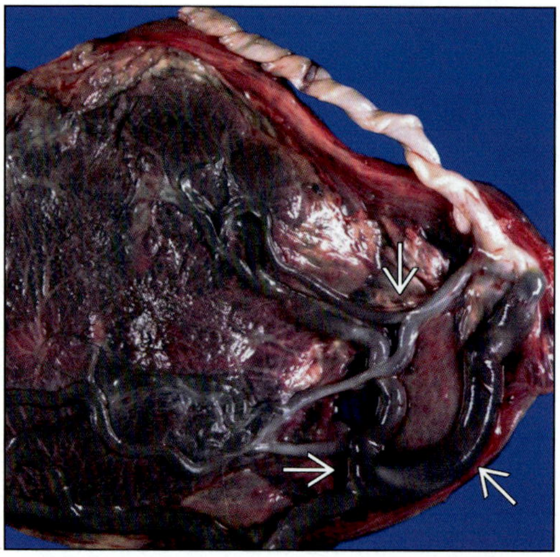

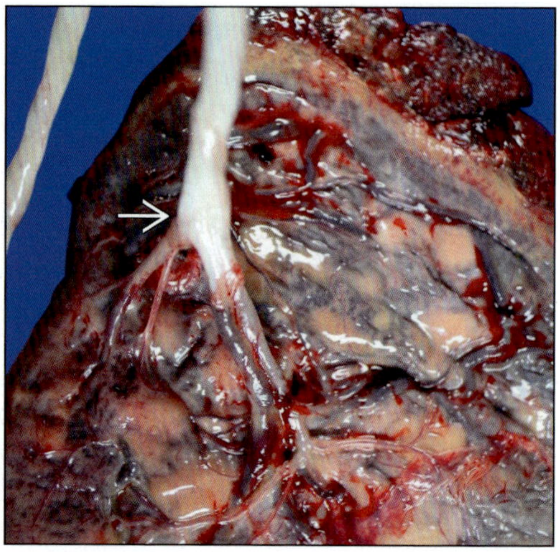

(Left) *Gross image shows vulnerable vessels ➡ in a velamentous insertion. Inspect closely for tears or thrombi and measure the length of the intramembranous course.* ***(Right)*** *In furcate cord insertion, the umbilical vessels branch ➡ like the tines of a fork before the cord inserts on the chorionic plate. Such vessels are vulnerable to compression or tearing.*

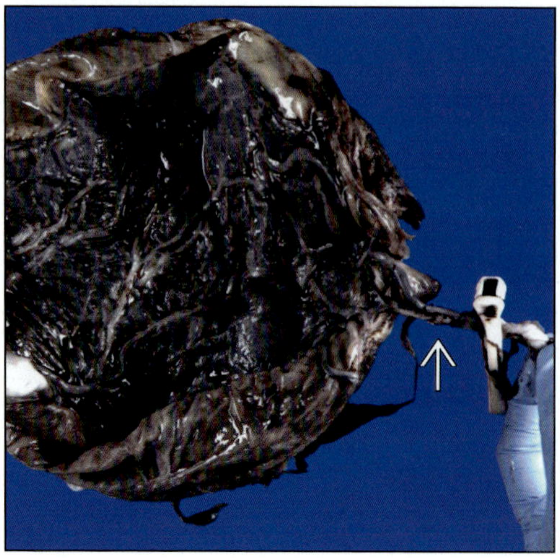

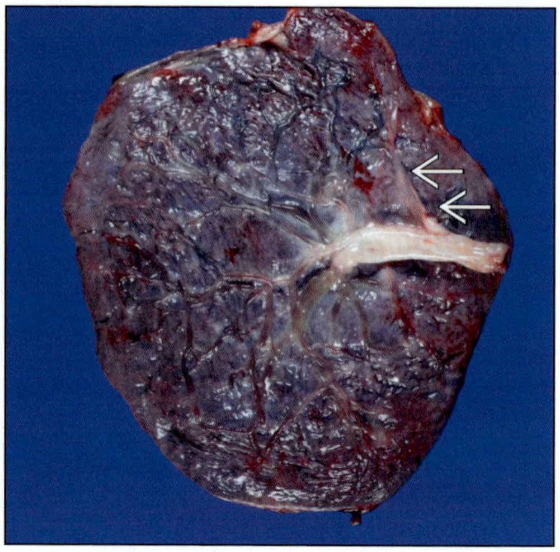

(Left) *The cord of this twin inserted in the membranes but branched ➡ before connecting with the membranous chorion. It is therefore both velamentous and furcate. Velamentous and marginal cord insertions are associated with discrepant growth in twins with the affected twin being smaller.* ***(Right)*** *In the amniotic web of the umbilical cord, an extension of amniotic membranes ➡ tether the cord to the chorionic plate. This may limit cord mobility and cause the cord to be functionally short.*

Microscopic Features

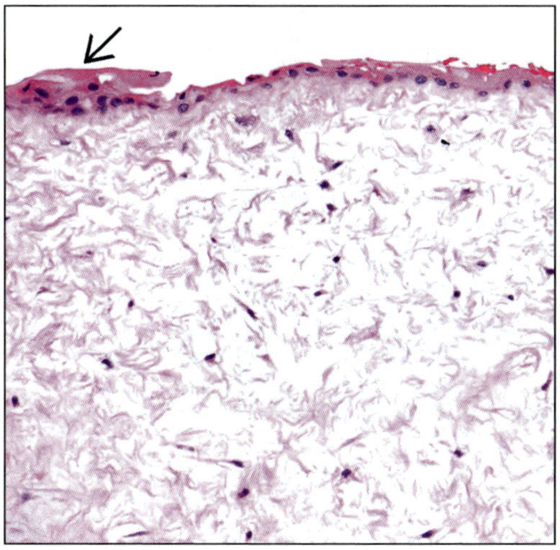

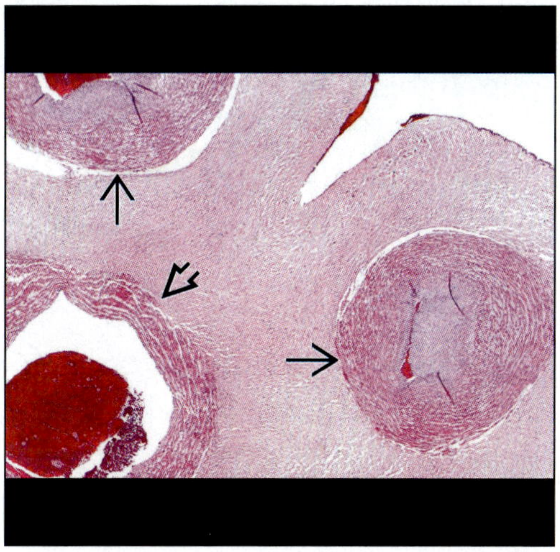

(Left) *The umbilical cord is covered by amniotic epithelium, an extension of fetal skin. The epithelium commonly becomes squamous →, particularly near the fetal umbilical insertion.* **(Right)** *The muscular layer of the 2 umbilical arteries → is thicker than that of the vein ⇨. The artery smooth muscle is arrayed in overlapping helices. The vein has circular and longitudinal layers. The cord contains no vasa vasorum; the vascular smooth muscle is nourished by the fetal blood.*

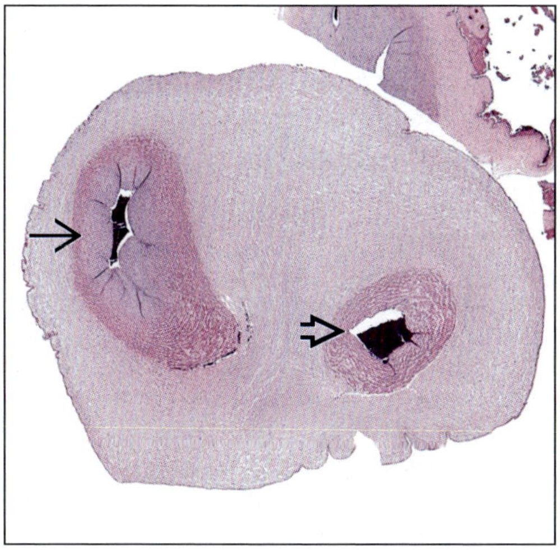

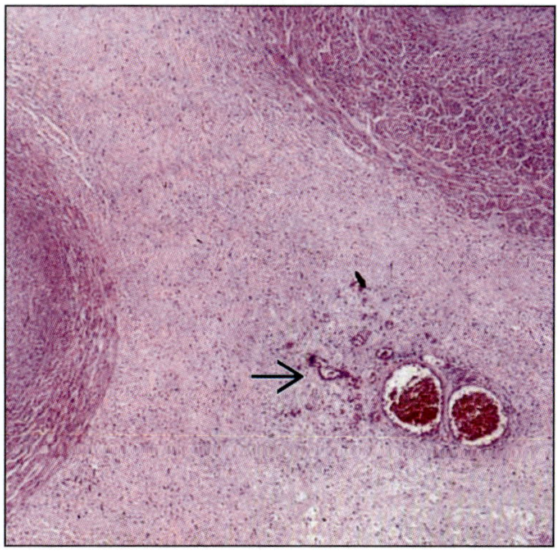

(Left) *A single umbilical artery should be confirmed microscopically. There is 1 umbilical artery → and 1 umbilical vein ⇨ present. This common anomaly has little clinical significance in the vast majority of newborns.* **(Right)** *These remnant vitelline vessels → accompanied the omphalomesenteric duct early in development. The multiple capillary channels are sometimes termed hemangioma of the cord, although they are not neoplastic and are unrelated to congenital hemangiomas.*

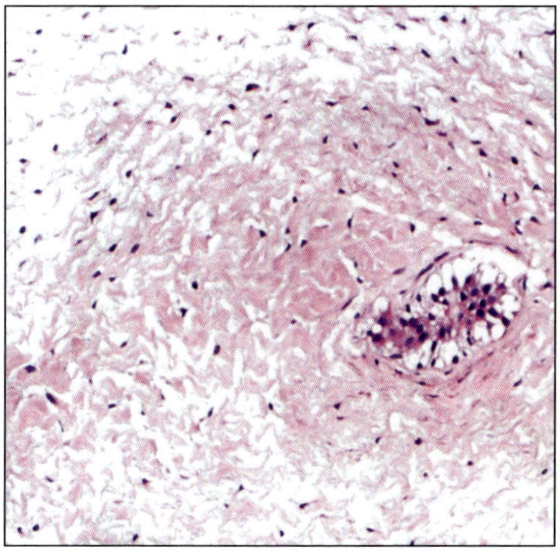

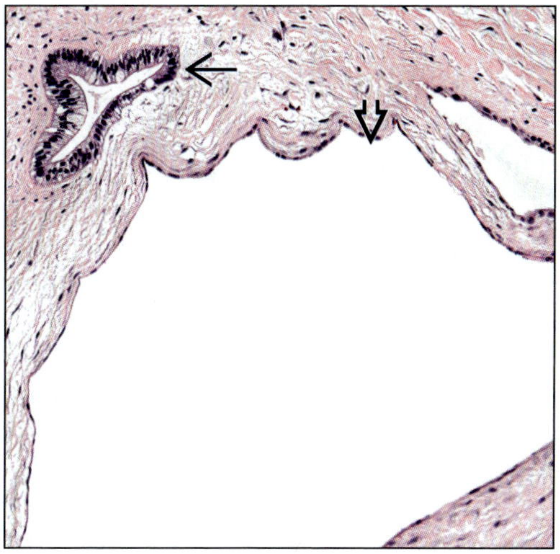

(Left) *Allantoic remnants are usually located between the 2 umbilical arteries. The epithelium is typically cuboidal or transitional. These are usually of no clinical significance. Rarely, large patent allantoic remnants communicate with a persistent urachus in the fetus. Urination into the cord may occur.* **(Right)** *This omphalomesenteric remnant → is accompanied by a large vitelline vessel ⇨. Omphalomesenteric duct remnants commonly have goblet cells and are located at the periphery of the cord.*

KNOTS

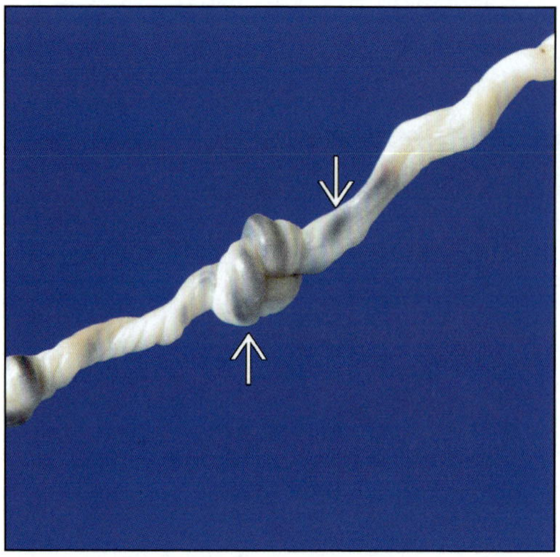

Gross image shows a tight, complex (2 loops) true knot of the umbilical cord with vascular congestion and dilation of the vessels ➡. This fetus was small for gestational age and had meconium-stained amniotic fluid at birth.

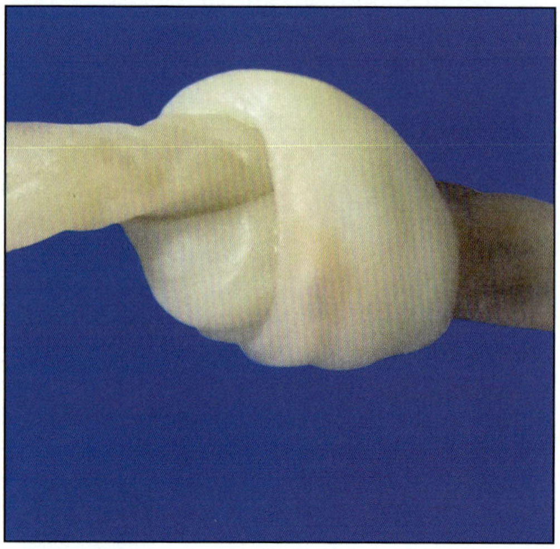

This image shows a tight, simple (1 loop) true knot of the umbilical cord. Note that there is no vascular congestion surrounding the knot. After untying the knot, there was underlying grooving of the cord.

TERMINOLOGY

Definitions

- True knot
  - Intertwining looped segment of umbilical cord that can lead to cord compression
- False knot (a.k.a. pseudoknot)
  - Appear to be knots but are truly the following
    - Focal accentuations of the vascular spirals
    - Local redundancies of umbilical vessels, commonly the vein (nodus spurious vasculosis)
    - Excessive amount of Wharton jelly present (nodus spurious gelatinous)

EPIDEMIOLOGY

Incidence

- 0.35-2.1% of umbilical cords contain a true knot
- True knots represent ~ 4% of all cord complications
- Equal frequency of true knots in fetal demise and term livebirth
- 0.1% of umbilical cords contain double true knots

ETIOLOGY/PATHOGENESIS

True Knot Formation

- Created by cord forming a loop with a diameter large enough to allow fetus to move through it
- Proposed to develop early in gestation when there is ample space for fetal movement and entanglement
  - Proposed to occur between 9 and 28 weeks gestation, after which cord length no longer increases significantly
  - Some narrow time period of knot formation to between 9 and 12 weeks gestation
- Depends on cord that is long enough to create a loop and factors that create more room, allowing for exaggerated fetal movement
- Proposed that knots can also result from descent of fetus through a loop of cord during labor
- Further axial movements by fetus, such as changes in lie and presentation, could result in tightening of knot or formation of a more complicated knot

Effects of True Knot Tightening

- Tightening of knot leads to compression of umbilical vessels with the following effects
  - Venous stasis and hypertension
  - Decreased venous return of oxygenated blood from placenta to fetus
  - Thrombosis in upstream fetal vasculature (chorionic vasculature &/or at site of knot)
- Tightening often occurs later in pregnancy secondary to increased traction on the umbilical cord due to
  - Fetal descent into pelvis or through birth canal
  - Membrane rupture with loss of cushioning effect of amniotic fluid

Deleterious Fetal Effects

- Depend on increased venous perfusion pressure
  - In vitro studies show increase in venous pressure required to perfuse umbilical vein; occurs with
    - Tightening of the knot
    - Increased number of knots in a single cord
    - Even a slack or loose knot
- Sublethal or lethal hypoxic fetal injury can result from true knots with
  - Complete umbilical blood flow obstruction
  - Critical reduction in umbilical blood flow associated with high venous pressure

Increased Risk of Fetal Vascular Compression Secondary to a True Knot

- During uterine contractions
- After rupture of membranes
- With greater size or bulk of knot
- With increased complexity of knot

False Knot Formation

- Etiology currently unknown
- Suggested to signify a temporal discrepancy of vascular growth with inadequate cord lengthening

CLINICAL IMPLICATIONS

Clinical Presentation

- True knots
  - Stillbirth or intrauterine fetal demise most devastating result of umbilical cord knot
  - Most fetuses with knots have a completely normal pregnancy and delivery without complications or sequelae
  - Fetuses have an increased risk during labor and delivery of
    - Nonreassuring fetal heart rate
    - Cord accidents at birth (cord prolapse or nuchal cord)
    - Cesarean delivery
    - Preterm delivery
    - Low Apgar score at 1 and 5 minutes
    - Meconium-stained amniotic fluid
    - Need for neonatal intensive care
  - Fetal distress during labor may be temporary with quick recovery soon after birth attributed to transient tightening of knot during delivery
  - Poor fetal growth or varying degrees of neurologic injury may occur with chronic intermittent knot tightening without complete obstruction
  - Controversial association with abnormal fetal venous pH and umbilical artery gas values
- False knots are typically of no clinical significance
  - Incidental findings during delivery
  - Often confused with true knots

Imaging Findings

- Prenatal diagnosis of true knot is rare and extremely difficult by ultrasound
- Larger &/or more complex knots are typically easier to visualize
- Knots do not have a characteristic prenatal ultrasonographic appearance
- Color Doppler &/or 3D ultrasonography may be more helpful than typical 2D ultrasound technique for detection

Risk Factors for True Knot

- Long umbilical cord
- Hypercoiled umbilical cord
- Male gender (secondary to longer cords in male fetuses)
- Polyhydramnios
- Small or small for gestational age fetus
- Monochorionic monoamniotic twin pregnancy (cord entanglement between twins)
- Prolonged gestation
- Amniocentesis during pregnancy (secondary to increased rate of fetal movement and uterine contractions)
- Grand multiparous mother (secondary to lax abdominal &/or uterine wall muscles)
- Maternal chronic hypertension
- Gestational diabetes or diabetes mellitus (secondary to increased risk of polyhydramnios)
- Advanced maternal age
- Maternal obesity
- Previous spontaneous abortion

Clinical Outcomes

- Most knots are not associated with adverse fetal outcomes
- Overall perinatal mortality rate of true knots: 8-11%
- 4x increased risk of stillbirth with true knot during pregnancy
  - In a population study, 2% of fetuses with true knots were stillborn, which accounted for 5% of all stillbirths of infants weighing > 2,500 g
  - Stillbirth secondary to true knots seen at all gestational ages
- 25% morbidity and mortality in association with double true knots
- False knots have no clinical sequelae described

MACROSCOPIC FINDINGS

General Features of True Knots

- Gross pattern of knots
  - Single or simple (1 loop)
  - Complex (> 1 overhand loop)
    - Figure-8 pattern (2 loops)
    - Loop around a fetal part with a half-hitch knot
  - Multiple (≥ 2 separate knots of 1 umbilical cord)
  - Knot between 2 umbilical cords in a monochorionic monoamniotic twin pregnancy secondary to entanglement of cords
- Indications of longstanding tight knot
  - Compression, grooving, and loss of Wharton jelly at site of knot
  - Cannot easily move or untie loops of knot with gentle tugging
  - Even when untied, unknotted cord curls and grooving persists
- Indications of true obstruction of umbilical cord by knot
  - Upstream (placental side) venous distention, congestion, and edema
  - Vascular distention may extend to upstream umbilical vein &/or chorionic plate vessels
  - Thrombus formation at site of knot &/or upstream thrombosis ± calcification of vessel thrombus (depending on chronicity)
- Tightness of knot does not necessarily indicate clinical significance without other suspicious features as the knot may have tightened transiently during delivery
- Indications of a newly formed or loose knot (typically not clinically significant)
  - No loss of Wharton jelly
  - No marked groove at site of knot
  - No curling of cord after untying

KNOTS

General Features of False Knots
- Can be quite large and complex, often bulbous
- Appears as a vascular protrusion or outpouching of Wharton jelly
- Can have redundancy of 1 umbilical vessel, commonly umbilical vein
- Do not cause compression of umbilical vessels; therefore, distention, congestion, &/or edema are not typically seen

Specimen Handling
- Document whether knot is tight or loose
- Document if congestion is present on either side of knot
- If possible, photograph knot showing distance from chorionic plate
- Untie knot and document whether it stays curled, implying chronicity (attempt only after documentation of true state with photography)
- Sections should be taken through knot after untying, or on either side of knot if left intact

MICROSCOPIC FINDINGS

General Features of True Knots
- Commonly have completely normal histology of umbilical cord
- If chronic fetal vascular obstruction occurs
  - Mural thrombus or complete occlusion of umbilical vein by thrombus can be seen
    - At site of knot or upstream (placental) umbilical vessels
    - In fetal chorionic or stem vessels
  - Umbilical and chorionic veins become thickened and may exhibit subendothelial, dome-shaped myxoid-appearing intimal protrusions
    - Associated with venous hypertension
    - Can have mural thrombi overlying these intimal protrusions
  - Villous stromal-vascular karyorrhexis or avascular villi may also be present in distal villous tree

General Features of False Knots
- Generally have a focal increase of Wharton jelly with normal histology of umbilical vessels
- May have a focal dilation of umbilical vessels &/or ≥ 2 umbilical veins in section
- Rarely can have a thrombus present

REPORTING CRITERIA

Include in Gross Description
- Location of true knot in relation to umbilical cord insertion into chorionic plate
- Whether true knot is tight or loose
- Number of knots &/or complexity of true knot
- If there is any vascular distention or congestion of umbilical vessels
- Gross evidence of thrombus formation at knot or any upstream location in umbilical cord or chorionic vessels
- After untying knot
  - Note whether it stays curled
  - Note if grooving or loss of Wharton jelly are seen
- Presence and number of false knots

Include in Final Diagnosis
- Presence of true knot and whether it is tight or loose
- Presence of a thrombus in umbilical, chorionic, or stem vessel
- Distal villous changes of fetal thrombotic vasculopathy
- Note false knots only if thrombus is present

SELECTED REFERENCES

1. Baergen RN: Umbilical cord pathology in surgical pathology clinics. In Baergen RN et al: Placental Pathology, An Issue of Surgical Pathology Clinics (The Clinics: Surgery). Vol 6, No 1. Philadelphia: Elsevier. 61-85, 2013
2. Räisänen S et al: True umbilical cord knot and obstetric outcome. Int J Gynaecol Obstet. 122(1):18-21, 2013
3. Benirschke K et al: Pathology of the Human Placenta. 6th ed. New York: Springer. 345-6, 2012
4. Rodriguez N et al: Three-dimensional high-definition flow imaging in prenatal diagnosis of a true umbilical cord knot. Ultrasound Obstet Gynecol. 39(2):245-6, 2012
5. Baergen RN: Manual of Pathology of the Human Placenta. 2nd ed. New York: Springer, 2011
6. Tantbirojn P et al: Gross abnormalities of the umbilical cord: related placental histology and clinical significance. Placenta. 30(12):1083-8, 2009
7. Tuxen AJ et al: Factors affecting umbilical venous perfusion during experimental cord knotting. Placenta. 26(10):753-7, 2005
8. Kraus FT et al: Atlas of Nontumor Pathology. Placental Pathology. Washington DC: American Registry of Pathology. 192-93, 2004
9. Airas U et al: Clinical significance of true umbilical knots: a population-based analysis. Am J Perinatol. 19(3):127-32, 2002
10. Hershkovitz R et al: Risk factors associated with true knots of the umbilical cord. Eur J Obstet Gynecol Reprod Biol. 98(1):36-9, 2001
11. Roberts RN: Combined simple and complex cord knots. Eur J Obstet Gynecol Reprod Biol. 62(1):131-3, 1995
12. Blickstein I et al: Predisposing factors in the formation of true knots of the umbilical cord--analysis of morphometric and perinatal data. Int J Gynaecol Obstet. 25(5):395-8, 1987

Gross Features

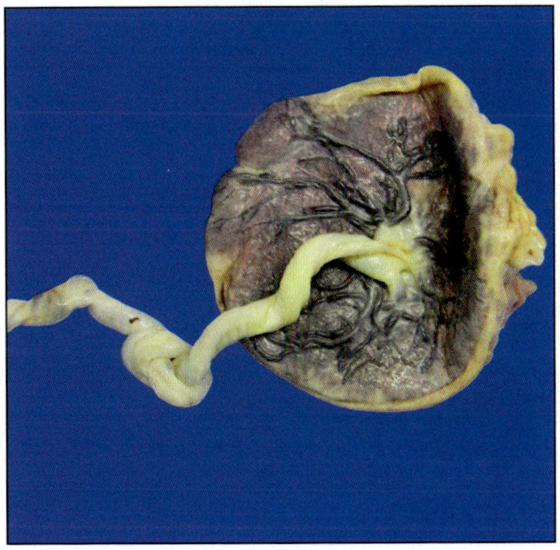

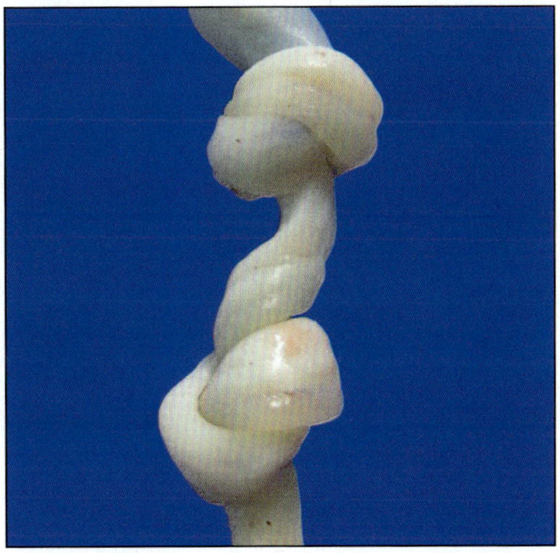

(Left) *Gross image shows a loose true knot located 11.5 cm from the insertion site in the chorionic plate. Note that there is no vascular congestion or compression of the underlying umbilical cord. This fetus did not suffer any clinical sequelae.* ***(Right)*** *Gross image shows 2 simple, tight true knots of a single umbilical cord. The pregnancy was complicated by oligohydramnios and 2-vessel umbilical cord. Histologically, a mural thrombus was identified in a stem villus.*

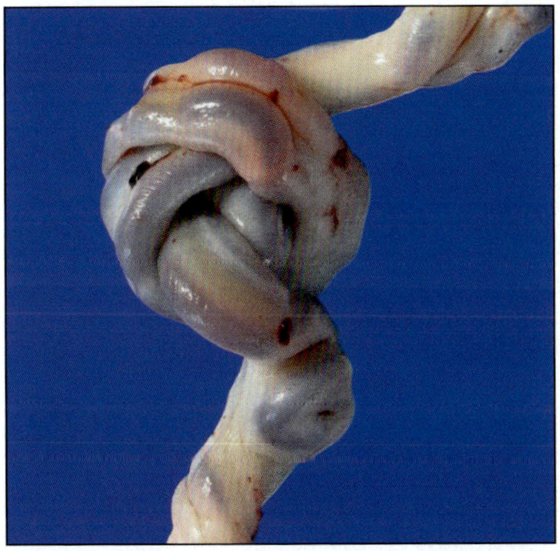

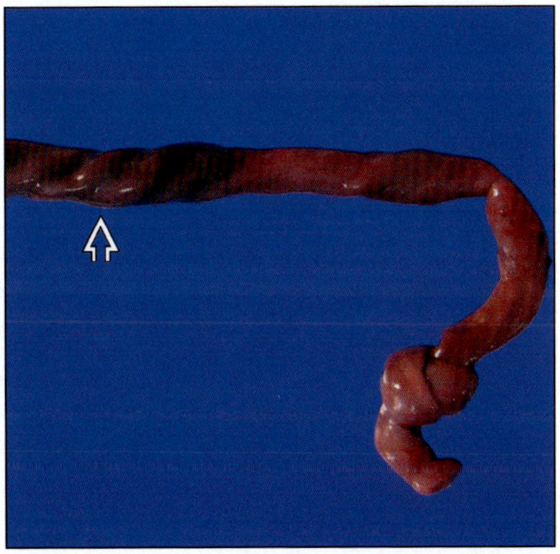

(Left) *Gross image shows a complex, multi-looped true knot with prominent vascular congestion. The fetus experienced distress during labor leading to C-section, suggesting transient tightening and vascular compression during labor may have occurred.* ***(Right)*** *Gross image shows a tight true knot of a stillborn infant with prominent congestion and vascular distention ➡. Thrombosis of the umbilical vein at the site of the knot was seen along with multiple thrombi of the chorionic vessels.*

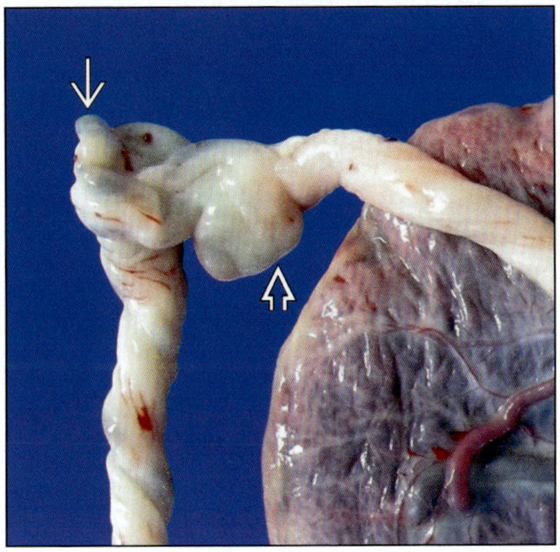

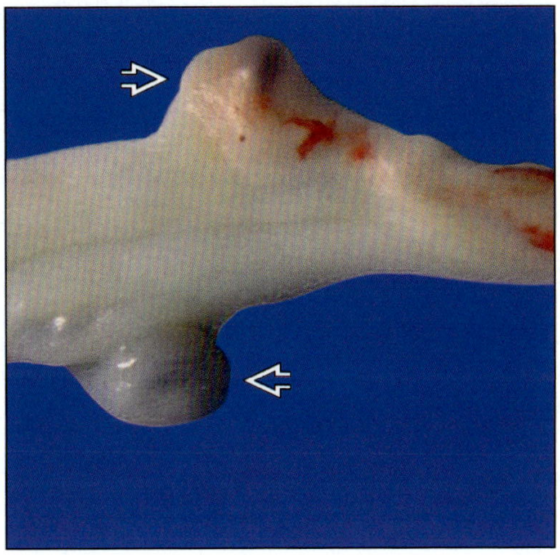

(Left) *Gross image shows a false knot (a.k.a. pseudoknot) with multiple protrusions of Wharton jelly ➡ and redundant vessels ➡.* ***(Right)*** *Gross image shows pseudoknots composed of vascular protrusions ➡, most likely redundant umbilical veins. Note that there is no congestion of the umbilical vessels proximal or distal to these protrusions. These false knots were found adjacent to a true knot, which is not an uncommon finding in umbilical cords with true knots.*

UMBILICAL CORD EDEMA AND THINNING

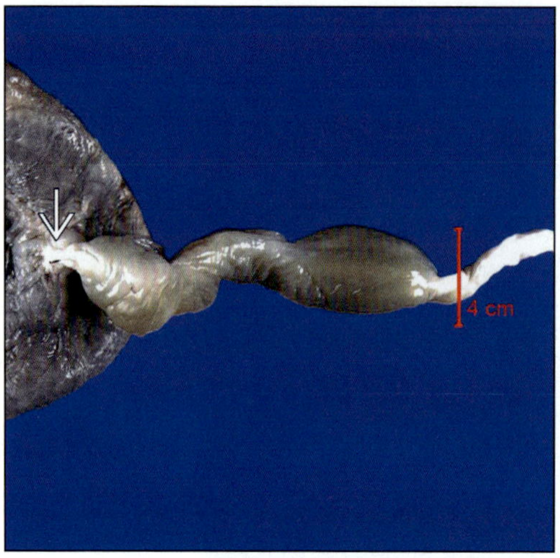

Massive localized edema is seen in this umbilical cord. Note the swollen and glistening surface of the cord with degeneration of Wharton jelly near the cord insertion site ➔.

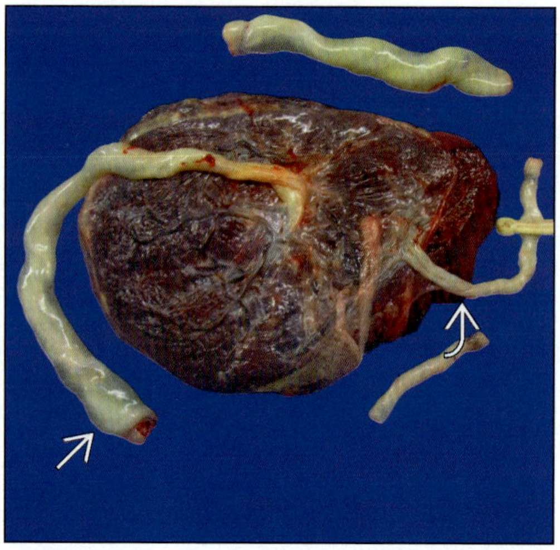

Monochorionic twin placenta has a thick ➔ and thin ➔ umbilical cord. The associated placental parenchyma shows unequal sharing, with the smaller cord associated with a smaller allocation.

TERMINOLOGY

Definitions

- Thick umbilical cord
  - Diameter is > 90th percentile for gestational age
    - Separate reference values are available for measurement by ultrasound in utero, gross evaluation, and on microscopic slides
  - Thickening may be focal or diffuse and is usually equated with edema of cord
- Thin umbilical cord
  - Diameter is < 10th percentile for gestational age
  - Thinning may be focal or diffuse
- Stricture
  - Sharply defined narrowed segment with decreased Wharton jelly &/or vascular constriction

EPIDEMIOLOGY

Incidence

- Thick cord
  - By definition, 10% of infants have excessively thick cords
  - Localized edema is rare
    - Often near fetal end
    - May be focal or multifocal
- Thin cord
  - By definition, 10% of infants have excessively thin cords
  - Stricture reported in
    - 5/1,369 deliveries (0.4%)
    - 9/297 spontaneous abortions (3%)

ETIOLOGY/PATHOGENESIS

Thick Cord

- Amount of Wharton jelly decreases near term
  - Cord reaches maximum diameter at 36 weeks
- Diffuse edema
  - Mechanism of edema similar to that of other tissues
    - Low oncotic pressure
    - Raised hydrostatic pressure
    - Increased water content (water content of edematous cords is 93.5%)
    - Leaky endothelium secondary to inflammation
- Localized swelling/edema
  - Effect of local injury
    - Meconium
    - Cord compression from entanglement, nuchal cord, or limb/body cord
    - Swelling between amniotic bands
    - Swelling on fetal side of tight knot (knots have blood back-up into placenta, not fetus)
  - Omphalocele at umbilicus
  - Cysts
    - Allantoic remnant cyst (1 in 200,000) may communicate with bladder and contain urine near fetal end
    - Omphalomesenteric duct cyst is common at fetal end of cord
    - Amniotic epithelial inclusion cyst
    - Mucoid degeneration: Bland pseudocyst filled with liquefied Wharton jelly without amniotic lining
  - Vascular lesions
    - Cord hemangioma
    - Cord hematoma: Accumulations of blood in Wharton jelly are often attributed to traumatic or mechanical damage
    - Idiopathic dilation of umbilical vein

Thin Cord

- Diffuse thinning
  - Due to significant decrease/loss of Wharton jelly volume, usually with decreased water content
    - Fetal volume depletion is secondary to longstanding uteroplacental underperfusion,

leading to decreased extracellular fluid/Wharton jelly
  - Due to overall decrease in cross-sectional area of umbilical cord vessels
    - Single umbilical artery
- Localized thinning
  - Focal reduction in diameter of fetal umbilical vessels
  - Segment of thinning may be associated with increased coiling
- Stricture
  - Most commonly found at fetal end of cord near umbilical insertion
    - Unclear if etiology is secondary to excessive coiling or due to a primary deficiency of Wharton jelly
  - Multiple strictures can be seen between helices in some cases of extreme overcoiling

CLINICAL IMPLICATIONS

Thick Cord

- Diffuse edema
  - Typically have normal outcome
  - More common in premature infants
  - Associated with
    - Gestational diabetes
    - Funisitis in amniotic fluid infection syndrome
    - Fetal hydrops
  - Associated with respiratory disorders in newborn
    - Transient respiratory distress and respiratory distress syndrome, likely related to gestational diabetes
- Localized edema
  - Umbilical cord remnant cysts
    - At umbilicus, must clinically exclude patent urachus or herniated fetal intestine
    - Large omphalomesenteric or allantoic cysts have separate clinical associations
    - Venous obstruction due to these conditions is suggested to be a cause of mucoid degeneration elsewhere in cord
  - Localized cysts noted on 3rd-trimester ultrasound are associated with multiple congenital anomalies, especially in cases of trisomy 18
    - Histology is not always described
    - Omphalocele present in some cases; others show only mucoid degeneration
  - Need to differentiate swelling of edema from hemorrhage
    - Umbilical cord hematomas are most commonly artifacts of cord clamping after birth
    - In true intrafunicular hemorrhage, perinatal mortality rate can be as high as 40-50% secondary to fetal blood loss or compression of umbilical vessels
  - May be due to mass-forming lesions of cord, such as hemangioma with its own clinical associations

Thin Cord

- Diffuse thinning
  - Complete absence of Wharton jelly is associated with fetal death in utero
  - Meconium-stained amniotic fluid is often present
  - Associated with
    - Preeclampsia
    - Intrauterine growth restriction
    - Fetal distress during labor
    - Single umbilical artery
    - Oligohydramnios
- Localized thinning and stricture
  - Associated with
    - Intrauterine fetal demise/macerated fetuses
    - Fetal intolerance to labor
  - Stricture
    - Can recur in subsequent pregnancies
    - Proposed to be a cause of nonimmune hydrops
    - Rarely occur in hypocoiled or normally coiled cords

MACROSCOPIC FINDINGS

General Features of Thick Cord

- Diffuse thickening
  - Cord appears diffusely swollen and glistening
- Focal thickening
  - Segment of cord appears swollen and often more translucent than adjacent segments
  - Transillumination for cysts or other lesions is recommended
- True hematoma
  - Red-purple, elongated, and fusiform throughout cord length, or focally, usually at fetal end
  - Hemorrhage replaces Wharton jelly on cut section
  - No clamping or puncture marks on exterior
- Artifactual cord hematoma
  - Can see clamp marks or puncture marks from cord sampling
  - May only displace Wharton jelly

General Features of Thin Cord

- Diffuse thinning
  - Single umbilical artery may be present
  - Tends to have lower coiling index
  - Associated with placental gross features of uteroplacental malperfusion and small for age placental weight
  - Associated with marginal insertion of umbilical cord
- Focal thinning and strictures
  - Associated with excessively long and hypercoiled cords
  - Rarely found in hypocoiled or normally coiled cords
  - Congestion and dilation of umbilical vessels may be seen
  - Umbilical vein may be severely compressed
  - Thrombi may be seen in umbilical vessels within or near strictured portion

Specimen Handling

- Note length and location of focal thickening or thinning of cord and presence of additional lesions identified on cut section

UMBILICAL CORD EDEMA AND THINNING

- If hemorrhage or hematoma is present, note extent and vessel involvement
  - Note associated puncture or clamp marks
    - If associated with clamp marks, unlikely to be any significance
    - If associated with puncture, need to assess whether there was cordocentesis in utero or after delivery
- Document significant associated findings, such as hematoma or other lesions with gross photograph

MICROSCOPIC FINDINGS

General Features of Thick Cord

- Diffuse edema
  - Typically, bland increase in amount of Wharton jelly ± increased mast cells and empty spaces without lining
  - Fetal inflammatory response (umbilical phlebitis, umbilical vasculitis, &/or funisitis) in amniotic fluid infection sequence
- Localized edema, depending on etiology, may manifest as
  - Bland degeneration of Wharton jelly (pseudocyst)
  - Degeneration of Wharton jelly with inflammation and possible thrombi of umbilical vessels
  - Effects of intense meconium deposition with rare pigmented macrophages, vascular necrosis, and thrombi
  - Hemangioma of cord
  - Cysts
    - Allantoic remnant cyst: Located between the 2 umbilical arteries and has a flattened to cuboidal epithelium
    - Omphalomesenteric duct cyst: Found near periphery of cord and lined by columnar cells similar to that seen in intestinal epithelium

General Features of Thin Cord

- Wharton jelly may be decreased with little separation of vessels
  - Rarely, it is completely absent
- Reduced cross-sectional area of umbilical vein
- Single umbilical artery may be present
- Stricture
  - Overall decreased Wharton jelly
  - Associated fetal large vessel thrombi
  - Villous capillary congestion
  - Compression &/or distension of umbilical vessels, especially vein
  - May see degeneration of umbilical vessels, usually with prolonged in utero demise to delivery interval

Method to Assess Cord Diameter From Histologic Sections

- Submit sections of umbilical cord from fetal end and placental end
- Measure 2 cord diameters at right angles to each other from each histologic section
- Average the 2 diameters
- In order to account for cord shrinkage caused by fixation and processing, a correction coefficient should be used
  - < 28 weeks = + 0.11 cm
  - > 28 weeks = + 0.17 cm
  - Proctor et al (2013) provide more specific cord diameter ranges

SELECTED REFERENCES

1. Baergen RN: Umbilical cord pathology. In Baergen RN et al: Surgical Pathology Clinics: Placental Pathology. Vol 6:1. Philadelphia: WB Saunders. 61-85, 2013
2. Proctor LK et al: Umbilical cord diameter percentile curves and their correlation to birth weight and placental pathology. Placenta. 34(1):62-6, 2013
3. Schaefer IM et al: Giant umbilical cord edema caused by retrograde micturition through an open patent urachus. Pediatr Dev Pathol. 13(5):404-7, 2010
4. Goynumer G et al: Umbilical cord thickness in the first and early second trimesters and perinatal outcome. J Perinat Med. 36(6):523-6, 2008
5. Ghezzi F et al: Sonographic umbilical vessel morphometry and perinatal outcome of fetuses with a lean umbilical cord. J Clin Ultrasound. 33(1):18-23, 2005
6. Emura T et al: Omphalocele associated with a large multilobular umbilical cord pseudocyst. Pediatr Surg Int. 20(8):636-9, 2004
7. Redline RW et al: Maternal vascular underperfusion: nosology and reproducibility of placental reaction patterns. Pediatr Dev Pathol. 7(3):237-49, 2004
8. Sepulveda W et al: Pseudocyst of the umbilical cord: prenatal sonographic appearance and clinical significance. Obstet Gynecol. 93(3):377-81, 1999
9. Babay ZA et al: A case of varix dilatation of the umbilical vein and review of the literature. Fetal Diagn Ther. 11(3):221-3, 1996
10. Benirschke K: Obstetrically important lesions of the umbilical cord. J Reprod Med. 39(4):262-72, 1994
11. Kero P et al: Colloid osmotic pressure of cord blood in relation to neonatal outcome and mode of delivery. Acta Paediatr Scand Suppl. 305:88-91, 1983
12. Coulter JB et al: Oedema of the umbilical cord and respiratory distress in the newborn. Br J Obstet Gynaecol. 82(6):453-9, 1975

Gross and Microscopic Features

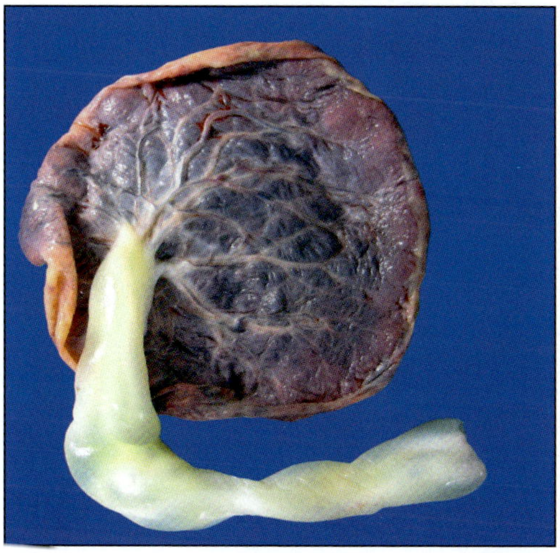

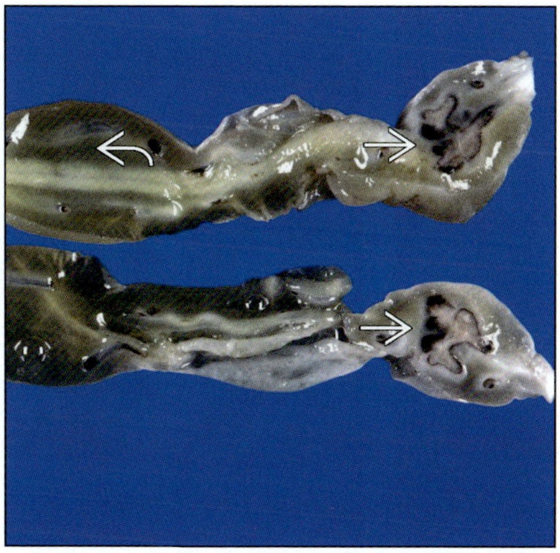

(Left) *This small placenta has a massively edematous, thick, swollen umbilical cord with a low coiling index. This severe edema was associated with hydrops of the fetus.* ***(Right)*** *Localized edema may be associated with a vascular malformation of the cord. Degeneration of Wharton jelly is also seen with brown discoloration of the gelatinous stroma.*

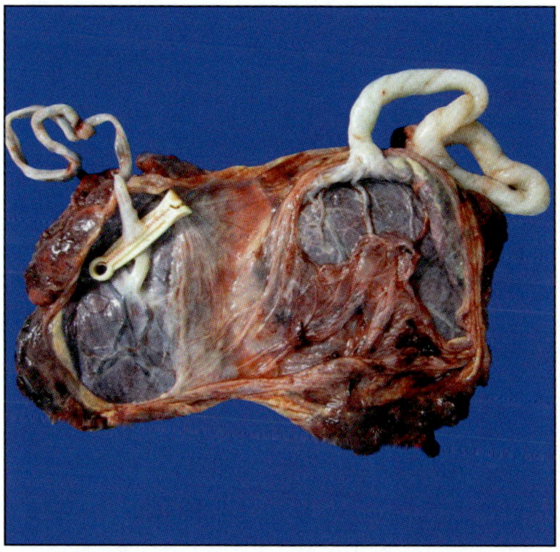

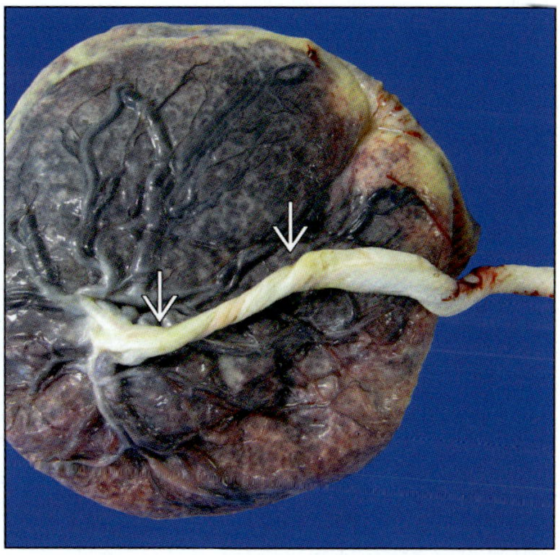

(Left) *Discordant fetal growth may be reflected in thick and thin cords, as in this dichorionic placenta.* ***(Right)*** *Segmental umbilical cord thinning is seen close to the placental insertion site. Note the decreased coiling as the cord widens away from the area of thinning.*

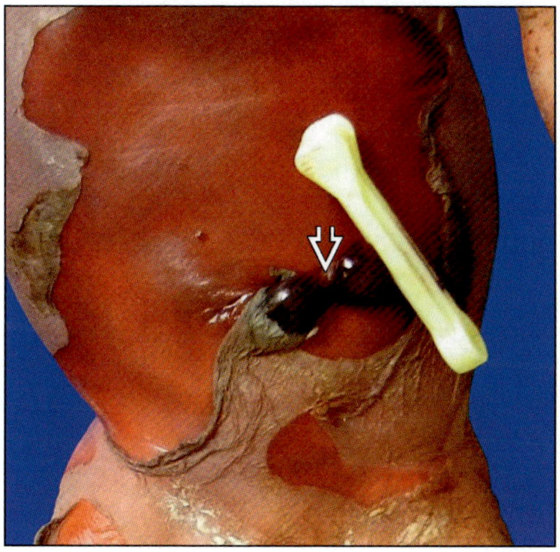

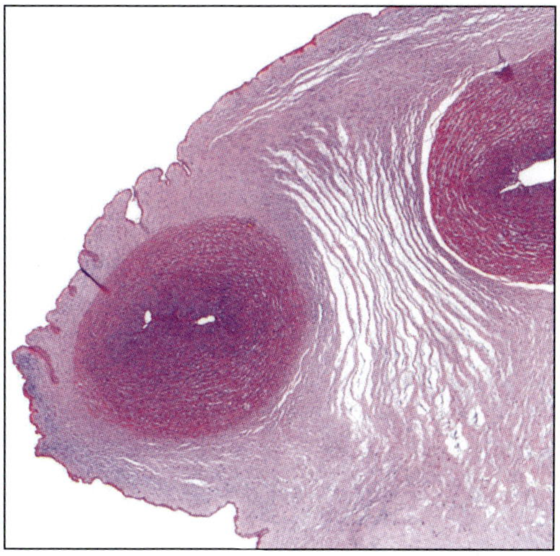

(Left) *A stricture is seen in the umbilical cord stump in this case of intrauterine fetal demise. The placental cord showed hypercoiling. At autopsy, the death was attributed to the lesion.* ***(Right)*** *In this thin umbilical cord, Wharton jelly is decreased. The substance of the cord appears blue-pink with minimal white space, and the vessels are close to the surface.*

HISTOPATHOLOGIC CHANGES OF UMBILICAL CORD

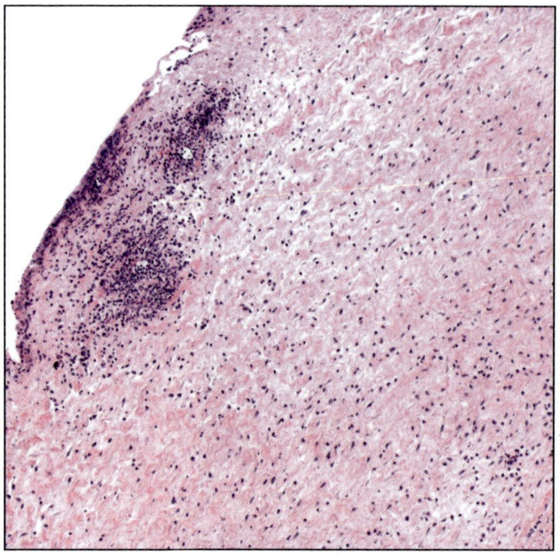

The term funisitis is very general; more specific terms have better clinical relevance. For example, peripheral funisitis (as depicted here) is strongly associated with congenital candidiasis.

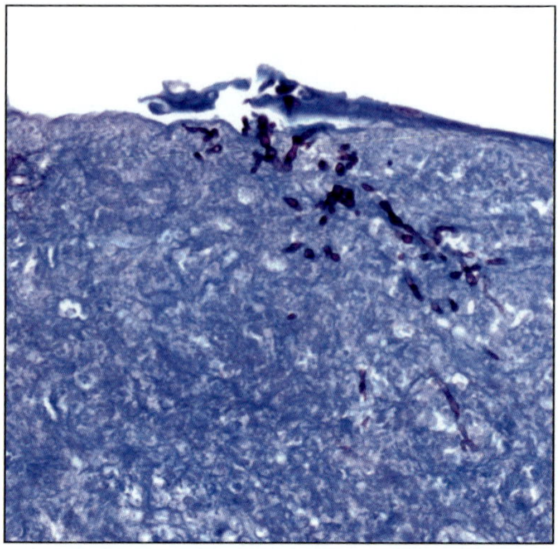

A PAS stain identifies the candidal organisms. The clinical team caring for the baby should be notified of such a result as a "critical value" in placental surgical pathology.

TERMINOLOGY

Definitions

- Umbilical phlebitis: Fetal inflammatory response
  - Neutrophils emanating from lumen to muscularis of umbilical vein
- Umbilical arteritis: Fetal inflammatory response
  - Neutrophils emanating from lumen to muscularis of umbilical artery
- Panvasculitis: Fetal inflammatory response involving vein and both arteries
- Funisitis: Fetal inflammatory response extending from vessels into Wharton jelly
- Peripheral funisitis: Accumulation of neutrophils beneath amniotic surface
- Fetal thrombotic vasculopathy: Occlusive or nonocclusive thrombi in umbilical cord, chorionic plate, or stem villous vasculature and associated distal villous changes
- Meconium-associated vascular necrosis: Necrosis of vascular smooth muscle in prolonged meconium exposure

Abbreviations

- Umbilical artery (UA)
- Umbilical vein (UV)
- Umbilical cord (UC)
- Fetal thrombotic vasculopathy (FTV)
- Meconium-associated vascular necrosis (MAVN)

INFLAMMATION OF CORD

Acute Inflammation

- Fetal inflammatory response to stimulus
  - Infection of amniotic fluid
    - Most common etiology
  - Chemical irritant, such as meconium
    - Must be localized to area of meconium changes, not associated with other changes of amniotic fluid infection sequence
  - Local injury
    - e.g., cordocentesis, UC prolapse
- Localization of inflammation correlates with acuity and severity of amniotic fluid infection
- Early response
  - Phlebitis
- Intermediate response
  - Arteritis
  - Panvasculitis
- Late response
  - Funisitis
  - Necrosis
  - Perivascular calcifications

Clinical Significance of Acute Umbilical Cord Inflammation

- Associated with
  - Clinical chorioamnionitis and microbial invasion of amniotic cavity
  - Higher cord blood IL-6 levels and fetal inflammatory response syndrome
  - Congenital sepsis in neonate
  - Decreased risk of respiratory distress syndrome in premature neonate
    - Chorioamnionitis appears to stimulate lung maturation in fetus, likely through endogenous steroids
  - *Ureaplasma urealyticum* and *Mycoplasma hominis*
    - Often present by PCR
    - May be associated with bronchopulmonary dysplasia

Peripheral Funisitis

- Virtually pathognomonic for *Candida* species
- May or may not be associated with congenital candidiasis in newborn

- *Candida* may not be clinically suspected if newborn does not have rash
- Finding of peripheral funisitis with fungi should prompt call to pediatrician/neonatologist regarding possibility of congenital candidiasis

Chronic Inflammation of Cord

- Very uncommon; suggests prolonged infection
- Numerous plasma cells suggest herpes simplex virus infection

Gross Changes in Umbilical Cord Inflammation

- Edema in severe inflammation of cord
- Chalky yellow-white concentric rings around vessels in severe necrotizing inflammation
- Yellow-white punctate lesions on cord surface in peripheral funisitis
  - Consider frozen section to demonstrate fungi quickly

Microscopic Changes in Umbilical Cord Inflammation

- Fetal acute inflammatory response
  - Neutrophils, migrating from vessel lumen through muscularis toward stimuli in amniotic fluid
  - Involves media of umbilical vein first, more commonly on fetal side of cord
  - Progresses to involve 1 or both umbilical arteries
  - Extends to Wharton jelly (funisitis) with prolonged inflammation
  - Becomes necrotizing, causing necrosis of vessel wall, and replacement of Wharton jelly by fibrin around vessels, usually with neutrophilic karyorrhexis
- Peripheral funisitis
  - May or may not have umbilical vasculitis
  - Neutrophils accumulate beneath amnion
  - Typically associated with fungal forms on GMS stain
- Chronic inflammation
  - Rare as fetal response
    - Numerous plasma cells should raise suspicion for congenital herpes simplex virus infection
- Response to noninfectious stimuli
  - Meconium deposition
    - Pigmented macrophages are rare in umbilical cord stroma
    - Chronic meconium exposure is usually required to cause inflammation in cord
    - Often associated with additional fetal and maternal inflammatory responses of amniotic fluid infection; look for evidence elsewhere
    - If present, fetal inflammatory response should be attributed to amniotic fluid infection, not solely meconium
  - Cordocentesis
    - May see few changes or evidence of organizing hemorrhage; reported that 20-30% of fetuses have hemorrhage from puncture site
    - Risk of fetal loss related to fetal thrombocytopenia and severity of fetal illness

Additional Placental Features

- Fetal inflammatory response in umbilical cord associated with
  - Acute chorioamnionitis (maternal inflammatory response)
  - Chorionic plate vasculitis (fetal inflammatory response)
  - Fetal thrombi (when fetal inflammation is severe or prolonged)
- Peripheral funisitis usually associated with
  - Microabscesses elsewhere on amniotic surface, with fungal organisms
  - May or may not have chorioamnionitis

VASCULAR LESIONS OF CORD

Umbilical Cord Thrombi

- ~ 1 in 1,000 deliveries
- More frequent in high-risk pregnancies (1 in 250)
- Incidence of vessel involvement
  - 71% UV alone
  - 11% UA alone
  - 18% artery and vein thrombosed
- Etiology reflected in Virchow triad
  - Blood stasis
    - Impediments to flow include cord compression, kinking of undercoiled cord, tight knots, strictures
    - Conditions that significantly slow blood flow, such as heart failure, excessively long cord, or increased resistance to flow in severely overcoiled cord
  - Vessel injury
    - Injury to endothelium from severe inflammation, MAVN, or vessel rupture
  - Hypercoagulable state
    - Increased red blood cells in gestational diabetes
    - 3rd spacing of intravascular volume
    - Genetic conditions that cause increased clotting
- Clinical significance
  - Mortality highest if both arteries occluded
  - Liveborn infants often have neonatal distress or die in newborn period
  - Survivors may have long-term sequelae such as neurologic injury
- Gross changes of cord thrombi
  - Brown-green discoloration of cord surface in area of thrombus or vascular necrosis
  - May see congestion on 1 side of lesion
  - Thrombus palpable and visible on cut section
  - Photograph clot as well as any associated gross lesions
  - Document associated abnormalities of umbilical cord
    - Excessively long or excessively short
    - Undercoiled or overcoiled
    - Abnormal cord insertion (marginal or velamentous)
    - Areas of flattening suggest compression by limb or body part
    - True knots

- Amniotic bands around cord
  - Look for associated changes in placenta
    - Chorionic plate thrombi
    - Pale areas of placental parenchyma corresponding to fetal thrombotic vasculopathy
- Microscopic changes of cord thrombi
  - Occlusive thrombus
    - In addition to thrombus filling the lumen, commonly see ischemic necrosis of vessel wall
    - Endothelial cells, myocytes depend on fetal blood for oxygen
    - If older lesion, may see calcification
  - Nonocclusive thrombus
    - Thrombus does not fill lumen, may see organization in vessel wall
    - Residual blood flow in part of vessel; vascular wall remains viable
    - Calcification in older lesion
    - Associated findings: Fetal inflammatory response to amniotic fluid infection, MAVN, iatrogenic cordocentesis changes

Meconium-Associated Vascular Necrosis

- ~ 1% of meconium-stained placentas
- Meconium deposition leads to myocyte apoptosis in portion of vessel wall underlying meconium staining
- Meconium substance on vascular smooth muscle causes vasoconstriction
- Clinical implications
  - Frequent cesarean section delivery due to fetal distress
  - Low Apgar scores
  - Acidemia on umbilical cord gases
  - Survivors may have long-term sequelae such as neurologic injury
- Gross changes of MAVN
  - Usually associated with subacute or chronic meconium staining
    - Dull-appearing, diffusely brown umbilical cord that is almost uniformly stained
  - May have linear ulceration overlying necrotic region of vessel
  - Associated gross changes
    - Large vessel thrombi in affected cord or chorionic plate
    - Pale parenchymal foci of fetal thrombotic vasculopathy
    - Multiple other placental pathologies, as fetal stress is associated with meconium passage
- Microscopic changes of MAVN
  - Hypereosinophilia of myocytes with pyknotic nuclei
  - Reactive and necrotic changes to amnion associated with meconium
  - Meconium-laden macrophages in cord stroma (rare) and membranes
  - May see occlusive or nonocclusive thrombi
  - May see acute and chronic inflammatory cells reacting to meconium
    - Distinguish from amniotic fluid infection by extent of inflammation, with amniotropism elsewhere
    - Meconium deposition and amniotic fluid infection frequently coexist

VASCULAR ANOMALIES OF CORD

Angioma

- Very rare, true incidence unknown
- Clinical associations
  - Large lesions may be associated with hydrops from high output cardiac failure
  - Rare case reported as arteriovenous malformation at fetal end of cord
    - Associated with lesional thrombi and DIC
    - Unclear if histology of this lesion differs from that most commonly described
  - ~ 1/3 with fetal or neonatal mortality, 1/3 with morbidity, and 1/3 with favorable outcome
  - Associated vascular malformation in neonate in subset of cases (port-wine stain)
- Gross features
  - Often associated with localized edema of umbilical cord
  - Reported greatest dimension ranges from 3-18 cm
  - Arise from 1 or both umbilical arteries
  - Most common at placental end of cord, in region of Hyrtl anastomosis (common connection between umbilical arteries near placental cord insertion site)
- Microscopic features
  - Irregular proliferation of capillaries separated by bundles of vascular smooth muscle
- Differential diagnosis
  - Persistence of vitelline vessels
    - Capillary channels form wreath around omphalomesenteric duct remnant
    - Usually lacks complexity of vascular malformation angioma
    - Abnormal vessels are in Wharton jelly, not smooth muscle/fibrous tissue
  - Intrafunicular hematoma
    - Dissection of fetal blood into Wharton jelly due to tearing of umbilical vessel (usually the vein)
    - Fetal blood in spaces resembles vascular malformation
    - No endothelial lining around blood collections
    - No smooth muscle/fibrous tissue component
    - Up to 50% perinatal mortality
    - May represent delivery artifact with no clinical significance

UMBILICAL CORD INJURY

Umbilical Cord Rupture

- Gross diagnosis
- Associated with
  - Short cords
  - Cords made functionally short due to limb/body entanglement
  - Cords ulcerated from meconium-associated vascular necrosis
  - Prolapsed cords

Grading and Staging of Fetal Inflammatory Response in Acute Chorioamnionitis

Diagnostic Category	Suggested Terminology	Definition
Stage 1	Umbilical phlebitis	Involves umbilical vein (&/or chorionic plate vessels)
Stage 2	Umbilical vasculitis (1 umbilical artery and vein) or umbilical panvasculitis (all 3 umbilical vessels)	Involves 1 or both umbilical arteries ± scattered neutrophils in Wharton jelly
Stage 3	Necrotizing funisitis, concentric umbilical perivasculitis	Concentric acute inflammation with karyorrhectic debris, eosinophilia of matrix ± mineralization
Grade 1 (mild-moderate)	No additional terminology	Scattered neutrophils beneath endothelium or in vascular smooth muscle, not confluent
Grade 2 (severe)	With a severe fetal inflammatory response	Confluent neutrophils beneath endothelium or in vascular smooth muscle with attenuation of vascular smooth muscle
Other patterns	Peripheral funisitis	Focal aggregates of neutrophils at the umbilical cord surface

Adapted from the Society for Pediatric Pathology Perinatal Section paper: Redline RW et al: Amniotic infection syndrome: nosology and reproducibility of placental reaction patterns. Pediatr Dev Pathol. 6(5):435-48, 2003.

    - Cords with severe necrotizing fetal inflammatory response
- Amniotic fluid may be port-wine colored due to fetal hemorrhage
- With prolonged duration, thrombus forms at rupture site and hemosiderin-laden macrophages are seen near rupture and in membranes
- Must exclude postdelivery avulsion of cord by communication with delivery attendants

Umbilical Cord Compression

- Grossly, compressed area appears discolored, macerated
    - Wharton jelly shows degenerative changes with loss of spaces, sometimes with cellular debris
- Microscopic changes are nonspecific and require correlation
- Umbilical vein most susceptible to compression
    - May see congestion of chorionic villi
    - Umbilical vein and chorionic plate veins may be dilated

SELECTED REFERENCES

1. Society for Maternal-Fetal Medicine (SMFM) et al: Fetal blood sampling. Am J Obstet Gynecol. 209(3):170-80, 2013
2. Goldenberg RL et al: The Alabama Preterm Birth Study: umbilical cord blood Ureaplasma urealyticum and Mycoplasma hominis cultures in very preterm newborn infants. Am J Obstet Gynecol. 198(1):43, 2008
3. Baergen RN: Cord abnormalities, structural lesions, and cord "accidents". Semin Diagn Pathol. 24(1):23-32, 2007
4. Egawa T et al: Ureaplasma urealyticum and Mycoplasma hominis presence in umbilical cord is associated with pathogenesis of funisitis. Kobe J Med Sci. 53(5):241-9, 2007
5. Lee SE et al: The intensity of the fetal inflammatory response in intraamniotic inflammation with and without microbial invasion of the amniotic cavity. Am J Obstet Gynecol. 197(3):294, 2007
6. Redline RW: Inflammatory responses in the placenta and umbilical cord. Semin Fetal Neonatal Med. 11(5):296-301, 2006
7. Sato Y et al: Umbilical arterial thrombosis with vascular wall necrosis: clinicopathologic findings of 11 cases. Placenta. 27(6-7):715-8, 2006
8. Daniel-Spiegel E et al: The association of umbilical cord hemangioma with fetal vascular birthmarks. Prenat Diagn. 25(4):300-3, 2005
9. Korkmaz A et al: Placental apoptosis in pregnancies with intrauterine meconium passage. Am J Perinatol. 22(3):133-8, 2005
10. Redline RW: Severe fetal placental vascular lesions in term infants with neurologic impairment. Am J Obstet Gynecol. 192(2):452-7, 2005
11. King EL et al: Myocytes of chorionic vessels from placentas with meconium-associated vascular necrosis exhibit apoptotic markers. Hum Pathol. 35(4):412-7, 2004
12. Redline RW et al: Amniotic infection syndrome: nosology and reproducibility of placental reaction patterns. Pediatr Dev Pathol. 6(5):435-48, 2003
13. Yoon BH et al: The relationship among inflammatory lesions of the umbilical cord (funisitis), umbilical cord plasma interleukin 6 concentration, amniotic fluid infection, and neonatal sepsis. Am J Obstet Gynecol. 183(5):1124-9, 2000
14. Qureshi F et al: Candida funisitis: A clinicopathologic study of 32 cases. Pediatr Dev Pathol. 1(2):118-24, 1998
15. Richards DS et al: Prenatal diagnosis of fetal disseminated intravascular coagulation associated with umbilical cord arteriovenous malformation. Obstet Gynecol. 85(5 Pt 2):860-2, 1995
16. Altshuler G et al: Meconium-induced umbilical cord vascular necrosis and ulceration: a potential link between the placenta and poor pregnancy outcome. Obstet Gynecol. 79(5 (Pt 1)):760-6, 1992
17. Altshuler G et al: Meconium-induced vasocontraction: a potential cause of cerebral and other fetal hypoperfusion and of poor pregnancy outcome. J Child Neurol. 4(2):137-42, 1989
18. Heifetz SA: Thrombosis of the umbilical cord: analysis of 52 cases and literature review. Pediatr Pathol. 8(1):37-54, 1988

HISTOPATHOLOGIC CHANGES OF UMBILICAL CORD

Fetal Inflammatory Response

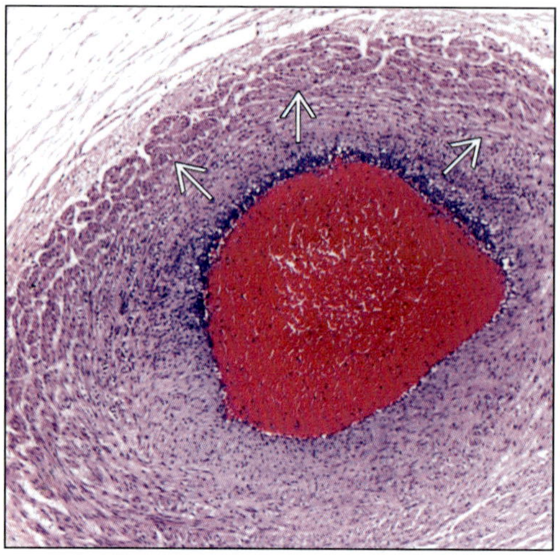
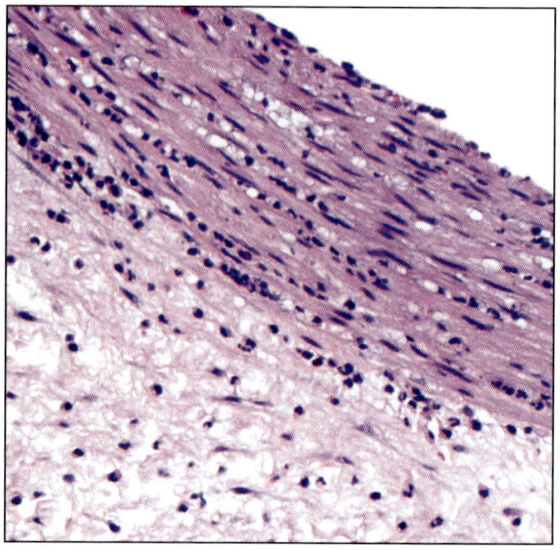

(Left) *In amniotic fluid infection, fetal inflammatory cells migrate toward* ➡ *the stimulus in the amniotic fluid.* ***(Right)*** *The fetal inflammatory response is graded and staged for better clinicopathologic correlation. This image shows a fetal inflammatory response at grade 1 (scattered neutrophils, not confluent), stage 2 (involving 1 or both umbilical arteries).*

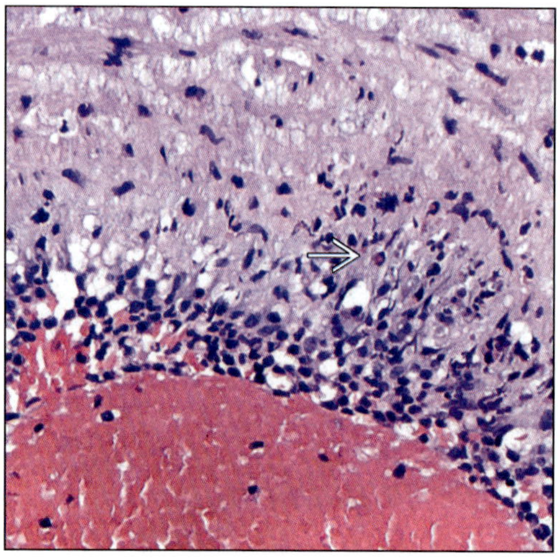
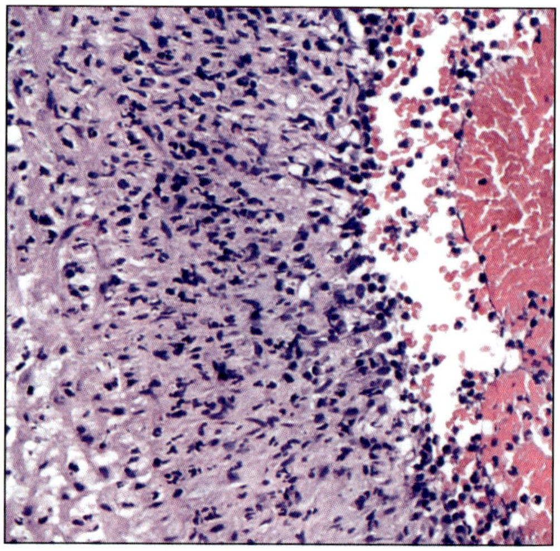

(Left) *The fetal inflammatory infiltrate is composed mostly of neutrophils with rare eosinophils* ➡*. The confluence of neutrophils makes this case a fetal inflammatory response grade 2 (severe). Involvement of the umbilical artery makes stage 2 (advanced).* ***(Right)*** *The confluence of neutrophils with attenuation of the vascular smooth muscle makes this a grade 2 (severe) fetal inflammatory response. It is stage 2 because it involves the umbilical artery.*

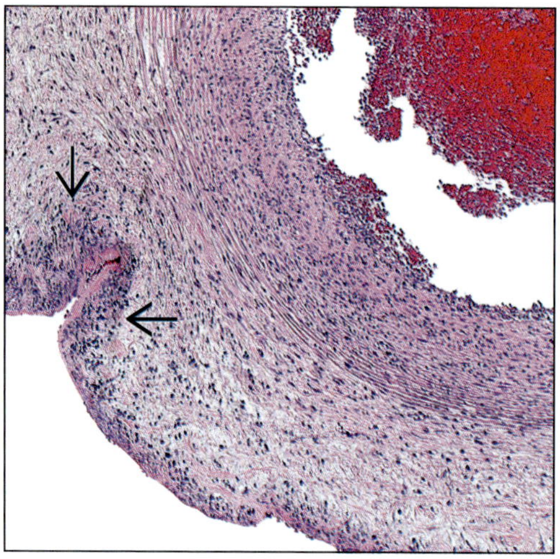
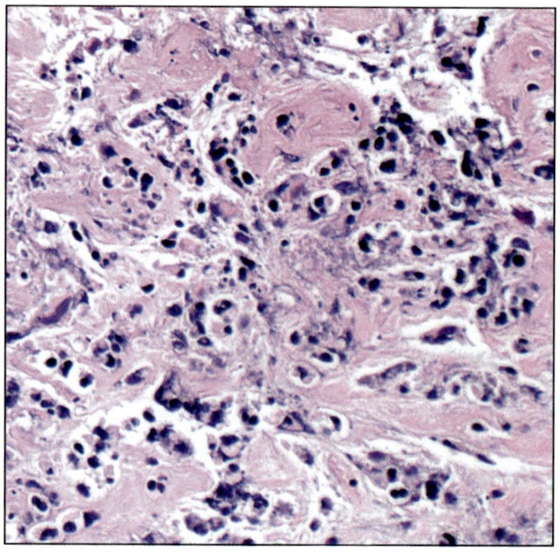

(Left) *The presence of concentric necrosis around the vessel makes this a grade 2 (severe), stage 3 (necrotizing funisitis) fetal inflammatory response. Also present is peripheral funisitis* ➡*. Branching hyphae of Candida were easily identified on GMS stain.* ***(Right)*** *This case of necrotizing funisitis also contains plasma cells. Plasma cells are uncommon in the cord. Longstanding bacterial infection may have plasma cells, but it is always prudent to exclude herpes simplex virus infection in such cases.*

Vascular Lesions of Cord

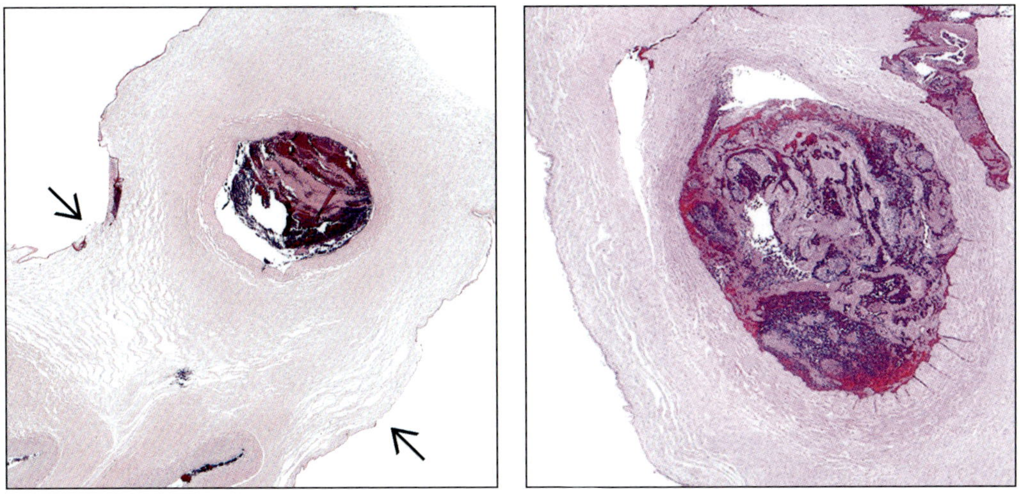

(Left) *This compressed area → of the cord shows an umbilical vein thrombus. Grossly, this region of flattened cord appeared macerated. These findings suggest compression from limb/body entanglement, such as a nuchal cord.* ***(Right)*** *Laminations attest to in vivo clot formation in this umbilical vein thrombus.*

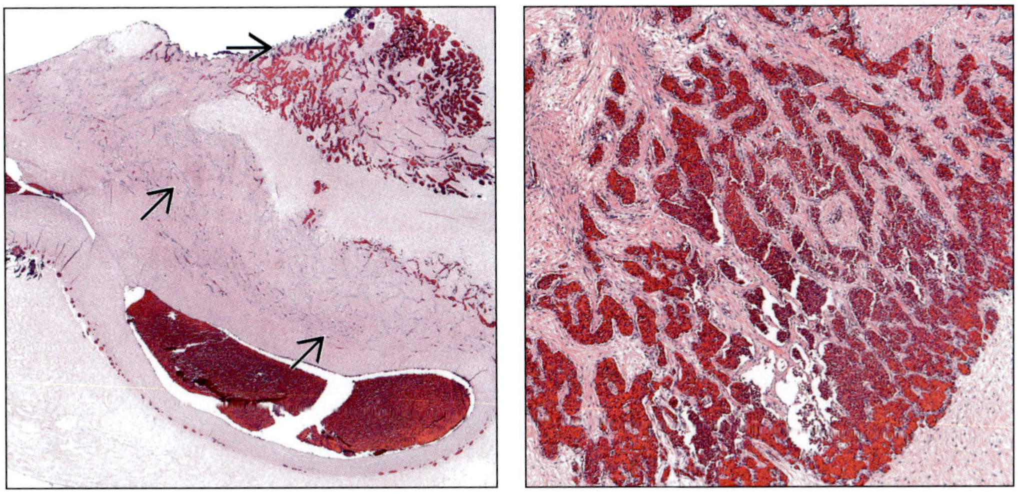

(Left) *Vascular malformations → of the cord (also termed angiomyxomas) are often associated with an umbilical artery.* ***(Right)*** *Unlike a cord hematoma from partial rupture, blood in these spaces of a vascular malformation is associated with endothelial cells and a branching fibromuscular stroma arising from the arterial smooth muscle.*

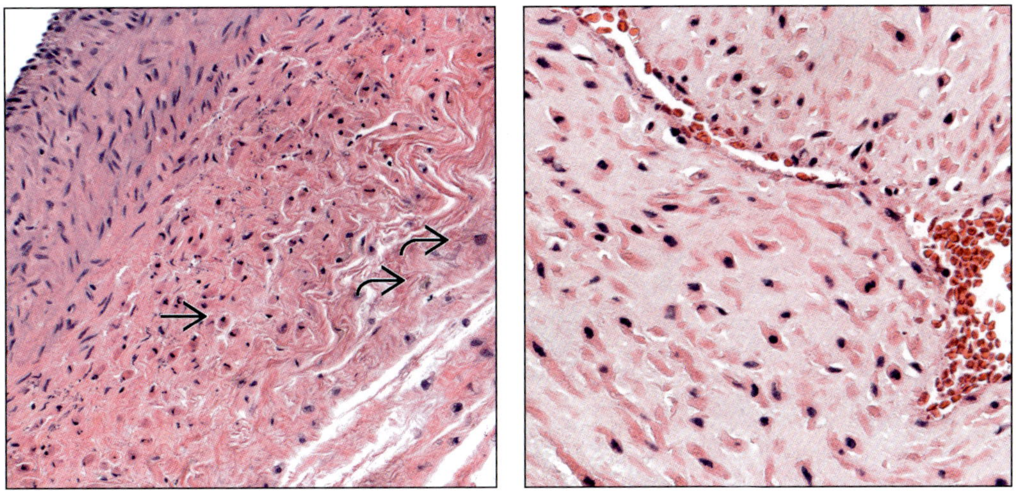

(Left) *Meconium-associated vascular necrosis is associated with prolonged heavy meconium exposure. The process begins from the outside in with individual smooth muscle cell apoptosis →. Occasional meconium-laden macrophages ↷ may be found.* ***(Right)*** *In contrast to the polarity of the change in meconium-associated vascular necrosis, the vascular smooth muscle pyknosis of prolonged in utero fetal demise is present throughout the muscularis.*

Extraplacental Membranes

GROSS EVALUATION AND NORMAL HISTOLOGY OF MEMBRANES

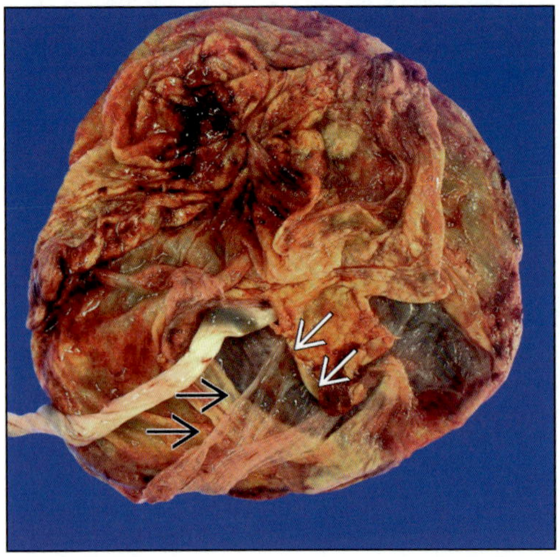

The placenta is often received with membranes "inside out." This image shows membranes in anatomic position. Note the thin, translucent amnion ⇨ partially separated from the thicker chorion and decidual layers ➡.

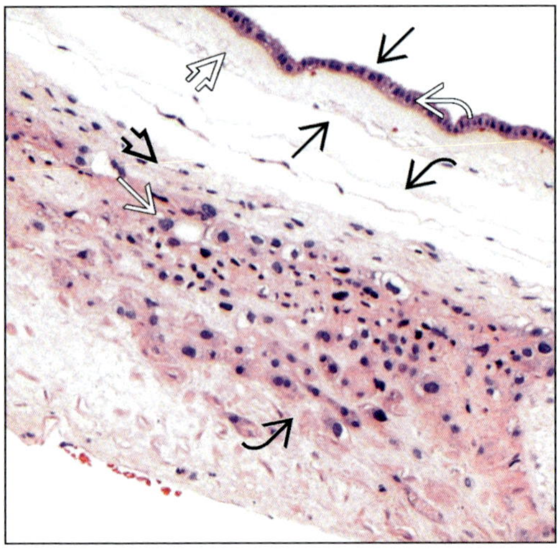

Layers include amnion ⇨ (amniotic epithelium with basement membrane ➡, connective tissue ➡), & chorion ⇨ (chorionic mesoderm ⇨, cellular chorion ➡ with intermediate extravillous trophoblast).

TERMINOLOGY

Definitions

- Extraplacental membranes: Amnion, chorion, and decidua extending from edge of placental disc
- Extrachorial placentation: Insertion of extraplacental membranes inside boundary of placental disc
- Chorion laeve: Membranous chorion
- Decidua capsularis: Layer of gestational endometrium overlying implanted conceptus
- Decidua parietalis: All decidua not overlying or underneath implanted conceptus

Synonyms

- Decidua parietalis and decidua vera

GROSS EVALUATION

Integrity

- Amnion normally loosely adherent to chorion
  - May slip entirely from chorion when edematous, but remains strongly attached to cord
- Amount of decidua present is variable
- Membranes excessively torn and shredded in hydropic placenta
- Torn membranes often discarded in delivery room

Color and Opacity

- Normal: Pink-white, variably translucent, glistening
- Chorioamnionitis: Usually yellow-white, opaque appearing
- Meconium: Variable with extent and chronicity
  - Recent: Blue-green, glistening, may have fresh meconium on surface
  - Subacute: Dark green-brown, slippery, and edematous
  - Chronic: Diffusely muddy brown (especially cord surface), dull appearing
- Retromembranous hemorrhage
  - Older hemorrhage is green-brown or yellow-tan on decidual side

Insertion

- Normal insertion of membranes at disc margin
  - Fusion of chorionic plate and basal plate at margin create inner boundary of intervillous space
- Extrachorial placentation, 2 types: Circumvallate and circummarginate
  - Circumvallate placenta: Important diagnosis
    - Membranes fold onto themselves, forming lip at junction of extraplacental membranes and chorionic disc
  - Circummarginate placenta
    - Membranes arise inside circumference of margin with flat junction
    - Thin fibrin ring may be present
    - Relatively common (6-20% of placentas)
    - No definite clinical significance

Measurements

- Distance from point of membrane rupture to disc margin
  - Only relevant in vaginal delivery with relatively intact membranes
  - Gives estimate of distance between placental implantation site and cervical os
  - Measurements < 2 cm suggest **placenta previa**
    - Placental implantation in lower uterine segment, with disc parenchyma overlying cervical os
    - ~ 1 in 2,500 gestations
    - Recognized clinically on ultrasound
    - Associated with marginal retroplacental hemorrhage, placenta accreta
    - May present with diffuse vaginal bleeding, premature labor
    - Risk of fetal exsanguination secondary to tearing of placental parenchyma
    - Partial placenta previa defined as disc edge within 2 cm of cervical os

SECTIONS TO BE SUBMITTED

Membrane Rolls

- 2 membrane rolls ideal for identification of significant pathology
- Multiple methods described; the following is useful for fresh or fixed tissue and involves tools present in most surgical pathology grossing stations
  - Instruments: Grooved forceps without teeth, 2 pins, cork board, scissors, and scalpel
  - Cut strip 2-4 cm in width perpendicular to site of rupture, leaving attachment to disc margin
  - Roll membranes around forceps grasping site of membrane rupture perpendicular to strip
  - Transfix roll to cork board at disc margin with 2 pins going through roll and center of forceps
  - Take 2 sections of roll, ~ 5 mm in width sectioning on either side of pins
  - Remove forceps, roll should remain intact
- If amnion stripped from chorion, submit representative sample separate from roll

MICROSCOPIC EVALUATION

Amnion

- Extension of fetal skin
- Normal histology
  - Single layer of cuboidal epithelial cells overlying basement membrane, adherent to connective tissue layer
  - Squamous metaplasia
    - May see full stratified squamous epithelium with keratinization
    - More common near term
    - More common near cord insertion
    - Excessive squamous metaplasia occurs with abrasion or trauma
  - When reactive, epithelium becomes tall and columnar

Chorion

- Normal histology composed of trophoblast and connective tissue
  - Inner cellular layer of chorionic mesoderm
  - Reticular layer
  - Pseudobasement membrane layer
  - Outer trophoblastic layer

Decidua

- Gestational endometrium, normal histology composed of
  - Decidual stromal cells
  - Spiral arteries
  - Veins
  - Endometrial glands: Uncommon in 3rd-trimester membranous decidua
  - Scattered lymphocytes and uterine NK cells

PLACENTAL DIAGNOSES FROM GROSS EXAM OF MEMBRANES

Placenta Membranacea

- Incidence
  - Rare (1 in 3,000-4,000 gestations)
- Etiology/pathogenesis
  - Extraplacental membranes fail to form
  - Chorionic villi covering early gestational sac do not regress
- Gross appearance
  - Cotyledons scattered throughout what should be membranes
  - Villous parenchyma diffusely thin (1-2 cm)
- Clinical associations
  - Vaginal bleeding
  - Placenta previa and accreta
  - Preterm delivery, fetal and neonatal morbidity
  - Should be suspected clinically, ensure membranes were not discarded at delivery

Circumvallate Placenta

- Incidence
  - Occurs in 1-2% of placentas
- Etiology/pathogenesis
  - Most likely marginal abruptions with fibrin accumulation
- Gross appearance
  - Membranes fold onto themselves forming lip at junction of extraplacental membranes and chorionic disc
- Microscopic findings
  - Fibrin, infarcted villi of margin folded over surface with doubled membranes
- Clinical associations
  - Intrauterine growth retardation
  - Intrauterine fetal demise
  - Low Apgar scores
  - Oligohydramnios
  - Placental abruption
    - Clinically described entity: Chronic abruption-oligohydramnios sequence (CAOS) with severe circumvallation
    - May have diffuse chorioamniotic hemosiderosis of membranes on microscopic examination

SELECTED REFERENCES

1. Ravangard SF et al: Placenta membranacea. Arch Gynecol Obstet. 288(3):709-12, 2013
2. Suzuki S: Clinical significance of pregnancies with circumvallate placenta. J Obstet Gynaecol Res. 34(1):51-4, 2008
3. Winters R et al: What is adequate sampling of extraplacental membranes?: a randomized, prospective analysis. Arch Pathol Lab Med. 132(12):1920-3, 2008
4. Ohyama M et al: Maternal, neonatal, and placental features associated with diffuse chorioamniotic hemosiderosis, with special reference to neonatal morbidity and mortality. Pediatrics. 113(4):800-5, 2004
5. Elliott JP et al: Chronic abruption-oligohydramnios sequence. J Reprod Med. 43(5):418-22, 1998

Graphic and Gross Features

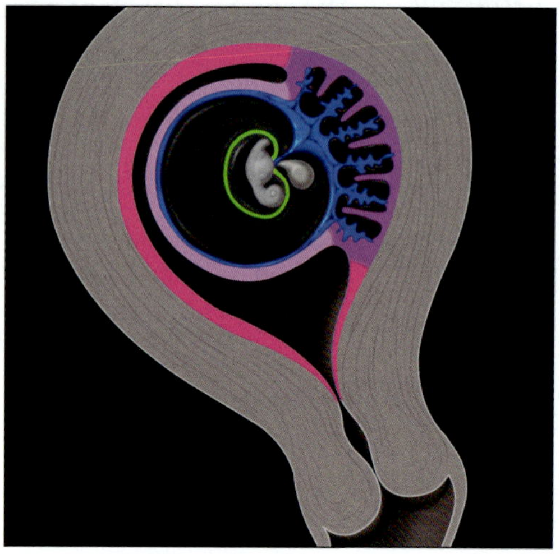

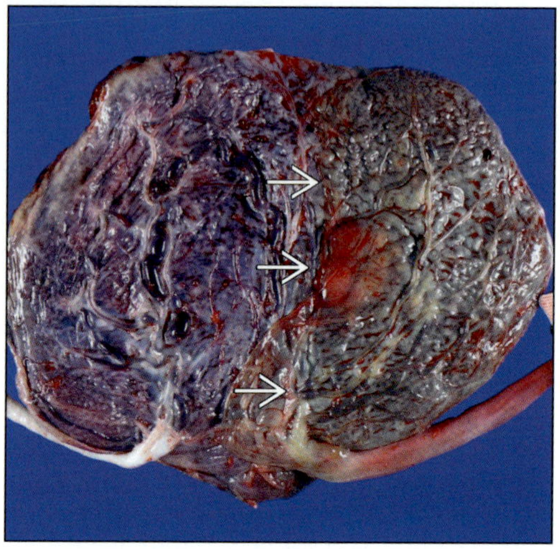

(Left) *The distinct membrane layers arise from early development. Amnion (green) surrounds the embryo. As the amniotic sac enlarges, amnion covers the cord and is apposed to the chorion (blue). The decidua capsularis (light pink) is the gestational endometrium overlying the conceptus. The rest of the decidua (fuchsia) eventually becomes apposed to the decidua capsularis.* ***(Right)*** *Gross exam includes noting the membrane color. The membranes of one twin are green →, suggesting meconium.*

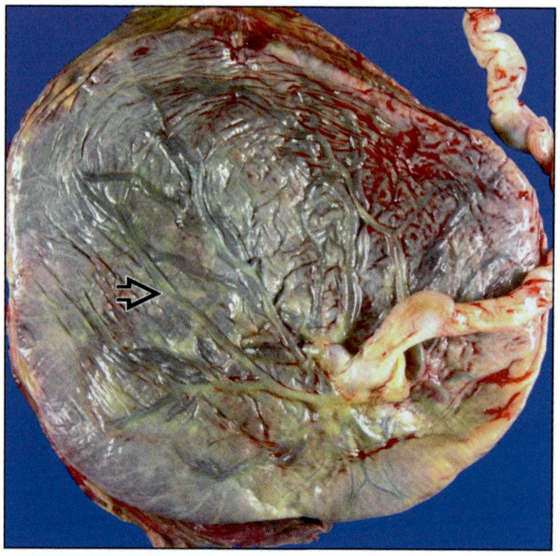

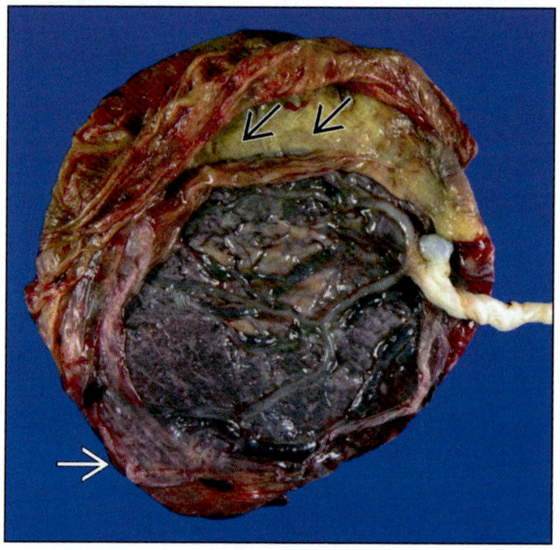

(Left) *Membrane opacity is best appreciated on the disc surface. The milky white opacity → here suggests amniotic fluid infection sequence.* ***(Right)*** *The point of membrane rupture → is assessed in vaginal deliveries. The shortest distance from the edge of the membranes to the disc insertion is measured. Values < 2 cm suggest a low-lying placenta. Note partial circumvallate insertion →.*

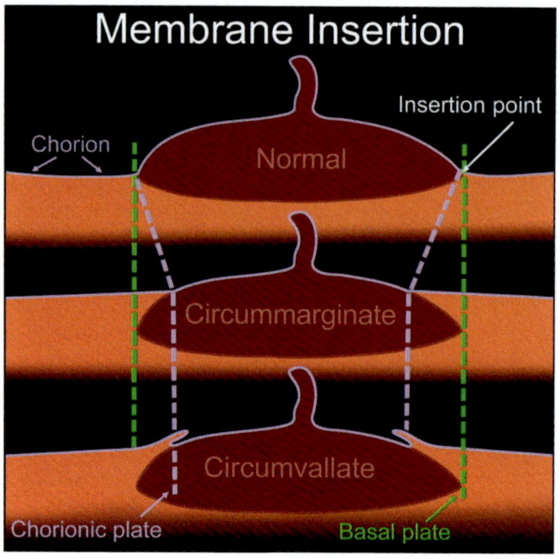

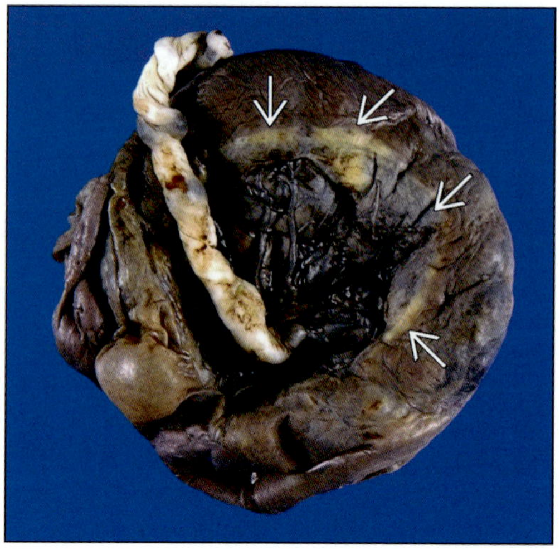

(Left) *Membranes normally insert at the disc margin, where the chorionic plate and basal plate meet. Circummarginate and circumvallate insertion types have the membranes arising from within the circumference of the disc (lavender line). Circummarginate insertion is flat; circumvallate insertion is raised by a fold.* ***(Right)*** *In circummarginate membrane insertion, a fibrin ring → delineates the site of membrane insertion inside the circumference of the disc margin. The insertion is flat.*

Gross and Microscopic Features

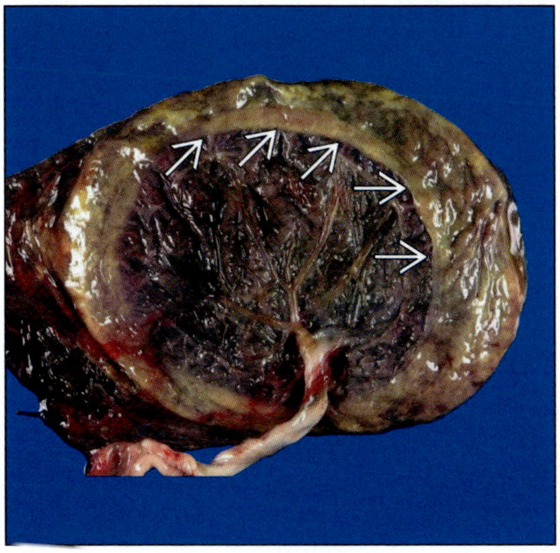

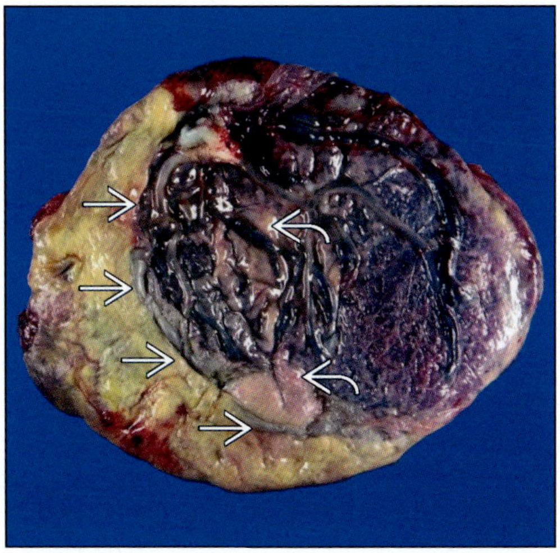

(Left) *Membrane insertion is circumvallate ➔ for 50% of the circumference and circummarginate for the remainder. The circumvallate insertion is raised from the surface, whereas the circummarginate portion is flat.* ***(Right)*** *Partial circumvallate membrane insertion ➔ is shown. The yellow discoloration suggests old hemorrhage and necrosis, consistent with chronic abruption. An older hematoma ➔ beneath the chorion is consistent with extension of a marginal hemorrhage.*

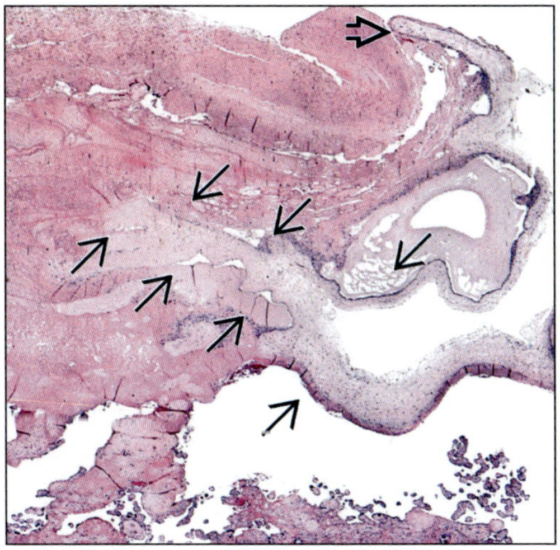

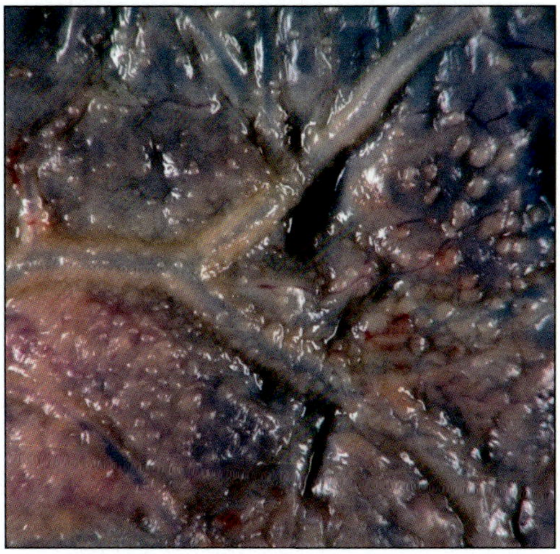

(Left) *The fold in circumvallate membrane insertion is easily seen microscopically. The membranes fold → over before the free edge ⇨ arises. Abundant old hemorrhage is present behind the membrane.* ***(Right)*** *Amnion nodosum is noted on gross exam. The amnion is covered in small whitish plaques, strongly associated with oligohydramnios. In oligohydramnios, fetal squames become too concentrated and deposit on the surface of the placenta.*

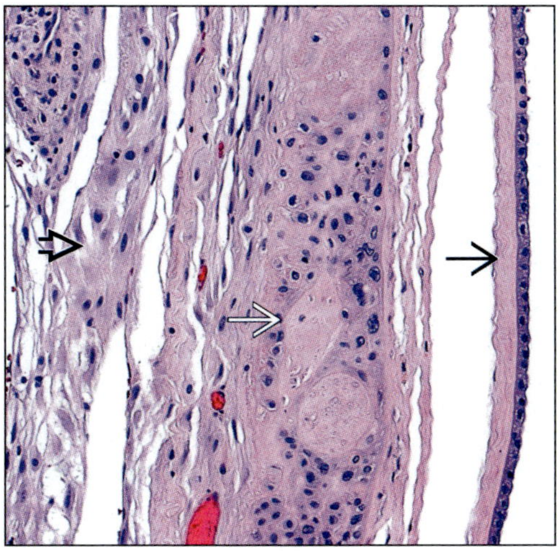

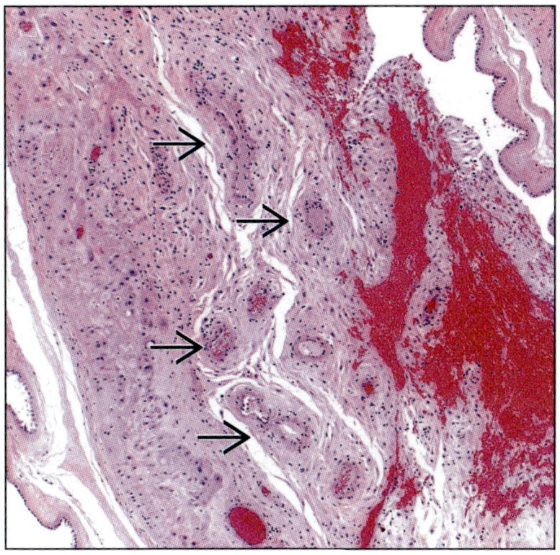

(Left) *Normal membrane histology is shown. The amnion epithelium → is low cuboidal, separated from the chorion by a space. The cellular chorion ➔ contains extravillous trophoblast as well as occasional regressed villi. The adherent decidua ⇨ is viable with scattered lymphocytes.* ***(Right)*** *The amount of decidua found in membrane rolls is variable. The membranous decidua is often the best place to observe maternal spiral arteries →.*

HISTOPATHOLOGIC CHANGES OF MEMBRANES

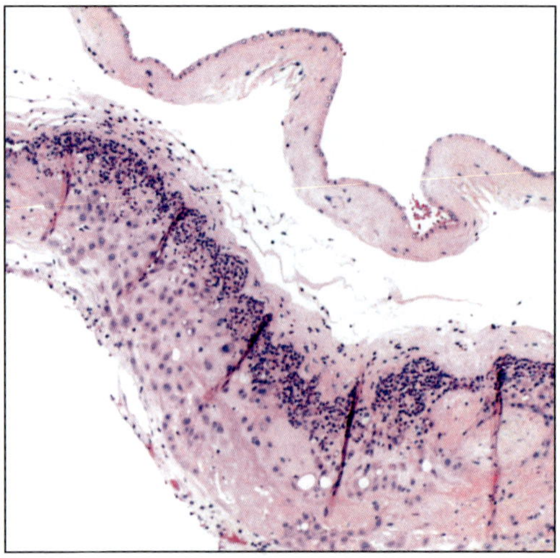

Chorioamnionitis is one of the most common placental pathologies. Precise terminology, with inclusion of grade and stage, allows better correlation with clinical outcomes.

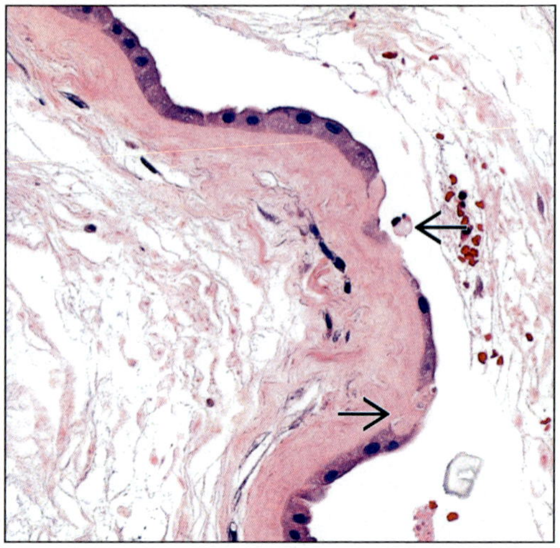

Meconium deposition in the placenta causes characteristic reactive and necrotic ⇒ changes in the amnion.

CONTENT

Scope of Discussion

- Changes of the amnion and chorion of placental membranes
- Membranous decidua discussed separately

CHANGES OF AMNION

Reactive Changes

- Low cuboidal epithelium of amnion becomes columnar or pseudostratified columnar
- Cytoplasm becomes vacuolated
  - Gastroschisis
    - Diffuse fine vacuolization of cells due to effect of gastric secretions in amniotic fluid

Amniocyte Necrosis

- Early
  - Loss of nuclear basophilia
- Later
  - Cell dropout
- Occurs in response to toxic substance (e.g., meconium, blood), or severe prolonged inflammation (necrotizing chorioamnionitis)

Edema

- Amnion slips from underlying chorion
- Basement membrane becomes thickened and eosinophilic
- Occurs with meconium, severe chorioamnionitis, fetal hydrops

Amnion Nodosum

- Deposition of fetal squames as nodules on surface of amnion
- Associated with oligohydramnios

Amniotic Bands

- Amnion separates from chorion during pregnancy, usually in 1st or early 2nd trimester
- Strips of amnion may twist around limbs or face causing amputations or malformations
- Cause of separation unclear; associations include maternal hyperglycemia, high-altitude pregnancies, and prior uterine surgeries

CHANGES OF CHORION

Changes in Chorionic Trophoblast Cell Number

- Usually decrease in number by term
- May proliferate as small cuboidal cells, or cuboidal vacuolated cells
- May be obscured or destroyed by acute (amniotic fluid infection sequence) or chronic (chronic chorioamnionitis) inflammation

Microscopic Chorionic Cysts

- Chorionic trophoblast cells secrete matrix-type fibrin-forming microscopic cysts filled with homogeneous-appearing pink fluid
- Microscopic chorionic cysts are a type of extravillous trophoblast cysts discussed separately

Chorionic Trophoblast Nuclear Pleomorphism

- Some degree of nuclear pleomorphism is common; may be related to tendency for extravillous trophoblast to become polyploid
  - Marked pleomorphism described in membranous chorionic trophoblast after cytotoxic chemotherapy

Chorion Nodosum

- Nodules of fetal squames embedded in chorionic mesenchyme

HISTOPATHOLOGIC CHANGES OF MEMBRANES

Grading and Staging of Maternal Inflammatory Response in Acute Chorioamnionitis

Category	Suggested Terminology	Definition
Stage 1: Early	Acute subchorionitis or chorionitis	Acute inflammation limited to the subchorionic space or membranous trophoblast, not extending into fibrous chorion
Stage 2: Intermediate	Acute chorioamnionitis	Diffuse or patchy acute inflammation of the fibrous chorion &/or amnion
Stage 3: Advanced	Necrotizing chorioamnionitis	Necrotizing acute inflammation of the chorion and amnion characterized by neutrophil karyorrhexis, amniocyte necrosis, &/or amnion basement membrane thickening or hypereosinophilia
Grade 1: Mild-moderate	(No additional descriptor recommended)	Scattered neutrophils, insufficient in extent to meet criteria for "severe"
Grade 2: Severe	Severe acute chorioamnionitis, **or** with subchorionic microabscesses	Confluent neutrophils (> 10 x 20 cells in extent); ≥ 3 isolated foci or in a continuous band

Excerpted from Redline RW et al: Amniotic infection syndrome: nosology and reproducibility of placental reaction patterns. Pediatr Dev Pathol. 6(5):435-48, 2003.

- Uncommon finding, only seen when chorion is exposed to fetal squames in amniotic fluid for a prolonged period of time
  - Early amnion rupture with amniotic bands, extraamniotic pregnancy, rarely in severe cases of amniotic fluid infection or meconium exposure when amnion has disintegrated

CHORIOAMNIONITIS

Acute Inflammation

- Hallmark of amniotic fluid infection
- Prominent cause of premature birth, especially in cases of premature rupture of membranes
- Frequently no association with clinical signs of chorioamnionitis, especially preterm
- Associated with ascending infection of membranes and amniotic fluid from genitourinary organisms
- Chorioamnionitis is a maternal inflammatory response, with migration of maternal neutrophils toward infected amniotic fluid
  - Maternal neutrophils migrate from intervillous blood space across chorionic plate and from decidual vessels across chorion and amnion
- Several grading systems exist, including 1 proposed by the Society for Pediatric Pathology Perinatal Section
  - Grading and staging system terminology aims to describe extent and severity of inflammation

Chronic Inflammation

- Usually lymphocytic, termed chronic chorioamnionitis
- Also a maternal inflammatory response but less commonly associated with infectious causes; usually associated with chronic villitis
- Associated with late preterm birth
- Numerous histiocytes in chorion underlying necrotizing acute inflammation is termed subacute chorioamnionitis
  - Associated with chronic lung disease in infants
  - Histologically and clinically distinct from chronic chorioamnionitis

PIGMENTED MACROPHAGES

Meconium

- Yellow-brown pigment found in amnion or chorion
- Characteristic reactive and necrotic changes in amnion

Diffuse Chorioamniotic Hemosiderosis

- Hemosiderin deposition in chorion and amnion of membranes and chorionic plate
  - Iron stain is positive
- Involves 1-2% of placentas submitted for pathologic examination
- Strongly associated with recurrent venous hemorrhage at margin of placenta (chronic abruption) as well as prematurity
  - Associated with circumvallate membrane insertion, chronic abruption-oligohydramnios sequence, and persistent pulmonary hypertension and pulmonary hypoplasia in neonate
- May have amnion necrosis, acute chorioamnionitis, subacute chorioamnionitis

SELECTED REFERENCES

1. Gundogan F and De Paepe ME: Ascending infection: acute chorioamnionitis. Surg Path Clinics. 6(1):33-60, 2013
2. Abellar RG et al: Effects of chemotherapy during pregnancy on the placenta. Pediatr Dev Pathol. 12(1):35-41, 2009
3. Park CW et al: The involvement of human amnion in histologic chorioamnionitis is an indicator that a fetal and an intra-amniotic inflammatory response is more likely and severe: clinical implications. Placenta. 30(1):56-61, 2009
4. Stanek J et al: Chorion nodosum: a placental feature of the severe early amnion rupture sequence. Pediatr Dev Pathol. 9(5):353-60, 2006
5. Redline RW et al: Amniotic infection syndrome: nosology and reproducibility of placental reaction patterns. Pediatr Dev Pathol. 6(5):435-48, 2003

HISTOPATHOLOGIC CHANGES OF MEMBRANES

Changes of Amnion and Chorion

*(**Left**) The vacuolation in gastroschisis is fine and diffuse. (**Right**) With meconium exposure, the vacuolation → is more coarse with greater variability in size than in gastroschisis. Traces of meconium pigment ⇨ can be seen in some vacuoles. This pigment tends to fade over time.*

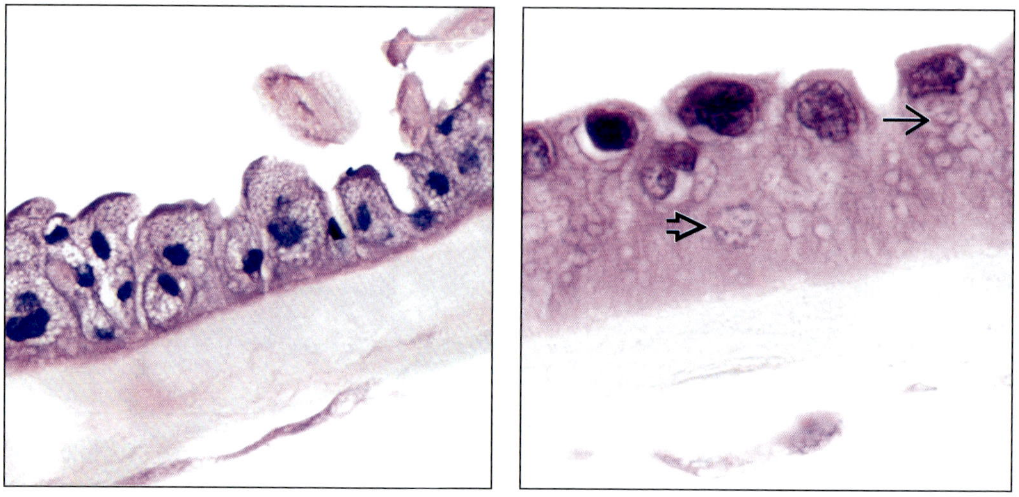

*(**Left**) In addition to vacuolation, the epithelium may become columnar or pseudostratified in reactive conditions. (**Right**) Meconium deposition is characteristically associated with reactive and necrotic changes in the amnion. The cells become columnar or pseudostratified → (reactive change) and lose nuclear basophilia ⇨ (necrotic change). Meconium pigment is present focally ↩.*

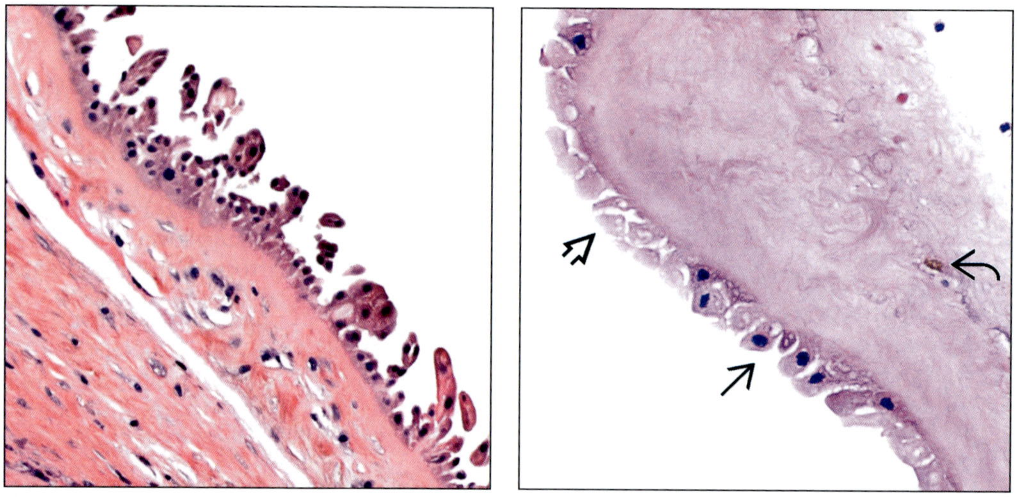

*(**Left**) Edematous amnion slips from the surface of the chorion and is difficult to sample in a membrane roll. It should be sampled separately. In edema, the amnion basement membrane is thickened and eosinophilic →. (**Right**) Amniotic bands are strips of amnion that have separated from the chorion and float in the amniotic fluid. They may constrict fetal body parts and cause malformations or amputations. The epithelium is commonly eroded → and the mesenchyme appears edematous ⇨.*

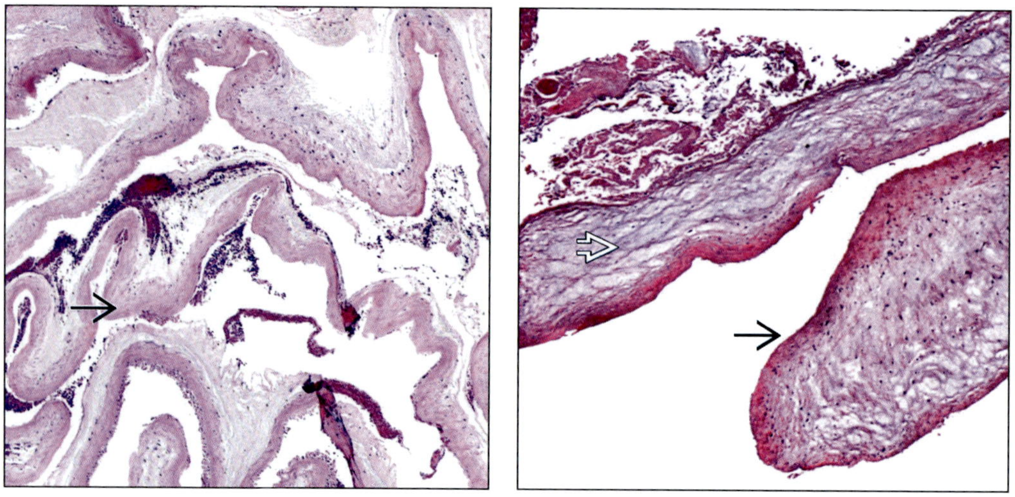

Chorionic Plate

GROSS EVALUATION AND NORMAL HISTOLOGY OF CHORIONIC PLATE

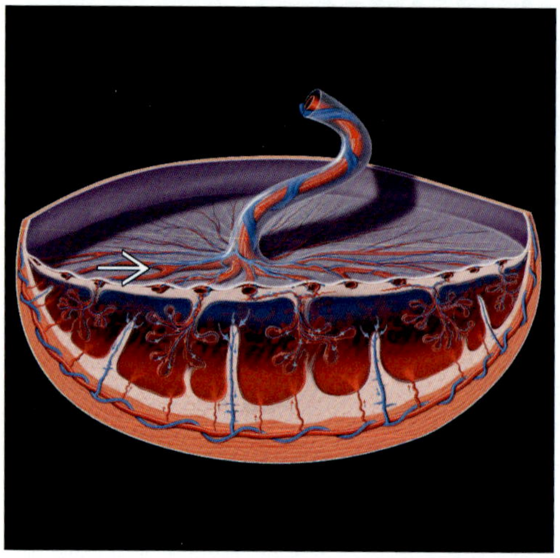

The chorionic plate (CP) vasculature ➡ carries fetal blood between the umbilical cord and villi. Deoxygenated blood from the umbilical arteries crosses over the oxygenated blood returning from fetal veins.

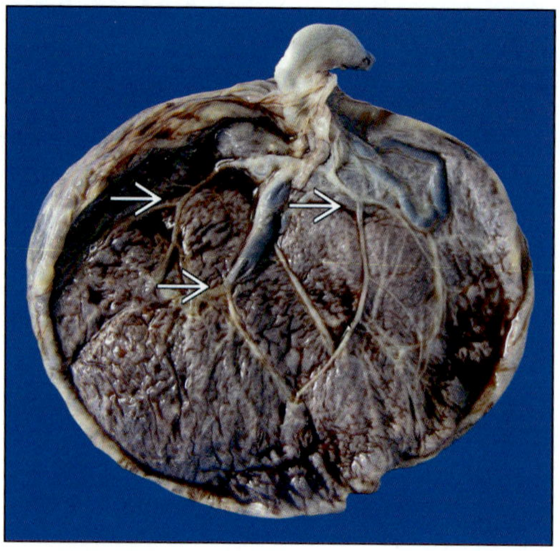

An important part of the gross examination of the chorionic plate focuses on the chorionic plate vasculature. This placenta displays a sparse distribution of CP vessels ➡, termed magistral.

TERMINOLOGY

Abbreviations

- Chorionic plate (CP)

Definitions

- CP forms fetal surface of placental disc
  - Distinct from
    - Chorion frondosum, which is placenta villous tissue proper of disc
    - Chorion laeve, which is **avascular** membranous portion of chorionic sac
- Chorionic plate vasculature
  - Represents the branches of umbilical vessels that extend onto the chorionic plate of placenta
  - Fetal in origin and carries only fetal blood

ETIOLOGY/PATHOGENESIS

Histogenesis

- CP development begins when 1st lacunae appear in syncytiotrophoblast layer (day 8 post conception)
- Fetal blood vessels of umbilical cord, chorionic plate, and proximal stem villi are derived from allantois via connecting stalk
  - These vessels establish contact with chorionic plate in 2nd month of gestation
    - They spread across chorionic mesoderm and enter proximal stem villi
    - Ultimately, they reach and connect to locally formed villous capillaries

MACROSCOPIC FINDINGS

Shape of Chorionic Plate

- Reflects shape of entire placental disc
- Most are round or oval
- ~ 10% of cases have variations of shape
  - Bilobed
    - 2-8% of placentas
    - ~ 2 equal-sized lobes are separated by membranes
    - Cord inserts in 1 of 2 lobes or in membranes
    - 2 lobes are connected by membranous vessels, vulnerable to compression, tear, and thrombosis
    - Both bilobed and succenturiate placentas are associated with implantation over regions with variable uterine perfusion (leiomyomas, cornu, cervical os)
  - Succenturiate lobes/accessory lobes
    - 5-6% of placentas
    - Similar to bilobed but with unequal-sized lobes
    - Cord usually inserts in larger lobe
    - 2 lobes are connected by membranous vessels, vulnerable to compression, tear, and thrombosis
    - Infarction or atrophy of smaller lobe is common
  - Placenta membranacea
    - Very rare
    - Nearly all of the fetal sac is covered by villous tissue; chorionic plate extends over all of what is usually extraplacental membranes
    - Typically, thin disc with limited villous growth
    - May have very large disc diameter with little to no attached free membranes
    - May appear as a small disc, with individual cotyledons scattered across free membranes
    - Can present clinically with 2nd-trimester vaginal bleeding and placenta previa
    - Often associated with abnormal implantation (placenta accreta, increta)
  - Placenta fenestra
    - Very rare
    - Chorionic plate has a defect within circumference
    - Underlying villous parenchyma is atrophied such that only tissue resembling free membranes is left covering the defect

- Atrophied region is likely due to implantation over a focal region of poor perfusion, such as a leiomyoma
- Differentiate from a missing cotyledon, which would have an irregular, torn-appearing surface on basal surface, or iatrogenic villous sampling after delivery
- Annular placenta (zonary)
  - Very rare
  - Disc is round or oval, villous parenchyma is distributed in a ring underneath the CP with a central thinned area
  - Large central atrophic zone may represent implantation over cervical os, with atrophy of central region not supported by decidua

Normal Gross Appearance and Physiology of CP Vessels

- Artery-vein pairs generally travel together on chorionic plate
- Arteries traverse over veins
- Chorionic arteries carry deoxygenated blood toward placental cotyledon (villous parenchyma)
- Chorionic veins carry oxygenated blood away from placental cotyledon and toward umbilical vein to fetus
- Muscular chorionic vessels can experience rhythmic contraction and are responsive to vasodilatory and vasoconstrictive mediators

Vascular Distribution Pattern

- Mechanisms that determine this pattern are not fully understood
  - Study of placental vasculature casts reveals 2 patterns of chorionic vessel branching
    - Dichotomous pattern: Symmetrical branching into 2 fairly similar daughter vessels
    - Monopodial pattern: Main, long mother tube that courses for a long distance with an almost constant diameter and has only small-diameter daughter tubes that branch off to the sides
  - Branching architecture is typically a combination of dichotomous and monopodial patterns
  - First 2-3 generations are always dichotomous

Patterns of Chorionic Vessel Coverage of Plate

- Disperse
  - Fine network of vessels that course from cord insertion and extend fairly evenly over CP, diminishing in diameter as they extend distally
    - Most common type is present in ~ 2/3 of placentas
    - Associated with centrally and paracentrally inserted umbilical cord
- Magistral
  - Less evenly distributed vessels with arteries that course to edge of placenta without diminishing in diameter
    - Less common type is present in ~ 1/3 of placentas
    - Associated with marginal and velamentous umbilical cord insertion
- Morphometric evidence that, compared with eccentric/marginal cord insertion, central cord insertion is associated with denser vascular coverage of chorionic plate

CP Vasculature in Twin Placentas

- Features of CP in fused dichorionic, diamniotic placentas
  - Dividing membrane is firmly attached to chorionic plate
  - Thickened ridge at attachment of dividing membrane to CP may be visible
  - Dividing membrane is thick and composed of 2 amnions and 2 fused chorions
  - Chorionic vascular territory for each twin terminates at dividing membrane with no anastomoses
- Features of CP in monochorionic, diamniotic placentas
  - Percentage of shared placental disc that belongs to each twin is determined by outlines of CP vasculature
  - Dividing membrane is **not** firmly attached to CP and may tear away easily
  - **No** thickened ridge at attachment of dividing membrane to CP is present
  - Dividing membrane is thin and composed of only 2 amnions
  - Chorionic vascular territory for each twin does **not** terminate at dividing membrane
    - Vessels of either twin can traverse beneath dividing membrane
  - Intertwin vascular connections may be visible on chorionic plate
    - Artery-to-artery connection: Superficial connection/anastomosis in which blood can be moved directly from artery of one twin into artery of other twin
    - Vein-to-vein connection: Superficial connection/anastomosis in which blood can be moved directly from vein of one twin into vein of other twin
    - Arteriovenous connection: Unpaired artery from one twin enters cotyledon adjacent to unpaired draining vein from other twin
  - Unique features of acardiac twin/twin reversed arterial perfusion
    - Large intertwin artery-to-artery connection with accompanying large vein-to-vein connection
    - Acardiac twin shows loss of direct vascular connections with placenta; no arteries enter cotyledons on chorionic plate

MICROSCOPIC FINDINGS

Chorionic Plate Layers

- Amnion
  - Loosely covers CP from ~ 17 weeks gestation
    - May detach when edematous
    - Can undergo similar changes as amnion of free membranes

GROSS EVALUATION AND NORMAL HISTOLOGY OF CHORIONIC PLATE

  - Component layers (epithelium, basement membrane, mesoderm, and spongy layer) same as in free membranes
- Chorionic mesoderm
  - Cellularity consists of fibroblasts and myofibroblasts set in connective tissue
  - Chorionic vessels course through this mesoderm
- Extravillous trophoblast
  - Reserve of cytotrophoblast capable of proliferation and migration into extravillous fibrin
  - Origin of Langhans fibrinoid and extracellular matrix at base of chorionic plate
  - May form cysts
    - Microscopic to grossly visible chorionic cysts
- Syncytiotrophoblast
  - Continuous with syncytiotrophoblast of stem villi
  - Often eroded early in development, replaced by fibrin
- Subchorionic fibrin
  - Becomes more prominent over gestation
  - Blood type fibrin
  - Attributed to turbulent flow of maternal blood as it reaches intervillous space below chorionic plate

Chorionic Plate Vasculature

- Chorionic veins and arteries are indistinguishable histologically
- Layers of vessel wall
  - Intima
    - Intimal thickening with myxoid-appearing protrusions into lumen is commonly seen (intimal cushion)
    - Intimal asymmetry may represent response to turbulent flow or increased vascular resistance
    - Should be considered thrombi only if fibrin cap &/or calcifications are present
  - Media
    - Smooth muscle layer of variable thickness
    - Asymmetric thinning of fetal side of wall is not uncommon
- Mural fibrin or calcification is not normal
- Mural inflammatory cells are not normal

REPORTING CRITERIA

Gross Examination

- Examination and description of intact appearance of CP vessels
  - Distribution of chorionic vasculature
  - Note any distended vessels or portions of vessels
  - Note any firm segments of vessels
  - Note any white discoloration or calcification of vessels
  - Note any disruption of vessels
- Examination and description of cut surface of vessels after serial sectioning of placenta
  - Note any distended vessels or portions of vessels
  - Note any white discoloration or layered appearance of vascular contents
  - Note any chalky mural calcifications
- Full thickness sections of placenta should include chorionic plate and representative chorionic vessels
- Gross features that should prompt additional sampling of chorionic vessels to attempt detection of abnormalities
  - Dilation of chorionic vessel with firm intraluminal contents, possible thrombosis
  - Firm segments of chorionic vessels with white discoloration
  - Cut surface of chorionic vessel with intraluminal mural or occlusive contents, possible thrombosis
  - Mural hemorrhage

SELECTED REFERENCES

1. Ravangard SF et al: Placenta membranacea. Arch Gynecol Obstet. 288(3):709-12, 2013
2. De Paepe ME et al: Correlation between cord insertion type and superficial choriovasculature in diamniotic-monochorionic twin placentas. Placenta. 32(11):901-5, 2011
3. Schwartz N et al: Placental morphologic features and chorionic surface vasculature at term are highly correlated with 3-dimensional sonographic measurements at 11 to 14 weeks. J Ultrasound Med. 30(9):1171-8, 2011
4. De Paepe ME et al: Placental markers of twin-to-twin transfusion syndrome in diamniotic-monochorionic twins: A morphometric analysis of deep artery-to-vein anastomoses. Placenta. 31(4):269-76, 2010
5. Suzuki S et al: Clinical significance of pregnancies with succenturiate lobes of placenta. Arch Gynecol Obstet. 277(4):299-301, 2008
6. Gordon Z et al: Anthropometry of fetal vasculature in the chorionic plate. J Anat. 211(6):698-706, 2007
7. De Paepe ME et al: Vascular distribution patterns in monochorionic twin placentas. Placenta. 26(6):471-5, 2005
8. Benirschke K: Remarkable placenta. Clin Anat. 11(3):194-205, 1998
9. Nordenvall M et al: Placental morphology in relation to umbilical artery blood velocity waveforms. Eur J Obstet Gynecol Reprod Biol. 40(3):179-90, 1991
10. Nordenvall M et al: Relationship between placental shape, cord insertion, lobes and gestational outcome. Acta Obstet Gynecol Scand. 67(7):611-6, 1988

Gross Features

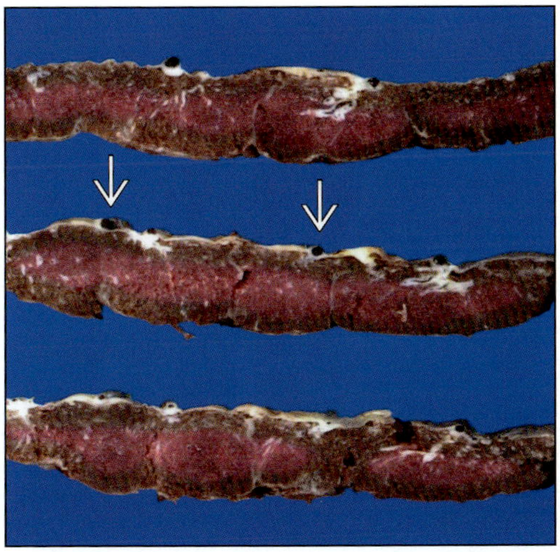

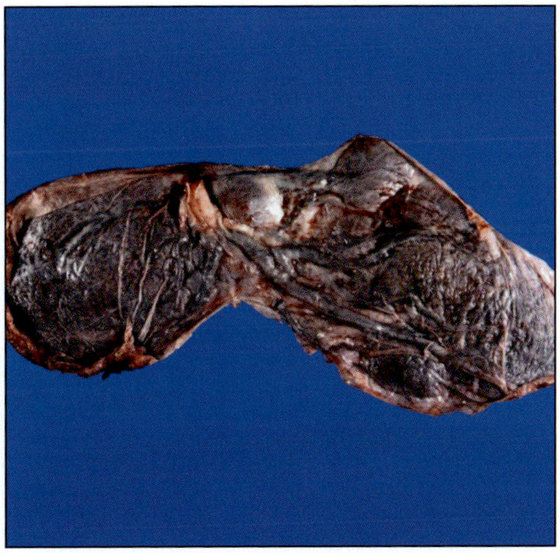

(Left) *Examination of the CP vasculature on a cut section shows the large fetal vessels on the upper edge of each slice ➡. This is an important opportunity to identify thrombi.* ***(Right)*** *Although it is usually round to oval, the chorionic plate, and therefore the placental disc itself, can have variant configurations, such as this bilobed placenta.*

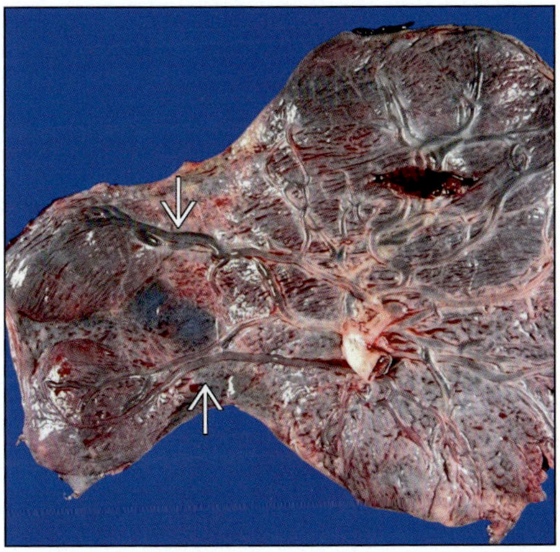

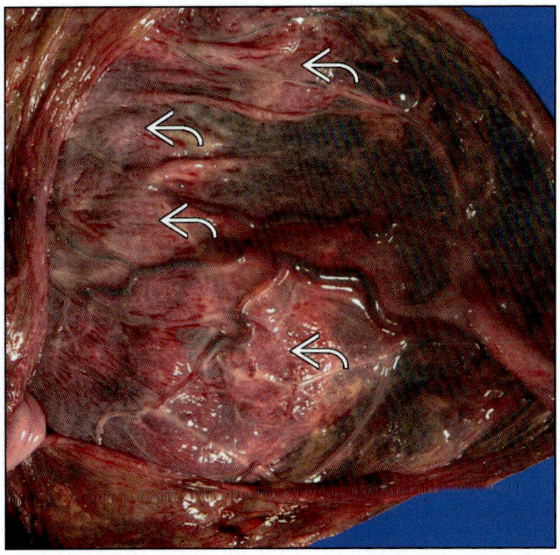

(Left) *This placenta has 2 accessory (succenturiate) lobes. Note that each are fed with branches of the chorionic plate vasculature ➡. These vessels can lie over the cervical os and present risk of fetal hemorrhage (vasa previa).* ***(Right)*** *Placenta membranacea is a rare abnormality. It may have a diffusely thinned disc with little to no membranes, or it may have cotyledons loosely scattered about the membranes ➡, as in this case.*

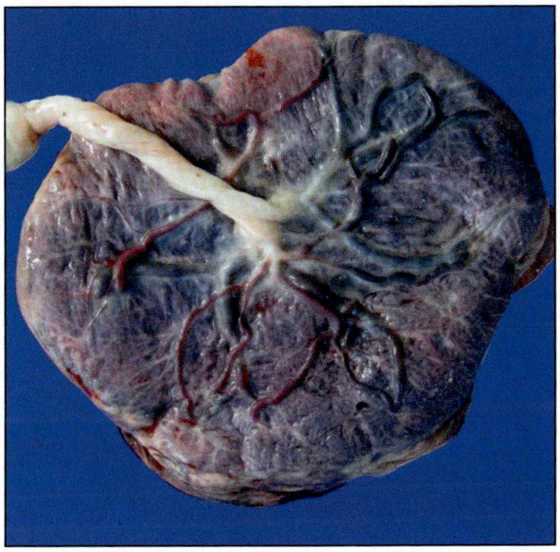

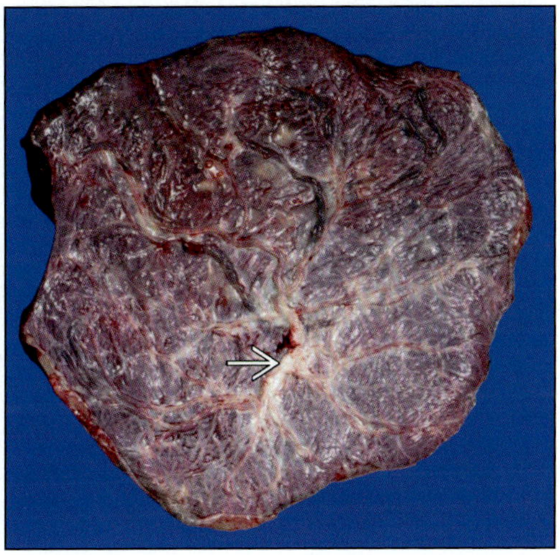

(Left) *Normal distribution of the CP vasculature shows fairly even coverage of the surface with CP vessels and a progressive decrease in size as they branch. Normal branching correlates with central or paracentral cord insertion.* ***(Right)*** *The fetal blood vessels form a disperse (normal) branching pattern on the chorionic plate of this trimmed placenta. Note the paracentral umbilical cord insertion ➡. The cord insertion site can be traced back from the CP vasculature when avulsed.*

GROSS EVALUATION AND NORMAL HISTOLOGY OF CHORIONIC PLATE

Gross Features

__(Left)__ Marginal umbilical cord insertions commonly have a magistral distribution of the chorionic plate vasculature. The large arteries course to the disc edge without diminishing significantly in diameter. __(Right)__ Similarly, velamentous cord insertions often have magistral vasculature. There are no precise measurements that discern magistral from normal. The appearance of large sparse vessels leaving large areas of the disc without CP vessels is consistent with the magistral pattern.

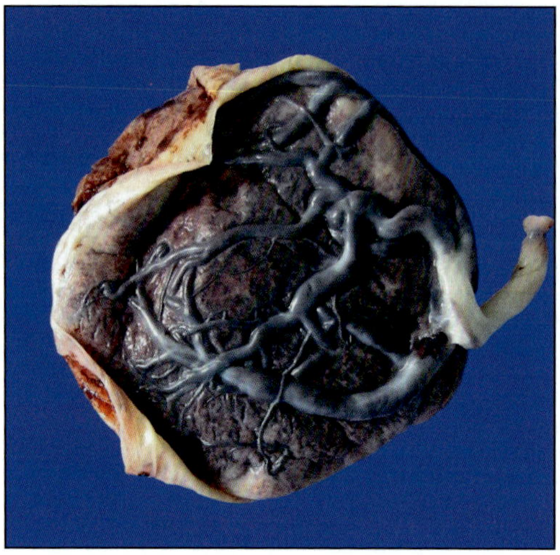

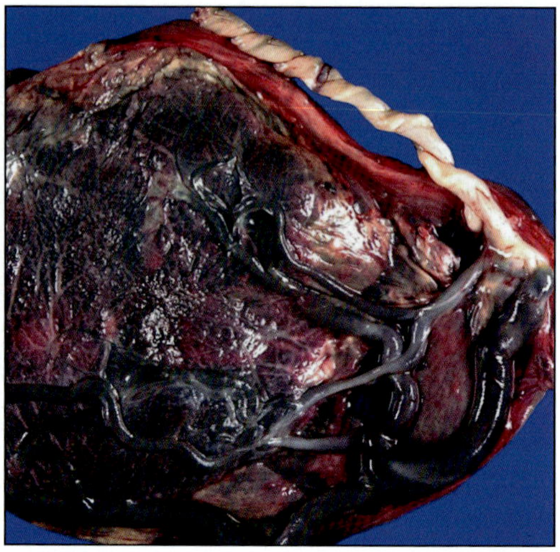

__(Left)__ This placenta also illustrates a magistral CP vascular distribution associated with a marginal cord insertion. __(Right)__ This placenta's chorionic plate shows several white and slightly distended veins → (arteries cross over them). Histology in this case showed several thrombi within these chorionic vessels. Also note that the umbilical cord is hypercoiled.

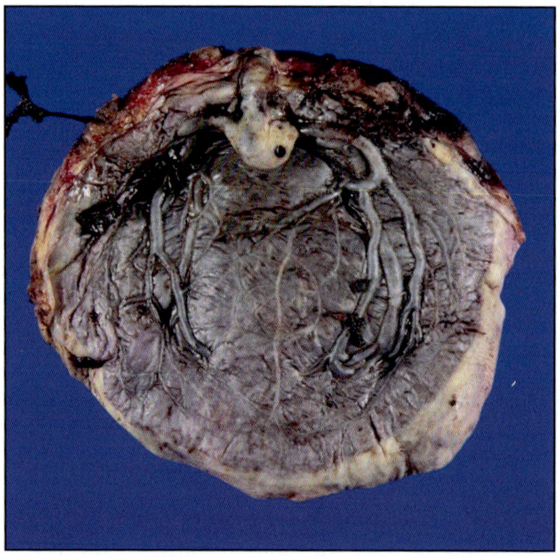

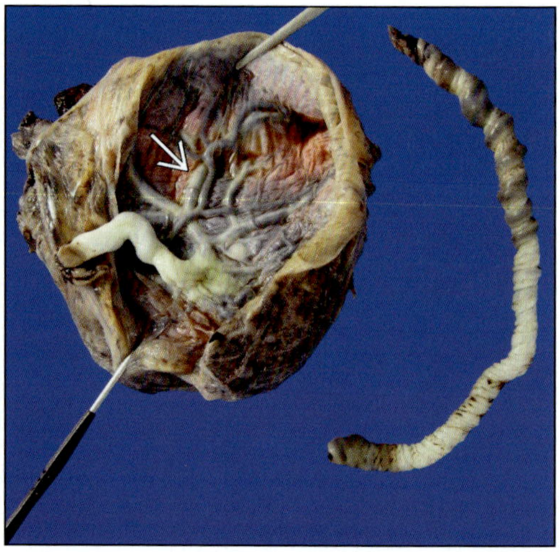

__(Left)__ The distal-most extent of the artery → enters the underlying cotyledon as a vein → of similar caliber emerges from the same spot →. Similar pairings are present all over the surface of the placenta. __(Right)__ This monochorionic twin placenta shows 1 cord with marginal insertion → (twin 1) and 1 with more paracentral insertion → (twin 2). The CP vasculature of twin 2 covers nearly 75% of the shared placental disc. A thrombus was confirmed in the firm white vessel of twin 2 →.

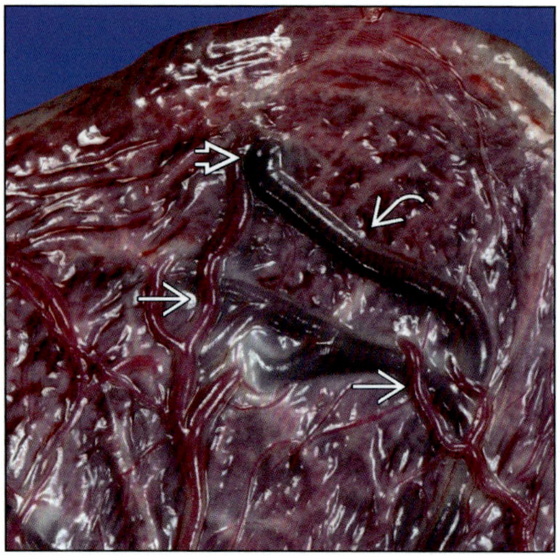

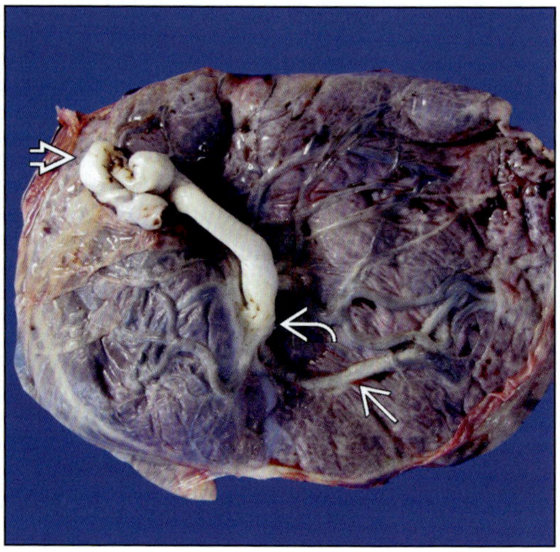

Microscopic Features

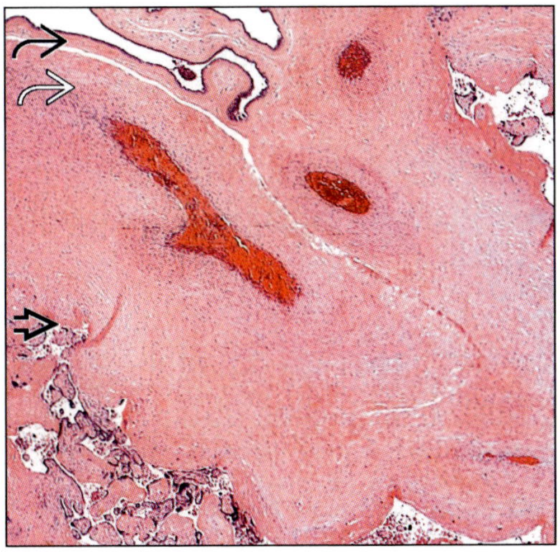

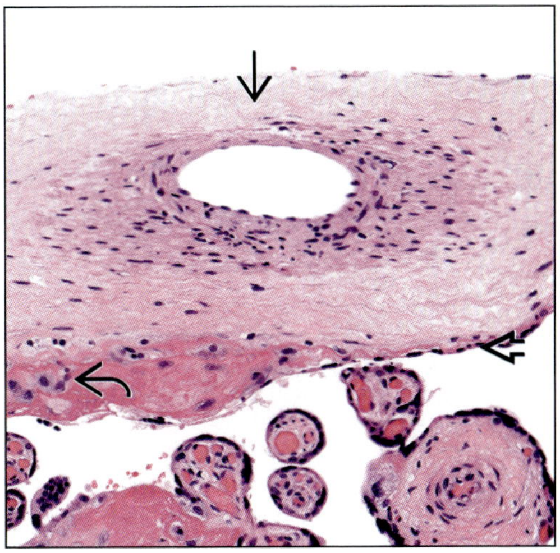

(Left) *At term, layers of chorionic plate that are distinguishable include amnion, chorionic mesoderm, and subchorionic fibrin.* ***(Right)*** *Amnion has slipped from the surface in this section of the chorionic plate. Chorionic plate vessel shows asymmetry of the wall, with thinning of the muscle on the side of the vessel closest to the amniotic sac. Also seen are extravillous cytotrophoblast cells in Langhans fibrinoid and the syncytiotrophoblast layer.*

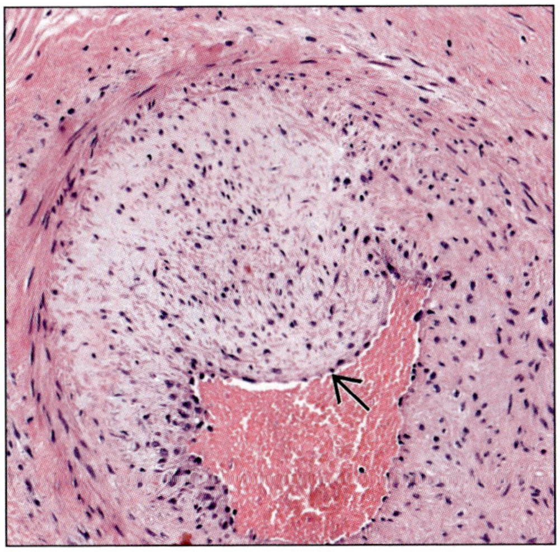

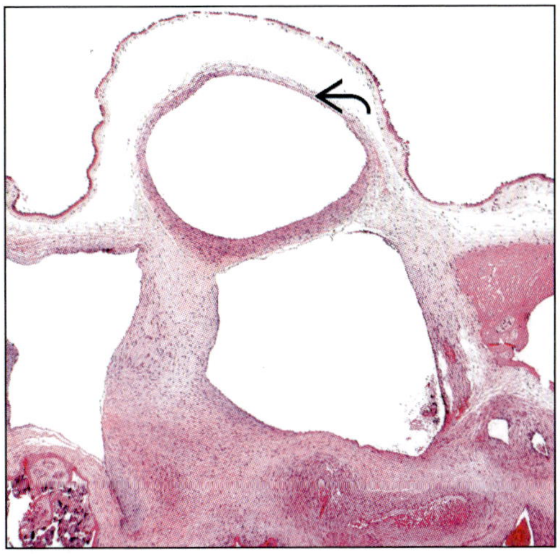

(Left) *CP vessel shows a myxoid intimal protrusion into the lumen. In this case, there is no endothelial disruption and a fibrin cap is not present.* ***(Right)*** *In this section of the CP, there is asymmetric thinning of the muscular wall on the top 1/2 of the superficial vessel. The arrangement suggests that this is an artery, overlying a vein, but such histologic designation is not reliable.*

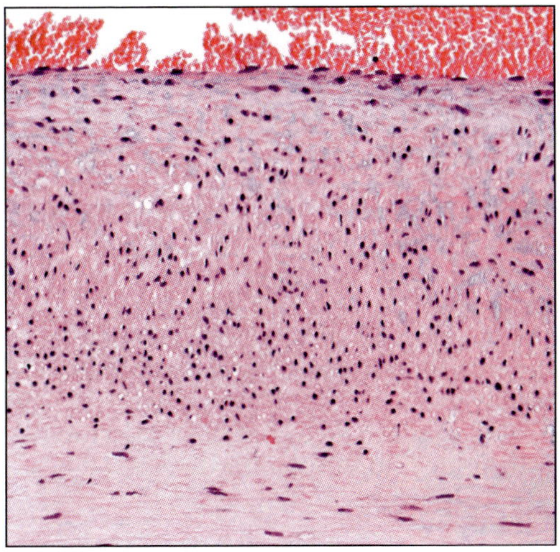

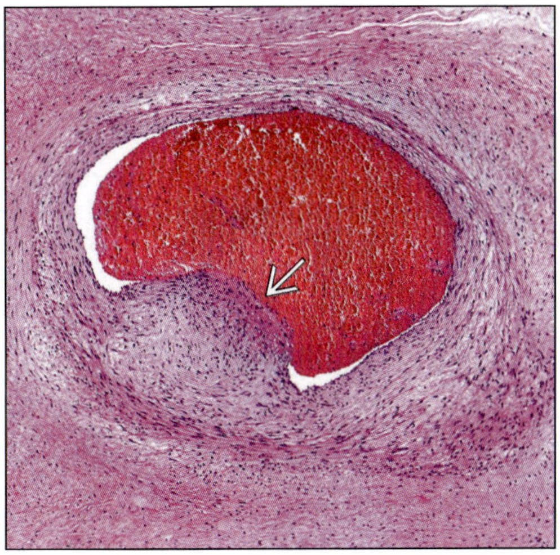

(Left) *The CP vessel wall typically has a thin endothelium overlying a thick media. There is no fibrointimal proliferation in this vessel.* ***(Right)*** *This CP vessel shows a myxoid intimal protrusion into the lumen and a fibrin cap, which is consistent with a mural fibrin thrombus.*

HISTOPATHOLOGIC CHANGES OF CHORIONIC PLATE

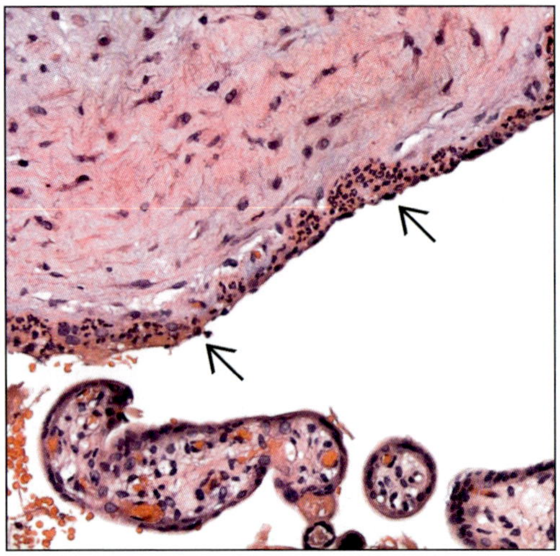

Acute subchorionitis is an early indication of amniotic fluid infection (AFI) ➔. Maternal neutrophils accumulate between the syncytiotrophoblast layer or subchorionic fibrin and chorionic plate (CP) connective tissue.

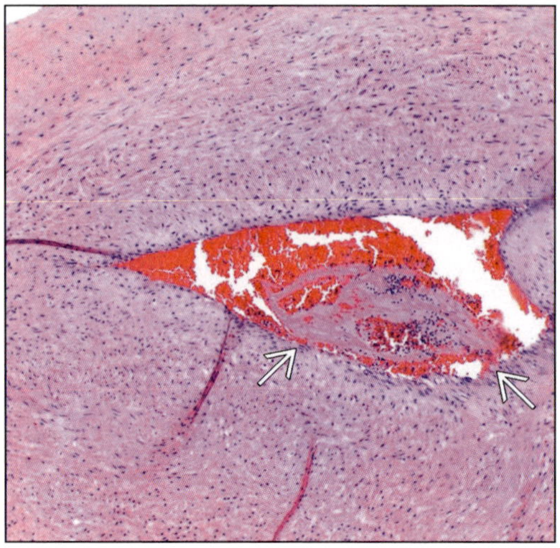

Recent chorionic plate vessel thrombi can be subtle as they are more rich in red blood cells. Focal attachment to the endothelium ➔ must be present to distinguish a thrombus from luminal fibrin.

TERMINOLOGY

Abbreviations

- Chorionic plate (CP)
- Amniotic fluid infection (AFI), amniotic fluid infection sequence (AFIS)
- Maternal inflammatory response (MIR), fetal inflammatory response (FIR)

MICROSCOPIC FINDINGS

Pigmented Macrophages

- Meconium
  - Meconium-laden macrophages may accumulate in CP
    - Dull, tan-brown pigment; iron stains negative
  - See reactive and necrotic changes, edema, in overlying amnion
  - See green to brown discoloration on gross exam
  - May see meconium-associated vascular necrosis in CP vasculature if meconium exposure is prolonged
- Diffuse chorioamniotic hemosiderosis
  - Hemosiderin-laden macrophages accumulate in CP
  - See brown, somewhat refractile pigment; iron stains positive
  - Associated with brown discoloration, marginal hemorrhage (chronic abruption), circumvallate membrane insertion on gross exam
  - Usually premature birth, with 2nd-trimester vaginal bleeding
    - May have chronic abruption-oligohydramnios sequence (CAOS), with respiratory failure in neonate

Acute Inflammation

- Acute subchorionitis
  - Sensitive site for detecting MIR to AFI
  - Aggregates of maternal neutrophils present beneath chorionic plate in subchorionic fibrin
    - Migrating from maternal intervillous blood space to chemoattractants in infected amniotic fluid
    - Confluent aggregates of ≥ 10 x 20 neutrophils are considered grade 2 (severe), fewer are grade 1
    - If MIR is limited to subchorionitis, stage is early (stage 1)
- Acute chorioamnionitis
  - Maternal neutrophils present in chorionic plate connective tissue
    - Usually see acute chorioamnionitis in free membranes as well
    - Confluent aggregates of ≥ 10 x 20 neutrophils are considered grade 2 (severe), fewer are grade 1
    - Indicates an intermediate stage of AFIS, MIR stage 2
- Necrotizing acute chorioamnionitis
  - Chorionic plate and membranes are severely inflamed, resembling abscess
  - See amnion necrosis, basement membrane hypereosinophilia, &/or karyorrhexis of neutrophils
    - Indicates late-stage MIR (stage 3)
  - Associated with prolonged, premature rupture of membranes
- Subacute chorioamnionitis
  - Infiltrate of histiocytes underlies superficial acute inflammation in CP
  - Usually seen with necrotizing acute chorioamnionitis
  - Associated with vaginal bleeding, chronic lung disease in infants with necrotizing and subacute chorioamnionitis
    - Diffuse chorioamniotic hemosiderosis also found with this histology; look for hemosiderin

Chorionic Vasculitis

- Fetal neutrophils migrate from CP vasculature toward stimuli in amniotic fluid

HISTOPATHOLOGIC CHANGES OF CHORIONIC PLATE

- Sensitive site to detect fetal inflammatory response to AFI
  - Grade 2 (severe) inflammation may be termed intense or marked chorionic vasculitis
  - If fetal inflammatory response is limited to CP vasculature, stage is early (FIR stage 1)
- May be complicated by thrombi
  - Strongly associated with neurologic impairment in affected neonate
- Mild CP vasculitis may be seen due to meconium effects alone but difficult to exclude AFI
  - Look for features of AFIS elsewhere

Chronic Inflammation

- Chronic chorionitis
  - Infiltrate of maternal lymphocytes and histiocytes in CP, usually in lower 1/2
  - Associated with chronic villitis of unknown etiology
  - May see basal chronic villitis in parenchyma and chronic chorioamnionitis in membranes
  - Rarely associated with hematogenous infections such as herpes simplex virus

Eosinophilic/T-Cell Chorionic Vasculitis

- Fetal T cells and eosinophils migrating from CP vasculature preferentially toward underlying intervillous space
- Rare finding, in ~ 0.2% of placentas submitted for pathologic examination
- Associated with chronic villitis of unknown etiology (VUE)
  - Most placentas with VUE will not have eosinophilic/T-cell vasculitis, but 30-40% of cases with eosinophilic/T-cell vasculitis will have associated chronic villitis
- Associated with fetal thrombi in affected vessel or elsewhere
  - Most placentas with fetal thrombi will not have eosinophilic/T-cell vasculitis, but 40% of cases with eosinophilic/T-cell vasculitis will have thrombi
- Clinical significance of isolated eosinophilic/T-cell vasculitis without other associated findings is unclear

CP Vessel Thrombi

- May be occlusive or nonocclusive, acute, subacute, or remote
  - Most commonly nonocclusive, with fibrin adhering to wall
  - With chronicity, develop mural calcification, become incorporated into vessel wall
    - May see patent lumen with fibrin and calcification in fibrointimal protrusion, indicates old, organized thrombus
- Look for associated villous changes of fetal thrombotic vasculopathy
  - Fibromuscular sclerosis or thrombi in stem villous vessels
  - Villous stromal vascular karyorrhexis or avascular villi
- Associations include severe CP vasculitis, extension from umbilical cord thrombi, hypercoiled cord, meconium-associated vascular necrosis

CP Vaso-Occlusive Changes

- Endothelial breakdown, extravasation of red blood cells, fibrous septation of lumen with organization into small, residual, multiple vascular channels
- Occurs with cessation of fetal blood flow or markedly reduced perfusion
  - Due to fetal demise, heart failure, or obstructed proximal flow
  - Similar changes described as "hemorrhagic endovasculosis"

Meconium-Associated Vascular Necrosis

- Severe, prolonged meconium deposition leads to apoptotic cell death of vascular smooth muscle
- Begins at site of meconium deposition on amniotic surface
- May be complicated by thrombi, likely impairs perfusion, even without thrombi
- Associated with pronounced meconium changes: Amnion edema and necrosis, numerous pigmented macrophages

Massive Dilatation of CP Vessel

- Dilatation of CP vessel > 4x neighboring vessels
- Attributed to marked congestion from umbilical cord obstruction
  - Look for gross cord lesions or venous thrombi that support cord obstruction
  - Look for villous congestion or intravillous hemorrhage
  - Look for thrombi, changes of fetal thrombotic vasculopathy in villous parenchyma

SELECTED REFERENCES

1. Katzman PJ et al: Eosinophilic/T-cell chorionic vasculitis and chronic villitis involve regulatory T cells and often occur together. Pediatr Dev Pathol. 16(4):278-91, 2013
2. Salas AA et al: Histological characteristics of the fetal inflammatory response associated with neurodevelopmental impairment and death in extremely preterm infants. J Pediatr. 163(3):652-7, 2013
3. Ryan WD et al: Placental histologic criteria for diagnosis of cord accident: sensitivity and specificity. Pediatr Dev Pathol. 15(4):275-80, 2012
4. Jacques SM et al: Eosinophilic/T-cell chorionic vasculitis: a clinicopathologic and immunohistochemical study of 51 cases. Pediatr Dev Pathol. 14(3):198-205, 2011
5. Wintermark P et al: Placental pathology in asphyxiated newborns meeting the criteria for therapeutic hypothermia. Am J Obstet Gynecol. 203(6):579, 2010
6. Ohyama M et al: Maternal, neonatal, and placental features associated with diffuse chorioamniotic hemosiderosis, with special reference to neonatal morbidity and mortality. Pediatrics. 113(4):800-5, 2004
7. Redline RW et al: Amniotic infection syndrome: nosology and reproducibility of placental reaction patterns. Pediatr Dev Pathol. 6(5):435-48, 2003

HISTOPATHOLOGIC CHANGES OF CHORIONIC PLATE

Microscopic Features

(Left) *In diffuse chorioamniotic hemosiderosis, pigmented macrophages contain hemosiderin ➔. This premature placenta had circumvallate membranes and old marginal hemorrhage.* ***(Right)*** *An iron stain demonstrates the numerous hemosiderin granules.*

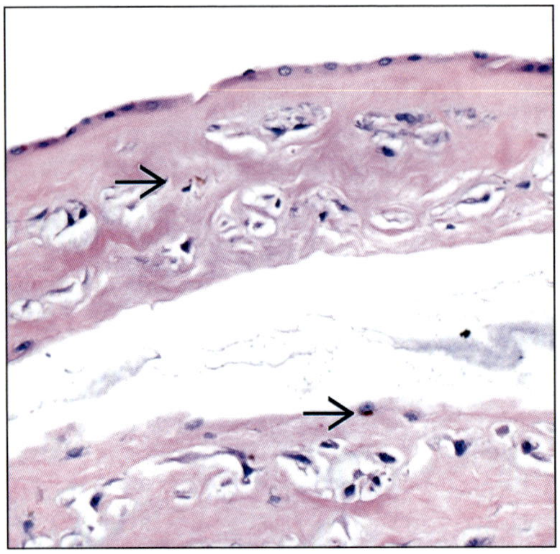

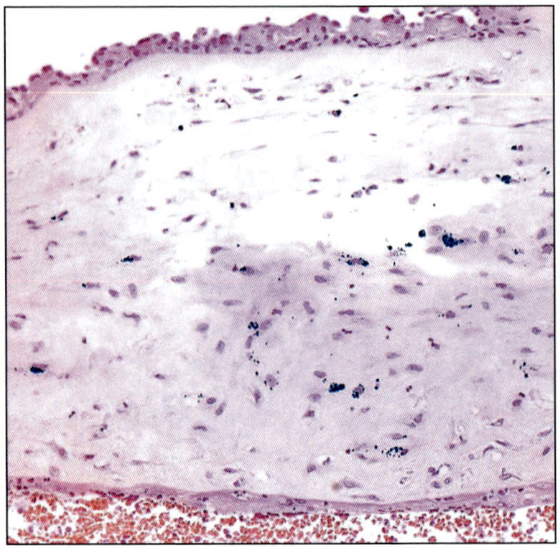

(Left) *In addition to the cord and membranes, the fetal and maternal inflammatory responses to AFI are evaluated in the CP. The maternal inflammatory response (MIR) ➔ is seen in subchorionic fibrin and connective tissue of the CP. The fetal inflammatory response (FIR) ⇨ is seen on the side of the CP vessel near the amniotic fluid.* ***(Right)*** *In prolonged necrotizing acute chorioamnionitis, a mononuclear cell infiltrate ⇨ can also be seen in the chorionic plate, termed subacute chorioamnionitis.*

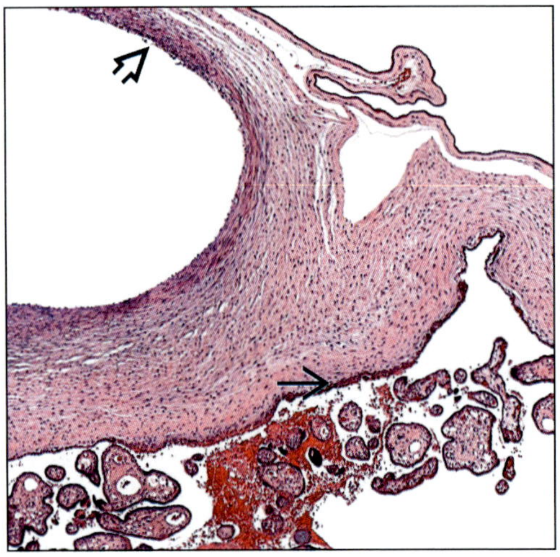

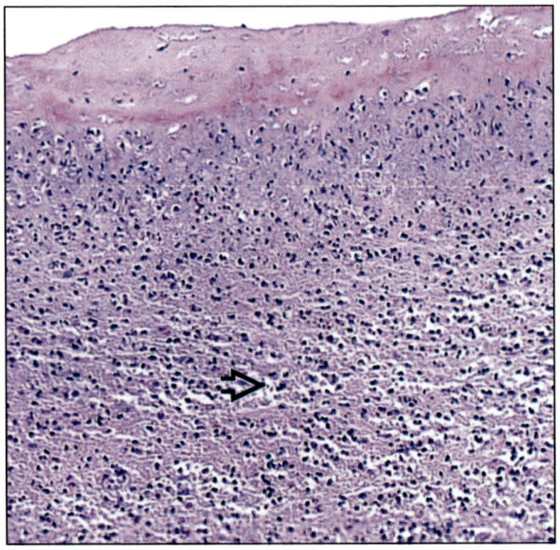

(Left) *The fetal inflammatory response can be subtle. Only scattered neutrophils and eosinophils are seen in the intima of this chorionic plate vessel ➔ (AFIS FIR grade 1, stage 1).* ***(Right)*** *This image of the amniotic side of a chorionic plate vessel shows scattered eosinophils. Eosinophils alone do not designate the infiltrate eosinophilic/T-cell vasculitis. Eosinophils are a frequent component of the very premature fetal inflammatory response to AFI.*

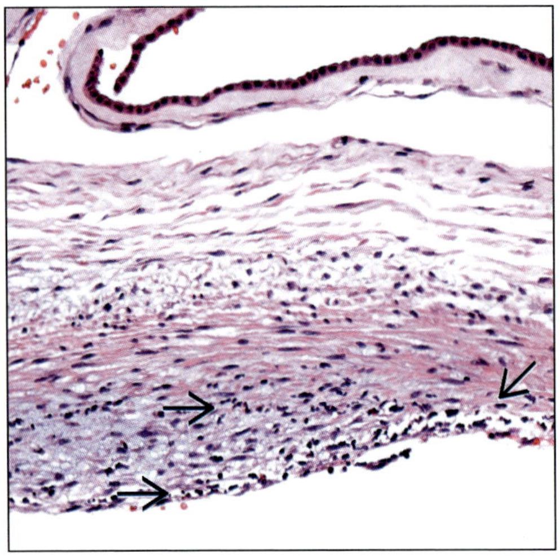

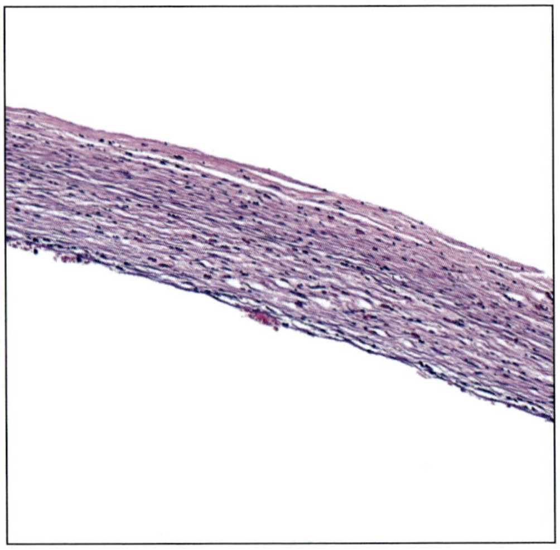

Microscopic Features

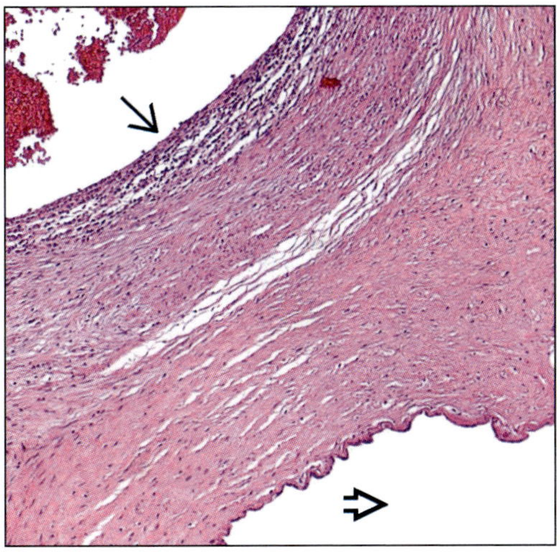
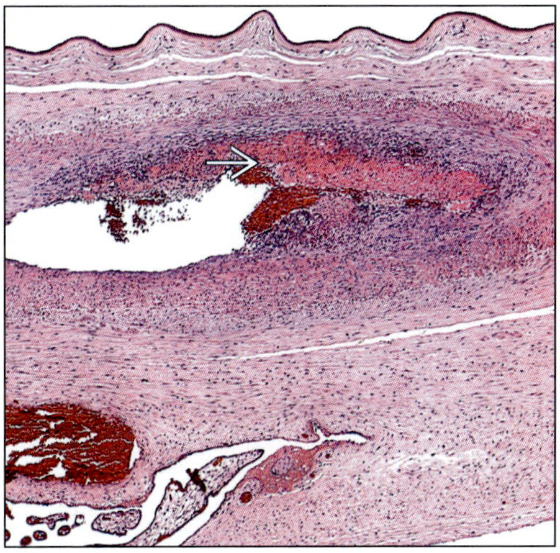

(Left) *This image shows true eosinophilic/T-cell vasculitis. The infiltrate ➔ of eosinophils and lymphocytes from the fetal blood is directed predominantly toward the underlying intervillous space ⇨.* ***(Right)*** *This image shows intense chorionic plate vasculitis complicated by thrombus formation ➡. This severe fetal inflammatory response is an ominous sign for neonatal morbidity and should not be missed.*

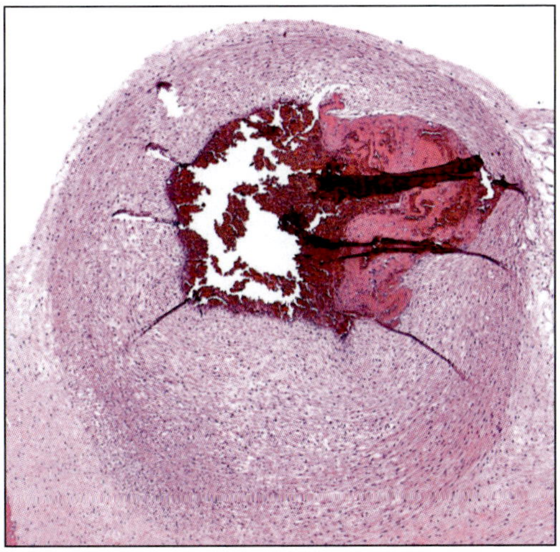
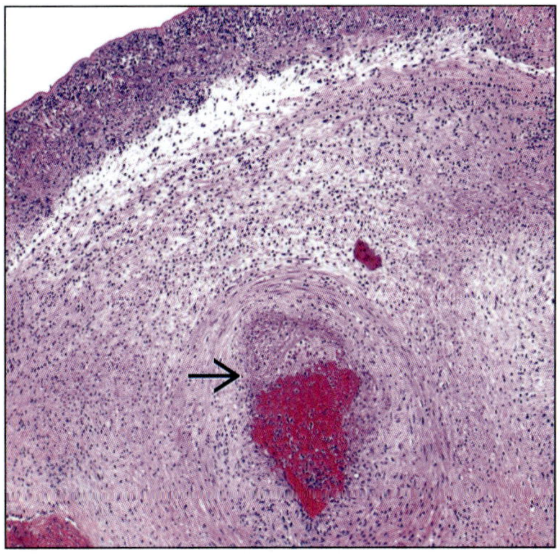

(Left) *This chorionic plate thrombus was associated with meconium deposition in the placenta. Vasospasm in response to toxic effects of meconium may have played a role in the pathogenesis.* ***(Right)*** *This chorionic plate vessel has undergone partial necrosis due to severe necrotizing chorioamnionitis affecting the chorionic plate. A thrombus ➔ has formed.*

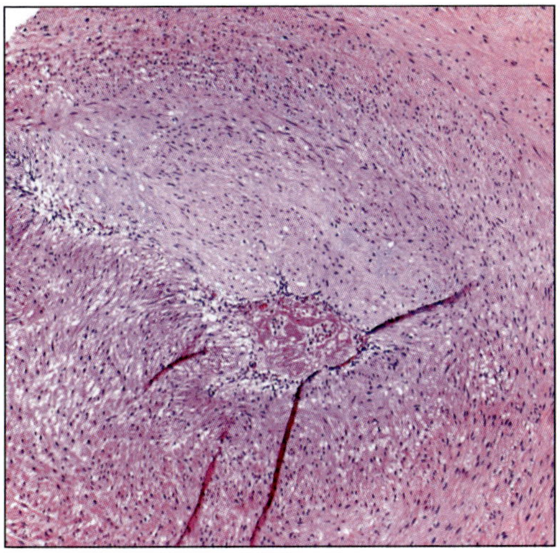
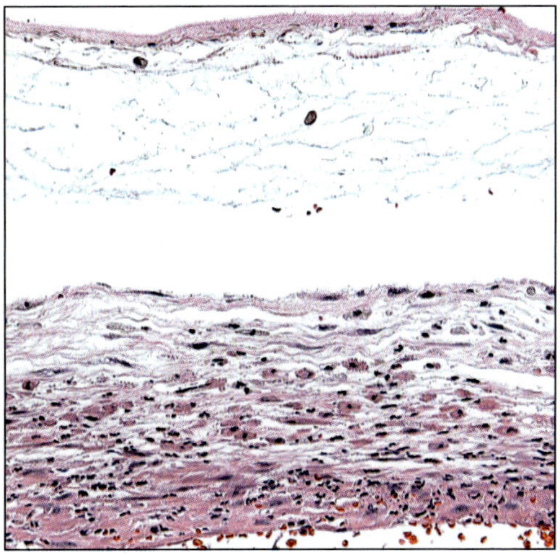

(Left) *This chorionic plate vessel thrombus from a twin placenta does not distend the vessel; instead, it appears collapsed, perhaps reflecting obstruction of arterial perfusion. With umbilical venous obstruction, the vessel may be markedly dilated.* ***(Right)*** *This section shows the amniotic aspect of a CP vessel with heavy meconium and meconium-associated vascular necrosis. The vascular smooth muscle cells closest to the site of deposition become apoptotic. CP vasculitis is present as well.*

Stem Villi

GROSS EVALUATION AND NORMAL HISTOLOGY OF STEM VILLI

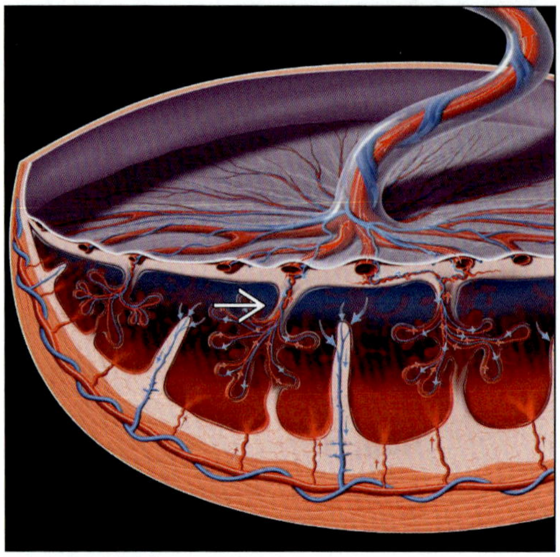

Stem villi ➡ take fetal blood to and from distal villi and chorionic plate vasculature, provide structural support, and, by anchoring to the basal plate, likely play a role in fetal regulation of intervillous space volume.

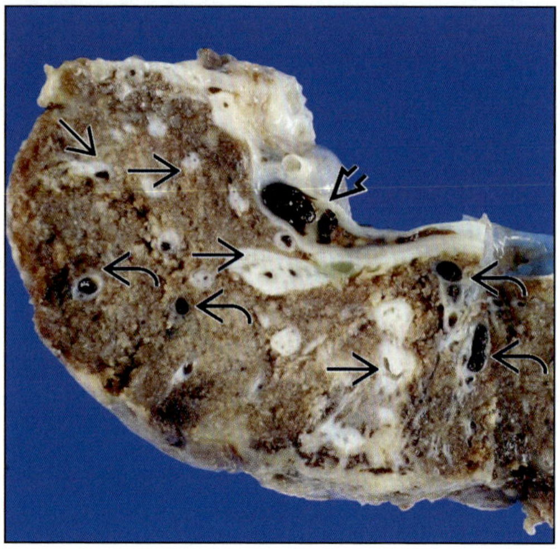

The numerous white foci containing vessels in the parenchyma are larger stem villi ➡. A subset ➡ show marked dilatation of 1 vessel with congestion, related to the chorionic plate thrombus ➡.

TERMINOLOGY

Definitions

- Stem villi: Placental villi containing muscular vessels and a dense fibrous stroma comprising > 1/2 the core connective tissue
  - Take fetal blood to and from distal villi and chorionic plate vasculature
  - Located in center of villous tree; can be likened to trunk
- Immature intermediate villi: Precursor chorionic villi that mature into stem villi
  - Reticulate stroma mixed with varying degrees of central compact fibrous stroma
    - By definition, dense fibrous stroma comprises < 1/2 the diameter

MACROSCOPIC FINDINGS

Normal Gross Appearance of Stem Villi

- Only largest stem villi are grossly visible
- Villous fibrous tissue appears as tan-white vertical streaks extending down from chorionic plate
- When in cross section, artery and vein may be visible

Stem Villous Abnormalities on Gross Exam

- Marked vascular dilatation ± thrombi
  - Usually seen in continuity with changes in a chorionic plate vessel
  - Marked vascular dilatation defined as lumen diameter that is 4x the neighboring vessels
  - Look for associated umbilical cord abnormalities and chorionic plate vessel thrombi or marked dilatation
  - Look for pale parenchymal foci of avascular villi resulting from fetal thrombotic vasculopathy
- Cysts
  - Cysts of stem villi usually only grossly visible in placental mesenchymal dysplasia (PMD)
  - Appear grape-like, similar to molar villi
  - PMD placentas may be a mosaic of cells with normal genomes and lesional diandrogenetic component
    - If lesional component comprises only minor population, gross changes may appear focal
- Chorangiomas
  - Commonly arise from stem villi under chorionic plate
    - Appear as oval, smooth, dark-red to tan-fibrous masses
    - Usually singular; may become more fibrous over time, appearing tan
  - Multifocal chorangiomatosis
    - Rarely described gross appearance with multiple golf-ball-sized lesions
    - Commonly associated with fetal anomalies and chromosomal abnormalities
    - Vascular proliferation thought to arise from peripheral capillary net of immature intermediate villi and early stem villi

MICROSCOPIC FINDINGS

Stem Villous Development and Histology

- Mesenchymal villi
  - Present from ~ 3 weeks post conception (5 weeks after last maternal menstrual period); abundant in 1st-trimester specimens and rare in 2nd- or 3rd-trimester placentas
  - Branching elongate villi with stroma of loose connective tissue containing polygonal cells, surrounded by cytotrophoblast and syncytiotrophoblast
  - Give rise to immature intermediate villi proximally in early gestation

Gross Pathology

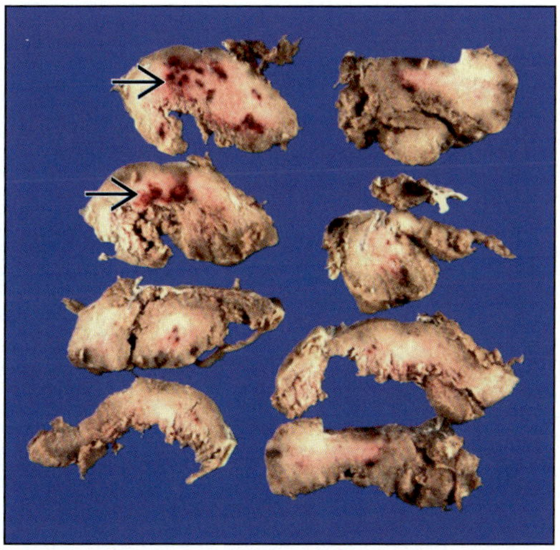

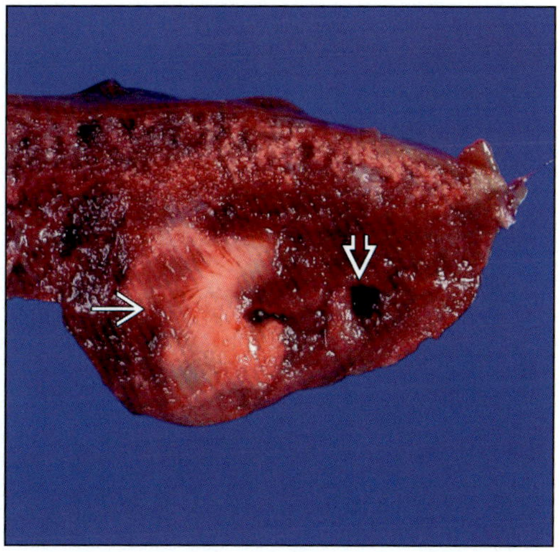

(Left) *Small foci of fetal-maternal hemorrhage* → *stand out from the edematous, pale parenchyma of this hydropic placenta.* ***(Right)*** *This tan lesion shows fine striations, consistent with laminations of an intervillous thrombus* ➡*. Also present is a benign flow void* ➡*.*

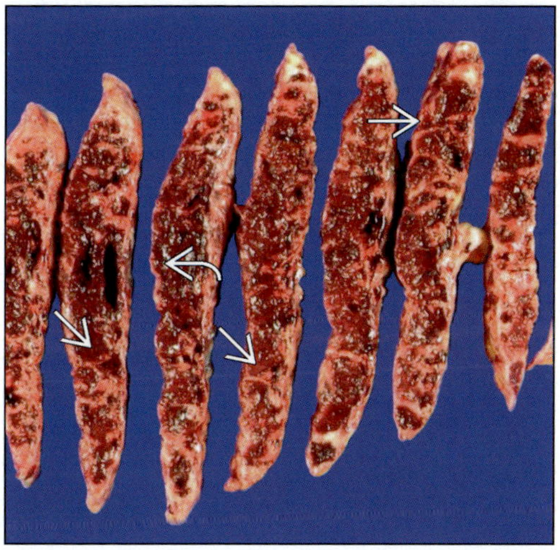

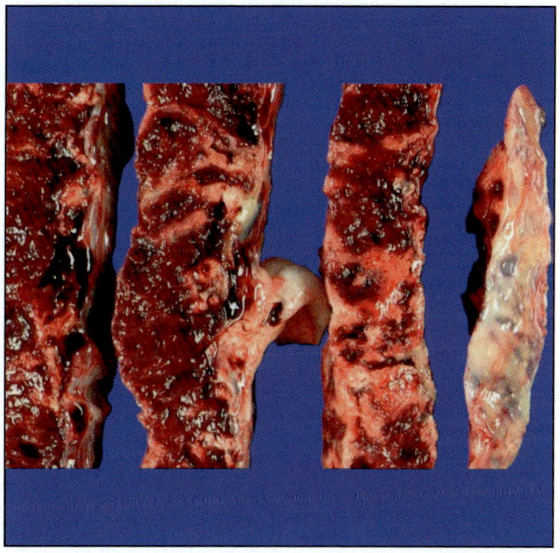

(Left) *These sections show a diffuse increase in fibrin, both crossing from chorionic plate to basal plate* ➡*, and localized at the basalis* ➡*, consistent with massive perivillous fibrin deposition.* ***(Right)*** *These slices provide a closer look at the unfixed appearance of increased perivillous fibrin. Tan-white strands cross the parenchyma.*

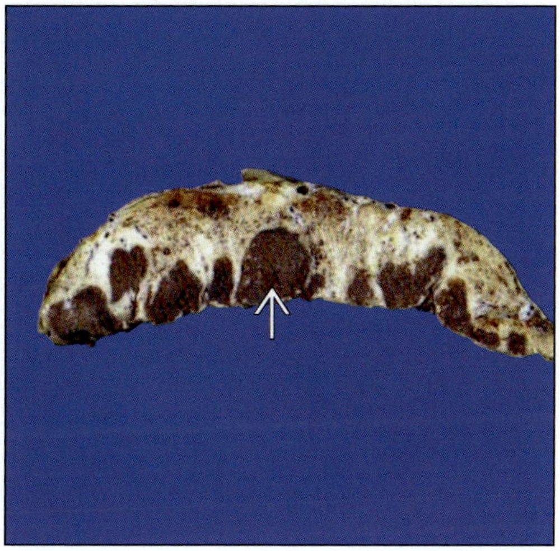

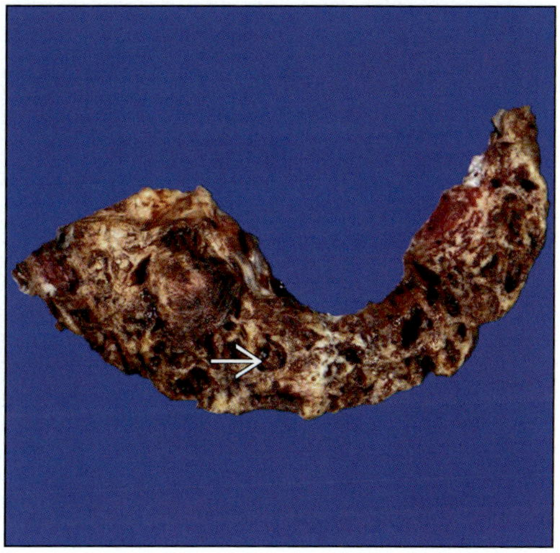

(Left) *After prolonged fixation, the contrast between pale fibrin and spared villous parenchyma* ➡ *is more stark.* ***(Right)*** *This case of massive perivillous fibrin deposition shows very little normal parenchyma after fixation. Small rounded nodules of remnant villous architecture* ➡ *are seen.*

GROSS EVALUATION AND NORMAL HISTOLOGY OF CHORIONIC VILLI

Normal Histology of 1st- and 2nd-Trimester Villi

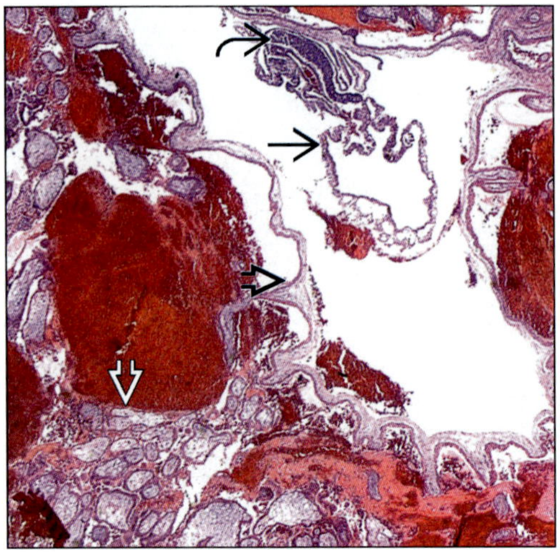

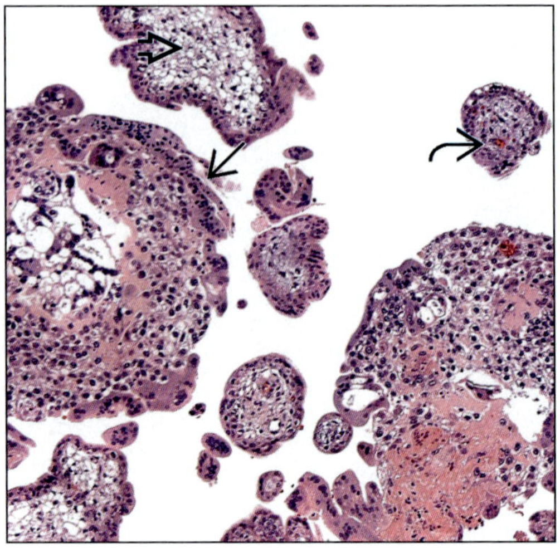

(Left) *The earliest villi form from the chorionic disc as projections into lakes of maternal blood. This image from an ectopic pregnancy shows an embryo ↷, yolk sac →, and chorionic plate ⇨ with primary, secondary, and tertiary villi ➡.* ***(Right)*** *The 1st-trimester villi continue the same process of villogenesis. Syncytiotrophoblast → is abundant, and the mesenchymal stroma is reticular with mostly polygonal stromal cells ⇨. Capillaries form in situ from the stroma ↷.*

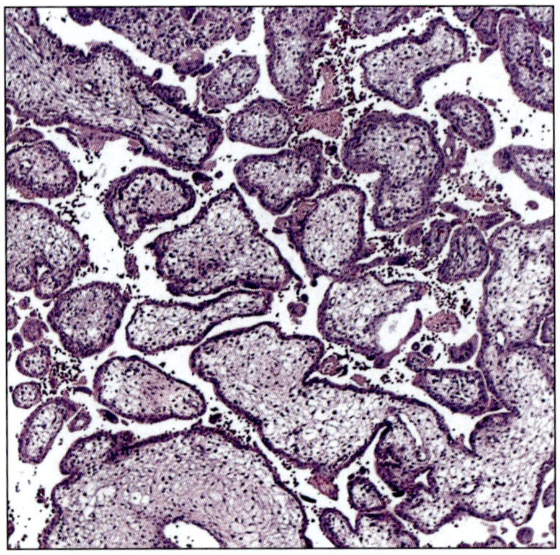

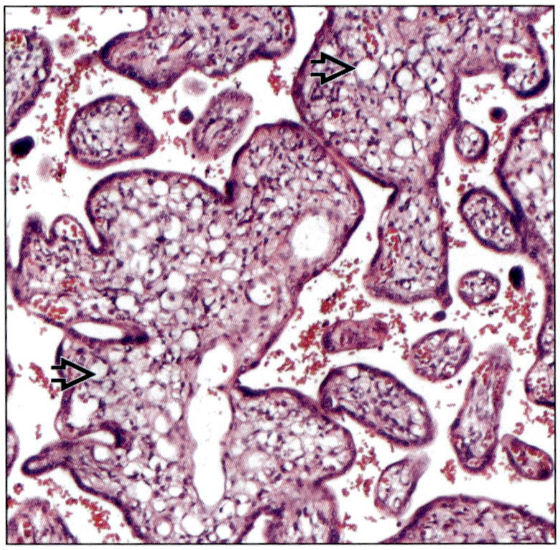

(Left) *These 1st-trimester villi have polygonal stromal cells in a loose mesenchyme. Similar-appearing mesenchymal villi may be seen throughout gestation in limited numbers. They are a source for further villogenesis.* ***(Right)*** *The 2nd-trimester placentas have numerous immature intermediate villi. These villi have a loose reticular stroma full of rounded spaces ⇨, many of which contain fetal macrophages (Hofbauer cells).*

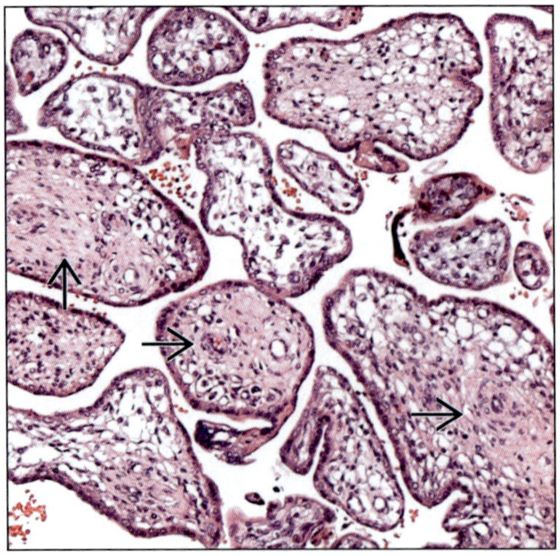

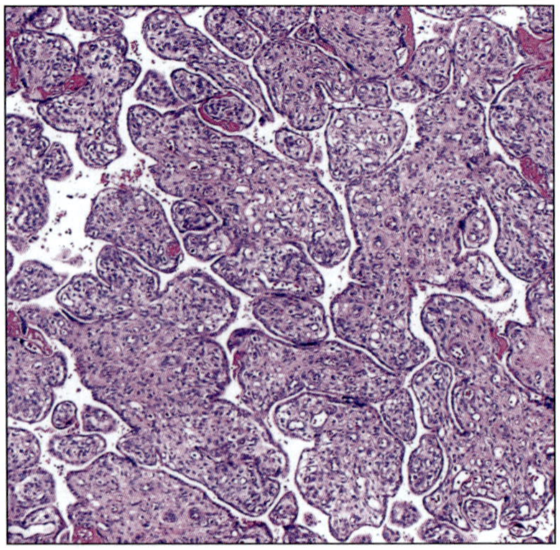

(Left) *These 2nd-trimester villi show maturation of the immature intermediate villi, with development of vascular smooth muscle and collagenization of the stromal core →.* ***(Right)*** *These 23-week-gestation villi are mostly immature intermediate villi with variable degrees of maturation. They lack the usually striking spaces at low power, an artifact of fixation.*

Normal Histology of 2nd- and 3rd-Trimester Villi

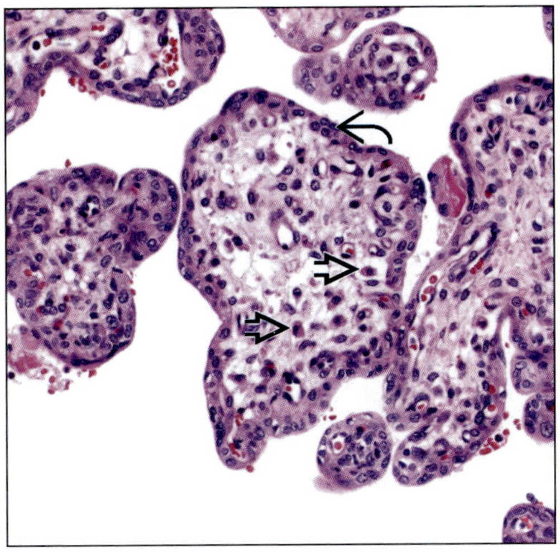

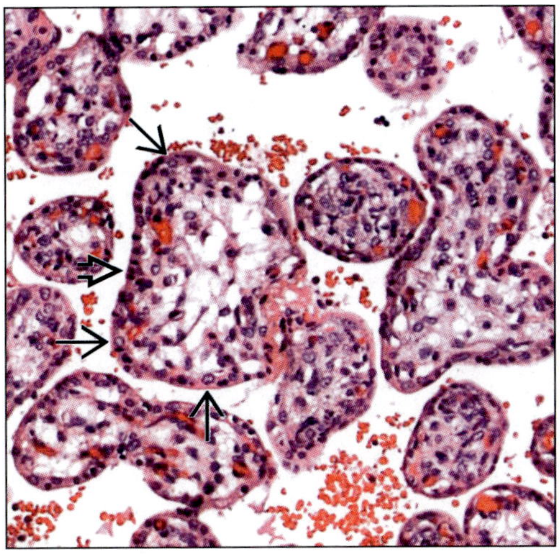

(Left) *This 27-week-gestation villus shows classic features of 2nd-trimester villi. Syncytiotrophoblast and cytotrophoblast nuclei* ↪ *are easily identified, as are Hofbauer cells* ⇨*. There are few stromal capillaries.* ***(Right)*** *Late in the 2nd trimester, groups of smaller villi resemble mature distal villi. However, fetal capillaries account for < 50% of the villous volume. Syncytiotrophoblast nuclei remain evenly spaced* ⇨*. The more vesicular cytotrophoblast nuclei* → *are seen.*

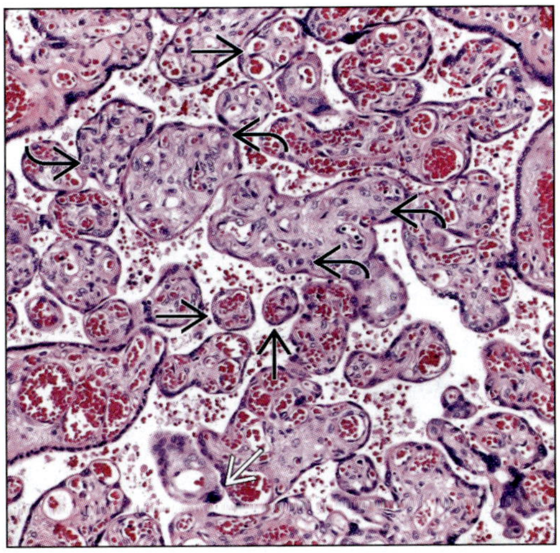

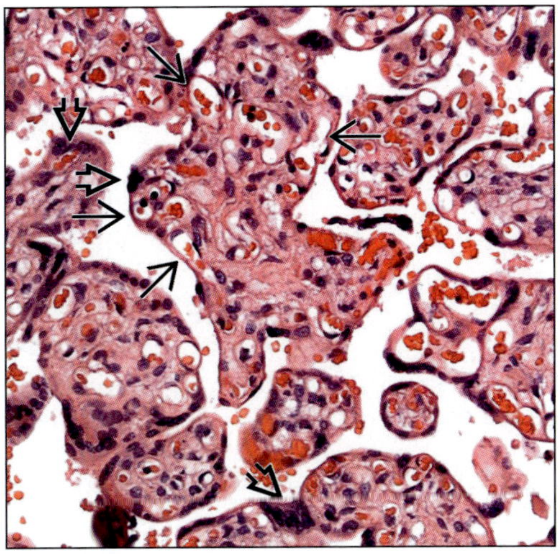

(Left) *Early in the 3rd trimester, distal villi are formed* →*. The larger immature villi have few vasculosyncytial membranes. Cytotrophoblast nuclei* ↪ *are visible, and < 20% of villi show syncytial knots* ➡*.* ***(Right)*** *Mature villi are optimized for gas and nutrient exchange. Syncytiotrophoblast nuclei are gathered into knots, and cytotrophoblast nuclei are rare, leaving the thin cytoplasm to form vasculosyncytial membranes* →*. Normal knots* ⇨ *barely rise above villous contour.*

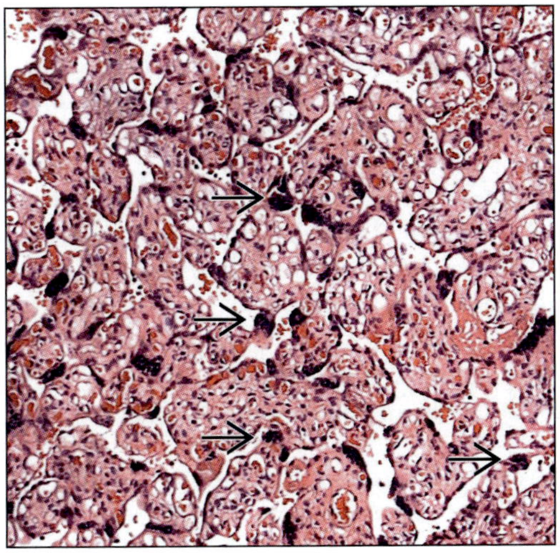

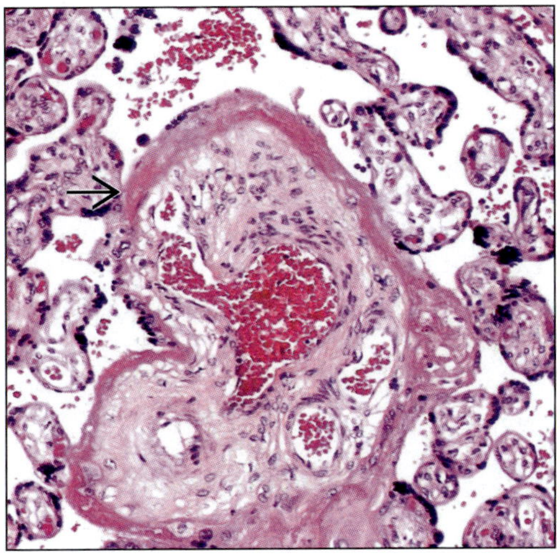

(Left) *These mature villi show bridging knots* → *joining adjacent villi. Standards for quantification of increased knots exclude bridging knots, and include only aggregates of > 5 syncytiotrophoblast nuclei that protrude above the villus contour.* ***(Right)*** *Another general feature of placental maturation is the presence of fibrin around stem villi. Over time, the syncytiotrophoblast layer becomes eroded and replaced by fibrin* →*.*

HISTOPATHOLOGIC CHANGES OF CHORIONIC VILLI

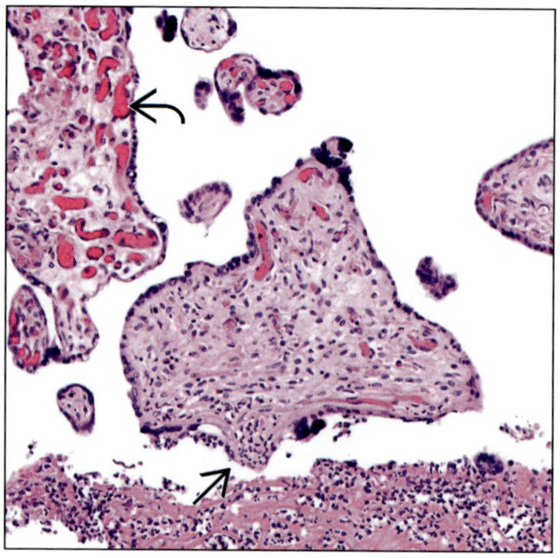

Acute villitis → is a rare but important finding, associated with fetal sepsis due to ascending infection (amniotic fluid infection sequence). These villi are also hypervascular (chorangiosis) →.

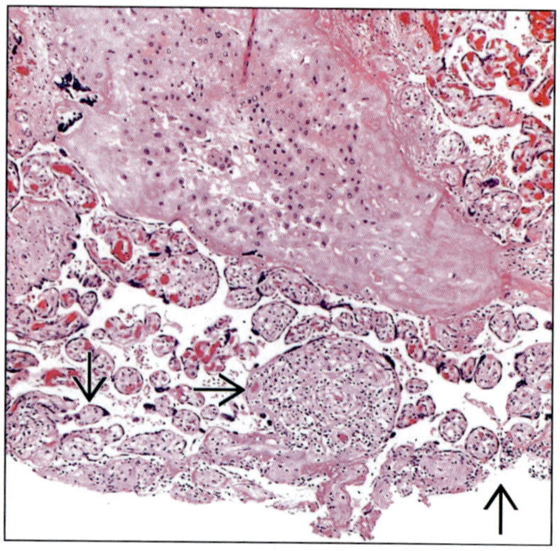

Chronic villitis → is a common finding. Most cases represent an abnormal maternal anti-fetal T-cell response, but 10% are associated with TORCH infections. Extensive lesions are clinically significant.

INFLAMMATION

Acute Villitis

- Accumulation of neutrophils in villus, usually between syncytiotrophoblast layer and stroma, usually focal, associated with fetal sepsis in amniotic fluid infection

Chronic Villitis

- Infiltrate of lymphocytes and histiocytes, rarely plasma cells
- May be focal or diffuse, basal or intraparenchymal
- May have associated chronic chorioamnionitis, fetal vasculopathy, or increased perivillous fibrin

DISORDERS OF VILLOUS MATURATION

Distal Villous Immaturity

- Failure to form appropriate numbers of distal villi in a mature placenta, villi appear larger than normal for GA and variably hypervascular

Villous Maturation Defect

- Failure to form sufficient vasculosyncytial membranes (VSMs) in mature distal villi
  - VSMs are areas of broad contact between a capillary and syncytiotrophoblast layer without intervening nucleus or connective tissue
    - Defined in mature placenta (after 34 weeks)
    - < 1 VSM per 4 small distal villi, on average, in a count of 10 HPF (400x)
- Seen in 6% of placentas after 34 weeks, associated with fetal demise around 38 weeks and hypercoiled umbilical cords, and appearance is similar to distal villous immaturity

Chorangiosis

- Too many capillaries per villus: > 10 capillaries per villus, in > 10 villi, in > 10 HPF

Distal Villous Hypoplasia

- Abnormal villous development with sparse, very small distal villi; similar-appearing areas are seen normally under chorionic plate and at placental margin
- Often associated with Tenney-Parker change, infarcts, maternal decidual vasculopathy

Increased Syncytial Knots

- Knots in > 20% of villi preterm (before 34 weeks) or 30% of villi at term (after 38 weeks) is pathologic and suggests placental ischemia (maternal malperfusion)
- Tenney-Parker change: Increased syncytial knots that stand out from villous surface as polypoid projections, often seen with distal villous hypoplasia

FETAL VASCULOPATHY

Villous Stromal-Vascular Karyorrhexis

- Distal villous lesion of fetal vascular obstruction, with karyorrhexis of fetal blood cells, endothelial cells, and stromal cells in a villus
- Similar lesions seen in fetal thrombotic vasculopathy, downstream of proximal chronic villitis, after fetal demise or in cases of severe fetal anemia

Avascular Villi

- Later distal villous lesion of fetal vascular obstruction, villi appear homogeneously pink and lack capillaries; syncytiotrophoblast layer is viable and affects groups of villi
- Similar lesions are seen in fetal thrombotic vasculopathy, downstream of proximal chronic villitis, after fetal demise

Intervillous Lesions and Other Changes

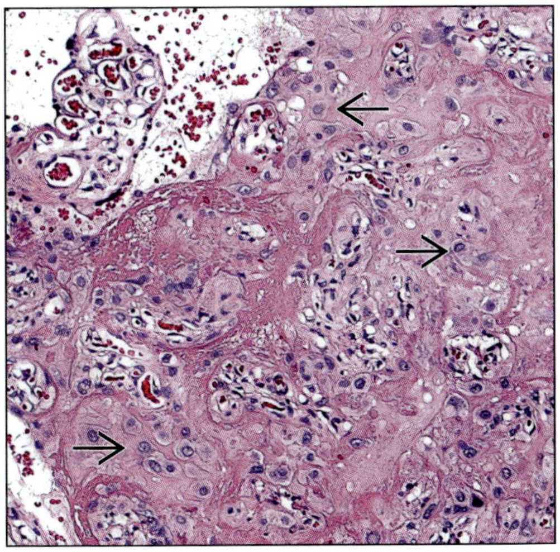
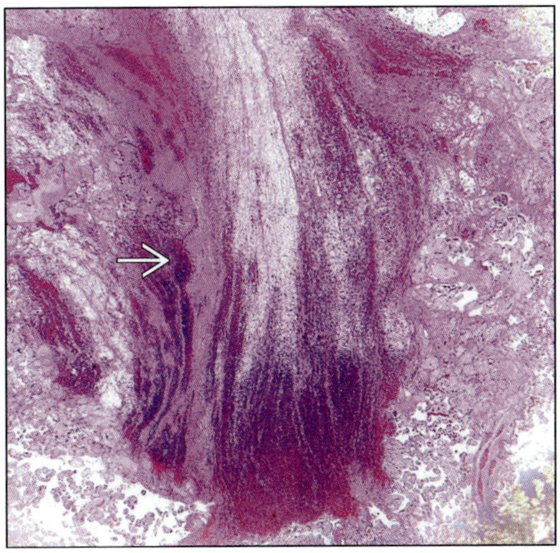

(Left) *Perivillous fibrin accumulates when the syncytiotrophoblast is injured or degenerates. In massive perivillous fibrin deposition, there are gross changes and EVTs ⇒ are numerous.* ***(Right)*** *Intervillous hemorrhage is a frequent cause of "tan lesions" on gross exam, commonly due to fetal-maternal hemorrhage ➡. The hemorrhage is confirmed as fetal by identification of NRBCs or with an immunohistochemical stain for fetal hemoglobin.*

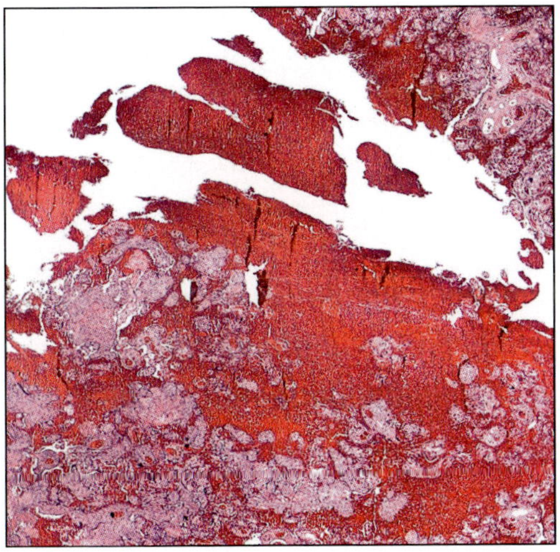
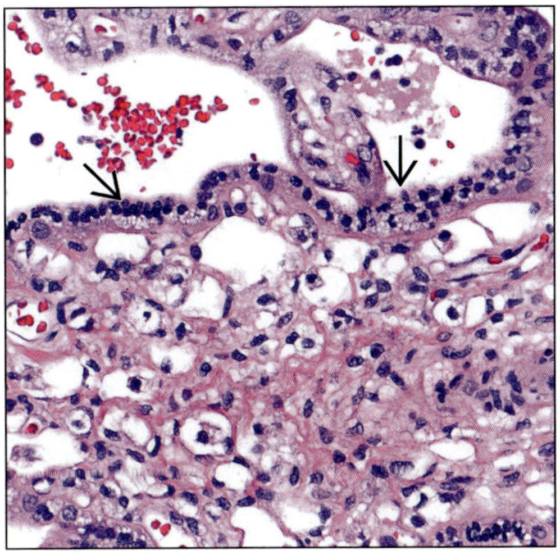

(Left) *This image shows dissecting intervillous hemorrhage separating populations of villi. This can be a histologic feature of acute placental abruption (retroplacental hemorrhage).* ***(Right)*** *The syncytiotrophoblast in this case shows cytoplasmic vacuolization ⇒. This uncommon change suggests a metabolic storage disease in the fetus and clinical correlation is imperative. Some liposomal drug formulations can cause similar changes.*

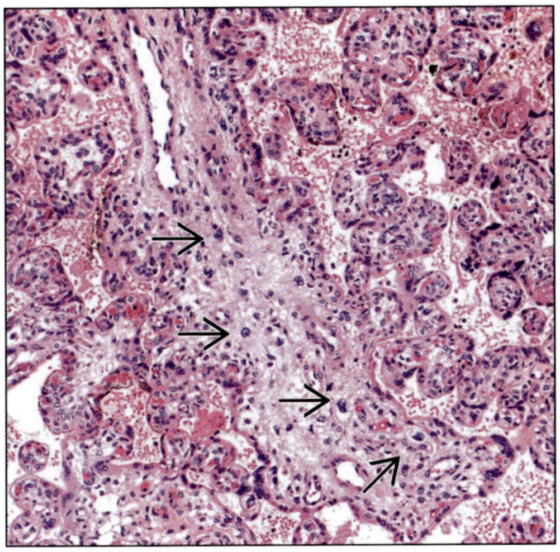
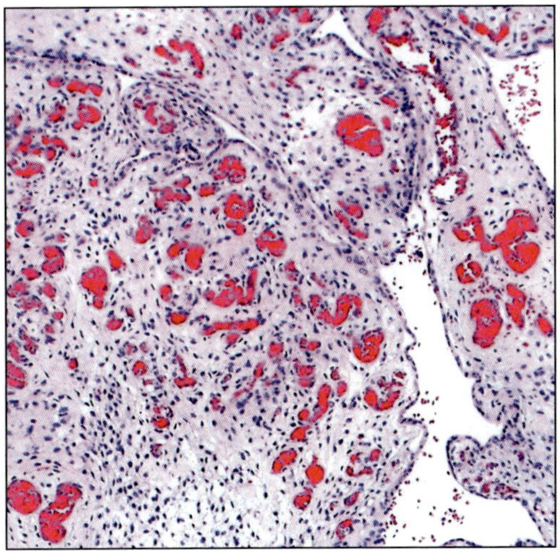

(Left) *Stromal cell cytomegaly ⇒ is an uncommon change associated with chromosomal abnormalities in some cases.* ***(Right)*** *Maze-like, irregular vascular proliferations are another dysplastic feature associated with chromosomal abnormalities. This image is from a case of placental mesenchymal dysplasia.*

Decidua

GROSS EVALUATION AND NORMAL HISTOLOGY OF DECIDUA

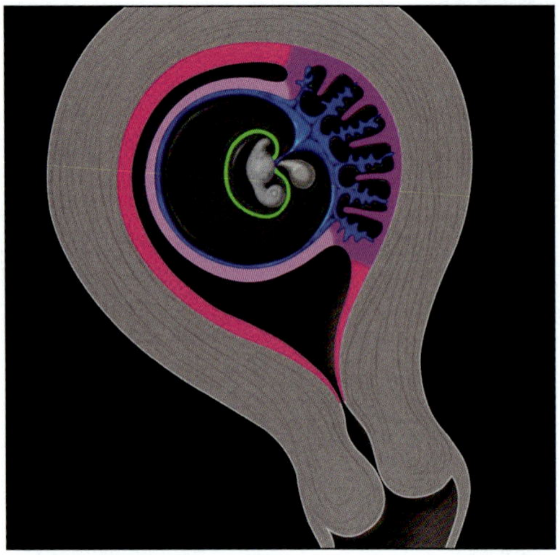

This diagram demonstrates the 3 types of decidua from early gestation. The decidua capsularis is in light pink, the decidua vera is in dark pink, and the decidua basalis is in purple.

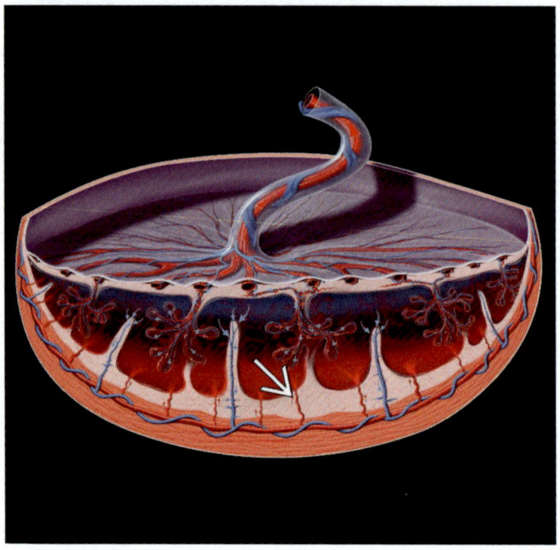

The decidua provides the only opportunity to evaluate maternal blood vessels ➔ in the delivered placenta. Vessels from all other sites are fetal. Maternal vessels are remodeled in pregnancy to optimize placental perfusion.

TERMINOLOGY

Definitions

- Decidua: Endometrium in pregnancy
  - Decidua capsularis: Decidua overlying implanted blastocyst; progressively atrophies as gestational sac enlarges; not distinguished after 22 weeks
  - Decidua vera, decidua parietalis: All decidual lining of uterine cavity except that of implantation site
  - Decidua basalis: Decidua underlying placenta at implantation site
- Marginal sinus: Region where decidua vera meets decidua capsularis at edge of placental disc and where uteroplacental veins open into intervillous space

Synonyms

- Decidua vera, decidua parietalis, and membranous decidua are synonyms

NORMAL FUNCTION OF DECIDUA

Facilitates Implantation

- Cytokines and cell surface molecules facilitate apposition, attachment, and penetration of blastocyst into gestational endometrium

Endocrine Function

- Decidual cells produce growth factors and cytokines that sustain embryo development

Immune Function

- Dendritic cells and uterine NK (uNK) cells migrate to decidua from 6th-11th week post conception
  - Influence stromal cell differentiation and interact with extravillous trophoblast in vascular remodeling

Facilitates Parturition

- Mechanical function
  - Latin root "deciduus" means "with tendency to fall off or shed"; decidua facilitates separation of placenta and membranes from uterus
    - Degenerative changes in upper decidua begin prior to labor and delivery in preparation for shedding
    - Absence of decidua leads to placenta accreta, increta, percreta wherein the placenta remains firmly attached to maternal tissues
- Endocrine function
  - Decidual prostaglandin production markedly increases during labor and plays a role in cervical ripening and myometrial contraction

MACROSCOPIC FINDINGS

Gross Appearance of Decidua

- Tan-yellow to gray tissue firmly adherent to membranes and basal surface of delivered placenta
  - Present in variable amounts, generally less in spontaneous term deliveries
- Decidua basalis vessels
  - Spiral arteries run perpendicular to surface in central placenta and more parallel at margins
    - Appear as punctate erosions
    - Estimated to number 0.5-1 per square centimeter of basal surface
  - Uteroplacental veins generally lay parallel to basal surface
    - Difficult to see; may appear as small white serpentine line segments

Pathologic Changes on Gross Examination

- Adherent blood clot
  - May be on basal surface, behind membranes, or at margin
    - Retroplacental hematoma may indent basal surface
  - Measure and weigh any well-formed hematomas

Decidual Vascular Remodeling in Pregnancy

Vasculature	1st Trimester	2nd Trimester	3rd Trimester	Postpartum
Spiral arteries of membranous decidua	Media thins out	Media remains thin	Media remains thin	Normal thickness resumes
Spiral arteries of decidua basalis	Extravillous cytotrophoblast cells invade wall and form luminal plugs; smooth muscle is replaced by fibrin	Lumen is enlarged and becomes patent; trophoblast cells embed in mural fibrin; 2nd wave of invasion goes deeper into arteries; ~ 1/3 of arteries invaded	All spiral arteries in central 2/3 are remodeled (90% of spiral arteries)	Placental bed vessels thrombose; trophoblasts in and near walls regress or die; smooth muscle regrows
Myometrial arteries	Media thins and lumen dilates	Arteries proximal to placental bed get remodeled with 2nd wave; all lumina remain dilated	Remodeling continues; vessel lumina remain dilated	Remodeled vessels thrombose; trophoblasts in and near walls regress or die; smooth muscle and elastica regrows; other lumina return to normal size; media thickens to pre-pregnant state
Veins	Lumen dilates	Veins underlying placental bed and at margins may have ingrowth of villi	Veins underlying placental bed may have ingrowth of villi; villous growth at margins facilitates lateral placental growth	Lumina return to normal size

- Shaggy red-brown myometrial fibers on basal surface
  - Indicate occult placenta accreta
  - Take sections of suspicious areas
- Incomplete basal cotyledons
  - Suggest possible incomplete removal of placenta
- Spiral artery thrombi in decidua basalis (rare)

MICROSCOPIC FINDINGS

Components of Decidua

- Endometrial stromal cells become decidual stromal cells under influence of progesterone
  - Polygonal stromal cells rich in glycogen and lipid
  - Proliferate and differentiate in pregnancy, become polyploid
  - Comprise 30% of cellularity in 1st trimester, 30-55% at term
- Immune cells
  - Uterine NK cells (uNK): 40% of cellularity in 1st trimester; 4-9% at term; secrete cytokines that aid in stromal cell differentiation and vascular remodeling
  - Macrophages and dendritic cells: 20% of cellularity in 1st trimester; 20-40% at term; aid in support of decidual function
  - T cells: 8-10% of cellularity in 1st trimester; 8-17% at term; play role in tolerance of fetal antigens
  - B cells and plasma cells: Very rare in normal pregnancy and comprise < 1% of decidual cells
- Vasculature
  - Spiral arteries
    - Have thinned walls in membranous decidua and do not undergo trophoblast-mediated vascular remodeling
    - Undergo trophoblast-mediated remodeling in decidua basalis for optimal uteroplacental perfusion
  - Veins do not undergo trophoblast-mediated remodeling and have dilated lumina with inconspicuous to absent smooth muscle
    - May see ingrowth of villi, especially at margins
- Extravillous cytotrophoblast (EVT) cells
  - Present at interface of membranous chorion or basal plate and decidua, stationary EVT cells secrete extracellular matrix, invasive EVT cells migrate to underlying tissues
  - Subset of invasive EVT cells remodels spiral arteries of decidua basalis (endovascular trophoblast); others remain outside of vessels (intermediate trophoblast)
- Multinucleated trophoblastic giant cells
  - Uncommon in normal decidual basalis; not seen in membranous decidua; thought to be derived from fusion of invasive EVT cells at end of their journey
- Glandular epithelium
  - Prominent in 1st-trimester specimens and uncommonly seen in delivered placental tissues
    - May show Arias-Stella reaction with nuclear enlargement and polymorphism as a result of polyploidy

SELECTED REFERENCES

1. Blois SM et al: Decidualization and angiogenesis in early pregnancy: unravelling the functions of DC and NK cells. J Reprod Immunol. 88(2):86-92, 2011
2. Whitley GS et al: Cellular and molecular regulation of spiral artery remodelling: lessons from the cardiovascular field. Placenta. 31(6):465-74, 2010
3. King A et al: Human uterine lymphocytes. Hum Reprod Update. 4(5):480-5, 1998
4. Dietl J et al: The decidua of early human pregnancy: immunohistochemistry and function of immunocompetent cells. Gynecol Obstet Invest. 33(4):197-204, 1992
5. Robertson WB et al: Uteroplacental vascular pathology. Eur J Obstet Gynecol Reprod Biol. 5(1-2):47-65, 1975

GROSS EVALUATION AND NORMAL HISTOLOGY OF DECIDUA

Gross Examination of Decidua

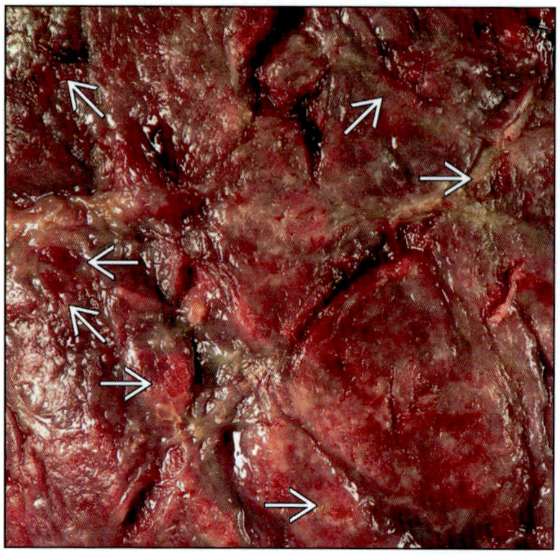
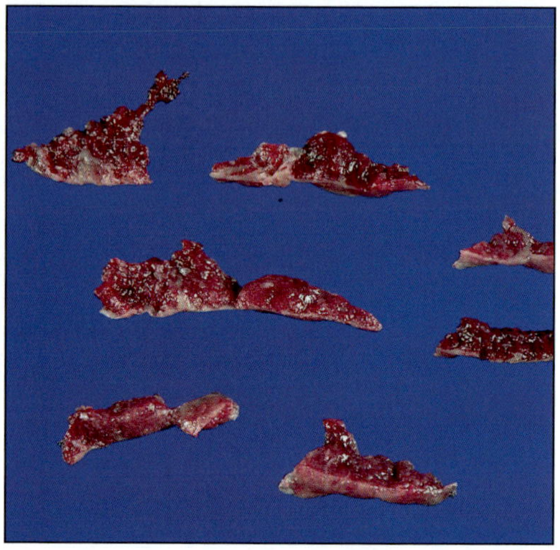

(Left) *Maternal decidual blood vessels appear as punctate or shallow erosions on basal surface. Small perpendicular wedge sections in these regions are useful for sampling them.* ***(Right)*** *These examples of decidua basalis wedge sections facilitate evaluation of basal spiral arteries. Several may fit in 1 cassette. Basal fibrin layer is thin; only rare decidual stromal cells will be seen. These sections are also useful for finding basal chronic villitis, increased basal perivillous fibrin, increased number of EVT cells, and plasma cells deciduitis.*

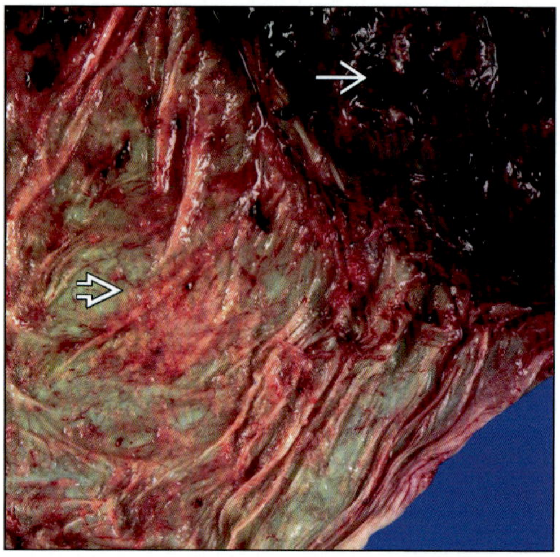
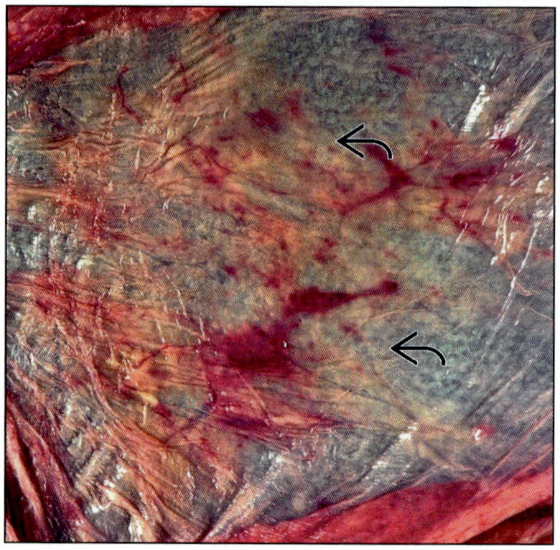

(Left) *Examination of the basal and membranous decidua provides an opportunity to evaluate the maternal vasculature. Viewed from the maternal side, the decidua is velvety tan-pink.* ***(Right)*** *Only a scant amount of residual decidua is seen behind the placental membranes in this image. As the amount of membranous decidua is variable, submission of 2 membrane rolls is ideal.*

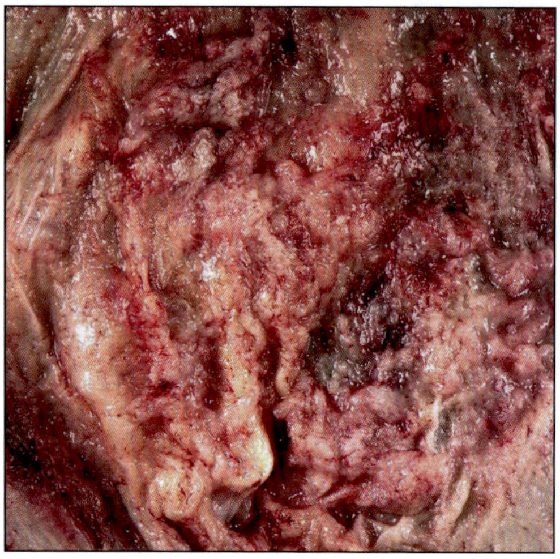
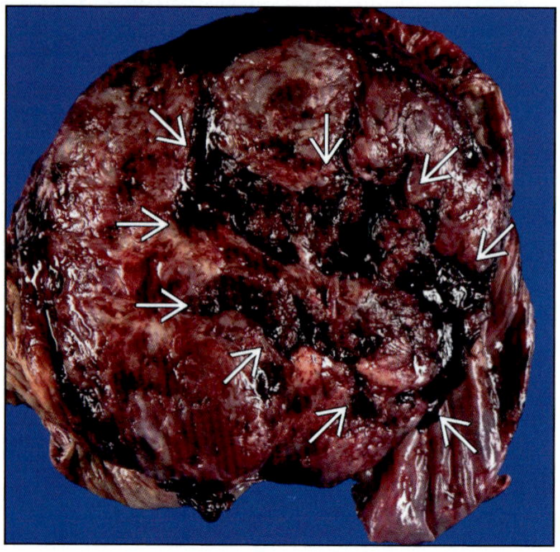

(Left) *In some specimens, membranous decidua is abundant, as seen in this image of the maternal surface of membranes. This is generally more common in nonspontaneous births.* ***(Right)*** *Retroplacental hemorrhage can be difficult to distinguish from nonspecific adherent blood. This case had a large marginal and retroplacental hemorrhage, which effaced and indented the parenchyma.*

Normal Decidual Histology

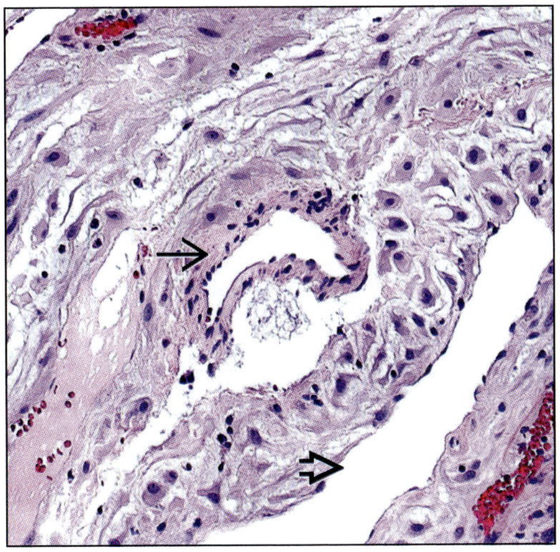

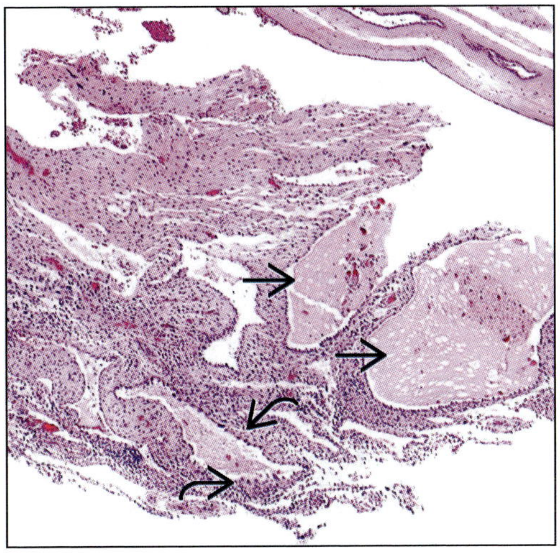

(Left) *This image shows a normal spiral artery →and vein ⇨ of the membranous decidua. Arteries of the membranes do not get remodeled by trophoblast, but the musculature should appear appropriately thin (< 1/3 the diameter of the vessel). The vein has minimal to no smooth muscle.* ***(Right)*** *Membranous decidua may be abundant in the preterm placenta. This image shows glands →, with focal Arias-Stella change ↷ characterized by hyperchromatic, enlarged nuclei.*

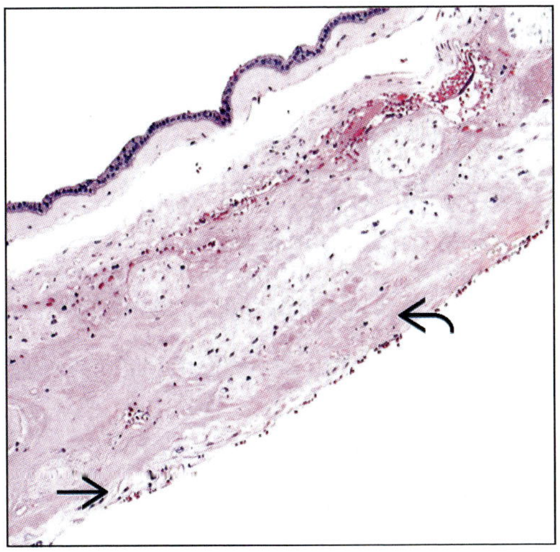

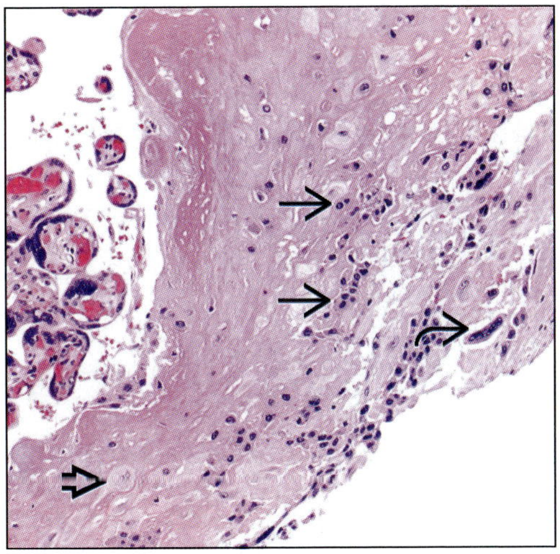

(Left) *Prior to labor and delivery, degenerative changes in the upper decidua ready the placenta and membranes for parturition. The membranes may only show fibrin ↷ with rare viable or necrotic residual decidual cells →.* ***(Right)*** *The basal surface may show minimal decidua, with mostly basal fibrin (Nitabuch fibrinoid) and EVT cells →. A multinucleate trophoblast cell ↷ is present. Rare decidual stromal cells ⇨ with pale nuclei and abundant cytoplasm are seen.*

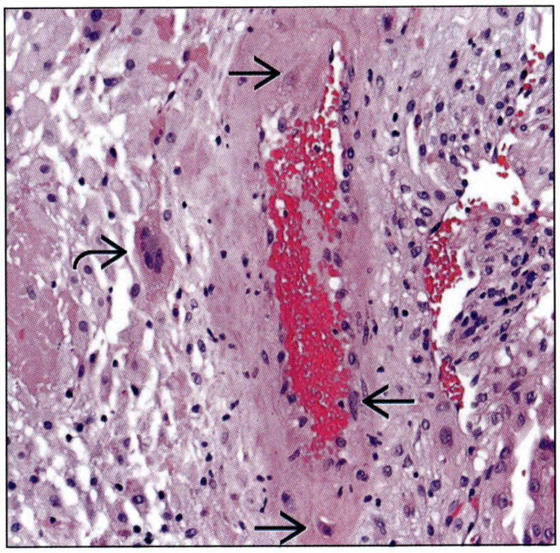

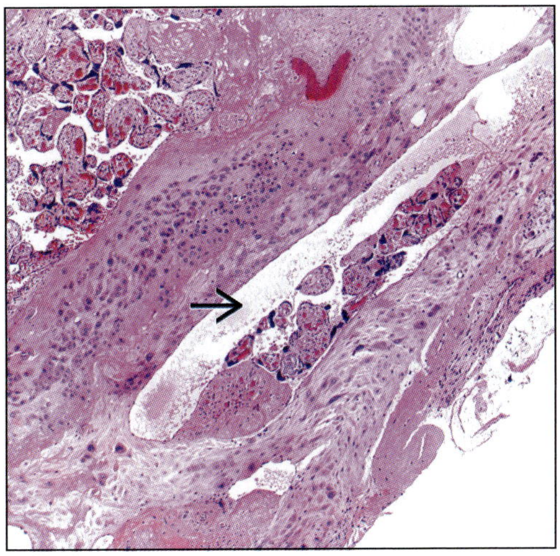

(Left) *This maternal spiral artery of the decidua basalis is adapted for pregnancy after trophoblast-mediated remodeling. The smooth muscle is replaced by fibrin → encasing occasional trophoblast cells. Also present is a multinucleate trophoblast cell ↷.* ***(Right)*** *Decidua basalis veins are not remodeled by trophoblast but may show extension of villi → into lumina. This is a normal mechanism of lateral placental growth and not evidence of placenta accreta.*

HISTOPATHOLOGIC CHANGES OF DECIDUA

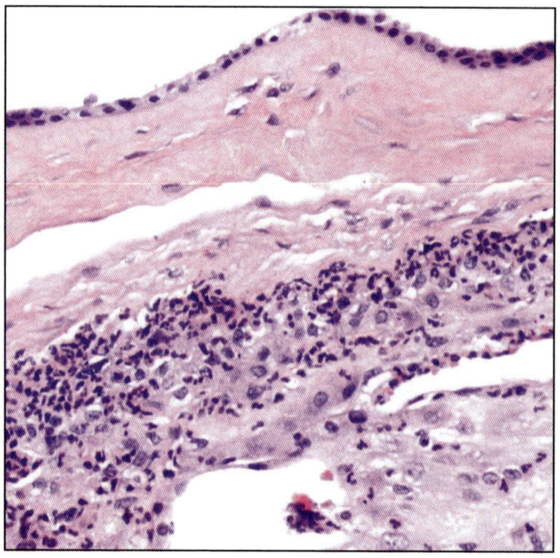

Acute deciduitis may be an early manifestation of the maternal inflammatory response to amniotic fluid infection (AFI). In AFI, maternal neutrophils migrate from decidual vessels toward the membranes.

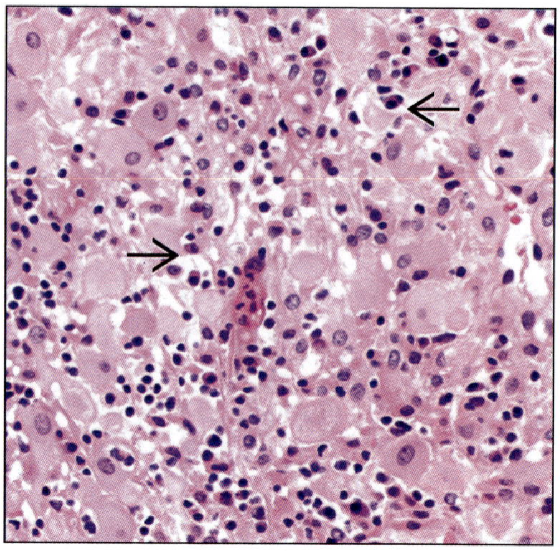

Although scattered lymphocytes are normal in the decidua, plasma cells ➔ are not. The presence of plasma cells suggests an abnormal immune environment and has numerous clinical associations.

ACUTE INFLAMMATION

Acute Deciduitis

- Maternal neutrophils in decidua
  - May be earliest maternal inflammatory response to amniotic fluid infection (AFI)
    - Neutrophils migrate from decidual vessels toward membranes and amniotic fluid
  - If limited to decidua without chorioamnionitis
    - Look for a fetal inflammatory response to further substantiate AFI sequence (AFIS)
    - Some cases of AFIS have a more robust fetal response than maternal response, e.g., group B *Streptococcus*
    - Diffuse decidual leukocytoclastic necrosis also has neutrophils

CHRONIC INFLAMMATION

Plasma Cell Deciduitis

- Presence of plasma cells and lymphocytes in decidua
  - Also termed chronic deciduitis
  - Lymphocytes are a normal constituent of decidua, but plasma cells are not
- Reflects abnormal immune environment; associations include
  - Chronic villitis of unknown etiology (VUE), especially basal VUE
  - AFIS
  - Hematogenous infections; look for additional changes
    - Cytomegalovirus
    - Herpes simplex virus
    - Syphilis
  - Preeclampsia, maternal decidual vasculopathy
  - Severe immune Rh isoimmunization
  - Unclear association with chronic endometritis
- May be seen in decidua basalis or membranous decidua
- Plasma cell deciduitis present in ~ 10% of preterm placentas

Perivascular Chronic Inflammation

- Prominent cuff of lymphocytes around maternal decidual vessels
  - Seen in some cases of preeclampsia
- Perivascular lymphocytes are normal in 1st trimester
  - Uterine NK cells coordinate vascular remodeling

NECROSIS

Laminar Decidual Necrosis

- Bland, band-like necrosis of upper decidua
  - Loss of decidual stromal cell and vascular cell nuclear basophilia
- May be physiologic change in preparation for parturition
  - May be normal at term, pathologic preterm
- Associated with intrauterine hypoxia in some studies but not in others
  - Discrepancy in significance may reflect gestational age

Diffuse Decidual Leukocytoclastic Necrosis

- Similar necrosis of decidua associated with karyorrhectic debris
  - ± neutrophils
- Associated with early preterm birth and preeclampsia
- Less commonly associated with positive amniotic fluid cultures or neonatal sepsis

MATERNAL DECIDUAL VASCULOPATHY

Incomplete Adaptation for Pregnancy

- Failure of maternal spiral arteries to undergo trophoblast-mediated vascular remodeling in decidua basalis
  - Presence of vascular smooth muscle in decidua basalis spiral arteries of central 2/3 placenta is diagnostic
  - Persistence of luminal trophoblast in 3rd-trimester decidua basalis spiral arteries suggests incomplete remodeling

Hypertrophic Vasculopathy

- Thickened vascular media in decidual spiral arteries
  - Wall thickness > 1/3 of vessel diameter is diagnostic
  - Associations
    - Hypertension, pregnancy-associated hypertensive disorders
    - Diabetes

Fibrinoid Necrosis

- Eosinophilic necrosis of vessel wall in membranous decidua or decidua basalis
  - Only unremodeled vessels are susceptible
  - Associated with preterm preeclampsia
  - May be complicated by thrombosis

Acute Atherosis

- Subintimal foamy macrophages in decidual vessel with fibrinoid necrosis
  - Only unremodeled vessels are susceptible
  - Associated with preterm preeclampsia
  - May be complicated by thrombosis

HEMORRHAGE

Retroplacental Hematoma

- Pathologic correlate of placental abruption
  - Hemorrhage in upper decidua basalis
  - Significance depends on amount of placental bed separated from maternal blood supply
  - Gross exam may show adherent clot with indentation of basal plate
  - Microscopic findings
    - Acute villous injury with intravillous hemorrhage
    - Wedge-shaped dissecting hemorrhage from basal surface into villous parenchyma in acute lesions
    - Recent or remote infarcts
    - Hemosiderin-laden macrophages
- Marginal abruption
  - May be chronic and repetitive throughout gestation
    - Attributed to venous bleeding at marginal sinus
  - Remote hemorrhage seen at margin, may extend behind placenta and membranes, circumvallate membranes
  - Clinical associations
    - Vaginal bleeding
    - Diffuse chorioamniotic hemosiderosis
    - Oligohydramnios
    - Preterm birth
    - Fetal growth restriction

Retromembranous Hemorrhage

- Adherent blood behind membranes is common and usually not significant
- Hemosiderin deposition in membranous decidua suggests chronicity
  - More common in preterm births
  - Associated with decidual necrosis
- Focal retromembranous hematomas may reflect amniocentesis sites

ABSENCE OF DECIDUA

Placenta Accreta, Increta, and Percreta

- Disorders of abnormal placental implantation in which placenta fails to separate from uterus
  - Characterized by an absence or deficiency of decidua
  - Placenta implants in myometrium or scar
  - Only fibrin and extravillous trophoblast separate villi from
    - Myometrium in placenta accreta, placenta increta
    - Serosa or adjacent organs in placenta percreta
- Associations all share deficiency of decidua
  - Implantation in lower uterine segment or cornua
  - Uterine scarring

Occult Placenta Accreta

- Basal myometrial fibers
  - May see shaggy red myometrial fibers attached focally to basal surface
  - Microscopically, myometrial fibers are adjacent to basal fibrin with no intervening decidua

SELECTED REFERENCES

1. Elsasser DA et al: Diagnosis of placental abruption: relationship between clinical and histopathological findings. Eur J Obstet Gynecol Reprod Biol. 148(2):125-30, 2010
2. Tantbirojn P et al: Pathophysiology of placenta creta: the role of decidua and extravillous trophoblast. Placenta. 29(7):639-45, 2008
3. Goldenberg RL et al: The Alabama Preterm Birth Study: diffuse decidual leukocytoclastic necrosis of the decidua basalis, a placental lesion associated with preeclampsia, indicated preterm birth and decreased fetal growth. J Matern Fetal Neonatal Med. 20(5):391-5, 2007
4. Stanek J et al: Occult placenta accreta: the missing link in the diagnosis of abnormal placentation. Pediatr Dev Pathol. 10(4):266-73, 2007
5. Goldenberg RL et al: The Alabama Preterm Birth Project: placental histology in recurrent spontaneous and indicated preterm birth. Am J Obstet Gynecol. 195(3):792-6, 2006
6. Stanek J et al: Laminar necrosis of placental membranes: a histologic sign of uteroplacental hypoxia. Pediatr Dev Pathol. 8(1):34-42, 2005
7. Redline RW et al: Maternal vascular underperfusion: nosology and reproducibility of placental reaction patterns. Pediatr Dev Pathol. 7(3):237-49, 2004
8. Salafia CM et al: Histologic evidence of old intrauterine bleeding is more frequent in prematurity. Am J Obstet Gynecol. 173(4):1065-70, 1995

HISTOPATHOLOGIC CHANGES OF DECIDUA

Microscopic Features

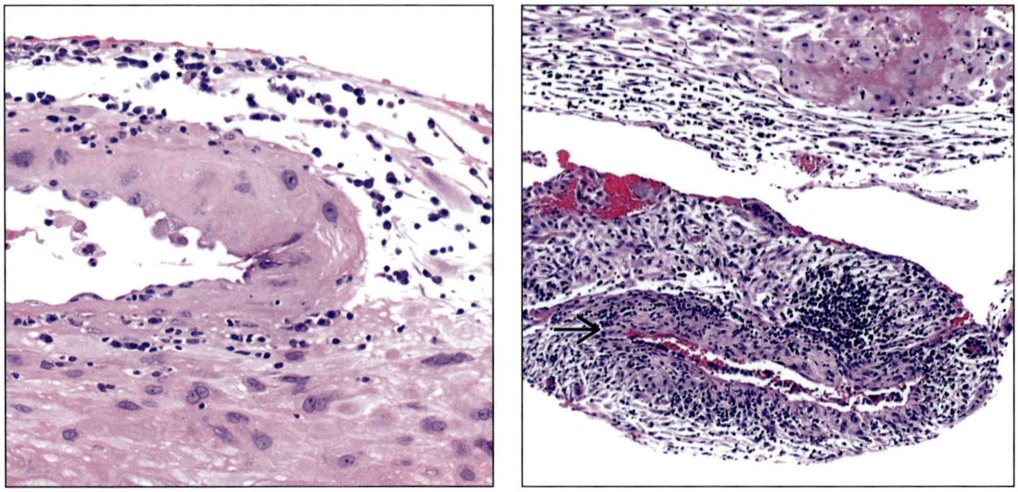

(Left) *Image of decidua basalis shows a spiral artery appropriately adapted for pregnancy and numerous surrounding plasma cells. The mother had recurrent preterm birth without further evidence of infection.* ***(Right)*** *This decidua basalis vessel has a prominent perivascular lymphoid infiltrate ➔, a finding sometimes seen in preeclampsia with other features of maternal decidual vasculopathy. As it resembles 1st-trimester changes, it may be a late attempt to remodel the vessel.*

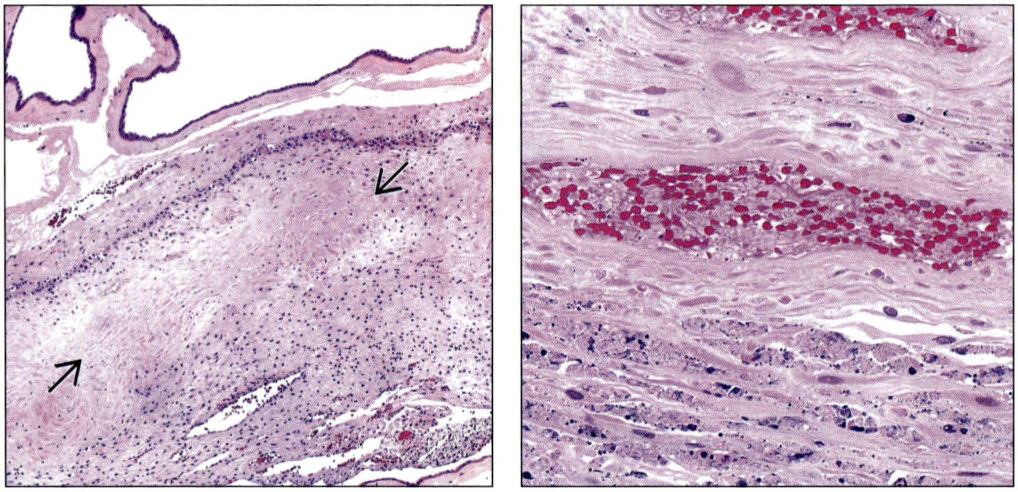

(Left) *Laminar decidual necrosis is a bland necrosis of the upper decidua ➔. It may be a normal physiologic finding at term, but pathologic preterm. Some experts attribute the finding to intrauterine hypoxia.* ***(Right)*** *Diffuse decidual leukocytoclastic necrosis is similar to laminar decidual necrosis, with the addition of karyorrhectic debris ± neutrophils. It is associated with preterm birth and preeclampsia.*

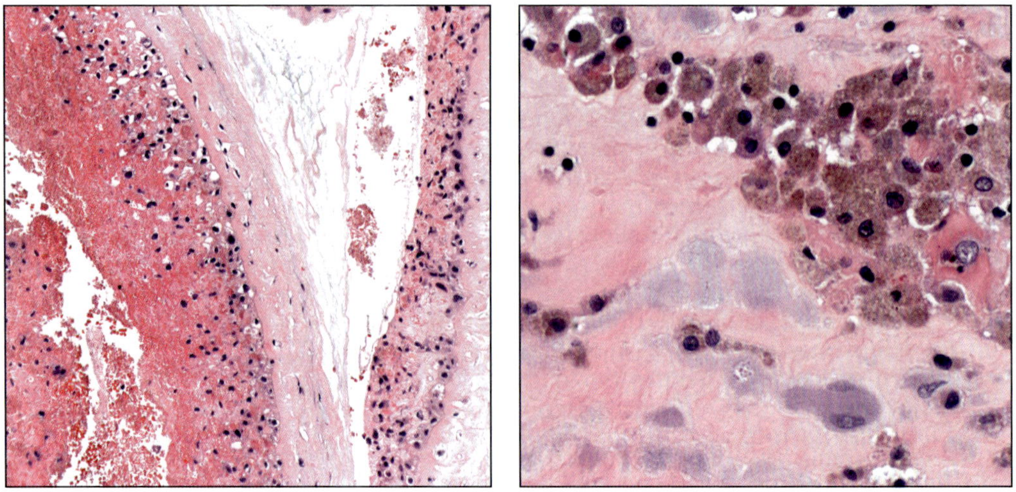

(Left) *Retromembranous hemorrhage is associated with decidual necrosis and extension of hemorrhage from a marginal abruption.* ***(Right)*** *Hemosiderin-laden macrophages impart chronicity to the hemorrhage. They are uncommonly found with retroplacental hematomas. Their presence has been associated with lesions that are 5-7 days old.*

Maternal Vasculopathy and Decidual Deficiency

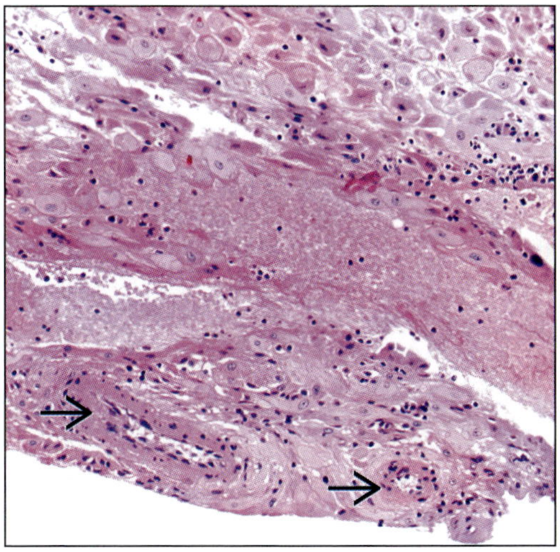
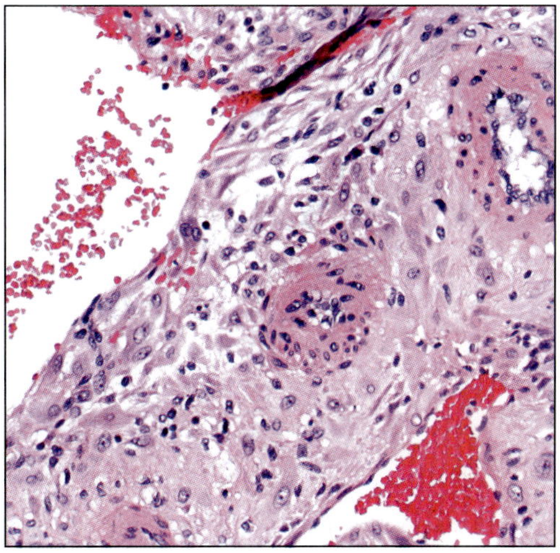

(Left) *Persistence of smooth muscle in decidua basalis spiral arteries* → *is pathologic. It represents a failure of trophoblast-mediated vascular remodeling. In addition to the resultant inconstant and reduced overall placental perfusion, this failure indicates dysfunction of the trophoblast or maternal immune cells.* ***(Right)*** *Hypertrophic maternal decidual vasculopathy is defined as a decidual vessel wall thickness > 1/3 of the total diameter.*

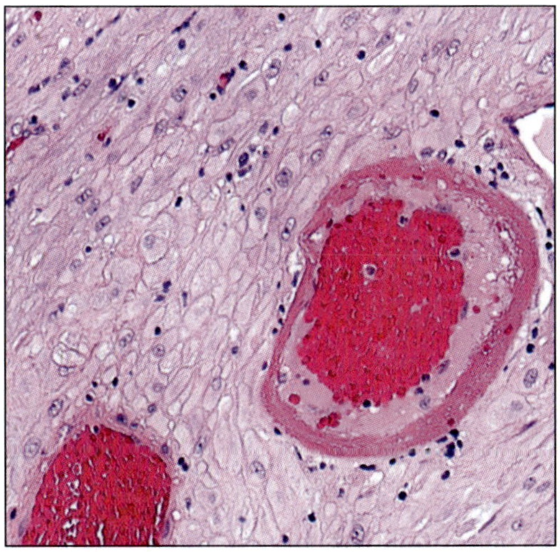
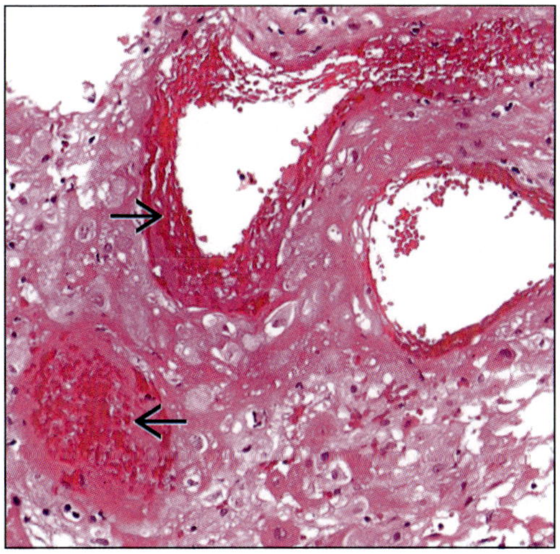

(Left) *Fibrinoid necrosis and acute atheromatous lesions are part of a spectrum of vascular injury seen in severe preterm preeclampsia. The necrotic vessel wall becomes intensely eosinophilic. In acute atheromatous lesions, foamy histiocytes accumulate beneath the endothelium.* ***(Right)*** *Thrombosis* → *may complicate fibrinoid necrosis of maternal decidual vasculopathy. Associated placental infarcts may be found.*

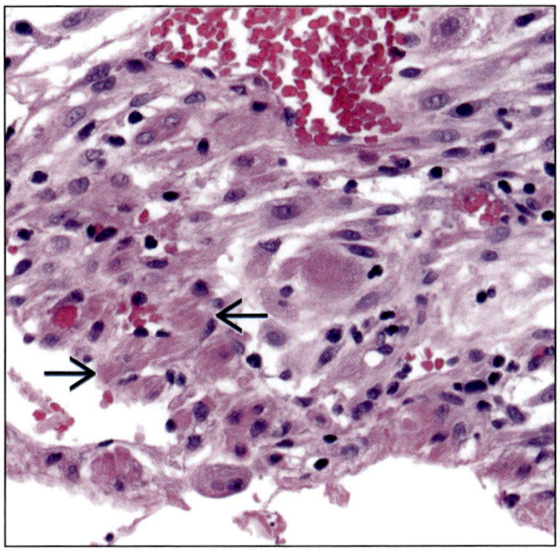
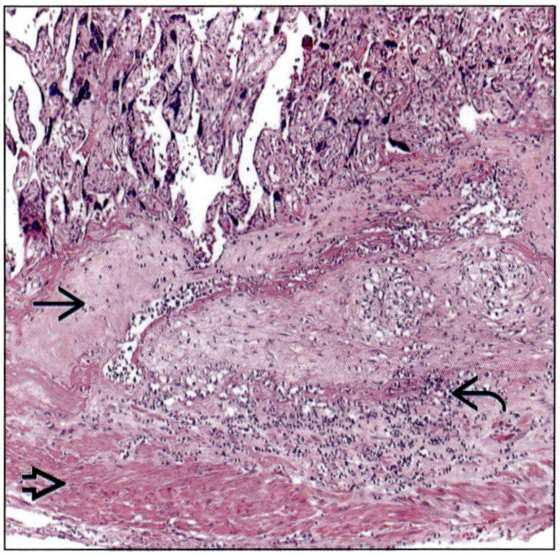

(Left) *In occult placenta accreta, myometrial cells* → *are found on the basal surface of the placenta, usually with a deficiency of decidual stromal cells. Potential causes include a submucosal leiomyoma.* ***(Right)*** *In this section of placenta increta, the placenta bed, with Nitabuch fibrin layer* →*, abuts the myometrium* ⇨ *without an intervening decidua. Abnormal placentation, such as placenta increta, is often associated with excessive chronic inflammation* ↩*.*

Meconium

MECONIUM-STAINED PLACENTA

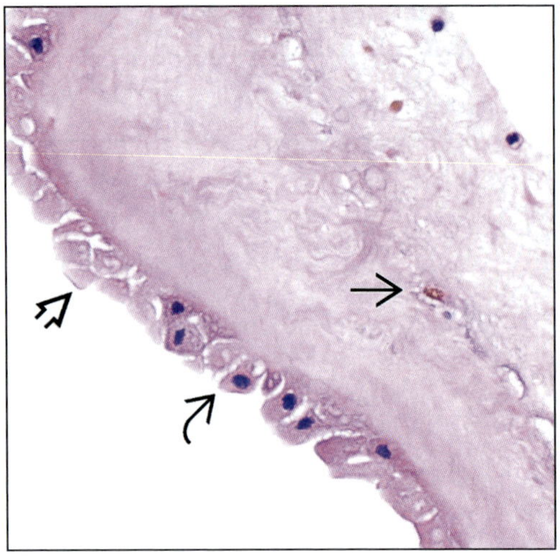

Meconium is toxic to amnion cells, inducing characteristic columnar change associated with vacuolation ⇾ and loss of nuclear basophilia ⇾. A yellow-brown meconium particle ⇾ is present.

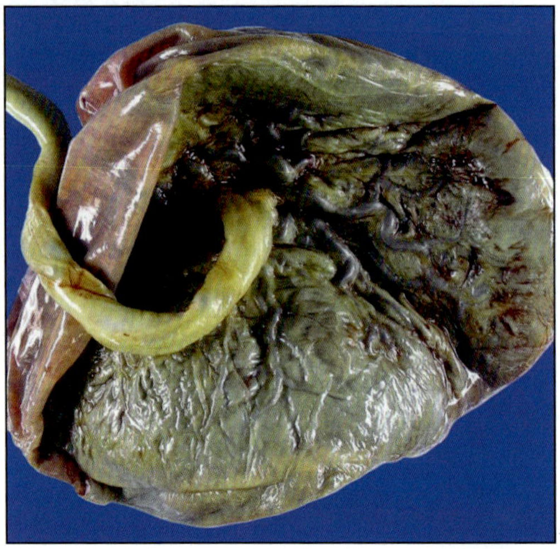

Gross photo shows diffuse bright green staining and a glistening appearance in recent meconium exposure.

TERMINOLOGY

Definitions

- Meconium: Early, dark green feces composed of intestinal secretions, mucus, lanugo, bile, and intestinal epithelial cells
- Meconium aspiration syndrome (MAS): Early-onset respiratory distress and persistent pulmonary hypertension in meconium-stained term or near-term infant
- Meconium-associated vascular necrosis (MAVN): Apoptosis of vascular smooth muscle underlying meconium deposition in chorionic plate or umbilical cord

EPIDEMIOLOGY

Prevalence of Meconium Staining

- 19% of term placentas, 31% of post-term placentas
- Very rare to see placental staining before 30 weeks gestation
- 9-16% of pregnancies have meconium-stained amniotic fluid noted at delivery

Incidence of MAVN

- ~ 1% of meconium-stained placentas demonstrate MAVN

ETIOLOGY/PATHOGENESIS

Meconium Passage In Utero

- Stimulated by hormone motilin
- Usually occurs in last month of pregnancy, more frequently in post term, and rarely in mid gestation
  - Some studies suggest fetal defecation is normal process from 2nd trimester throughout gestation
- Controversial association with fetal distress
  - Proposed association with preceding fetal distress and hypoxia
    - Other studies show no association with tocograms or fetal pH
    - May reflect complications of post-term infant
  - Meconium staining is not usually only pathologic change in cases with poor outcomes
    - Likely contribution from other processes such as chorioamnionitis, fetal thrombotic vasculopathy, or extensive chronic villitis

MAVN

- Prolonged meconium exposure is toxic to vascular smooth muscle cells of chorionic plate and umbilical cord
- Meconium causes vasoconstriction, even in absence of MAVN

CLINICAL IMPLICATIONS

MAS

- Affects 2% of infants born with meconium-stained amniotic fluid

MAVN

- Associated with CNS injury and significant neonatal morbidity and mortality

MACROSCOPIC FINDINGS

General Features

- Note color, consistency, and extent of staining on cord and membranes
  - Color ranges from bright green to muddy brown
  - Amnion may be edematous and slippery
- Follow routine protocol with particular attention to the possibility of ulcerations &/or thrombi of umbilical cord and chorionic plate vasculature

MECONIUM-STAINED PLACENTA

Chronicity of Meconium Staining, Gross Appearance and Associations

Chronicity	Gross Features	Clinical Outcomes	Placental Pathology
Acute	Blue-green discoloration, glistening surface, particulate slimy meconium present	Usually normal	Few associated placental lesions except low level of acute chorioamnionitis
Subacute	Slippery edematous membranes, dark discoloration	Outcomes of combined subacute and chronic: Lower 5 minute Apgar scores, umbilical artery acidosis	Pathologies of combined subacute and chronic: Associated with fetal thrombi, infarcts, acute chorioamnionitis, chronic villitis, MAVN
Chronic	Dull appearance, diffuse muddy staining, cord stained		

MAVN = meconium-associated vascular necrosis. Adapted from Benirschke et al: Anatomy and Pathology of the Placental Membranes. In Benirschke et al: Pathology of the Human Placenta. 6th ed. New York: Springer-Verlag. 275, 2012; Kaspar HG et al: The placenta in meconium staining: lesions and early neonatal outcome. Clin. Exp. Obst. & Gyn. 27(1): 63-6, 2000.

MICROSCOPIC FINDINGS

Meconium Staining

- Characteristic changes in amnion
  - Alternating areas of columnar reactive change with vacuolation and necrosis with loss of nuclear basophilia
  - May see globular pigment in amniotic epithelium
- May see mild chemical chorioamnionitis
  - Occasional neutrophils only
    - Note that meconium may promote bacterial growth; amniotic fluid infection is frequently present
- Meconium-laden macrophages found in amnion, chorion, and sometimes decidua
  - Depth of their presence implies chronicity
  - Distinguish from hemosiderin-laden macrophages with Prussian blue stain
  - Luna-Ishak stain will positively stain bile with greenish hue to confirm meconium if needed
  - Immunohistochemical stain recently described for meconium: Zinc coproporphyrin I

DIFFERENTIAL DIAGNOSIS

Diffuse Chorioamniotic Hemosiderosis

- Most important distinction from meconium because it has its own clinical significance
- See hemosiderin deposition, from phagocytosis of lysed red cells
  - Dark yellow to brown pigment
- Does not have typical reactive and necrotic changes of amnion
- Usually associated with chronic abruption, circumvallation
- Prussian blue stain will identify iron in hemosiderin-laden macrophages

Other Pigments

- Other pigments that may be seen in placenta
  - Hematoidin
    - Brown pigment similar to bilirubin
    - Found at sites of prolonged blood accumulation, like old hemorrhages
    - Does not react with iron stain
  - Lipofuscin
    - Yellow to light brown pigment
    - Noted after 32 weeks gestation
    - Will not have characteristic amniotic changes associated with meconium
  - Melanin
    - Described with prolonged rupture of membranes
    - Associated with dermatopathic conditions in fetus
    - Similar distribution as meconium pigment, positive Masson-Fontana stain
  - Formalin pigment
    - Fixation artifact, often with acid or alkaline formalin solution and prolonged fixation
    - Black dots formed from degradation of hemoglobin
    - Found in areas of blood, e.g., around vessels of villi
    - No characteristic amnion changes as in meconium; distribution not similar to meconium

SELECTED REFERENCES

1. Benirschke et al: Anatomy and Pathology of the Placental Membranes. In Benirschke et al: Pathology of the Human Placenta. 6th ed. New York: Springer-Verlag. 275, 2012
2. Furuta N et al: Immunohistochemical detection of meconium in the fetal membrane, placenta and umbilical cord. Placenta. 33(1):24-30, 2012
3. Poggi SH et al: Variability in pathologists' detection of placental meconium uptake. Am J Perinatol. 26(3):207-10, 2009
4. Kaspar HG et al: The placenta in meconium staining: lesions and early neonatal outcome. Clin Exp Obstet Gynecol. 27(1):63-6, 2000
5. Holcberg G et al: Vasoconstrictive activity of meconium stained amniotic fluid in the human placental vasculature. Eur J Obstet Gynecol Reprod Biol. 87(2):147-50, 1999
6. Burgess AM et al: Inflammation of the lungs, umbilical cord and placenta associated with meconium passage in utero. Review of 123 autopsied cases. Pathol Res Pract. 192(11):1121-8, 1996
7. Altshuler G et al: Meconium-induced umbilical cord vascular necrosis and ulceration: a potential link between the placenta and poor pregnancy outcome. Obstet Gynecol. 79(5 (Pt 1)):760-6, 1992
8. Altshuler G et al: Meconium-induced vasocontraction: a potential cause of cerebral and other fetal hypoperfusion and of poor pregnancy outcome. J Child Neurol. 4(2):137-42, 1989
9. Miller PW et al: Dating the time interval from meconium passage to birth. Obstet Gynecol. 66(4):459-62, 1985

MECONIUM-STAINED PLACENTA

Gross Features

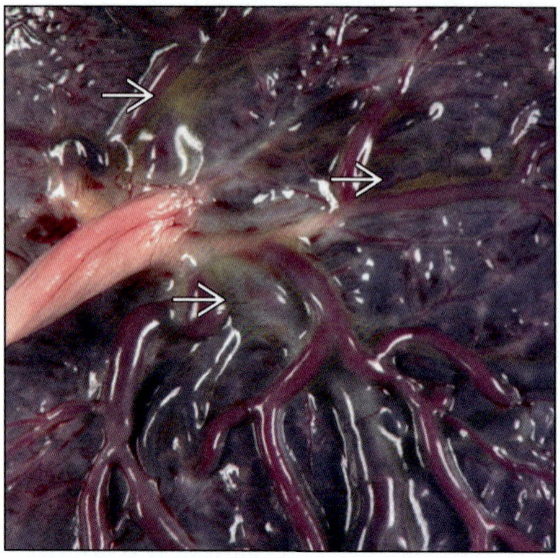

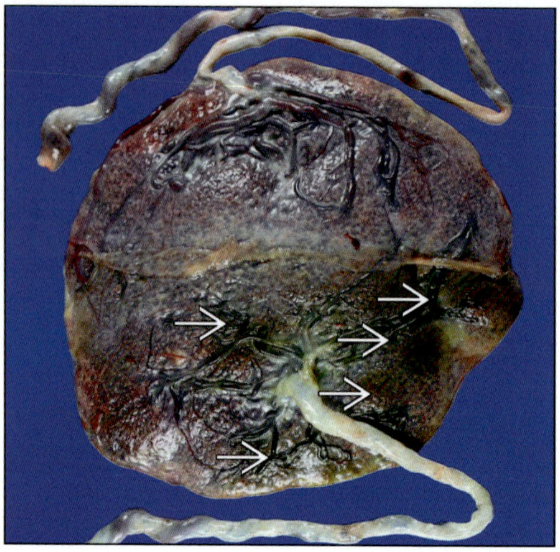

(Left) *Acute meconium deposition appears as a focal green-yellow discoloration* ➔. *Note the overall glistening appearance. The amnion remains attached to the surface.* ***(Right)*** *Comparison of the chorionic plate in a monochorionic diamniotic twin placenta shows that the recent meconium soilage* ➔ *is limited to the amniotic sac of the lower twin.*

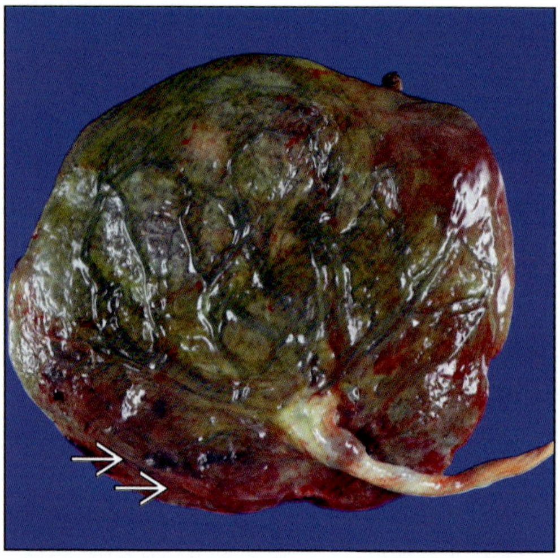

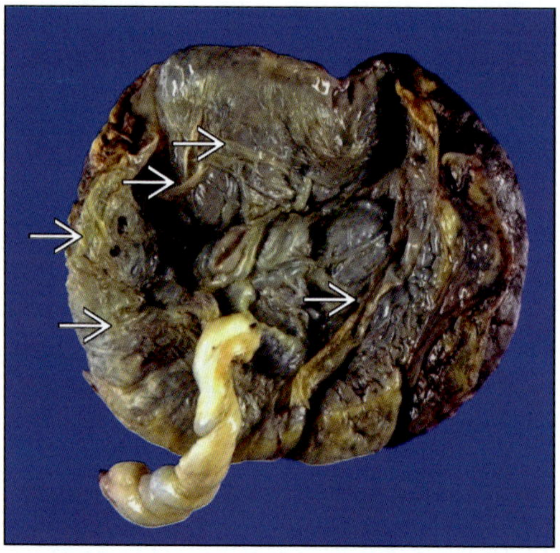

(Left) *Subacute meconium exposure is shown. The green-yellow discoloration is more diffusely distributed. Folds in the amnion* ➔ *on the surface of the chorionic plate attest to edema and slippage of the amnion.* ***(Right)*** *Subacute/chronic meconium exposure after formalin fixation is shown. The placenta and cord are diffusely yellow-brown stained. The crinkles and folds on the surface* ➔ *indicate that the edematous amnion has slipped from the dull-appearing chorionic plate surface.*

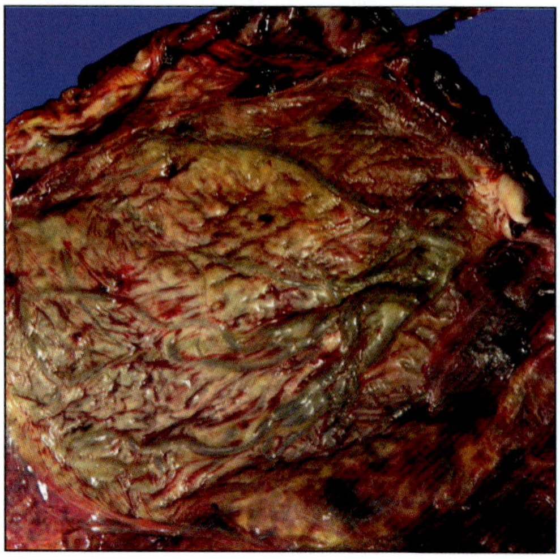

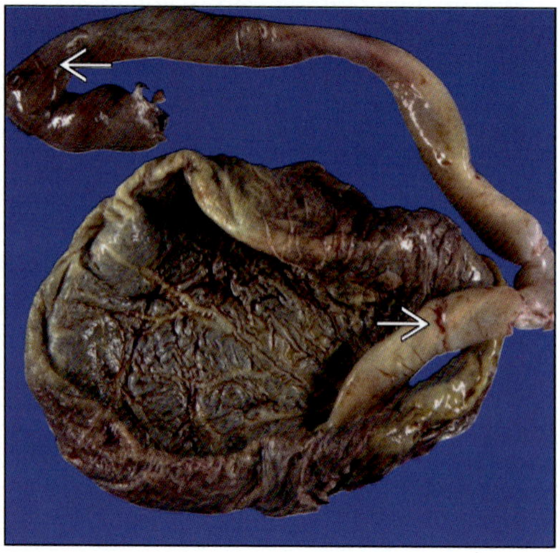

(Left) *Subacute/chronic meconium exposure with chorioamnionitis shows diffuse tan-brown staining and opacity surrounding the chorionic plate vasculature. Amniotic fluid infection sequence often complicates meconium spillage in the amniotic fluid.* ***(Right)*** *Chronic meconium exposure in a formalin-fixed placenta is shown. The cord and membranes are diffusely stained and appear dull. Careful inspection of the cord for ulcerations* ➔ *is warranted, as meconium-associated vascular necrosis occurs in this setting.*

Microscopic Features

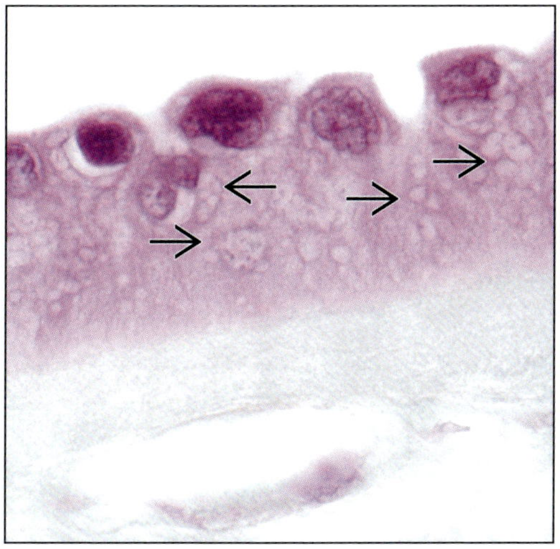

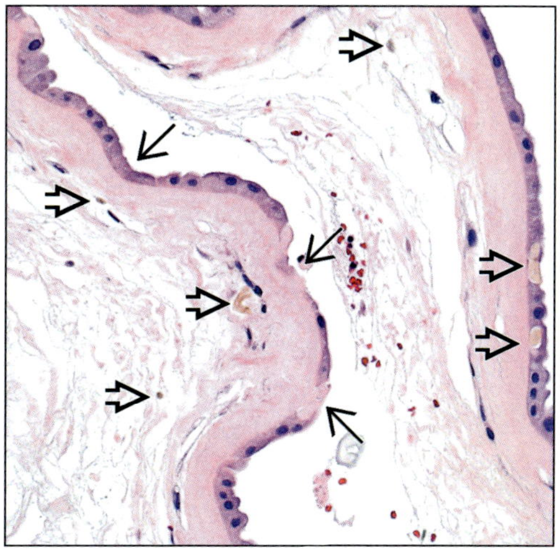

(Left) *Reactive changes in the amnion are shown. The normally cuboidal epithelium becomes columnar or pseudostratified, with coarse cytoplasmic vacuolation →. The basement membrane remains mostly invisible at this early stage.* ***(Right)*** *As exposure progresses, the amnion becomes edematous. Foci of the amnion epithelium lose nuclear basophilia →. Globular particles of meconium → may be found. The basement membrane becomes dense and eosinophilic.*

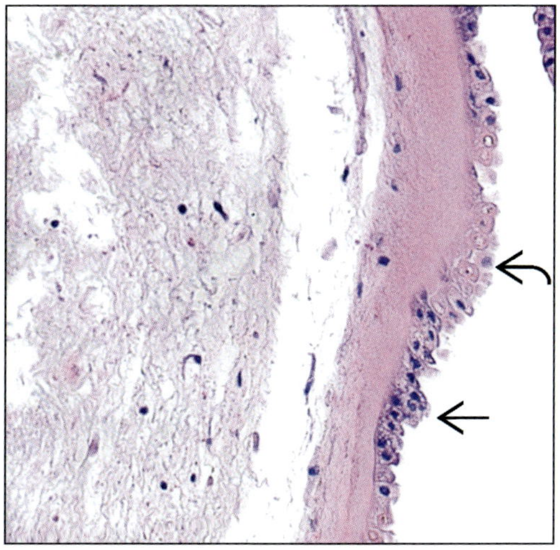

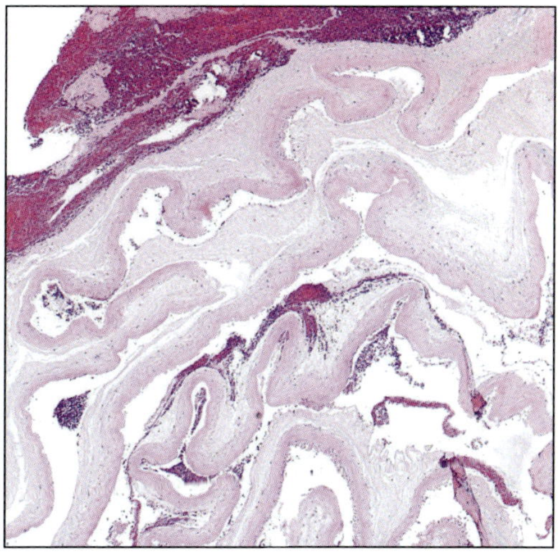

(Left) *Reactive → and necrotic → changes in the amnion epithelium are shown. The basement membrane is thick and pink. The underlying connective tissue appears "dirty."* ***(Right)*** *Diffuse amnion necrosis and edema in prolonged meconium exposure are shown. Nuclear basophilia of the amnion epithelial cells is mostly lost. The membranes are edematous with striking eosinophilia of the basement membrane.*

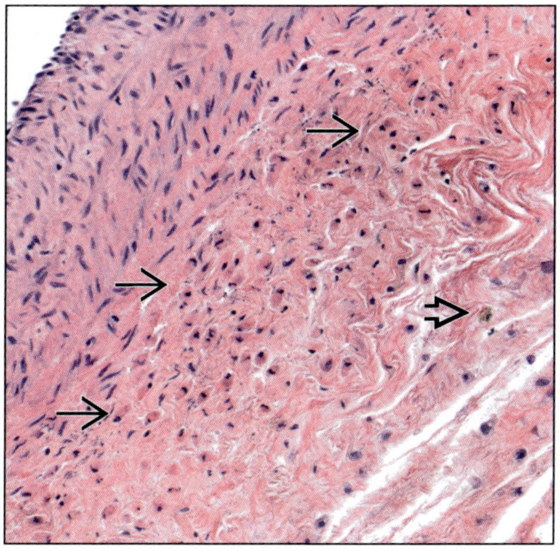

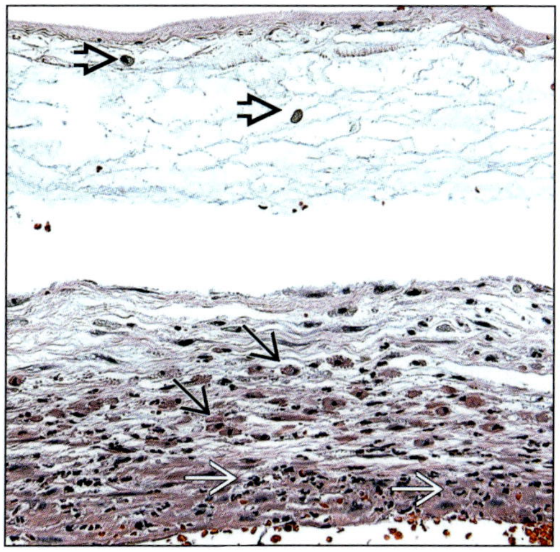

(Left) *Meconium-associated vascular necrosis (MAVN) occurs on side of vessel nearest to amnion. Vascular smooth muscle cells lose connectivity, round up, and become pyknotic →. Note pigmented macrophages →.* ***(Right)*** *MAVN in chronic meconium staining is shown. Individual vascular smooth muscle cells → become polygonal and apoptotic. Meconium particles → are seen in media and above in edematous amnion. Fetal inflammatory response is evidenced by neutrophils →.*

Amniotic Fluid Infection Sequence

AMNIOTIC FLUID INFECTION SEQUENCE (MATERNAL AND FETAL INFLAMMATORY RESPONSE)

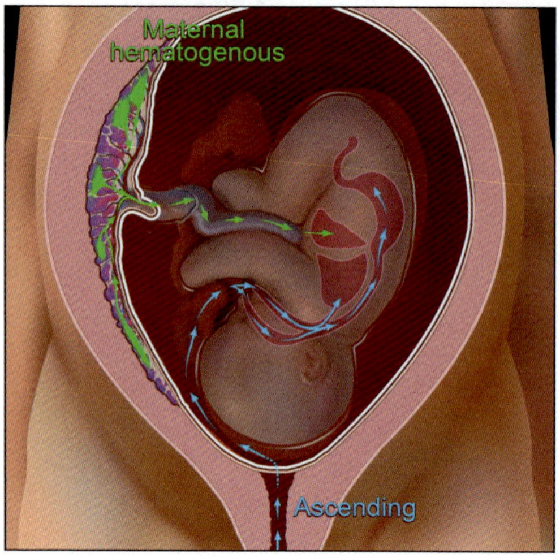

In utero infection is acquired in 2 ways: Ascending from the maternal genitourinary tract, and hematogenous from the maternal bloodstream. Amniotic fluid infection is typically an ascending infection.

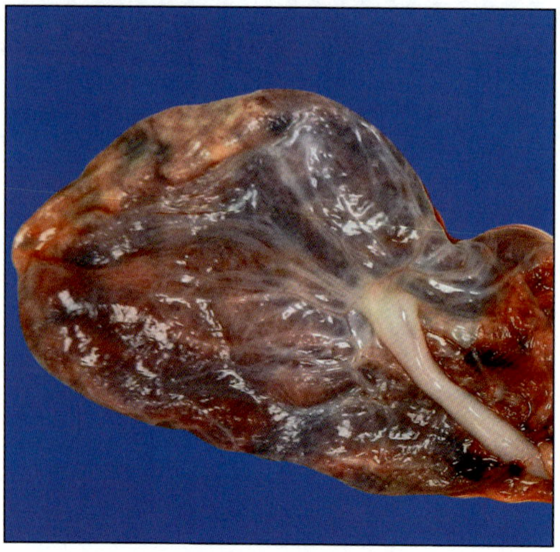

Acute chorioamnionitis is rarely a gross diagnosis. This placenta has only slightly cloudy membranes but significant histologic inflammation. A foul odor may accompany the infected membranes.

TERMINOLOGY

Abbreviations

- Amniotic fluid infection sequence (AFIS)

Definitions

- Describes progression of maternal and fetal inflammatory responses to ascending infection of amniotic cavity by cervicovaginal flora
- Maternal inflammatory response (MIR): Maternal neutrophils reacting to stimuli in amniotic fluid
  - Grade 1 (mild, moderate): Defined as not severe
  - Grade 2 (severe): At least 10x20 confluent neutrophils located between chorion and decidua in at least 3 foci or in a continuous band
  - Stage of involvement reflects progression of inflammation from maternal decidual vessels or at the subchorionic maternal intervillous space, through chorion to amnion with eventual necrosis of the tissue and fragmentation of the neutrophils
- Fetal inflammatory response (FIR): Fetal neutrophils reacting to infected amniotic fluid; response is directed from umbilical cord or chorionic plate vessels toward amnion (amniotropic)
  - Grade 1 (mild, moderate): Defined as not severe
  - Grade 2 (severe): Near confluent neutrophils with attenuation of vascular smooth muscle
  - Stage of involvement reflects progression of inflammation from fetal vessels of cord and chorionic plate vessels toward stimuli in amniotic fluid
    - Fetal inflammation is usually noted initially in veins but progresses to involve arteries
    - Fetal inflammation may include a variable number of eosinophils

ETIOLOGY/PATHOGENESIS

Infectious Agents

- Convention accepts that acute chorioamnionitis is a maternal inflammatory reaction to an infectious agent
  - Most common organisms are genital mycoplasmas, e.g., *Ureaplasma urealyticum*
  - Also associated with AFIS are *Streptococcus agalactiae*, *Escherichia coli*, *Fusobacterium* spp., *Gardnerella vaginalis*, group B *Streptococcus*, *Staphylococcus*, *Propionibacterium*, *Peptostreptococcus*, *Pseudomonas*, *Proteus*, *Klebsiella*, and *Candida* spp.
- Hematogenous infections of placenta are less commonly associated with maternal and fetal inflammatory response patterns of AFIS, and usually involve direct infection and inflammation of the villi ± fetal vasculitis

CLINICAL ISSUES

Presentation

- Clinical chorioamnionitis is defined as maternal fever of > 38 °C (100.4 °F) plus 2 or more of the following
  - Maternal (> 110) or fetal (> 160) tachycardia
  - Uterine tenderness
  - Foul vaginal discharge
  - Maternal leukocytosis (WBC > 15,000 $10^3/\mu L$ or WBC > 12,500 $10^3/\mu L$ with > 85% polys)
- 66-75% of women with significant inflammation within membranes are asymptomatic
- Chorioamnionitis is more frequent in preterm placentas
  - 40-50% < 27 weeks, 15% at 28-36 weeks, 2-10% of term placentas
  - Preterm placentas are more likely to initially have chorionic plate vasculitis as a fetal response
  - Term placentas are more likely to initially have inflammation of umbilical cord as a fetal response

AMNIOTIC FLUID INFECTION SEQUENCE (MATERNAL AND FETAL INFLAMMATORY RESPONSE)

Key Facts

Terminology
- Amniotic fluid infection sequence (AFIS)
  - Describes progression of maternal and fetal inflammatory responses to ascending infection of amniotic cavity by cervicovaginal flora
- Maternal inflammatory response is reflected in acute subchorionitis and chorioamnionitis
- Fetal inflammatory response is reflected in umbilical vasculitis and chorionic plate vasculitis

Clinical Issues
- 66-75% of women with significant inflammation within membranes are asymptomatic
- Chorioamnionitis is etiology of nearly 40% of all preterm deliveries
- Relatively small amount of inflammation in decidua or chorion may cause preterm labor

Microscopic Pathology
- Maternal inflammation progresses from decidua or subchorionic space into chorion, then into amnion
- Neutrophils in attached membranes may be of fetal origin, extending from fetal vessels
- Fetal inflammation is usually noted initially in umbilical vein, progresses to involve arteries and chorionic plate vessels
- Severe inflammation and necrosis of decidua is frequently associated with midgestation abruption

Diagnostic Checklist
- The more severe and higher the inflammation is within membranes, the more likely there will be neonatal sepsis

Treatment
- Once inflammatory cascade is activated, it cannot be stopped or reversed by antibiotics or tocolytics
- Antibiotics to reduce risk of fetal and maternal sepsis

Prognosis
- Chorioamnionitis is etiology of nearly 40% of all preterm deliveries, especially preterm premature rupture of membranes
- Chorioamnionitis may result in dysfunctional uterine contractions and ↑ incidence of cesarean section, ↑ risk for postpartum hemorrhage due to uterine atony
- FIR is associated with FIR syndrome with neonatal morbidity and risk of neurologic injury, especially preterm
  - Mechanisms of neuronal injury include cytokines, ischemia, and toxic injury by bacterial products or actual infection
- Chorioamnionitis is commonly associated with meconium passage

MACROSCOPIC FEATURES

General Features
- Maternal inflammation of membranes
  - Chorioamnionitis is rarely recognized grossly
  - Subacute chorioamnionitis has opaque yellow-white membranes
- FIR in umbilical cord or chorionic plate vessels is rarely identified grossly
  - Necrotizing funisitis has a thick layer of necrotic calcified debris in cord, resulting in "barber pole" appearance

MICROSCOPIC PATHOLOGY

Histologic Features
- Description of severity and location of inflammation with attention to both maternal and fetal responses provides more clinically useful information
  - Many grading and staging systems exist
    - Little agreement on how many neutrophils are needed to warrant chorioamnionitis diagnosis
    - Most clinical significance occurs with "severe" grades, except group B streptococcal infection
  - Organisms are rarely identified within membranes
    - Their presence indicates heavy colonization
- MIR to AFIS
  - Acute deciduitis: Neutrophils in decidua parietalis
    - Neutrophils marginate in decidual vessels, migrating into decidua
    - Inflammation appears first in decidua overlying cervical os
    - Severe inflammation and necrosis of decidua is frequently associated with midgestation abruption
  - MIR stage 1: Acute subchorionitis, acute chorionitis
    - Extraplacental membranes: Patchy to diffuse neutrophils in cellular or fibroblastic chorion
    - Chorionic plate: Neutrophils marginate in subchorionic fibrinoid and extend into chorion
  - MIR stage 2: Acute chorioamnionitis
    - Acute inflammation above cellular chorion, may or may not extend into amnion
  - MIR stage 3: Necrotizing acute chorioamnionitis
    - Amniocyte necrosis and neutrophil karyorrhexis, thickening and hypereosinophilia of amnion basement membrane
  - Subacute chorioamnionitis
    - Amniocyte necrosis with heavy mixed inflammatory infiltrate, extensive karyorrhexis, histiocytic infiltrate in underlying chorion
- FIR to AFIS
  - Inflammation is oriented toward amniotic fluid, not circumferential around vessel
  - Granulocytes initially marginated beneath endothelium, then extend into muscle and out into Wharton jelly or chorionic plate connective tissue
  - Severe fetal vasculitis may be complicated by thrombi, an ominous finding for neonatal morbidity
  - FIR stage 1
    - Umbilical phlebitis

AMNIOTIC FLUID INFECTION SEQUENCE (MATERNAL AND FETAL INFLAMMATORY RESPONSE)

Mode of Placental and Fetal/Neonatal Infection				
Infectious Agent	Maternal Hematogenous	Ascending	Intrapartum	Postnatal
Bacteria				
Group B *Streptococcus*	Rare	Very common	Very common	Rare
Escherichia coli	Rare	Frequently		
Listeria	Very common	Rare		
Treponema	Very common			
Viruses				
Cytomegalovirus	Very common	Rare	Very common	Very common
Herpes simplex virus	Rare	Rare	Very common	Frequently
HIV	Rare	Rare	Frequently	Rare
Parvovirus B19	Frequently			
Varicella-zoster virus	Rare		Frequently	Frequently
Enterovirus				Frequently
Parasites				
Toxoplasmosis	Frequently			
Trypanosoma cruzi (Chagas)	Frequently			
Malaria	Rare			
Fungi				
Candida		Frequently	Rare	Rare
Coccidioides immitis	Rare			

    - Chorionic plate vasculitis
  - FIR stage 2
    - Umbilical arteritis
  - FIR stage 3
    - Concentric umbilical perivasculitis: Neutrophils surround 1 or more umbilical vessels in Wharton jelly
    - Subacute necrotizing funisitis: Heavy inflammation with extensive karyorrhexis, ± fine calcifications

ANCILLARY TESTS

Placental Cultures
- Rarely positive and frequently contaminated with vaginal flora; organisms may be difficult to culture

Gram or Other More Specific Stains
- May be helpful in organisms visible on routine H&E

DIFFERENTIAL DIAGNOSIS

Chronic Chorioamnionitis
- Less commonly due to amniotic fluid infection
  - More commonly associated with chronic villitis of unknown etiology

T-Cell Lymphocytic and Eosinophilic Vasculitis
- Fetal chorionic plate vasculitis oriented toward intervillous space, not amnion

DIAGNOSTIC CHECKLIST

Clinically Relevant Pathologic Features
- Final diagnosis should state "amniotic fluid infection sequence" followed by bullets indicating component maternal and fetal response findings with full histologic terminology, grade, and stage

Pathologic Interpretation Pearls
- The more severe and higher the inflammation is within the membranes, the more likely there will be neonatal sepsis

SELECTED REFERENCES

1. Park CW et al: The involvement of human amnion in histologic chorioamnionitis is an indicator that a fetal and an intra-amniotic inflammatory response is more likely and severe: clinical implications. Placenta. 30(1):56-61, 2009
2. Redline RW et al: Amniotic infection syndrome: nosology and reproducibility of placental reaction patterns. Pediatr Dev Pathol. 6(5):435-48, 2003
3. Ohyama M et al: Re-evaluation of chorioamnionitis and funisitis with a special reference to subacute chorioamnionitis. Hum Pathol. 33(2):183-90, 2002
4. Kim CJ et al: Umbilical arteritis and phlebitis mark different stages of the fetal inflammatory response. Am J Obstet Gynecol. 185(2):496-500, 2001

AMNIOTIC FLUID INFECTION SEQUENCE (MATERNAL AND FETAL INFLAMMATORY RESPONSE)

Microscopic Features

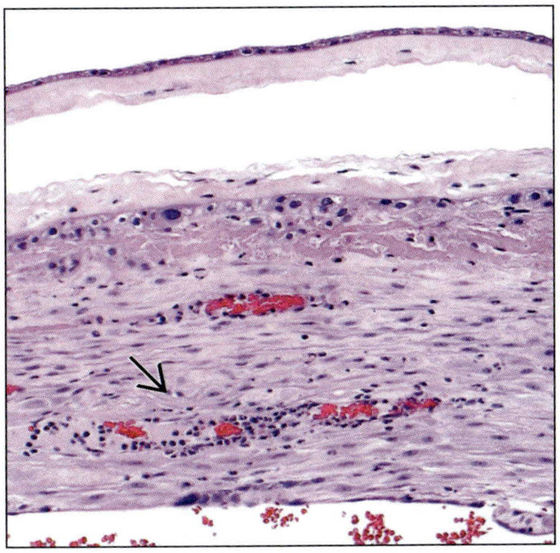

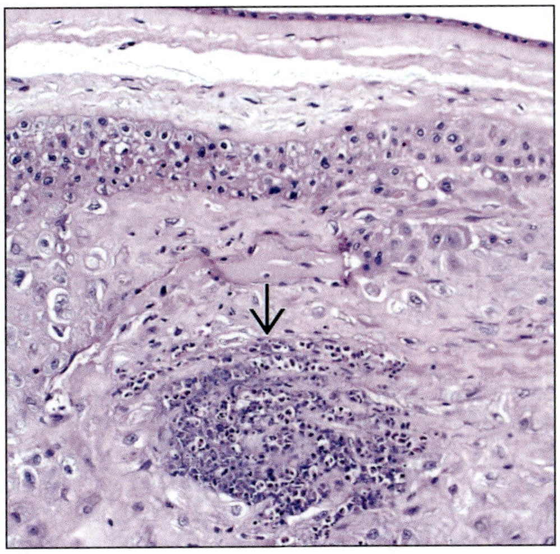

(Left) *The earliest stage of the maternal response is margination of maternal neutrophils within small vessels → in the decidua parietalis (mild, acute deciduitis).* ***(Right)*** *Small areas of acute inflammation with necrosis → are frequently found in the decidua and may not always indicate infection, but they have been described as "wear and tear" and possibly have a role in the onset of labor. In some cases, inflammation may be a reaction to bland decidual necrosis.*

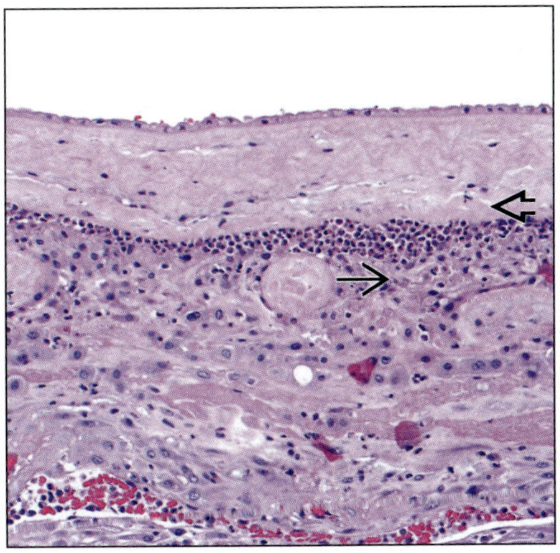

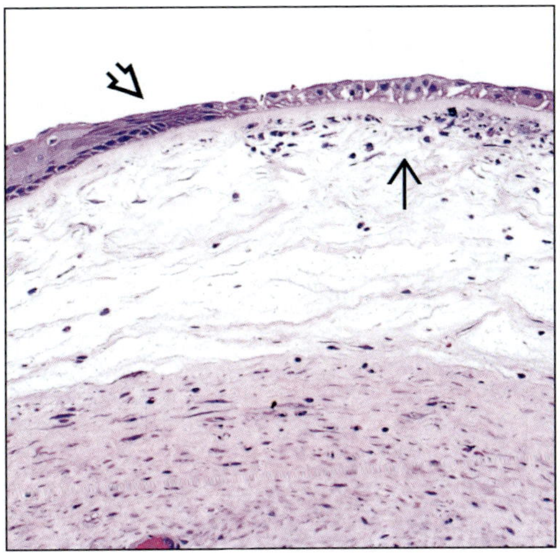

(Left) *Maternal neutrophils respond to chemotactic factors in the amniotic fluid and frequently marginate between cellular → and fibroblastic ⇨ chorion. The density of the connective tissue may impede further migration. This image shows moderate acute chorioamnionitis (maternal inflammatory response grade 1, stage 2).* ***(Right)*** *Neutrophil chemotaxis → toward substances within the amniotic fluid (amniotropic) is blocked by squamous metaplasia ⇨. The amnion is edematous.*

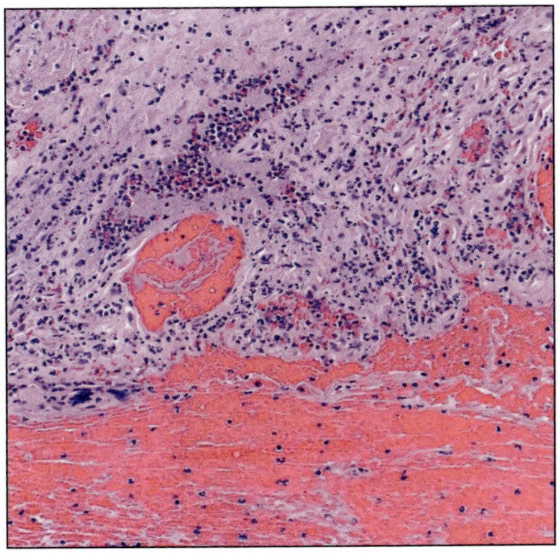

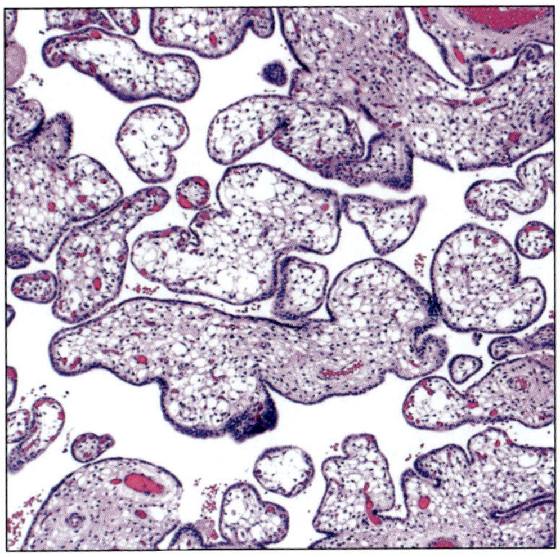

(Left) *Acute placental abruption occurring between 16 and 24 weeks gestation is commonly associated with chorioamnionitis. Decidual necrosis secondary to maternal vasculopathy associated with preeclampsia generally occurs after 24 weeks gestation.* ***(Right)*** *Villous edema may be seen in the setting of acute chorioamnionitis and abruption.*

AMNIOTIC FLUID INFECTION SEQUENCE (MATERNAL AND FETAL INFLAMMATORY RESPONSE)

Microscopic and Gross Features

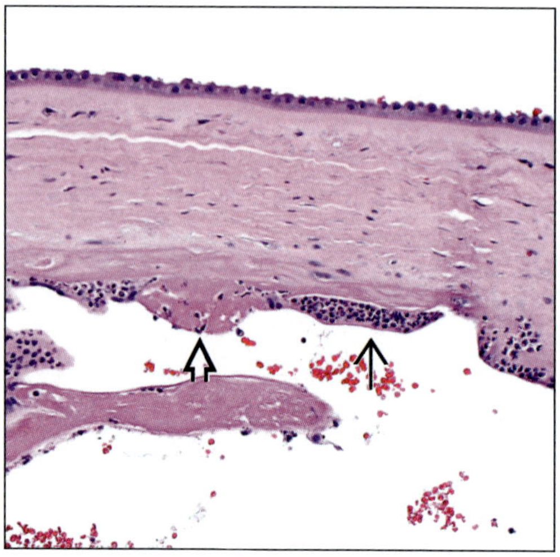

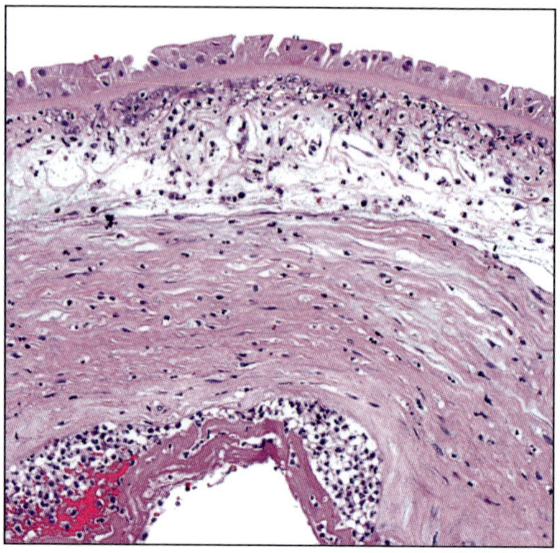

(Left) *This section of the chorionic plate shows maternal neutrophils ➔ marginated in the subchorionic fibrin ⇨ (acute subchorionitis). This is a sensitive site for detecting amniotic fluid infection sequence (AFIS).* ***(Right)*** *These membranes of the chorionic plate show full thickness inflammation, with thickening and eosinophilia of the amnion basement membrane, and karyorrhexis of neutrophils. The diagnosis is necrotizing acute chorioamnionitis (maternal inflammatory response stage 3, grade 2).*

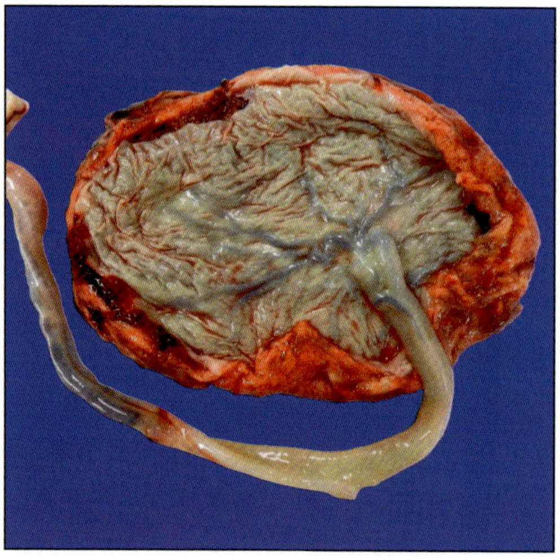

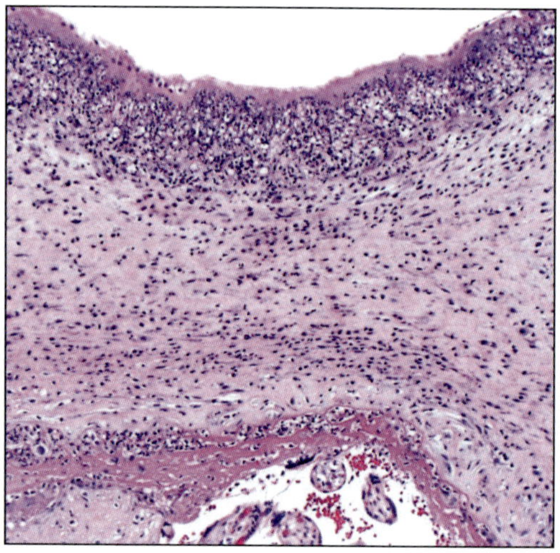

(Left) *A premature placenta with opaque membranes is characteristic of subacute necrotizing chorioamnionitis. The umbilical cord is also discolored, suggestive of funisitis.* ***(Right)*** *Subacute necrotizing chorioamnionitis is characterized by a heavy layer of necrotic neutrophils in the amnion, with necrosis of the amnion epithelium, and increased mononuclear cells in the chorion below. This type of inflammation is believed to be present for up to 2 weeks prior to delivery.*

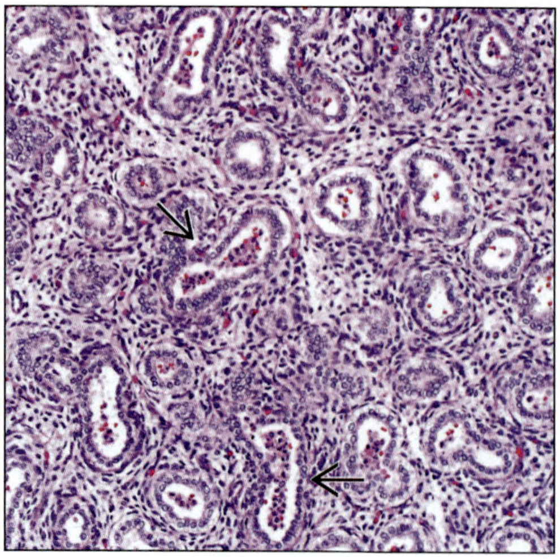

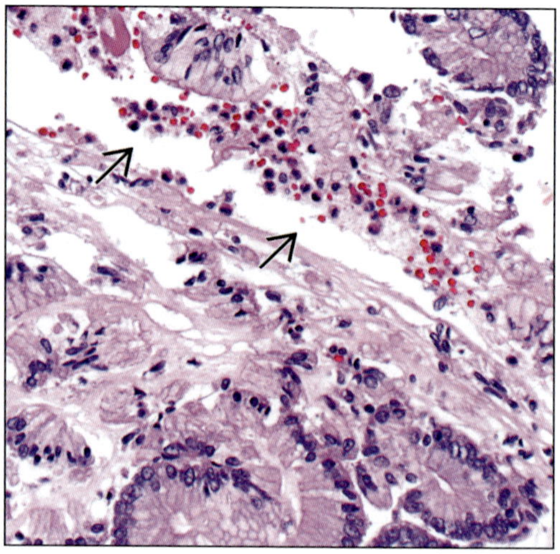

(Left) *H&E of premature lungs show neutrophils in the airways ➔. Breathing movements bring debris from the amniotic cavity into the airways. The neutrophils are mostly fetal in origin. This is termed congenital pneumonia.* ***(Right)*** *The fetal swallowing mechanism is more robust than breathing in very immature fetuses and the inflammation ➔ may be more apparent in the stomach than in the lungs. These findings support AFIS as a cause of fetal demise vs. a postmortem event.*

Microscopic and Gross Features

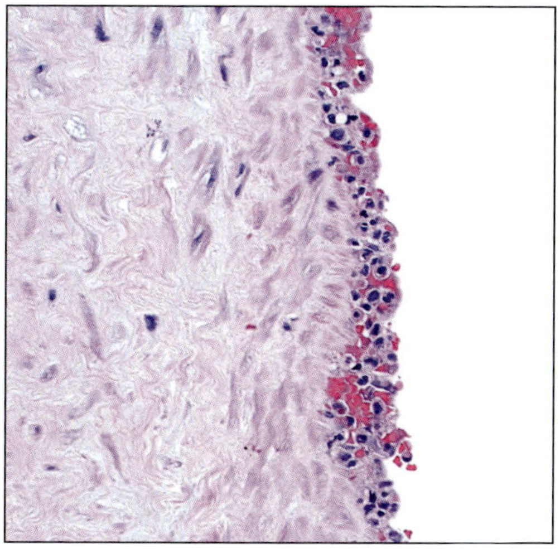

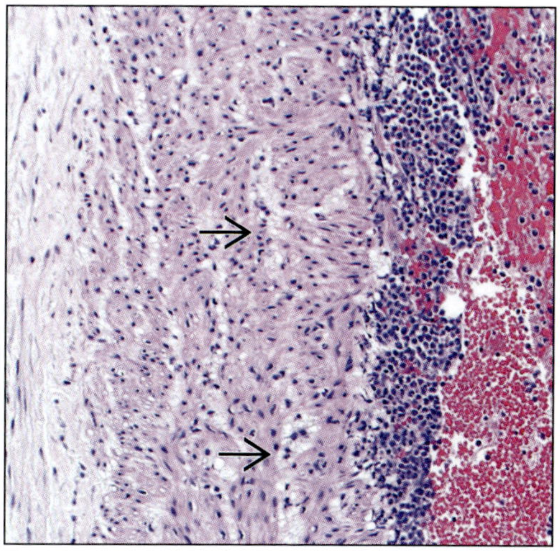

(Left) Margination of the fetal neutrophils beneath the endothelium is the earliest feature of a fetal inflammatory response. Usually, this first occurs within the umbilical vein or a chorionic plate vessel. Inflammation of the umbilical arteries is usually a later feature. *(Right)* Extremely heavy margination of neutrophils in the umbilical vein seen here is associated with extension of the neutrophils out into the muscular wall of the vessel (phlebitis).

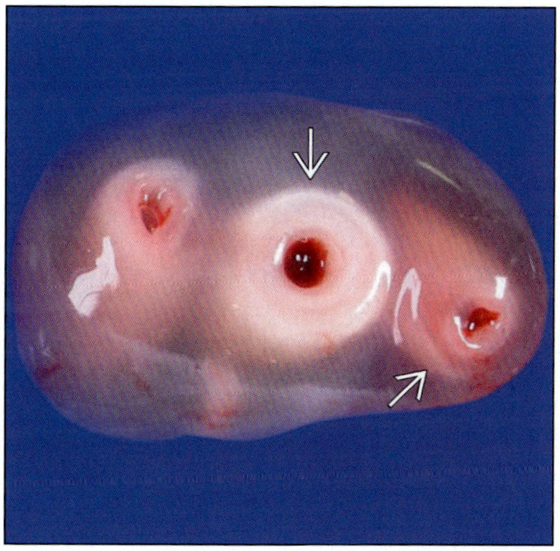

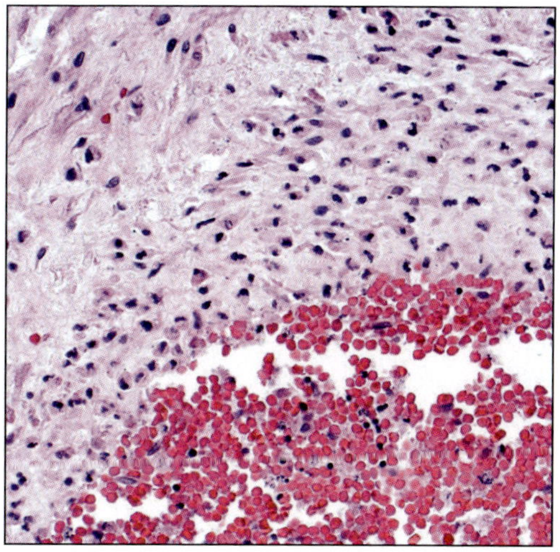

(Left) This section of umbilical cord from a premature delivery has marked edema of Wharton jelly and white exudate partially around the vessels, which represents concentric perivasculitis. *(Right)* This section of umbilical cord is from a moderately macerated fetus and shows pseudofunisitis. Degenerative changes of vascular smooth muscle nuclei resemble neutrophils. The fetal inflammatory response is usually minimal in pre-viable fetuses.

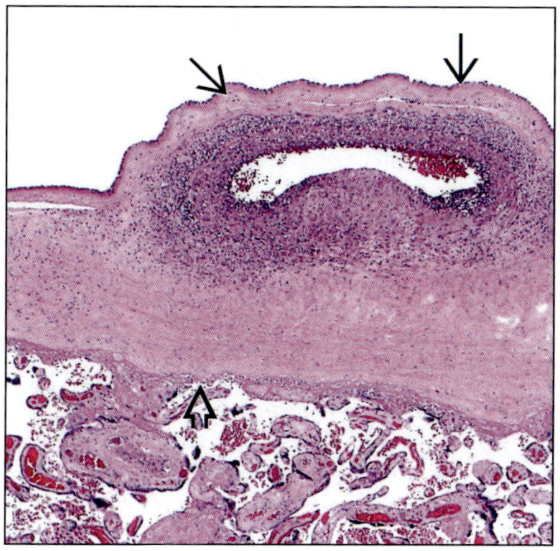

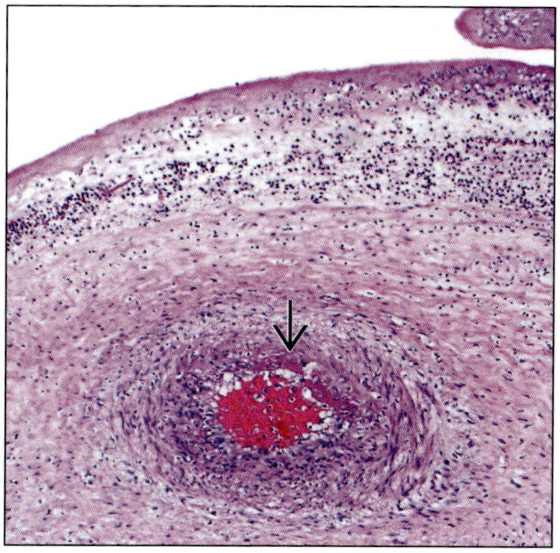

(Left) Chorionic plate vasculitis exemplifies the fetal response. Note that there is very little maternal inflammation within the membranes or marginated at the subchorionic space. Discordance between fetal and maternal inflammation may be seen in group B Streptococcus infection. *(Right)* This case of necrotizing acute chorioamnionitis with severe chorionic plate vasculitis is complicated by a nonocclusive fibrin thrombus in the fetal vessel, an ominous finding.

GROUP B *STREPTOCOCCUS*

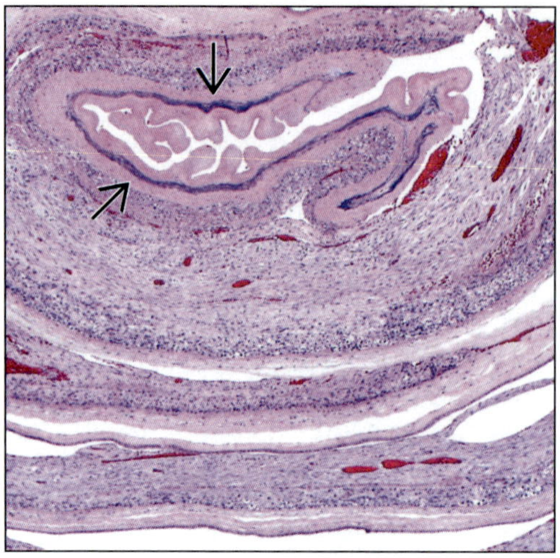

Heavy colonization ⇒ with group B streptococcal (GBS) infection is seen in membranes at zone of membrane rupture. Women without immunity commonly feature no or minimal maternal inflammatory response.

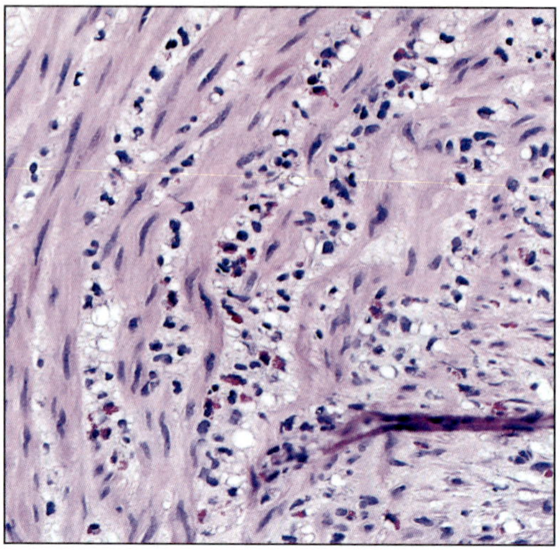

Moderate fetal inflammation of the umbilical vein is present with numerous eosinophils. Fetal eosinophils have been described in GBS but may also be a feature of extreme prematurity.

TERMINOLOGY

Abbreviations

- Group B *Streptococcus* (GBS)

ETIOLOGY/PATHOGENESIS

Infectious Agents

- *Streptococcus agalactiae* (GBS)
  - 9 serotypes, 5 of which cause majority of neonatal disease
    - Ia, Ib, II, III, and V
- Small gram-positive cocci, usually found in pairs or short chains
- In culture, it has mucoid white colonies with β-hemolysis
- Type-specific antibodies provide immunity
- Normally found in lower gastrointestinal tract
- Colonization of genitourinary tract occurs in 15-40% of women, majority of whom are asymptomatic
  - 40-50% recurrence of colonization in subsequent pregnancies
- Transmission of GBS from mother to fetus
  - Most often from ascending infection (amniotic fluid infection)
  - Less commonly from colonization at time of delivery
  - Rarely acquired postnatally
- Capsular polysaccharides shield organism from complement-mediated destruction
  - Allows GBS to multiply in bloodstream

CLINICAL ISSUES

Presentation

- Leading cause of neonatal sepsis in most years (alternates with *E. coli*)
- 50% of infants born to colonized mothers are colonized at birth and 1% develop GBS disease
- Heavy colonization, prematurity, prolonged rupture of membranes, and clinical chorioamnionitis are all associated with increased risk for neonatal disease
- Early-onset disease is invasive and occurs within < 7 days of life
  - Usually result of ascending infection (amniotic fluid infection)
  - Most present within 1st hours of life; also results in fetal demise
  - Sepsis (without source), neutropenia, respiratory distress, pneumonia, and, rarely, meningitis
  - Incidence: 0.4-1.4/1,000 live births
- Late-onset disease is diagnosed between 7 days and 3 months
  - Usually result of acquisition during birth
  - Bacteremia, meningitis, or focal infections such as osteomyelitis, septic arthritis, or cellulitis
  - Incidence: 0.3/1,000 live births

Laboratory Tests

- Centers for Disease Control and Prevention (CDC) recommends screening of all pregnant women between 35 and 37 weeks gestation
  - Rectal and vaginal swabs submitted for cultures or DNA testing
- Rapid assays (e.g., PCR) may be used for unscreened women presenting in preterm labor

Treatment

- Guidelines for screening and intrapartum treatment of GBS colonization during pregnancy have been established by consensus of American Academy of Pediatrics (AAP), American College of Obstetricians and Gynecologists (ACOG), and CDC
- Intrapartum antibiotics are effective in preventing early-onset disease but do not affect late-onset disease

GROUP B *STREPTOCOCCUS*

Key Facts

Etiology
- *Streptococcus agalactiae* (group B *Streptococcus* [GBS])
- Small gram-positive cocci, usually found in pairs or short chains
- In culture, it has mucoid white colonies with β-hemolysis
- Colonization of genitourinary tract occurs in 15-40% of women, majority of whom are asymptomatic
  - 40-50% recurrence of colonization in subsequent pregnancies

Clinical Issues
- GBS is leading cause of neonatal sepsis in most years (alternates with *E. coli*)
- 50% of infants born to colonized mothers are colonized at birth and 1% develop GBS disease
- Early-onset disease is invasive and occurs within < 7 days of life
  - Usually result of ascending infection
- Late-onset disease is diagnosed between 7 days and 3 months
  - Usually result of acquisition during birth
- Intrapartum antibiotics are effective in preventing early-onset disease but do not affect late-onset disease

Microscopic Pathology
- GBS is frequently associated with minimal or no maternal inflammatory reaction
- GBS is associated with heavy colonization and large numbers of bacteria in 40% of cases
- Fetal inflammatory response may be significantly more robust than maternal inflammatory response

Prognosis
- Early-onset disease: 4-15% mortality
- Late-onset disease: 0-6% mortality

IMAGE FINDINGS

Radiographic Findings
- Early-onset disease results in nonspecific changes on infant radiographs; very similar to hyaline membrane disease

MACROSCOPIC FEATURES

General Features
- Chorioamnionitis may be associated with thickened, cloudy, white to yellowish green membranes
  - No gross features are specific for GBS

MICROSCOPIC PATHOLOGY

Histologic Features
- Frequently associated with minimal or no maternal inflammatory response
  - 38-75% have histologic chorioamnionitis
- Associated with heavy colonization and large numbers of bacteria in 40% of cases
- Fetal inflammatory response may be significantly more robust than maternal inflammatory response
  - Funisitis is present in 27-58% of cases
  - Fetal inflammatory response may include large numbers of eosinophils
- Villous edema, a nonspecific feature of amniotic fluid infection sequence, may be present
- Acute villitis may be present, usually in cases with fetal sepsis

ANCILLARY TESTS

Immunohistochemistry
- Helpful when cultures are not available

DIFFERENTIAL DIAGNOSIS

Other Streptococcal Organisms
- Other *Streptococcus* species are usually associated with severe histologic chorioamnionitis

Staphylococcus aureus
- Methicillin-sensitive and methicillin-resistant *Staphylococcus aureus* are rare causes of chorioamnionitis

DIAGNOSTIC CHECKLIST

Pathologic Interpretation Pearls
- Heavy bacterial colonization of membranes with minimal maternal inflammation

SELECTED REFERENCES

1. Tudela CM et al: Intrapartum evidence of early-onset group B streptococcus. Obstet Gynecol. 119(3):626-9, 2012
2. Verani JR et al: Prevention of perinatal group B streptococcal disease--revised guidelines from CDC, 2010. MMWR Recomm Rep. 59(RR-10):1-36, 2010
3. De Paepe ME et al: The histologic fetoplacental inflammatory response in fatal perinatal group B-streptococcus infection. J Perinatol. 24(7):441-5, 2004
4. Novak RW et al: Significance of placental findings in early-onset group B streptococcal neonatal sepsis. Clin Pediatr (Phila). 24(5):256-8, 1985

GROUP B *STREPTOCOCCUS*

Microscopic Features

(Left) *Only a light sprinkling of bacteria → in the membranes is present in this case without a maternal inflammatory response. This is consistent with heavy GBS colonization but could be easily overlooked.* ***(Right)*** *Gram stain of the same section of membranes shows numerous gram-positive cocci →. Gram stains rarely show organisms that are not visible on routine H&E stains.*

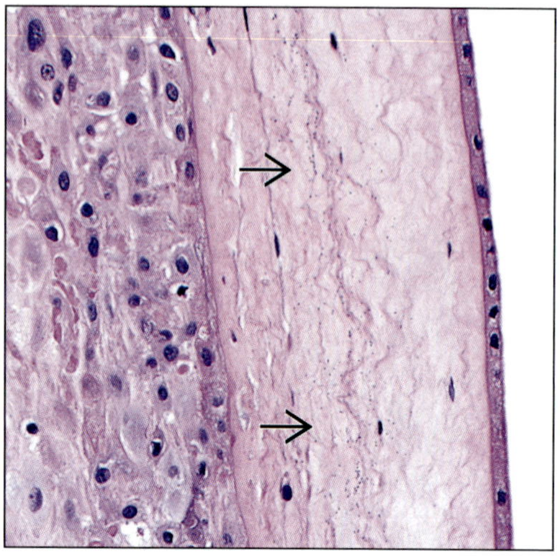

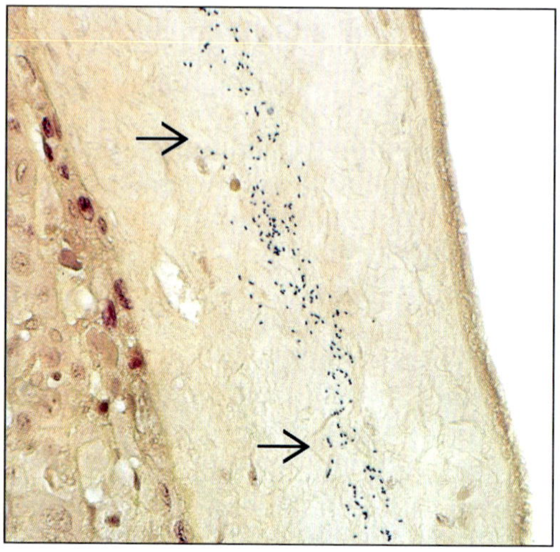

(Left) *Immunohistochemistry is very useful in confirming that these organisms are GBS. This may be useful for monitoring in subsequent pregnancies.* ***(Right)*** *In this case of chorioamnionitis, a single GBS colony → is found beneath the amnion epithelium.*

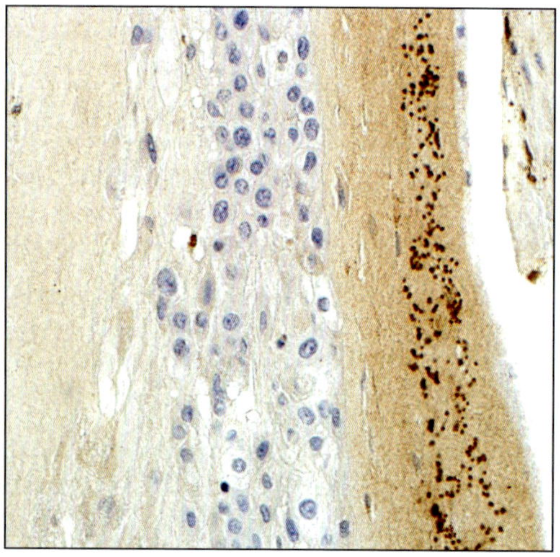

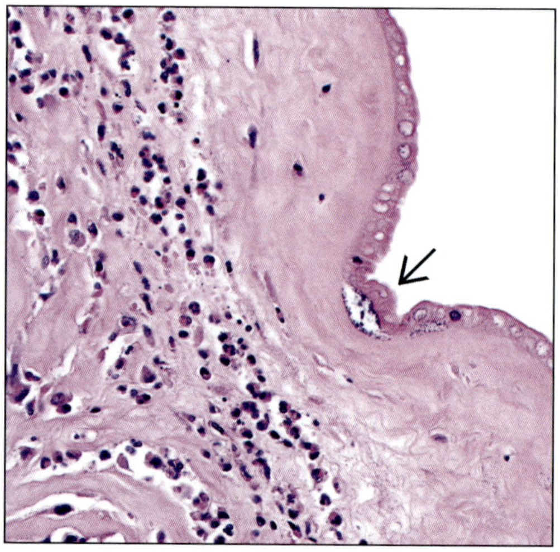

(Left) *The presence of acute villitis → heralds fetal sepsis. Large numbers of GBS bacteria ⇨ are present within fetal vessels.* ***(Right)*** *Gram stain shows numerous gram-positive bacteria ⇨ within the fetal stem vessels. This stem villus also shows acute villitis →.*

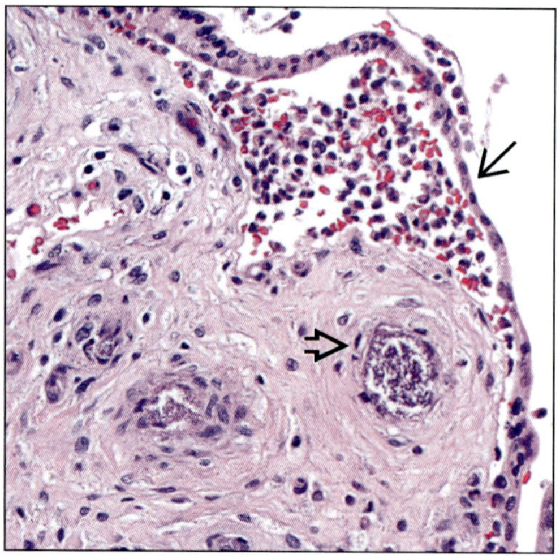

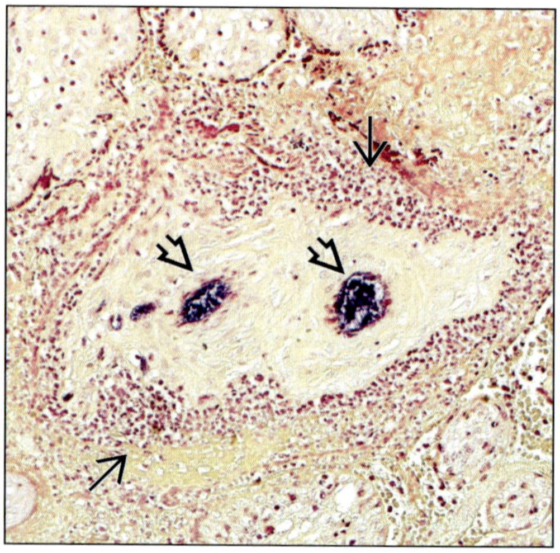

MACROSCOPIC FEATURES

General Features

- *Listeria* associated with multiple parenchymal micro- or macroabscesses
  - Amniotic fluid generally appears meconium stained (even in extremely premature deliveries unlikely to pass meconium)
- Other organisms have nonspecific features of chorioamnionitis
- Some organisms, such as *E. coli*, result in foul or feculent odor

MICROSCOPIC PATHOLOGY

Histologic Features

- Most of these bacteria have been implicated in acute chorioamnionitis but have no specific histologic features
  - Regardless of organism, extreme prematurity has high incidence of subacute necrotizing chorioamnionitis
- Maternal sepsis and shock
  - May be associated with severe chorioamnionitis
  - May have large number of neutrophils and fibrin present in maternal intervillous space
  - May have large number of bacteria in intervillous space without a maternal or fetal inflammatory response
- *Staphylococcus*
  - Fetus may show skin pustules, lung abscesses with increased incidence of pneumothorax and empyema, rarely osteomyelitis
- *Listeria monocytogenes*
  - Placenta
    - Heavy colonization, possibly due to enhanced replication or impaired clearance
    - Chorioamnionitis with large number of organisms, extracellular and intracellular in amnion epithelium; funisitis
    - Acute villitis with micro- or macroabscesses
  - Fetus
    - Early-onset disease, widespread microabscesses in skin, lungs, liver, adrenal gland, spleen, and heart (endocarditis)
    - Acute cutaneous abscesses (granulomatosis infantisepticum), with large number of neutrophils and organism
    - Late-onset disease, meningitis
- *Fusobacterium* spp.
  - Placenta
    - Associated with severe acute necrotizing or subacute necrotizing chorioamnionitis
    - Very thin, long, filamentous rods, usually vertically oriented within amnion epithelium and connective tissue; difficult to see on H&E
  - Fetus may show necrotizing pneumonia
- *Mycobacterium tuberculosis*
  - Organisms rarely found in placenta
  - May have granulomatous villitis with multinucleated giant cells
  - AFB stains should be performed on all sections

ANCILLARY TESTS

Histochemistry

- Gram stain
  - May be helpful in cases wherein bacteria are seen on routine stains

DIAGNOSTIC CHECKLIST

Clinically Relevant Pathologic Features

- Fetal bacterial infection may be responsible for 8-21% of stillbirths

Pathologic Interpretation Pearls

- Bacteria are rarely seen, and when present, usually indicates heavy infection or lack of antibiotic therapy

SELECTED REFERENCES

1. Capoccia R et al: Ureaplasma urealyticum, Mycoplasma hominis and adverse pregnancy outcomes. Curr Opin Infect Dis. 26(3):231-40, 2013
2. Centers for Disease Control and Prevention (CDC): Vital signs: Listeria illnesses, deaths, and outbreaks--United States, 2009-2011. MMWR Morb Mortal Wkly Rep. 62(22):448-52, 2013
3. Leli C et al: Microbial and vaginal determinants influencing Mycoplasma hominis and Ureaplasma urealyticum genital colonization in a population of female patients. Infez Med. 21(3):201-6, 2013
4. Monari F et al: Fetal bacterial infections in antepartum stillbirth: a case series. Early Hum Dev. 89(12):1049-54, 2013
5. Rowe JH et al: Listeria monocytogenes cytoplasmic entry induces fetal wastage by disrupting maternal Foxp3+ regulatory T cell-sustained fetal tolerance. PLoS Pathog. 8(8):e1002873, 2012
6. Teixeira AB et al: Neonatal listeriosis: the importance of placenta histological examination-a case report. AJP Rep. 1(1):3-6, 2011
7. Han YW et al: Term stillbirth caused by oral Fusobacterium nucleatum. Obstet Gynecol. 115(2 Pt 2):442-5, 2010
8. Bakardjiev AI et al: Listeria monocytogenes traffics from maternal organs to the placenta and back. PLoS Pathog. 2006 Jun;2(6):e66. Erratum in: PLoS Pathog. 2(7):e80, 2006
9. Hutto C et al: Congenital and Perinatal Infections: A Concise Guide to Diagnosis. From Totowa: Humana Press, 2006
10. Jones B et al: Escherichia coli: a growing problem in early onset neonatal sepsis. Aust N Z J Obstet Gynaecol. 44(6):558-61, 2004
11. Negishi H et al: Staphylococcus aureus causing chorioamnionitis and fetal death with intact membranes at term. A case report. J Reprod Med. 43(4):397-400, 1998
12. Topalovski M et al: Listeriosis of the placenta: clinicopathologic study of seven cases. Am J Obstet Gynecol. 169(3):616-20, 1993
13. Altshuler G et al: Fusobacteria. An important cause of chorioamnionitis. Arch Pathol Lab Med. 109(8):739-43, 1985

OTHER BACTERIAL AND MYCOBACTERIAL SPECIES

Escherichia coli

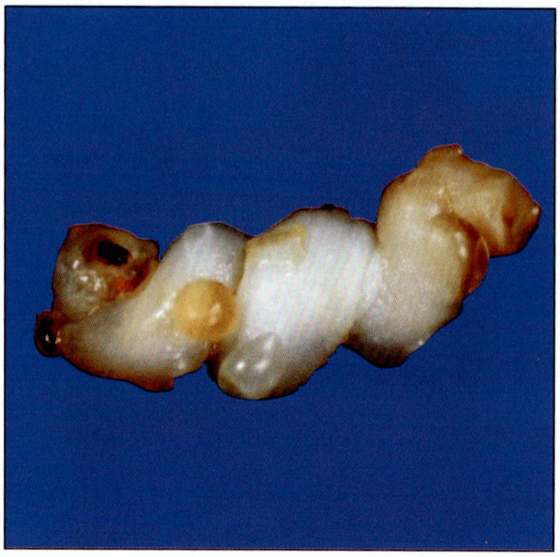

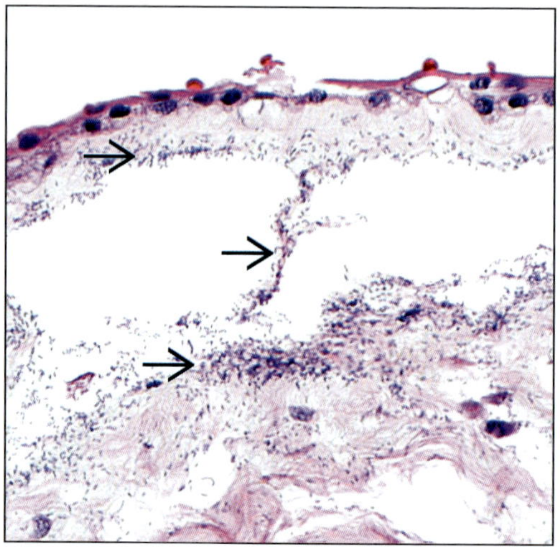

(Left) *Umbilical cord from a midgestation loss shows clear fluid-filled vesicles due to E. coli infection.* ***(Right)*** *H&E section from an umbilical cord vesicle shows numerous rod-shaped bacteria →, consistent with E.coli. Note that there is no inflammatory response, a feature not uncommon in extreme prematurity.*

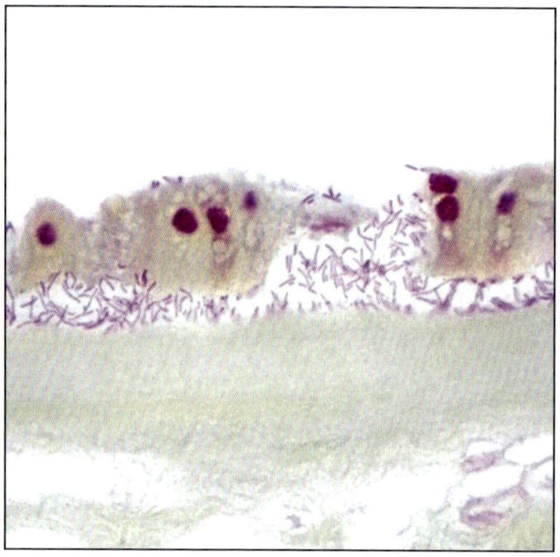

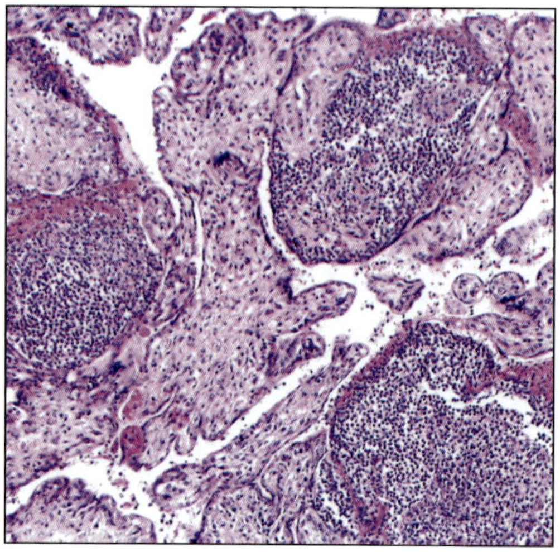

(Left) *Amnion epithelium hosts a large number of gram-negative rods, consistent with E. coli.* ***(Right)*** *Acute villitis may occur with E. coli, often in maternal sepsis with pyelonephritis. The placenta is directly infected through the maternal bloodstream.*

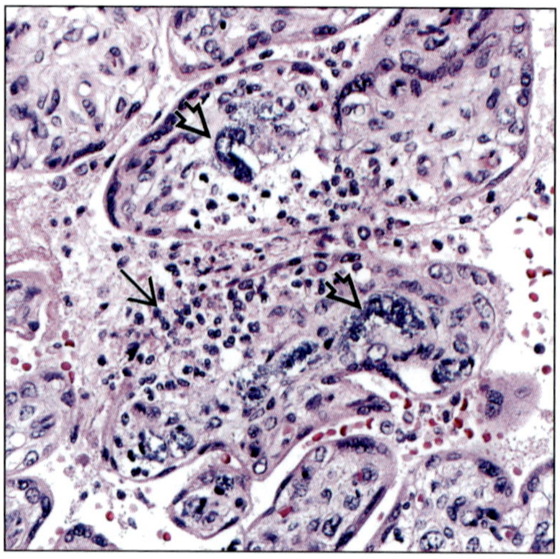

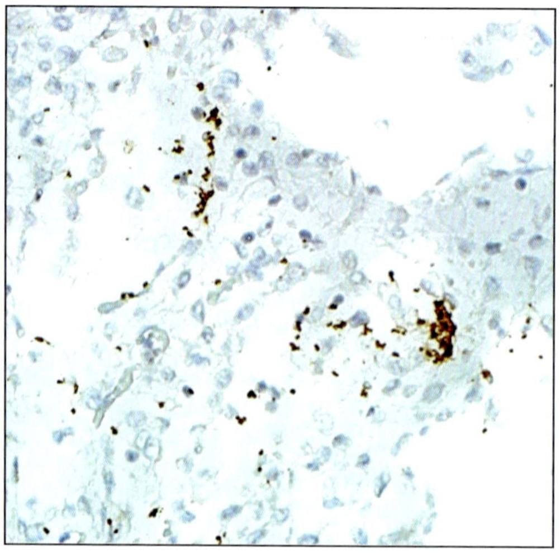

(Left) *Fetal sepsis is associated with acute villitis →. In this case, a large number of organisms are present in the fetal capillaries ⇨. This type of fetal sepsis usually occurs in extreme prematurity.* ***(Right)*** *H&E section of the lung from a case of E. coli chorioamnionitis shows that a large number of rod-shaped organisms are positive with the immunohistochemistry stain specific for E. coli. This may be useful in cases wherein autopsy cultures were not obtained.*

Listeria monocytogenes

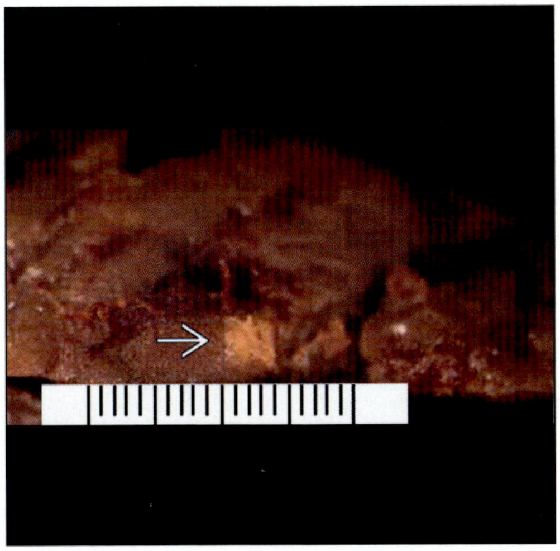

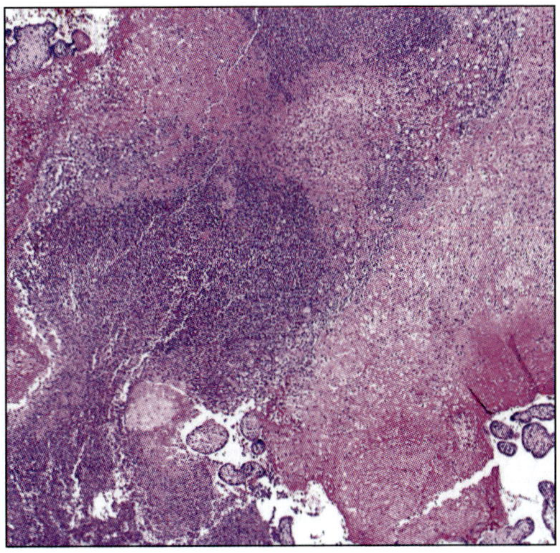

(Left) *Gross photograph of the maternal surface of the placenta shows a light-yellow microabscess* ➔ *due to Listeria.* ***(Right)*** *H&E shows the microscopic appearance of a placental Listeria abscess.*

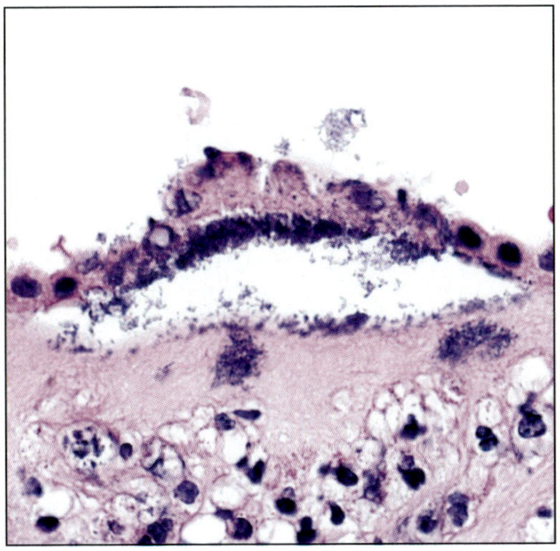

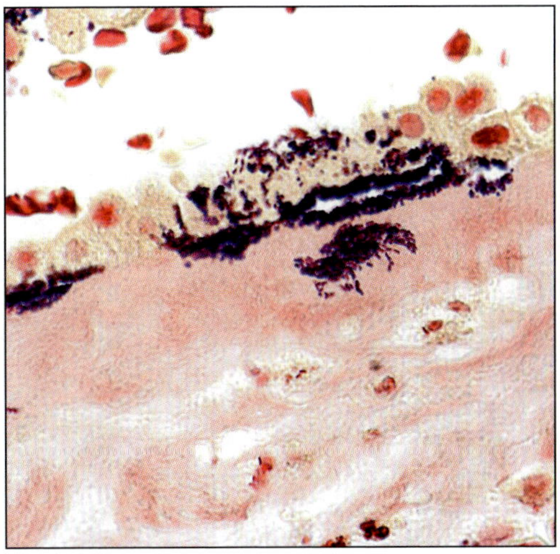

(Left) *This case of Listeria shows a large number of bacteria within the amnion. Heavy colonization is commonly seen with Listeria but can be seen with other microorganisms as well.* ***(Right)*** *Gram stain of the Listeria organisms shows gram-positive coccobacilli. Listeria may be mistakenly called gram-positive cocci or overgrowth of diphtheroids.*

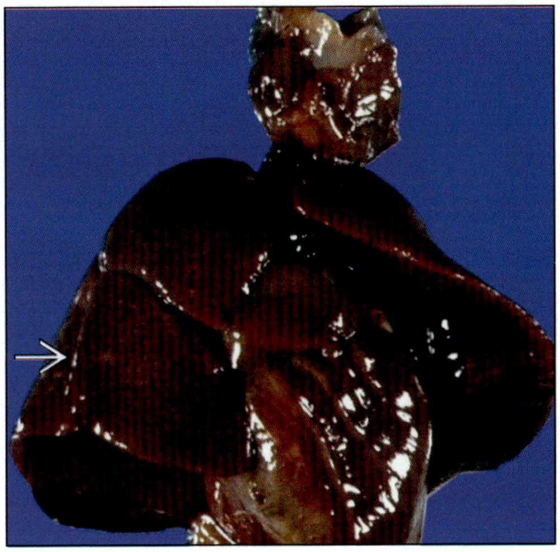

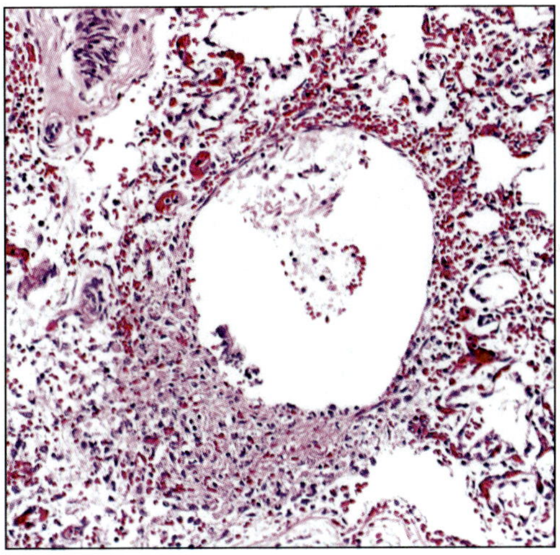

(Left) *Fetal lung at autopsy shows subtle microabscesses* ➔ *of Listeria in lung parenchyma.* ***(Right)*** *Microscopic exam shows congenital necrotizing pneumonia secondary to Listeria. Similar lesions are found in the liver and skin.*

OTHER BACTERIAL AND MYCOBACTERIAL SPECIES

Fusobacterium spp.

*(**Left**) Fusobacterium is a very long, thin filamentous bacterium → usually found vertically oriented in the amnion. It is associated with severe chorioamnionitis. (**Right**) Fusobacterium is gram negative but generally poorly staining. The bacteria are visible in this section because of the large number of bacteria that are localized in the amnion epithelium →.*

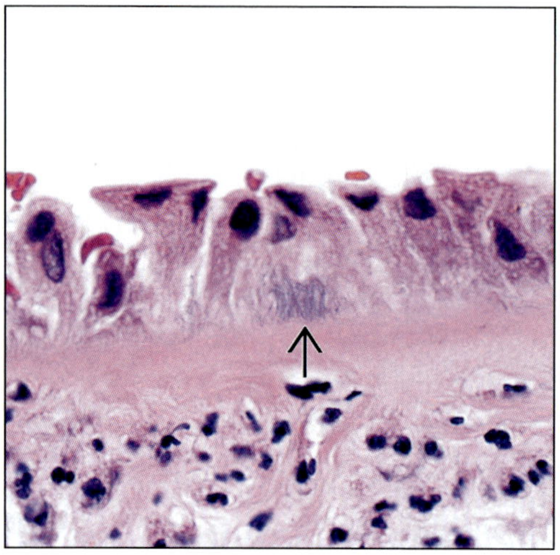

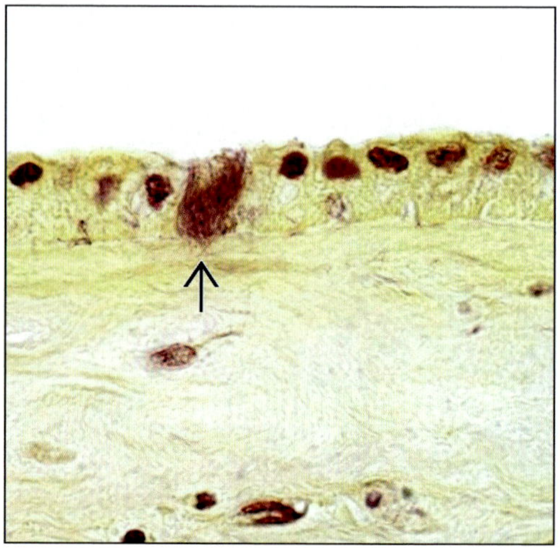

*(**Left**) Subacute necrotizing chorioamnionitis is associated with extreme prematurity. Fusobacterium species are a frequent causative organism. In this image, they impart a hairy appearance to the amnion →. (**Right**) Warthin-Starry stain is very useful in highlighting the organisms within the amnion and subamniotic connective tissue.*

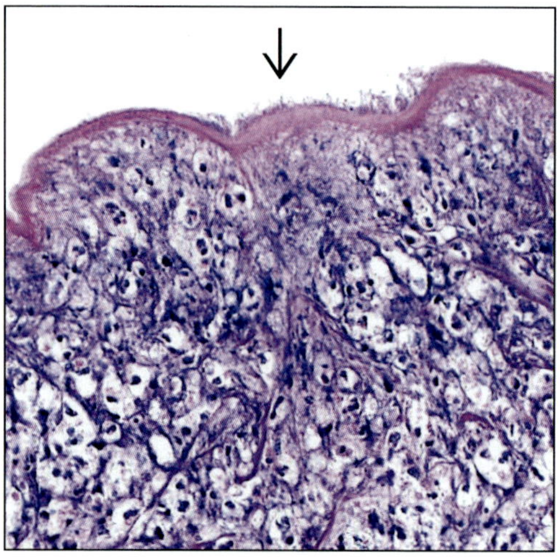

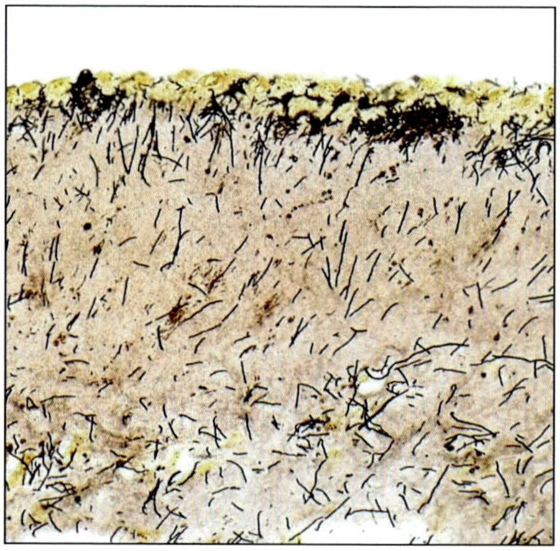

*(**Left**) This section shows monochorionic, diamniotic dividing membranes with Fusobacterium infection in twin A →, but not in twin B ⇨. Because twin A is usually located closer to the cervix, its amniotic sac is more susceptible to ascending infection than that of twin B. (**Right**) Gram stain shows mixed infection with gram-negative filamentous Fusobacterium spp. → and gram-positive cocci ⇨. Fusobacterium is a frequent component of polymicrobial infections.*

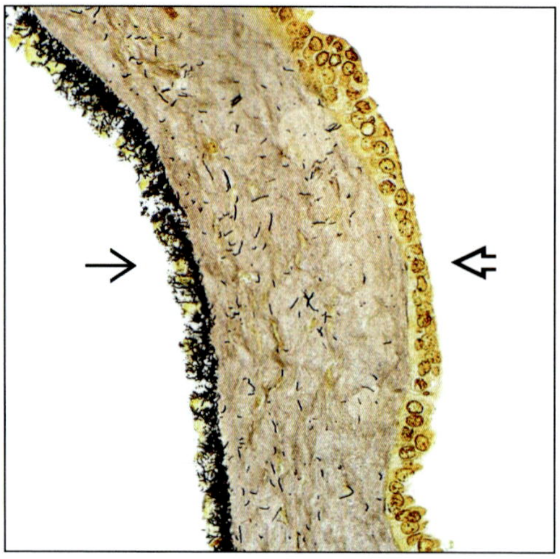

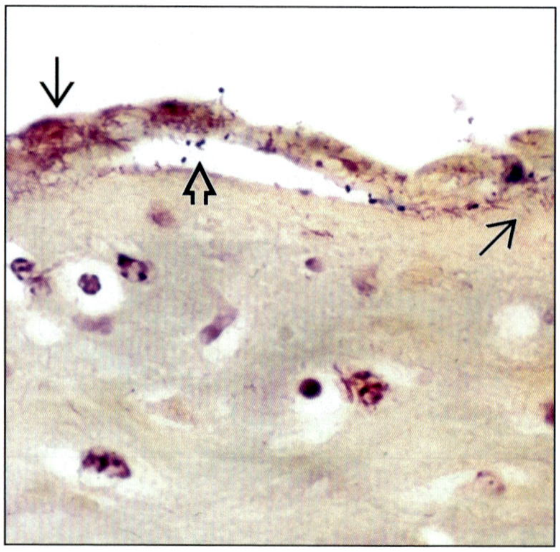

Chorioamnionitis in Candida Infection

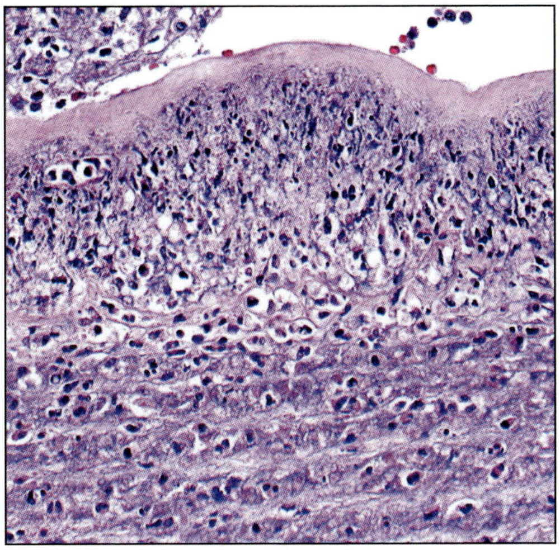

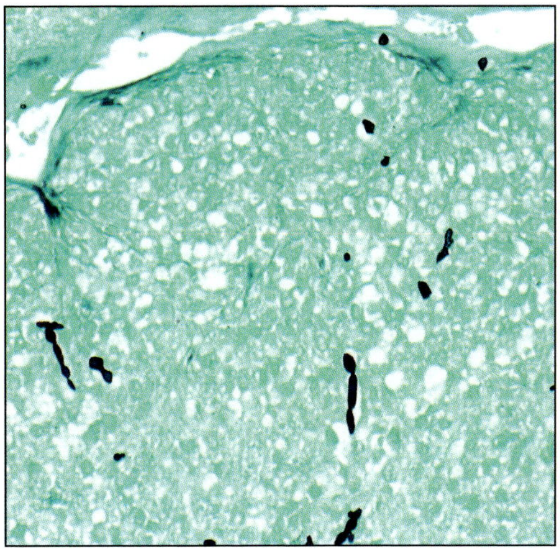

(Left) *Candida albicans may rarely be associated with chorioamnionitis, which can be severe.* ***(Right)*** *Candida albicans-associated chorioamnionitis rarely has significant numbers of yeast and pseudohyphae in the membranes, even in the presence of severe chorioamnionitis.*

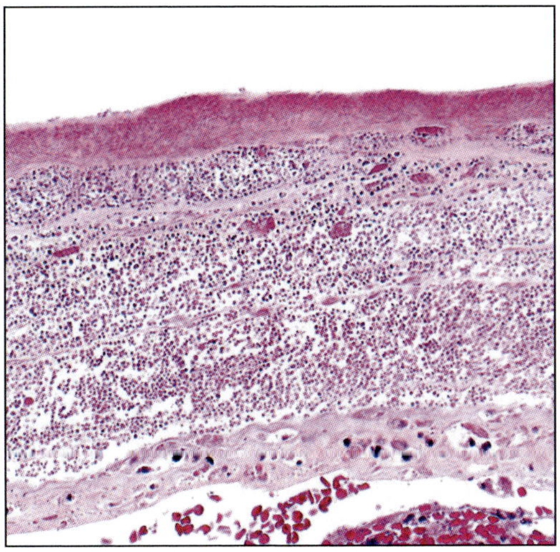

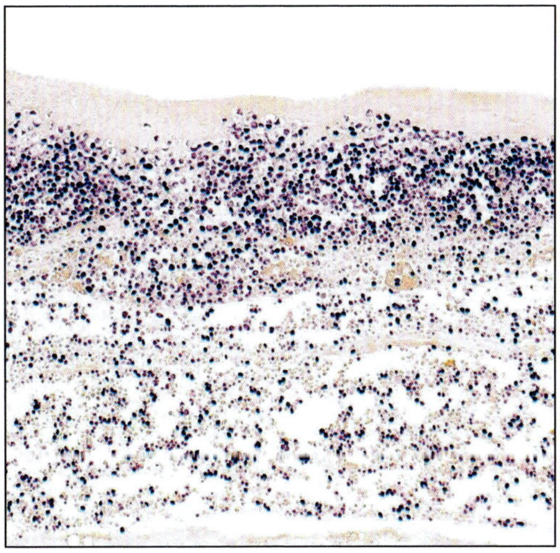

(Left) *Candida glabrata does not form pseudohyphae and is often found in large numbers in the membranes, but it is rarely associated with funisitis.* ***(Right)*** *Candida glabrata is gram positive, as are all fungi. The absence of pseudohyphae may be misdiagnosed as a coccoid bacterium.*

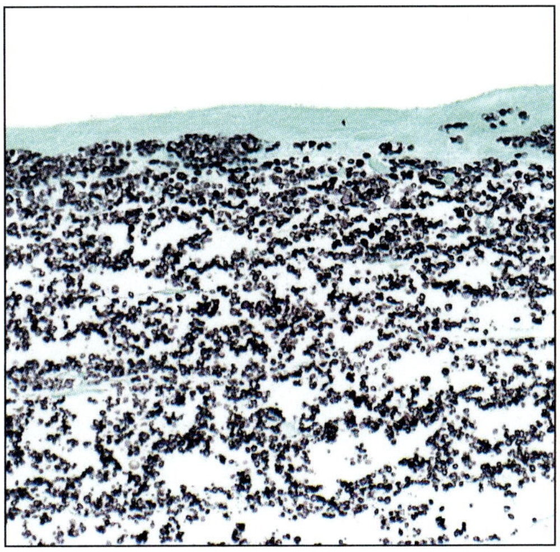

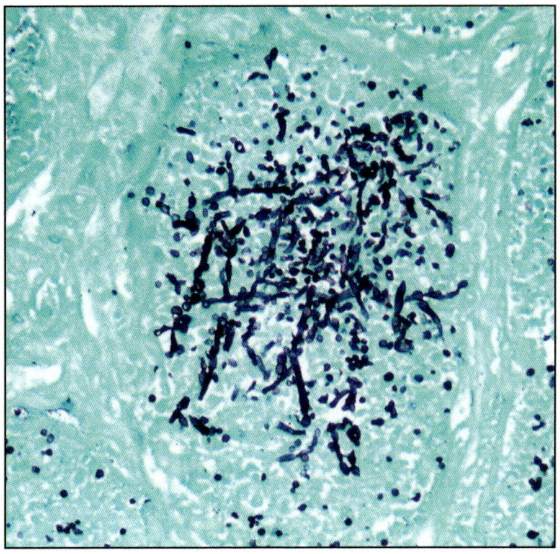

(Left) *Candida glabrata is positive with GMS stain, as are all fungi. Bacteria may also be weakly positive with GMS, but the yeast are significantly larger.* ***(Right)*** *This is a section of kidney from a case of disseminated candidiasis. With dissemination, the organisms may form colonies that can be misdiagnosed as true fungus. Rare true hyphae may be seen, but pseudohyphae and yeast will always be present as well.*

Placental Infections With Villitis and Other Findings

CYTOMEGALOVIRUS

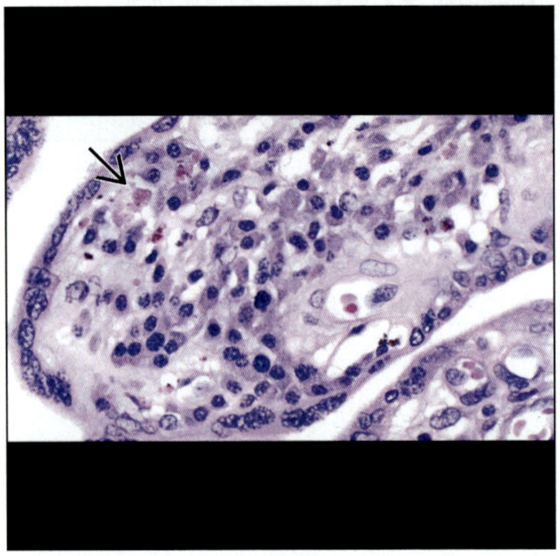

Classic cytomegalovirus (CMV) histopathology includes lymphoplasmacytic villitis with hemosiderin →.

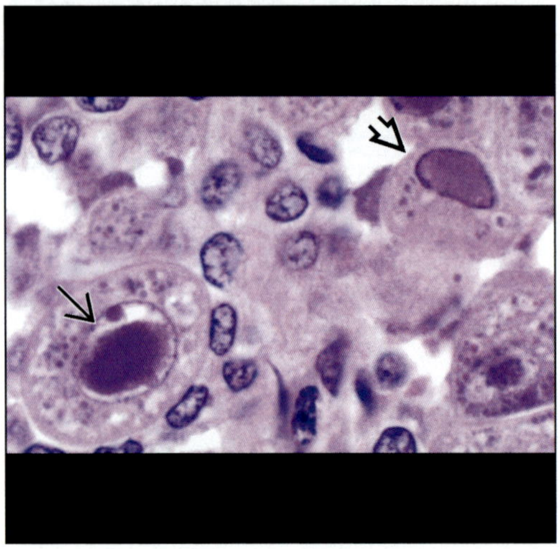

This shows both Cowdry type A → and Cowdry type B ⇒ intranuclear inclusions, in addition to the basophilic cytoplasmic inclusions in the renal tubules in a case of congenital CMV infection.

TERMINOLOGY

Abbreviations

- Cytomegalovirus (CMV)

ETIOLOGY/PATHOGENESIS

Infectious Agents

- CMV is most common congenital viral infection, occurring in 1-2% of newborns
- Congenital CMV may be transmitted from mother to child in 3 ways
  - In utero vertical transmission across placenta (hematogenous spread)
    - 30-50% of pregnant women during primary CMV infection
    - 1-3% of women with reactivation of CMV
  - Intrapartum transmission by cervical secretions
    - Women with primary or reactivated CMV infection may shed virus from cervix
    - 50% of women shedding virus from cervix will infect baby during vaginal delivery
  - Postpartum transmission through breast milk
    - 30-70% of women with primary or reactivated CMV infection shed virus in breast milk
- CMV antibody-negative women have 1-2% risk of primary CMV infection during pregnancy

CLINICAL ISSUES

Presentation

- CMV is a leading cause of brain injury and sensorineural hearing loss in children
- 85-90% of infected infants are asymptomatic
  - 10-17% of asymptomatic infants have unilateral or bilateral deafness
- Symptoms
  - Central nervous system manifestations include
    - Meningoencephalitis
    - Chorioretinitis
    - Hydrocephalus
    - Microcephaly
    - Periventricular calcifications
  - Systemic symptoms include
    - Hepatosplenomegaly
    - Anemia
    - Neutropenia
    - Thrombocytopenia
    - Petechiae
    - Purpura

Treatment

- Drugs
  - Intravenous ganciclovir for symptomatic infants
  - Oral valganciclovir is currently under investigation

Prognosis

- Mortality for symptomatic congenital CMV is ~ 30%
- Infection acquired earlier in gestation, especially < 20 weeks, has worse outcome
  - Associated with premature birth, hydrops, intrauterine growth restriction (IUGR), and intrauterine fetal demise (IUFD)

MACROSCOPIC FEATURES

General Features

- Placenta may be hydropic
- Fetus may have
  - Symmetric growth restriction (if acquired early in gestation)
  - Hydrops
  - Hepatosplenomegaly
  - Microcephaly

CYTOMEGALOVIRUS

Key Facts

Etiology

- CMV is most common congenital viral infection, occurring in 1-2% of newborns
- Congenital CMV may be transmitted vertically in utero, at time of delivery by cervical secretions, or through breast milk

Clinical Issues

- CMV is a leading cause of brain injury and sensorineural hearing loss in children
- 85-90% of infected infants are asymptomatic
- Central nervous system involvement includes meningoencephalitis, chorioretinitis, microcephaly, hydrocephalus, and periventricular calcifications
- Infected infants may have pancytopenia with hepatosplenomegaly, petechiae, and purpura
- Prematurity, hydrops, intrauterine growth restriction (IUGR), and intrauterine fetal demise (IUFD) with early in utero infection

Microscopic Pathology

- Lymphoplasmacytic villitis
- Avascular villi with hemosiderin-laden macrophages
- Rare viral inclusions in Hofbauer cells and endothelium
- Eosinophilic necrotic debris in villi with suspicious viral inclusions

Ancillary Tests

- Immunohistochemistry for CMV is very useful in confirming diagnosis

MICROSCOPIC PATHOLOGY

Histologic Features

- Lymphoplasmacytic villitis
- Avascular villi with hemosiderin-laden macrophages
- Viral inclusions in Hofbauer cells and endothelium
  - May be rare
- Eosinophilic necrotic debris in villi with suspicious viral inclusions
  - Eosinophilic debris is usually immunoreactive for CMV

ANCILLARY TESTS

Immunohistochemistry

- Anti-CMV antibodies against immediate-early, early, or late viral antigens available
- Can be useful in confirming diagnosis
  - Sensitivity is not 100%
  - If lymphoplasmacytic villitis is present, urine culture or other studies of neonate for CMV may be warranted

PCR

- PCR for CMV on formalin-fixed paraffin-embedded tissue may be more sensitive than immunohistochemistry

DIFFERENTIAL DIAGNOSIS

Other Viral Infections

- Other viruses of herpes family will have similar intranuclear inclusions, but only CMV has intracytoplasmic inclusions

Fetal Thrombotic Vasculopathy

- May occur in conjunction with CMV infection, especially when villitis affects proximal stem villi

Neonatal Alloimmune Thrombocytopenia

- May have lymphoplasmacytic villitis
- Congenital CMV should be clinically excluded with cultures

DIAGNOSTIC CHECKLIST

Pathologic Interpretation Pearls

- CMV should always be considered when there is lymphoplasmacytic villitis

SELECTED REFERENCES

1. Folkins AK et al: Diagnosis of congenital CMV using PCR performed on formalin-fixed, paraffin-embedded placental tissue. Am J Surg Pathol. 37(9):1413-20, 2013
2. Iwasenko JM et al: Human cytomegalovirus infection is detected frequently in stillbirths and is associated with fetal thrombotic vasculopathy. J Infect Dis. 203(11):1526-33, 2011
3. Demmler-Harrison GJ: Cytomegalovirus. In Feigin RD et al: Feigin & Cherry's Textbook of Pediatric Infectious Diseases. 6th ed. Philadelphia: Saunders. 2,022-43, 2009
4. Chou D et al: Cytomegalovirus infection of trophoblast cells elicits an inflammatory response: a possible mechanism of placental dysfunction. Am J Obstet Gynecol. 194(2):535-41, 2006
5. McDonagh S et al: Patterns of human cytomegalovirus infection in term placentas: a preliminary analysis. J Clin Virol. 35(2):210-5, 2006
6. Althaus J et al: Chronic villitis in untreated neonatal alloimmune thrombocytopenia: an etiology for severe early intrauterine growth restriction and the effect of intravenous immunoglobulin therapy. Am J Obstet Gynecol. 193(3 Pt 2):1100-4, 2005
7. Ozono K et al: Diagnosis of congenital cytomegalovirus infection by examination of placenta: application of polymerase chain reaction and in situ hybridization. Pediatr Pathol Lab Med. 17(2):249-58, 1997

Microscopic Features

__(Left)__ Lymphoplasmacytic villitis may be focal, as seen in this case of an asymptomatic baby with a positive urine culture for CMV. __(Right)__ More florid lymphoplasmacytic villitis may be seen with abundant hemosiderin.

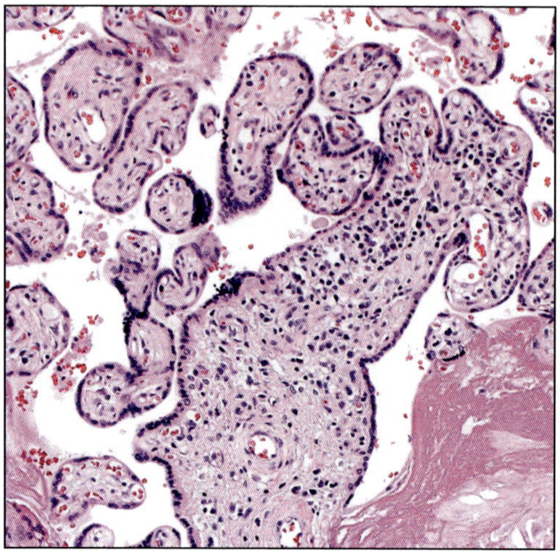

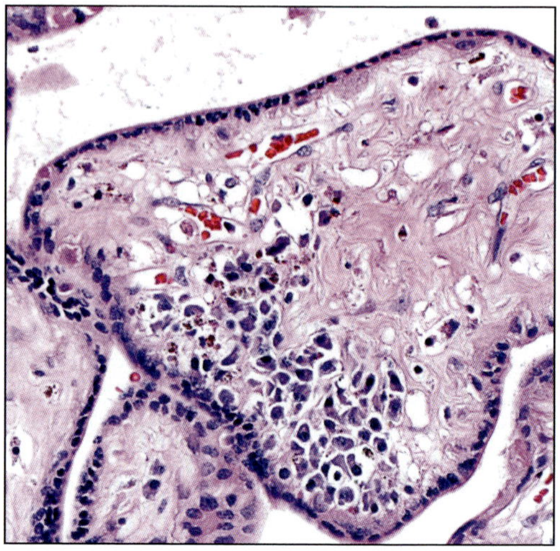

__(Left)__ Iron stain is positive within Hofbauer cells in avascular villi without residual inflammation. __(Right)__ Granulomatous villitis is unusual in CMV placentitis. This case is from an HIV(+) patient who had reactivation of CMV during pregnancy.

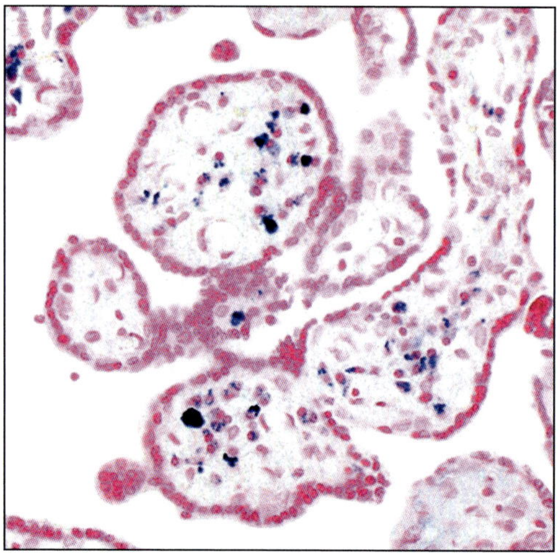

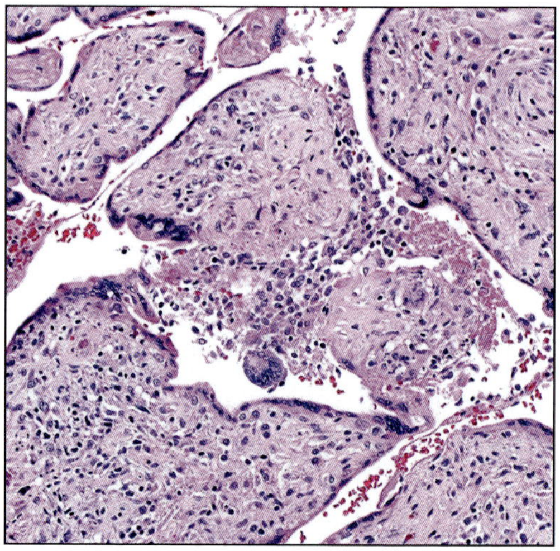

__(Left)__ Numerous characteristic CMV inclusions are noted in the Hofbauer cells and capillary endothelium of this villus without significant inflammation. __(Right)__ Immunohistochemistry may identify numerous CMV(+) cells that are not suspected on the routine H&E stains.

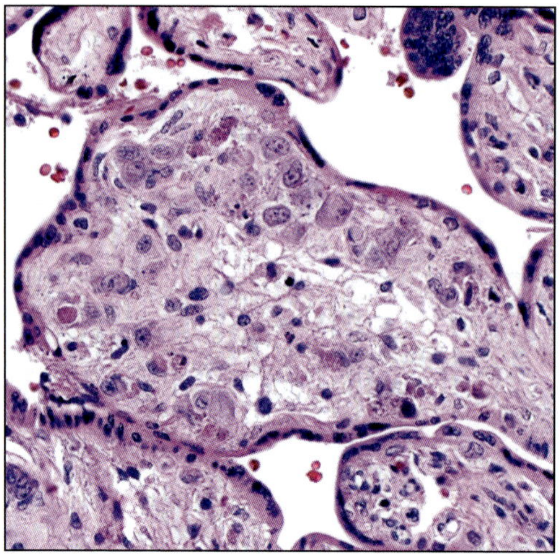

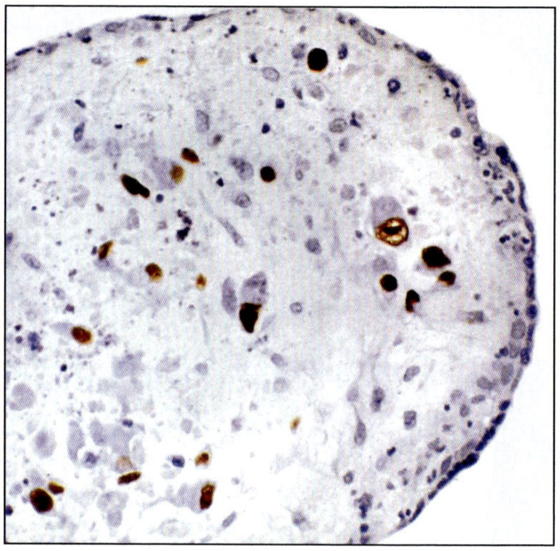

Microscopic Features

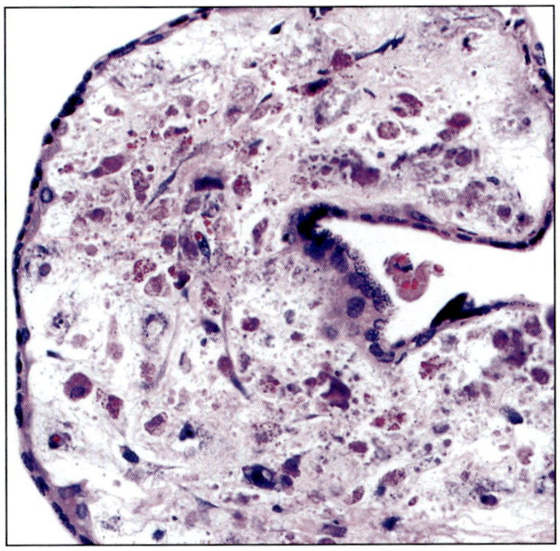

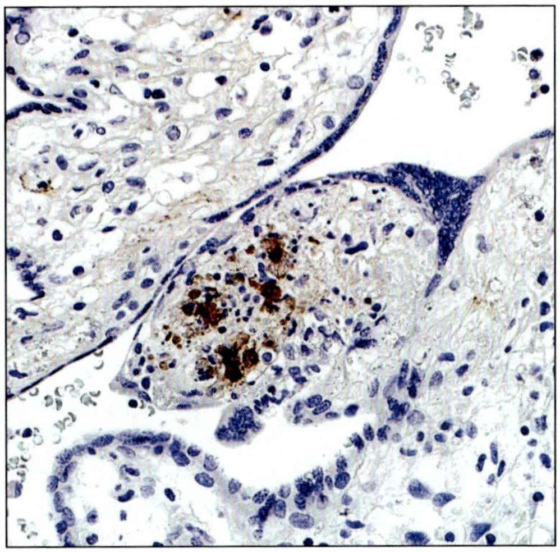

(Left) *Villi may show stromal necrosis with abundant eosinophilic debris that may calcify in some cases. Some cells appear suspicious for viral inclusions.* ***(Right)*** *Immunohistochemistry for CMV will highlight the debris and confirm the presence of the virus in suspicious cells.*

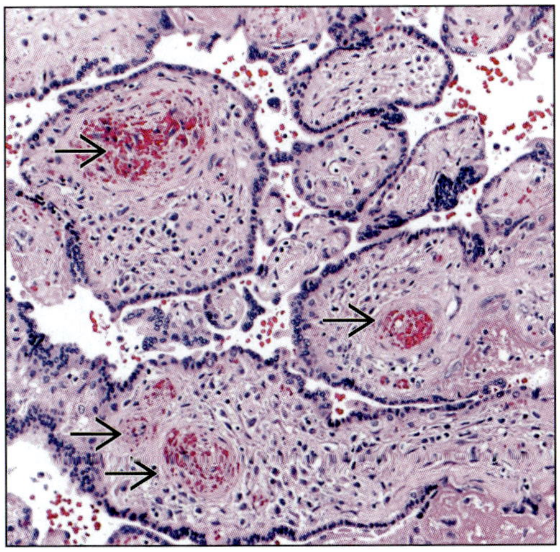

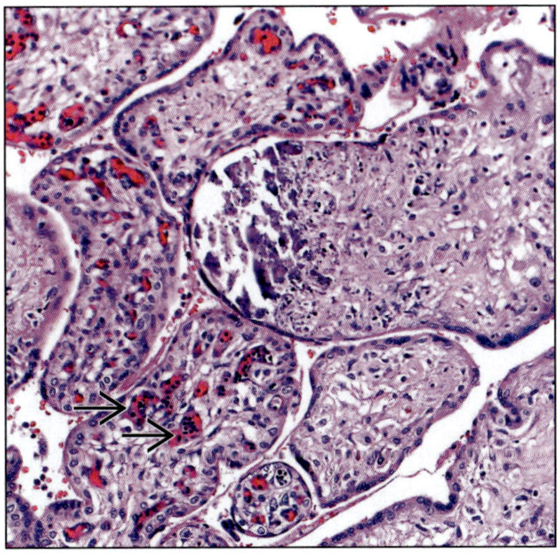

(Left) *CMV infection may be associated with extensive fetal vascular occlusion* ➔ *characterized by loss of endothelial integrity, red blood cell extravasation, and septation. This could result from proximal chronic villitis of stem villi as in villitis of unknown etiology, or possibly from viral infection of the endothelium.* ***(Right)*** *A calcified, avascular, inflamed villus is found adjacent to normal-appearing villi with marked fetal erythroblastosis* ➔.

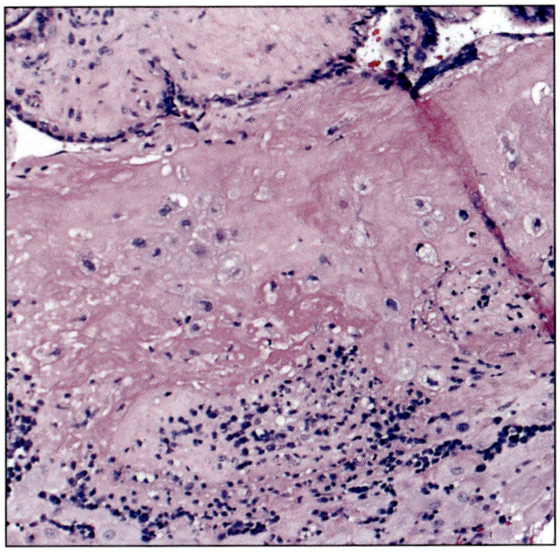

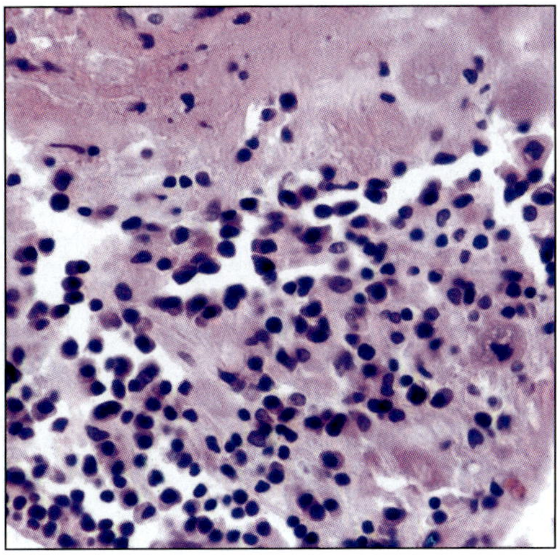

(Left) *The placental basal plate may have significant chronic inflammation.* ***(Right)*** *Lymphoplasmacytic deciduitis may be seen in CMV, but this feature is much less specific for CMV infection than lymphoplasmacytic villitis.*

CYTOMEGALOVIRUS

Features of Congenital CMV

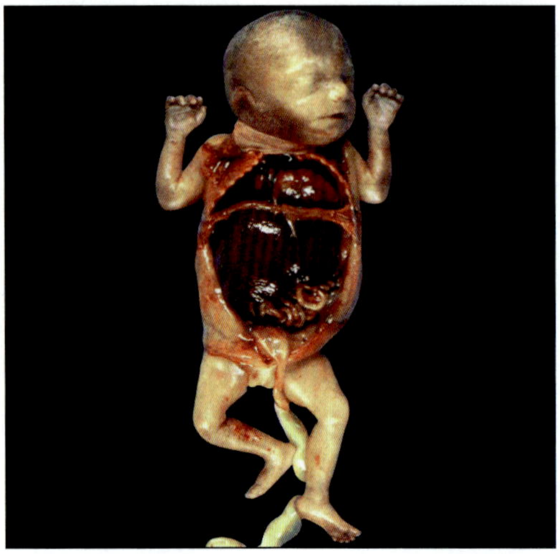

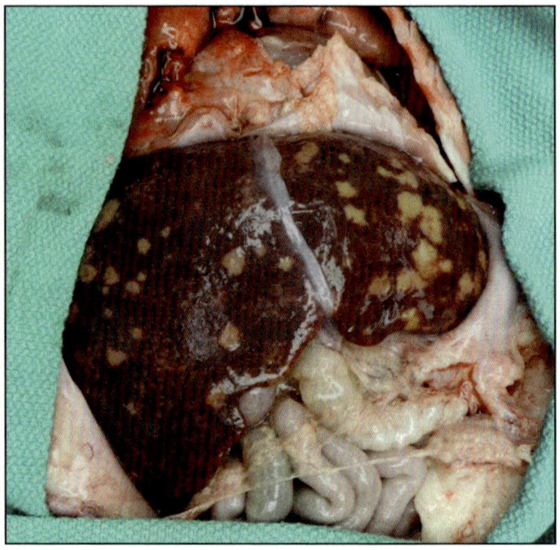

(Left) *There is massive hepatomegaly in this mildly hydropic previable fetus with congenital CMV infection.* ***(Right)*** *This neonate had symptomatic congenital CMV and survived for 4 months with persistent viremia despite antiviral therapy. The liver is markedly enlarged and shows numerous white areas of remote hepatic necrosis.*

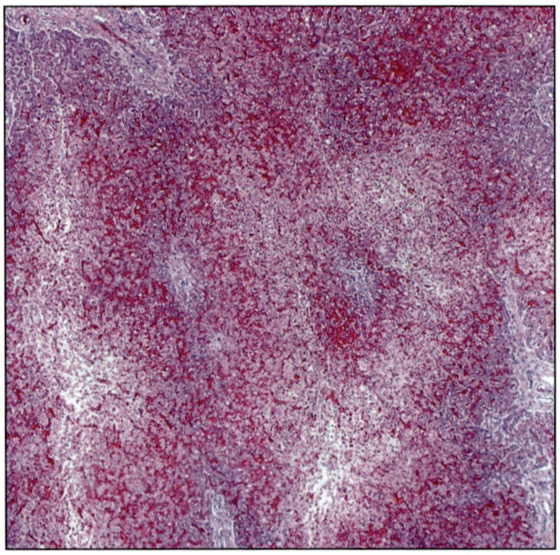

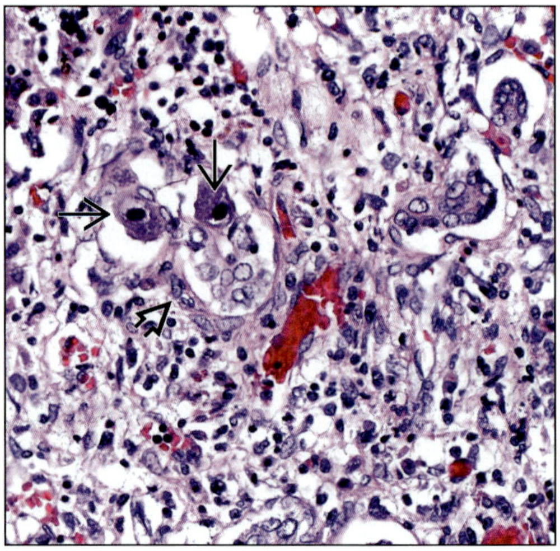

(Left) *Congenital CMV may cause massive hepatic necrosis. CMV inclusions are usually visible in biliary epithelium.* ***(Right)*** *Numerous CMV inclusions ⇨ may be seen within the liver bile duct epithelium ⇨.*

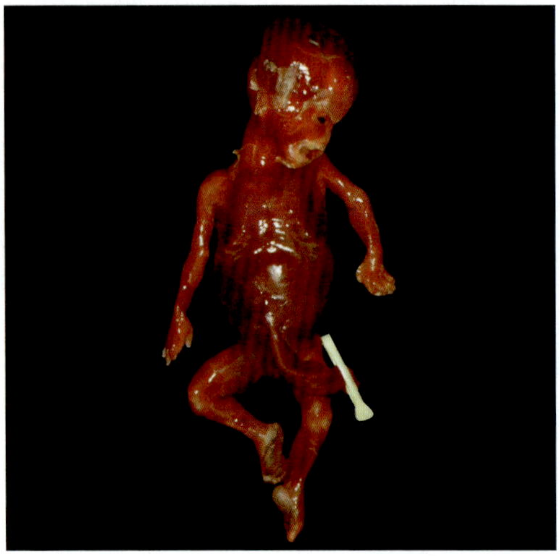

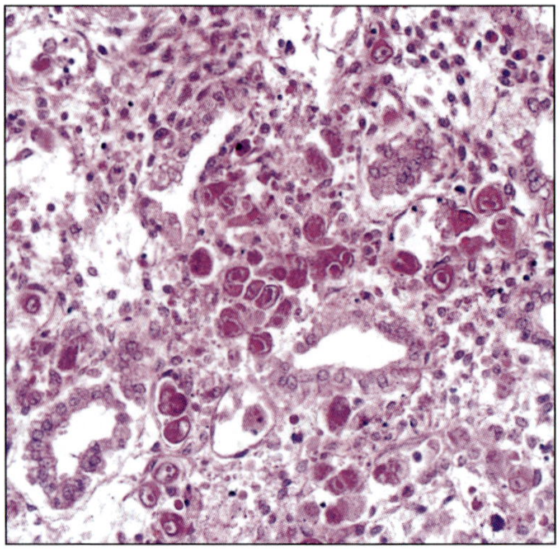

(Left) *Severely macerated fetus was found to have CMV infection on microscopic examination.* ***(Right)*** *Microscopic examination of tissues from macerated fetuses can be very useful, as in this case, which shows numerous CMV inclusions in lung tissue that is otherwise mostly devoid of nuclear chromatin basophilia.*

Brain Findings With Congenital CMV

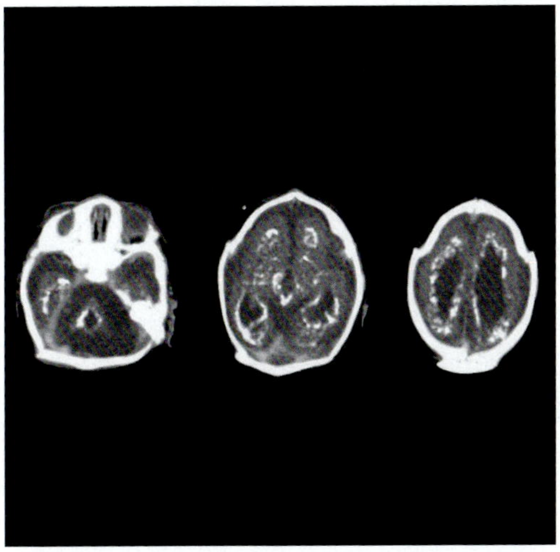

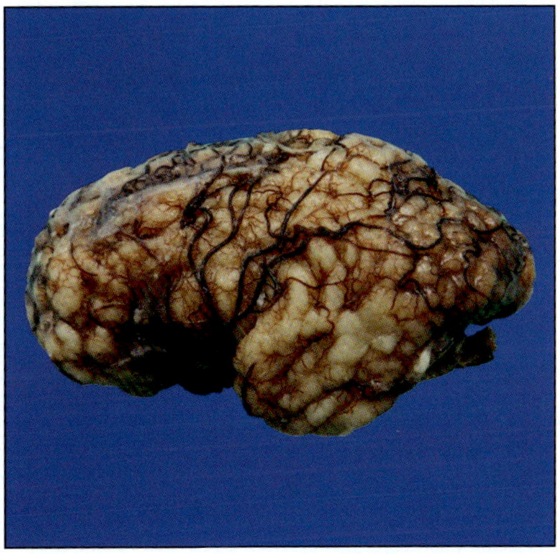

(Left) *CT scan shows hydrocephalus with periventricular calcifications in a case of congenital CMV.* ***(Right)*** *Central nervous system (CNS) involvement with congenital CMV may show microencephaly with polymicrogyria, as in this case of demise at 36 weeks gestation.*

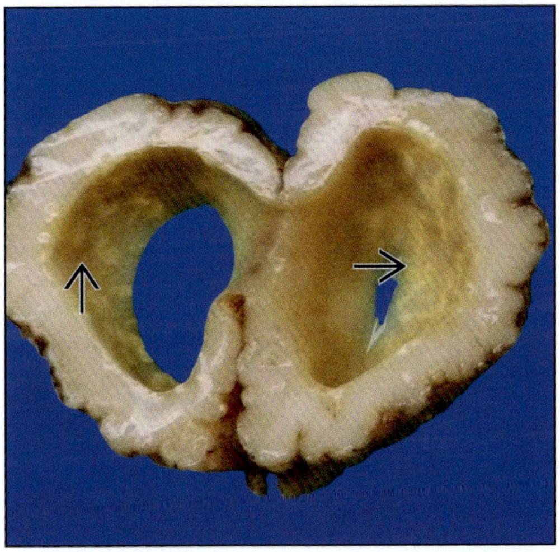

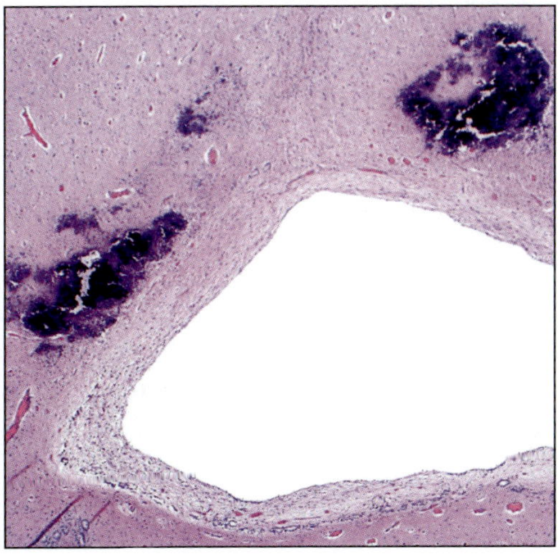

(Left) *Hydrocephalus may be seen with congenital CMV, as in this case with multiple yellow subependymal calcifications →.* ***(Right)*** *Microscopic examination of the 4th ventricle shows periventricular block-like calcification.*

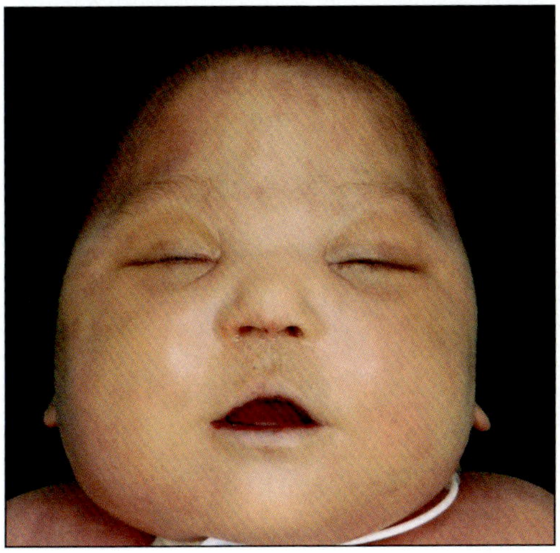

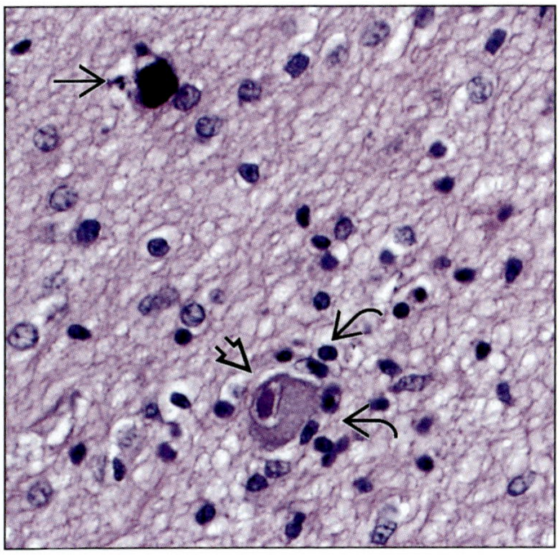

(Left) *This baby, who survived 4 months with congenital CMV, shows severe microcephaly.* ***(Right)*** *This section of brain from the periventricular area shows microcalcification → and a CMV inclusion cell ⇨ that is partially surrounded by microglial cells ↪, forming a type of microglial nodule.*

PARVOVIRUS B19

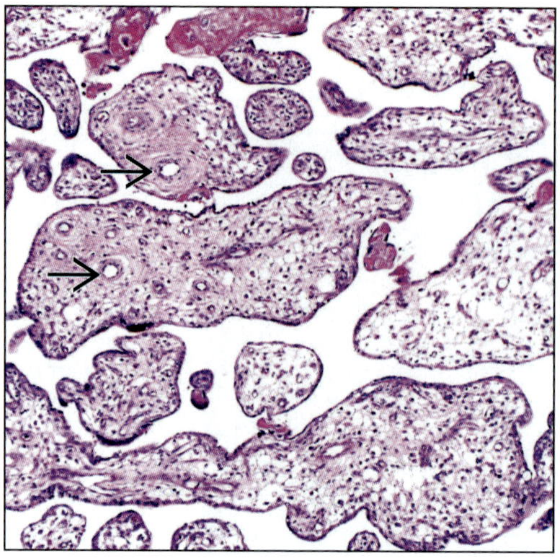

Diffuse villous edema is seen in this case of parvovirus infection. Fetal blood spaces are mostly empty ⇒, which is consistent with fetal anemia.

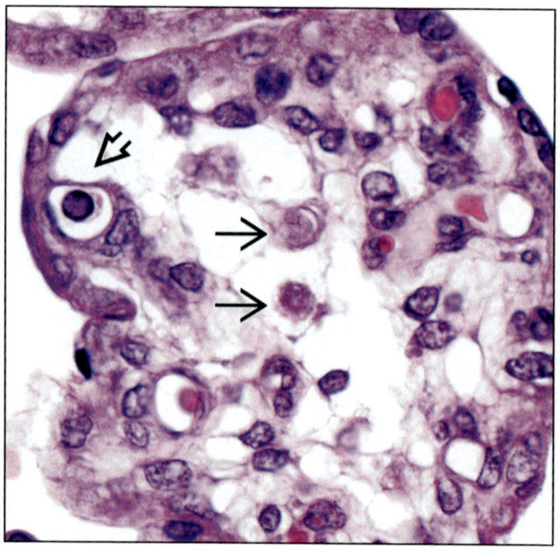

This edematous villus shows a characteristic intranuclear parvovirus inclusion in a nucleated red blood cell ⇒. A nonspecific feature of villous edema is prominent Hofbauer cells ⇒.

ETIOLOGY/PATHOGENESIS

Infectious Agents

- Parvovirus B19 is a single-stranded DNA member of Parvoviridae family and is species specific
  - Globoside or erythrocyte P antigen is necessary for infection of host cell
    - Present on surface of syncytiotrophoblast and cytotrophoblast, erythroid precursors, red cells, some megakaryocytes, endothelial cells, and fetal myocardium

CLINICAL ISSUES

Presentation

- Erythema infectiosum, also called 5th disease, initially described as the 5th viral exanthem in childhood
  - In children
    - Petechial eruption in glove or stocking pattern with truncal reticular erythema and "slapped cheek" appearance
  - In adults
    - Asymptomatic
    - Violaceous plaques of nodules, firm flesh-colored papules, papular and eczematous eruptions
    - Transient aplastic crisis
    - Arthritis
  - Winter/spring epidemics
- Maternal parvovirus infection during pregnancy
  - ~ 50% of women are at risk for infection; 1% incidence of seroconversion during pregnancy
    - Once women have seroconverted, antibodies are protective for life
  - Vertical transmission occurs in 33% of women with primary infection during pregnancy
    - Fetus may develop nonimmune hydrops approximately 4 weeks after exposure
    - 15% of nonimmune hydrops are due to parvovirus
  - Nonimmune hydrops fetalis due to parvovirus
    - Virus infects erythroid precursors
    - Shortened red blood cell survival with hemolysis and erythroid hypoplasia
    - Severe fetal anemia results in high cardiac output failure
    - Parvovirus may also infect myocardium, contributing to cardiac dysfunction
  - Maternal serum α-fetoprotein (MSAFP) may be elevated due to fetal hydrops

Treatment

- No specific treatment for parvovirus
  - Intrauterine transfusion may be done for fetal anemia
  - Immune globulin is used in immunoincompetent individuals

Prognosis

- 5-10% of in utero infections result in lethal hydrops
  - Infection during 2nd trimester is associated with greatest risk for hydrops
  - 1st trimester is associated with lower risk
  - 3rd trimester is associated with very low risk
- Resolution of hydrops may occur with or without intrauterine transfusion

MACROSCOPIC FEATURES

General Features

- Placenta is large, pale, and friable

MICROSCOPIC PATHOLOGY

Histologic Features

- Placenta

PARVOVIRUS B19

Key Facts

Etiology

- Parvovirus B19 is a single-stranded DNA member of Parvoviridae family
- Infection of fetal erythroid precursors and myocardial cells may lead to hydrops fetalis with severe fetal anemia

Clinical Issues

- Parvovirus during pregnancy may result in nonimmune hydrops fetalis 4-6 weeks post exposure
- Vertical transmission occurs in 33% of women during primary infection
- Severe fetal anemia results in high cardiac output failure
- 15% of nonimmune hydrops are due to parvovirus
- 5-10% of in utero infections result in lethal hydrops

Microscopic Pathology

- Placenta
  - Marked villous edema
  - Increased fetal nucleated red blood cells, many with intranuclear basophilic or eosinophilic inclusions
  - Usually without significant chronic villitis
- Fetal findings
  - Liver is most severely affected
  - Bone marrow is hypocellular

Diagnostic Checklist

- Marked increase in nucleated red blood cells (erythroblastosis fetalis) associated with hydropic placenta should prompt a search for parvovirus inclusions

---

  - Increased nucleated red blood cells (NRBCs), many with intranuclear basophilic or eosinophilic inclusions
  - Diffuse villous edema
  - Increased number of T lymphocytes within villi, but usual findings of chronic villitis are not present
- Fetal organs
  - Liver is most severely affected
    - Erythroid hyperplasia
    - Atypical giant pronormoblasts; cell nonpermissive for viral replication
    - Moderate to marked hemosiderosis
    - Rarely giant cell transformation of hepatocytes and fibrosis
  - Bone marrow is hypocellular
  - Myocarditis may be difficult to distinguish from circulating NRBCs with viral inclusions

ANCILLARY TESTS

Immunohistochemistry

- Immunostain for parvovirus is very useful for confirming viral inclusions in NRBCs

DIFFERENTIAL DIAGNOSIS

Erythroblastosis Fetalis Due to Immune-Mediated Hemolysis

- Lacks viral inclusions in NRBCs
- Severe autolysis may result in pseudoinclusions in any condition
  - Immunohistochemistry for parvovirus on fetal organs in addition to placenta may be useful

Myeloid Proliferations of Down Syndrome

- May present in utero with hydrops, numerous nucleated precursor hematopoietic cells in peripheral blood
- Greater variety of precursor cell types (e.g., myeloid precursors, megakaryoblasts) than in parvovirus

Fetal Hydrops Due to Chronic Maternal Fetal Transfusion

- May see numerous erythroblasts in villous capillaries
- No viral inclusions
- Find evidence of fetal blood in maternal intervillous blood space
  - Confirm fetal-maternal transfusion by Kleihauer-Betke stain on maternal blood

DIAGNOSTIC CHECKLIST

Pathologic Interpretation Pearls

- Marked increase in NRBCs (erythroblastosis fetalis) associated with hydropic placenta should prompt a search for parvovirus inclusions

SELECTED REFERENCES

1. Al-Buhtori M et al: Viral detection in hydrops fetalis, spontaneous abortion, and unexplained fetal death in utero. J Med Virol. 83(4):679-84, 2011
2. Young NS et al: Parvovirus B19. N Engl J Med. 350(6):586-97, 2004
3. Jordan JA et al: Placental cellular immune response in women infected with human parvovirus B19 during pregnancy. Clin Diagn Lab Immunol. 8(2):288-92, 2001
4. Jordan JA et al: Globoside expression within the human placenta. Placenta. 20(1):103-8, 1999
5. Essary LR et al: Frequency of parvovirus B19 infection in nonimmune hydrops fetalis and utility of three diagnostic methods. Hum Pathol. 29(7):696-701, 1998
6. Boley TJ et al: Parvovirus infection in pregnancy. Semin Perinatol. 17(6):410-9, 1993

PARVOVIRUS B19

Microscopic and Gross Features

(Left) *These villi show a marked increase in fetal nucleated red blood cells → (erythroblastosis fetalis).* ***(Right)*** *Immunohistochemistry confirms the presence of parvovirus within many cells in the fetal capillaries.*

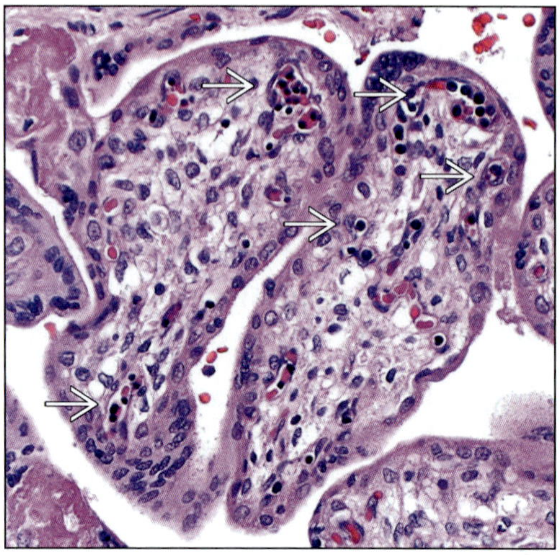

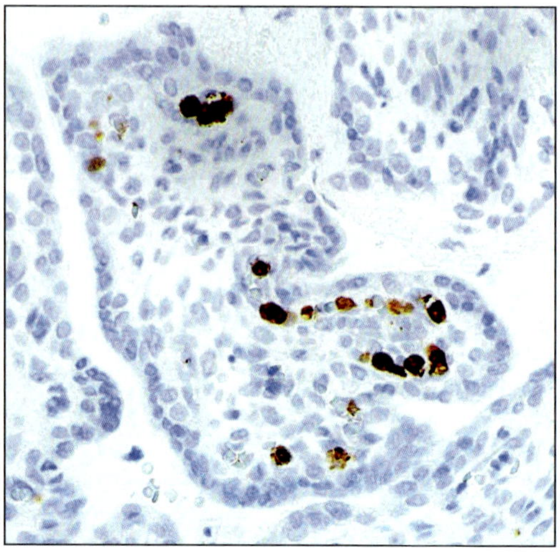

(Left) *Previable fetus with hydrops secondary to parvovirus infection is shown.* ***(Right)*** *Erythropoiesis is increased and left shifted in the fetal liver. Viral inclusions include those of abnormally large erythroid precursors with nuclear clearing → and smaller normoblasts with glassy eosinophilic inclusions →. There is increased → granular iron in the hepatocytes and Kupffer cells due to rapid turnover of red blood cells.*

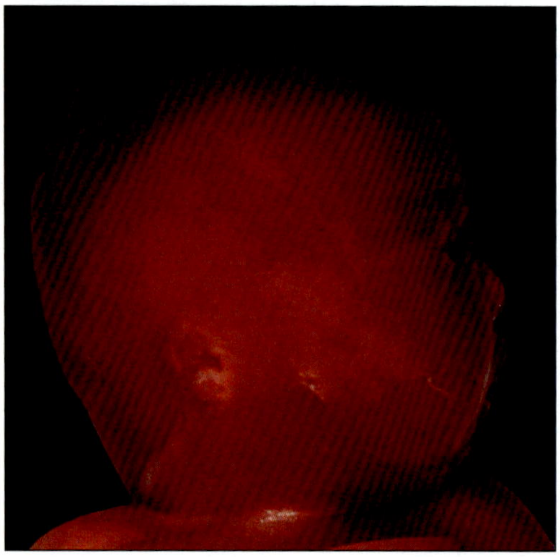

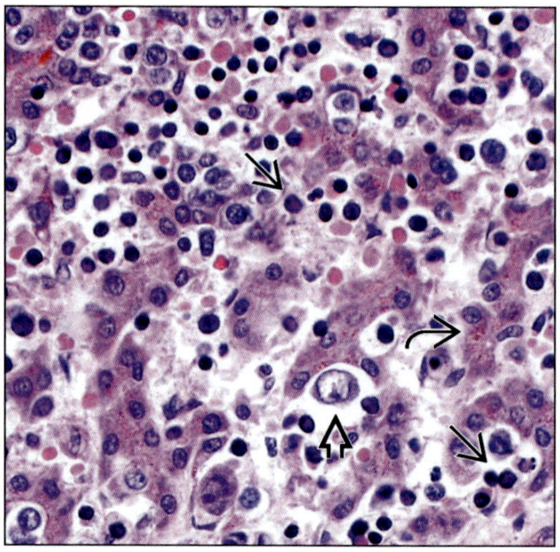

(Left) *This very thin section of liver shows characteristic parvovirus inclusions → in nucleated red blood cells and iron → in hepatocytes. Iron will also be present in Kupffer cells.* ***(Right)*** *On this immunohistochemical stain for parvovirus, the majority of erythroid precursor cells are positive.*

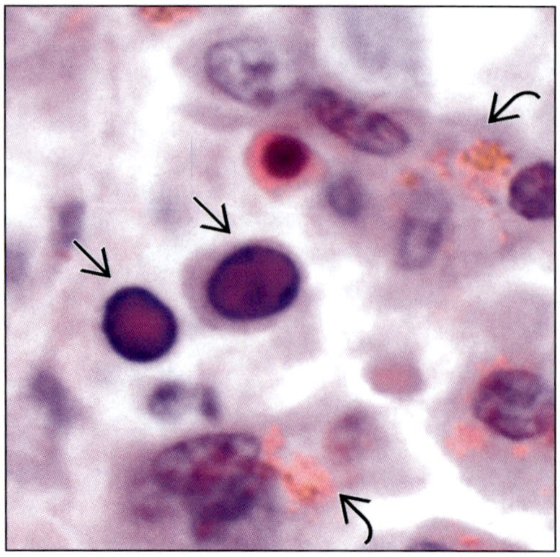

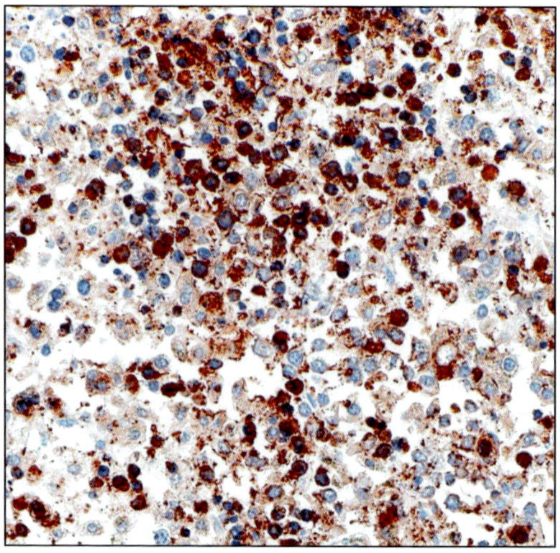

Microscopic Features

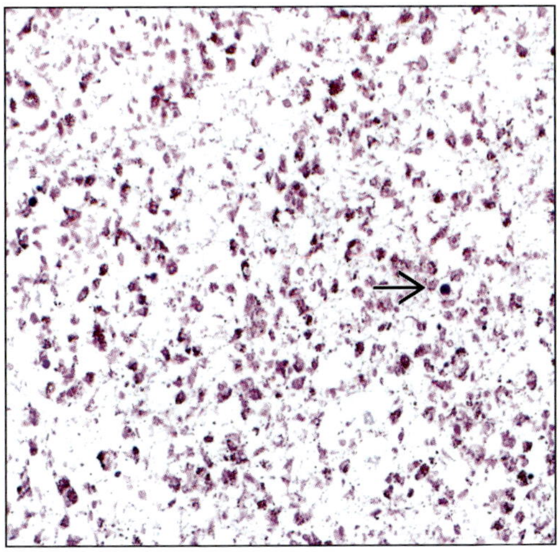
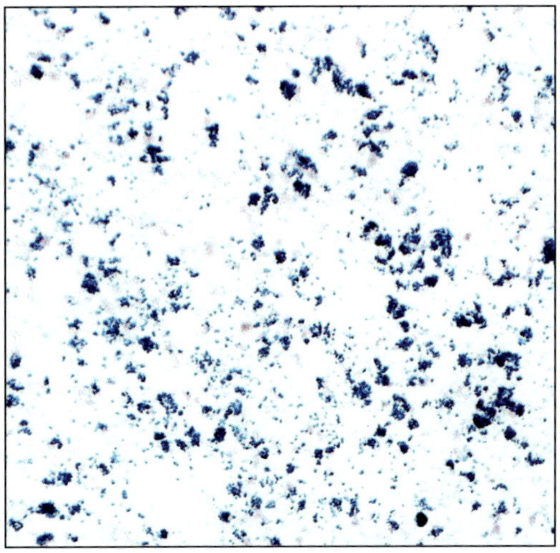

(Left) *In this severely macerated fetal liver, cytologic detail is very poorly preserved. Pigment is present, which could represent either iron or formalin pigment. A rare intact cell shows a possible viral inclusion* ⇒. ***(Right)*** *The same fetal liver shows diffuse positive iron staining.*

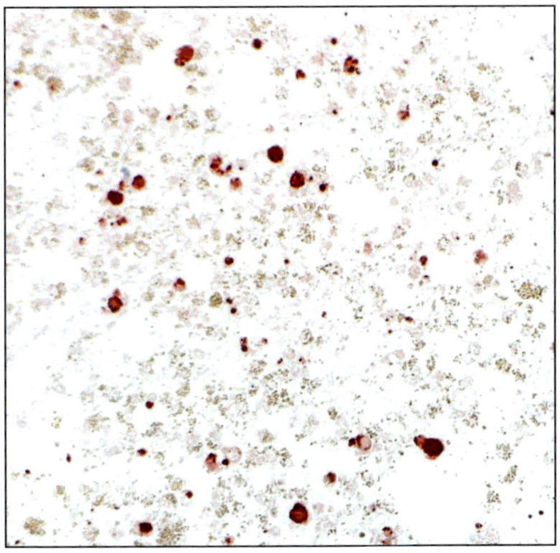
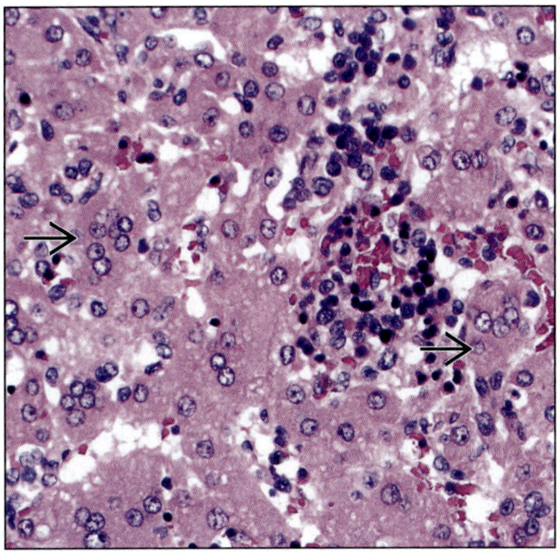

(Left) *The same fetal liver is positive with immunohistochemistry for parvovirus.* ***(Right)*** *A rare finding with congenital parvovirus is giant cell transformation of hepatocytes* ⇒.

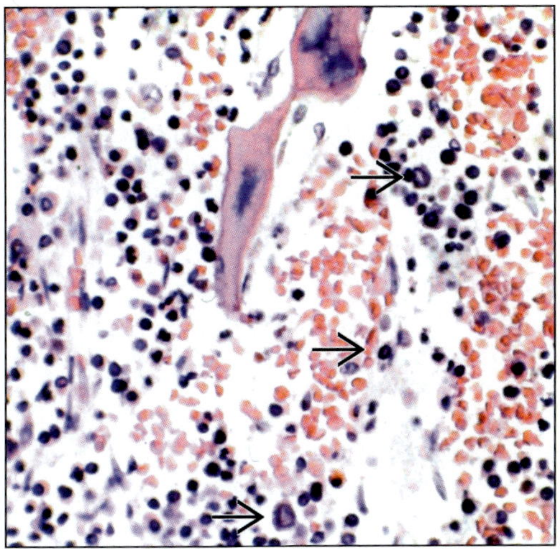
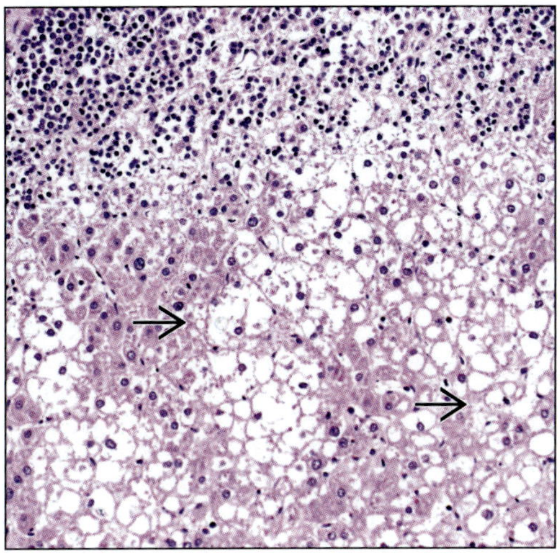

(Left) *The 2nd-trimester bone marrow is often hypocellular as hematopoiesis is still extensive in the liver. Intranuclear parvovirus inclusions are seen* ⇒. ***(Right)*** *This adrenal gland shows massive accumulation of lipid in the fetal cortex* ⇒. *This feature of in utero hypoxic stress was noted in all cases of parvovirus that were examined. It probably reflects the severe fetal anemia.*

HERPES SIMPLEX VIRUS

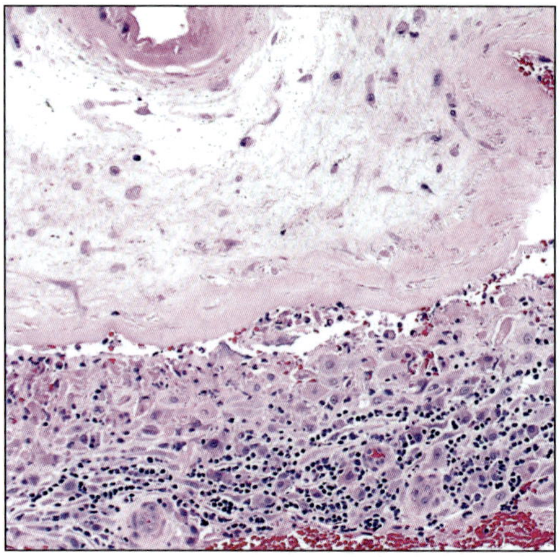

H&E section of the free membranes shows lymphocytic deciduitis, necrotic amnion, and necrotic stromal cells, consistent with an ascending herpes simplex virus (HSV) infection.

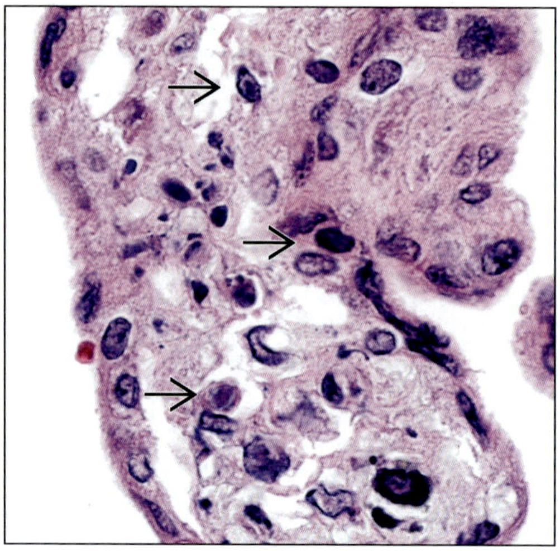

H&E stain shows chronic villitis with stromal cells that have characteristic HSV viral inclusions ⇒, consistent with hematogenous transplacental spread of the virus.

TERMINOLOGY

Abbreviations

- Herpes simplex virus (HSV)

Types

- Herpes simplex virus type 1 (HSV1)
- Herpes simples virus type 2 (HSV2)
- Skin, eyes, mouth (SEM) mucocutaneous type of neonatal herpes simplex virus infection

ETIOLOGY/PATHOGENESIS

Infectious Agents

- HSV1 and HSV2
  - Herpes simplex virus is a double-stranded DNA, enveloped virus

Placental Cells Susceptible to HSV Infection

- HSV entry mediators are decreased on villous syncytiotrophoblast and invasive trophoblast
- Villous mesenchymal cells, endothelium, and mast cells are permissive to infection
- Fetal membrane mesenchymal stromal cells are permissive to HSV infection

CLINICAL ISSUES

Epidemiology

- Incidence
  - 20-30% of the general population is HSV2 seropositive
  - 1% incidence of HSV2 seroconversion during pregnancy
  - Maternal antibodies to HSV1 are slightly protective against primary HSV2 infection
  - Incidence of HSV2 in placental samples by PCR reported as high as 9% in asymptomatic women
- Congenital/neonatal infection
  - Incidence
    - 1 per 1,500-5,000 births
  - Vast majority of infections are acquired at time of vaginal delivery during primary maternal infection
    - Risk for transmission during primary infection is 30-50%
    - Risk for transmission during recurrent infection is 5%
    - Majority of women who transmit virus to infant are asymptomatic
  - Infection is rarely acquired as an ascending infection
  - Only 5% of infection is transmitted through the placenta during maternal viremia
- Postnatal exposure to herpetic lesions, often from family members, can be source of neonatal infection
  - Direct orogenital suction of bleeding penile wound at time of circumcision (Orthodox Jewish practice) has been associated with neonatal infection

Presentation

- Transplacental infection
  - Skin
    - Early lesions are denuded or ulcerated
    - Older lesions appear as hypopigmented scars
  - Liver failure with coagulopathy and hepatic encephalopathy
  - Microcephaly
  - Hydrocephalus
  - Hydranencephaly
- Intrapartum and postpartum infection
  - Mucocutaneous infection accounts for 42% of neonatal herpes simplex virus
    - Clustered vesicles with erythematous base, bullae, pustules, erythematous macular exanthem
    - Eye involvement is keratoconjunctivitis, which can progress to chorioretinitis
    - Only 10% have mouth lesions
    - Presents at 11 days

HERPES SIMPLEX VIRUS

Key Facts

Etiology

- HSV2 is agent in 75% of congenital/neonatal cases
- Incidence of neonatal HSV: 1 per 1,500-5,000 births
- Presence of maternal antibodies to HSV1 is slightly protective against primary HSV2 infection
- Vast majority of neonatal HSV is acquired at time of vaginal delivery during primary infection
- HSV is rarely acquired as ascending infection
- Only 5% of congenital/neonatal HSV is transplacental acquisition
- Postnatal exposure to herpetic lesions, usually from family members, may also infect infant

Clinical Issues

- Mucocutaneous infection (SEM) accounts for 42% of neonatal HSV
- Disseminated infection accounts for 23% of neonatal HSV
- Encephalitic type of infection accounts for 35% of neonatal HSV
- Sepsis, irritability, temperature instability, fever unresponsive to antibiotics, shock
- May have markedly elevated lactic acid and ammonia suggestive of inborn error of metabolism

Microscopic Pathology

- Rarely associated with necrotizing villitis
- Rare HSV inclusions seen in villi, umbilical cord, and membranes
- Liver: Geographic coagulative necrosis with large number of multinucleated giant cells with intranuclear inclusions
- Adrenal gland: Cortical necrosis with calcifications

- Disseminated infection accounts for 23% of neonatal herpes simplex virus; usually presents with nonspecific signs and symptoms that involve liver, adrenal glands, lungs, and brain
  - Sepsis
  - Irritability
  - Temperature instability
  - Fever unresponsive to antibiotics
  - Shock
  - Respiratory distress
  - Pneumonitis
  - Apnea
  - Hepatosplenomegaly
  - Jaundice
  - Bleeding diathesis or disseminated intravascular coagulation
  - Seizures
  - Presents at 11 days
  - Patients rarely have skin lesions
  - May have markedly elevated lactic acid and ammonia suggestive of inborn error of metabolism
- Encephalitic form accounts for 35% of neonatal herpes simplex virus
  - Rarely present with skin lesions
  - May present in association with disseminated disease or SEM
  - Presents later at 16 days

Treatment

- Drugs
  - Currently, acyclovir is best available anti-herpes simplex virus drug

Prognosis

- Disseminated form of disease is rarely treated in time
  - Mortality is 57% with treatment
  - 61% of survivors have neurodevelopmental abnormalities
- Encephalitic form of disease
  - Untreated central nervous system disease has 50% mortality
  - Mortality with treatment is 15%
  - 64% of survivors have long-term neurodevelopmental sequelae
- SEM disease has 0% mortality if treated
  - Risk for multiple skin recurrences
  - Can progress to CNS or disseminated disease
- HSV2 has a worse prognosis

MACROSCOPIC FEATURES

General Features

- Placenta
  - Usually completely normal
- Fetus
  - Cutaneous lesions
  - Hepatosplenomegaly
    - Liver: Miliary distribution of necrotic yellow-white lesions, often with erythematous rim
  - Adrenal gland
    - Areas of cortical necrosis and calcifications

MICROSCOPIC PATHOLOGY

Histologic Features

- Viral infection results in cell swelling with cell death and hemorrhagic necrosis
- Placenta
  - Usually completely normal
  - Rarely associated with necrotizing lymphoplasmacytic villitis
  - Rarely associated with chronic inflammation around fetal vessels, variably rich in plasma cells
  - Rare herpes simplex virus inclusions seen in villi, umbilical cord, and membranes
  - Ascending HSV infection may be associated with lymphocytic chorioamnionitis and chronic vasculitis of chorionic plate vessels in amniotropic pattern
- Fetus
  - Liver

- Geographic coagulative necrosis with large number of multinucleated giant cells with intranuclear inclusions
  - Adrenal gland
    - Cortical necrosis with calcification
  - Lungs
    - Necrotizing pneumonitis

Cytologic Features

- Herpes simplex virus infection has
  - Multinucleated giant cells
  - Nuclear molding
  - Ground-glass chromatin
  - Thickened nuclear membrane
- Cowdry type A
  - Usually found in older lesions
  - Large eosinophilic intranuclear inclusion surrounded by a halo "owl eye"
- Cowdry type B
  - Usually found early or primary infections
  - Smudged nuclei
  - Intranuclear eosinophilic inclusion that pushes the chromatin to the nuclear membrane, without a halo

DIFFERENTIAL DIAGNOSIS

Other Members of Herpesvirus Family

- Have similar intranuclear inclusion and cause tissue necrosis
  - Cytomegalovirus
  - Varicella-zoster virus
  - Adenovirus

Other Infectious Agents Causing Vesicular Eruptions in Neonate

- *Staphylococcus*
- *Treponema*
- *Candida*
- *Listeria*

Noninfectious Agents Causing Vesicular Eruptions in Neonate

- Erythema toxicum
- Pustular melanosis
- Urticaria pigmentosa
- Incontinentia pigmenti
- Neonatal lupus
- Epidermolysis bullosa
- Langerhans cell histiocytosis

DIAGNOSTIC CHECKLIST

Pathologic Interpretation Pearls

- Always consider HSV infection in infant who has fever and is unresponsive to antibiotics
- Ascending HSV may show lymphoplasmacytic chorioamnionitis with necrosis of amnion and chorion
- Always rule out HSV when plasma cell funisitis or numerous plasma cells in necrotic membranes are seen
- Hematogenous HSV may show minimal inflammation
- May see necrosis of villous trophoblast and stromal cells

SELECTED REFERENCES

1. Finger-Jardim F et al: Herpes simplex virus: prevalence in placental tissue and incidence in neonatal cord blood samples. J Med Virol. 86(3):519-24, 2014
2. Avanzi S et al: Susceptibility of human placenta derived mesenchymal stromal/stem cells to human herpesviruses infection. PLoS One. 8(8):e71412, 2013
3. Centers for Disease Control and Prevention (CDC): Neonatal herpes simplex virus infection following Jewish ritual circumcisions that included direct orogenital suction - New York City, 2000-2011. MMWR Morb Mortal Wkly Rep. 61(22):405-9, 2012
4. Bale JF et al: Herpes Simplex Virus Infections of the newborn. Curr Treat Options Neurol. 7(2):151-156, 2005
5. Chatterjee A et al: Severe intrauterine herpes simplex disease with placentitis in a newborn of a mother with recurrent genital infection at delivery. J Perinatol. 21(8):559-64, 2001
6. McGann KA: Herpesvirus infection in the fetus and neonate: epidemiology and clinical manifestations. Sem Pediatr Inf Dis. 8(3):136-50, 1997
7. Heifetz SA et al: Necrotizing funisitis and herpes simplex infection of placental and decidual tissues: study of four cases. Hum Pathol. 25(7):715-22, 1994
8. Altshuler G: Pathogenesis of congenital herpesvirus infection. Case report including a description of the placenta. Am J Dis Child. 127(3):427-9, 1974

Microscopic Features

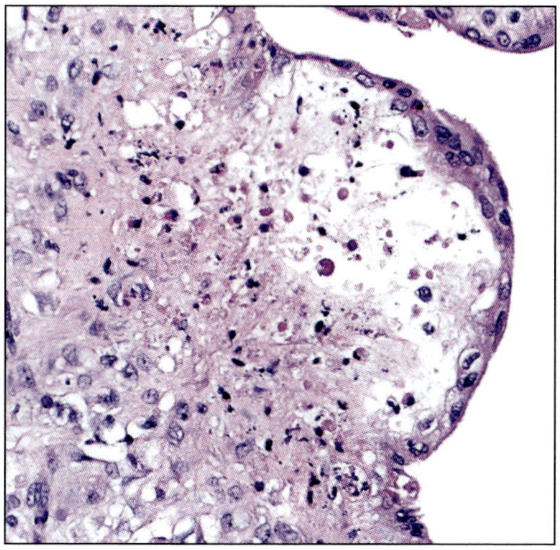
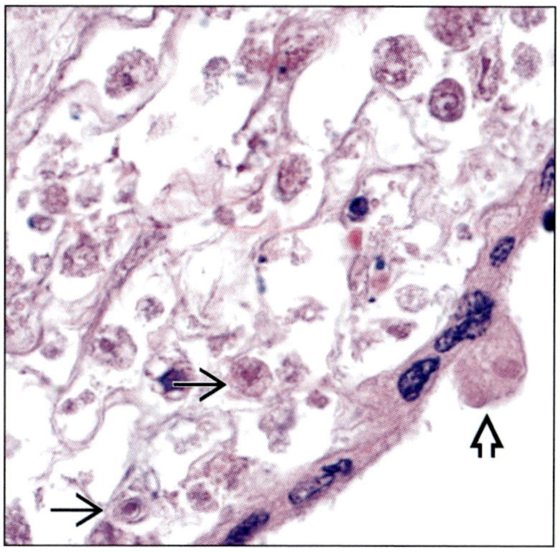

(Left) *Transplacental infection may show active necrotizing villitis, usually lymphoplasmacytic.* ***(Right)*** *Villitis with necrotic Hofbauer cells → and syncytiotrophoblast ⇨ with inclusions suspicious for herpes simplex virus are consistent with hematogenous transplacental HSV infection.*

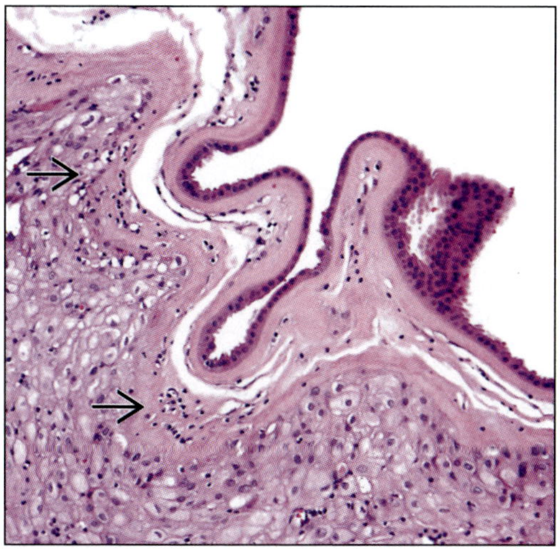
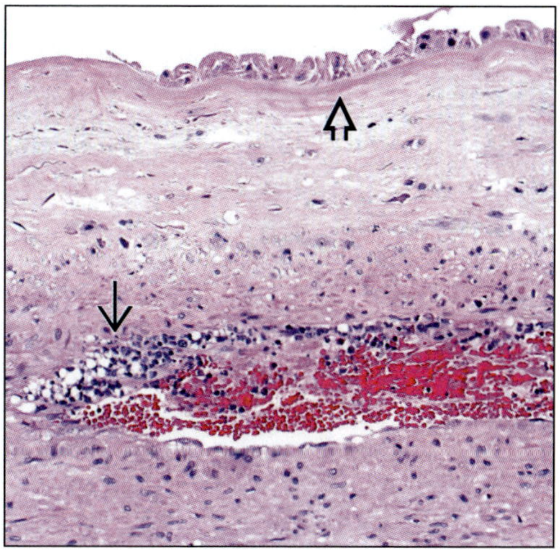

(Left) *Ascending herpes simplex virus infection may be associated with mild lymphoplasmacytic chorioamnionitis of the free membranes →.* ***(Right)*** *Chronic inflammation → of a chorionic plate vessel in an amniotropic pattern is also suggestive of an ascending HSV infection. Note the associated degeneration of the amnion epithelium ⇨.*

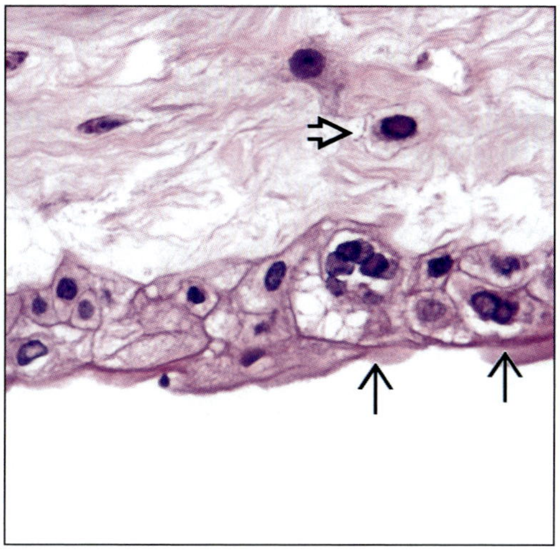
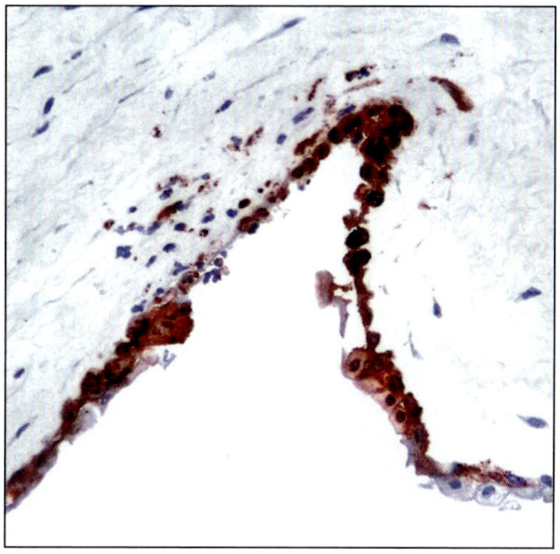

(Left) *Amniotic surface of the umbilical cord with multinucleated giant cell → and stromal cell containing intranuclear inclusion ⇨ is characteristic of herpes simplex virus.* ***(Right)*** *Amnion surface of the umbilical cord has numerous amniocytes and subamniotic stromal cells positive for herpes simplex virus by immunohistochemistry.*

HERPES SIMPLEX VIRUS

Neonatal Disseminated HSV Infection

(Left) *H&E of lung shows diffuse alveolar damage with hyaline membranes* → *and chronic pneumonitis* ⇨ *from ascending herpes simplex virus.* ***(Right)*** *H&E of lung shows intraalveolar fibrin, chronic inflammation, hyaline membranes, and numerous herpes simplex virus inclusions* →.

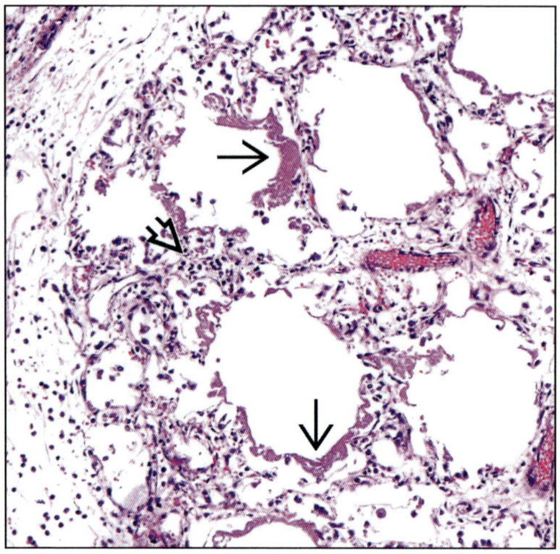

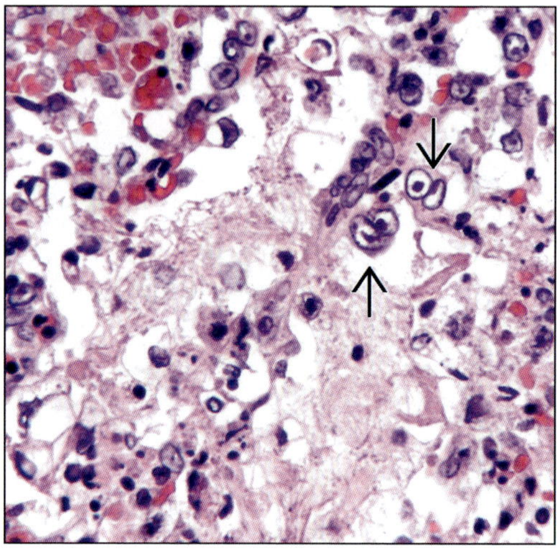

(Left) *Gross photo of transplacental herpes simplex virus shows multiple pinpoint areas of necrosis and calcification within the adrenal cortex.* ***(Right)*** *H&E shows adrenal cortex with focal necrosis* → *that contains abundant organisms on immunohistochemistry.*

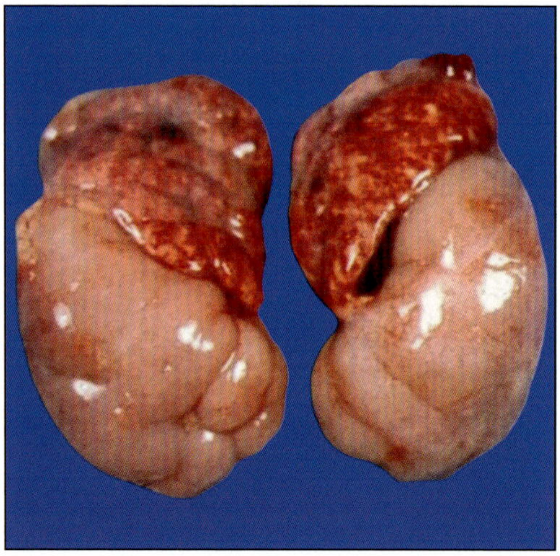

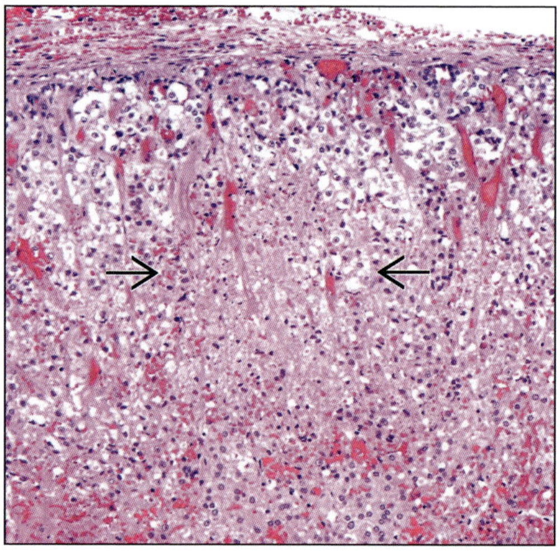

(Left) *Congenital disseminated herpes simplex virus is shown. Multiple punched-out skin lesions contain multiple organisms, which would be highly infectious.* ***(Right)*** *Transplacental herpes simplex virus infection results in marked necrosis of the brain, which is not the typical temporal lobe involvement seen in older children and adults.*

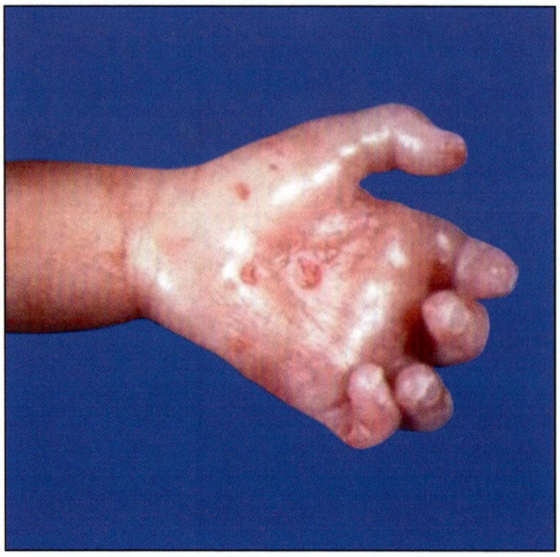

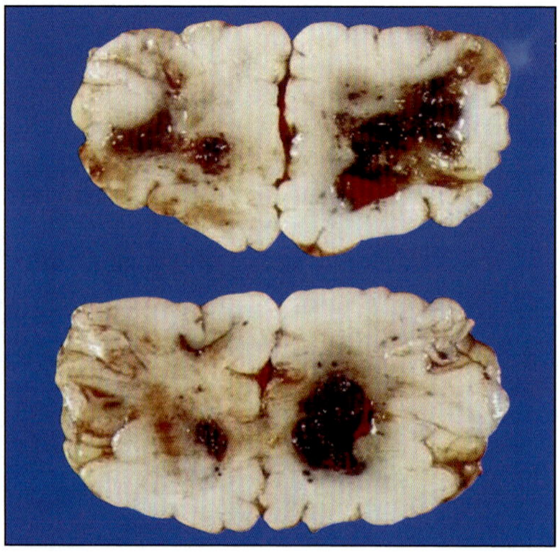

Neonatal Disseminated HSV Infection

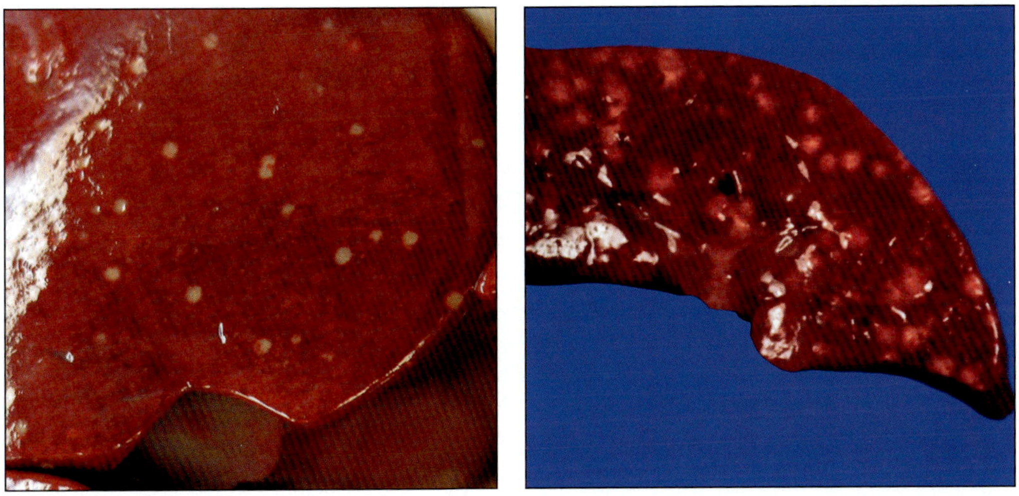

(Left) *This liver has multiple yellow-white, slightly depressed necrotic lesions.* ***(Right)*** *Cut surface of the liver demonstrates multifocal necrosis. The central yellow-white areas of necrosis are surrounded by hyperemia.*

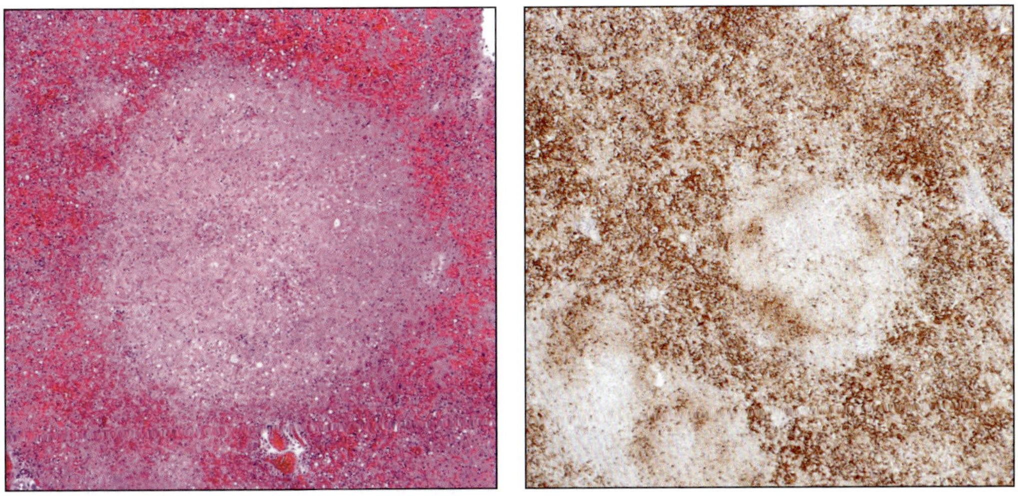

(Left) *H&E section of the liver with disseminated HSV shows an area of coagulative necrosis with acute hemorrhage at the interface.* ***(Right)*** *Immunohistochemistry for HSV is diffusely positive in the residual hepatic parenchyma but negative in the central area of necrosis.*

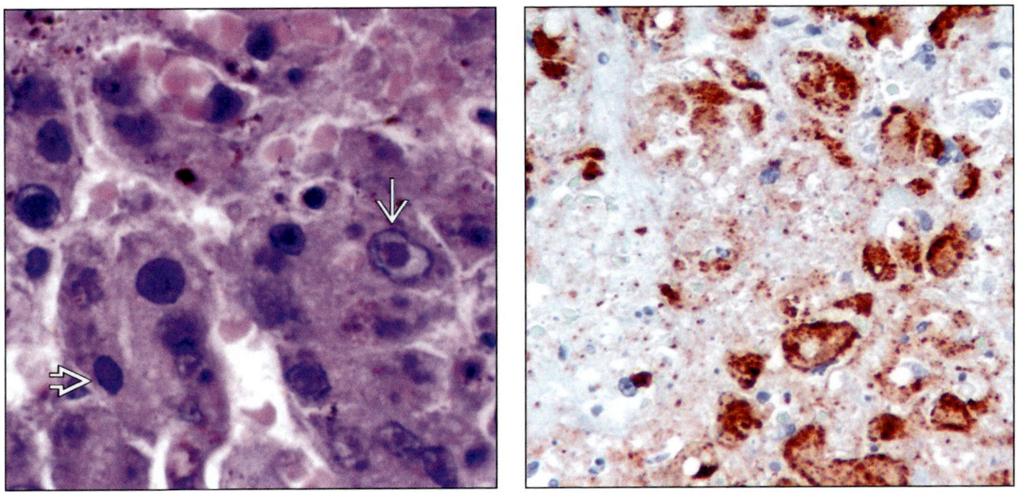

(Left) *H&E shows hepatocytes with Cowdry type A ➔ and Cowdry type B ⇨ intranuclear inclusions of herpes simplex virus.* ***(Right)*** *Immunohistochemistry for HSV may be positive within nuclei of the hepatocytes. Necrosis often results in leaky nuclear membranes, resulting in diffuse positivity in the cytoplasm of the hepatocytes.*

OTHER VIRUSES

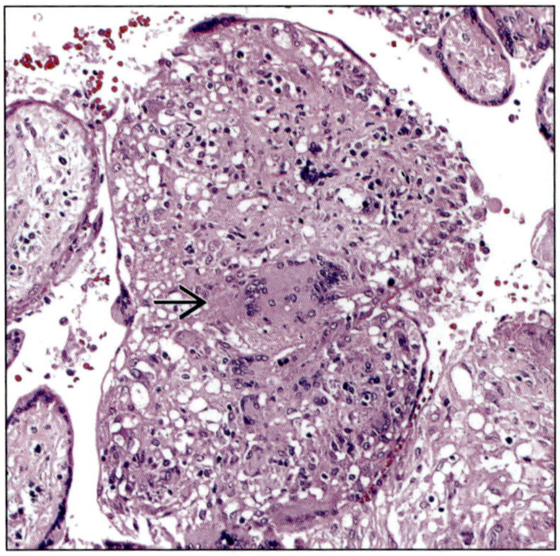

Granulomatous villitis with lymphocytes and Langhans-type multinucleated giant cells ➔ is seen in this case of congenital varicella-zoster virus (VZV) infection occurring in the 1st trimester.

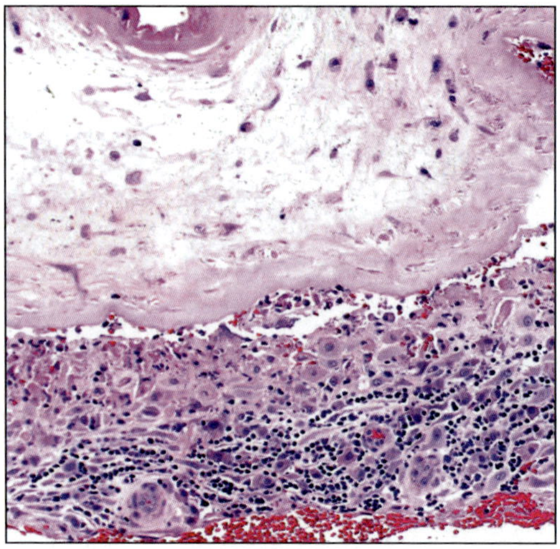

A significant lymphocytic or lymphoplasmacytic deciduitis may be seen in women with viral syndrome shortly prior to delivery. This case is associated with herpes simplex virus.

TERMINOLOGY

Abbreviations

- Human herpesvirus (HHV)
  - Varicella-zoster virus (VZV)
  - Epstein-Barr virus (EBV)
  - HHV types 6-8 (HHV-6, HHV-7, HHV-8)
- Human papillomavirus (HPV)
- HIV type 1 (HIV-1)
- Lymphocytic choriomeningitis virus (LCMV)

Definitions

- Vertical transmission
  - Transmission of virus from mother to fetus
- Villitis
  - Inflammation of chorionic villi may be lymphocytic ± plasma cells and histiocytes, granulomatous, or, rarely, neutrophilic
    - Inflammatory cells are predominately maternal T lymphocytes invading villous stroma
- Fetal inflammatory response
  - Usually acute and rarely chronic inflammation emanating from fetal vessels of placenta or umbilical cord
    - Inflammatory cells are usually neutrophils, rarely lymphocytes, histiocytes, or plasma cells
    - Eosinophils may be a prominent component, associated with neutrophils and, less commonly, lymphocytes

ROUTES OF VERTICAL TRANSMISSION

Intrauterine, Transplacental, or Ascending

- Virus must traverse several barriers to infect fetus from maternal viremia
  - Trophoblast, villous stroma, capillaries
- Trophoblast cells are highly resistant to viral infection
  - Attenuate viral replication by induction of autophagy
- Viruses may infect placenta from implantation site endometrium
- Virus present within vagina or cervix may ascend to infect amniotic fluid

Intrapartum

- Via exposure to infected blood or secretions during delivery

Postnatal

- Through physical contact or breast milk

CLINICAL IMPLICATIONS

Clinical Presentation

- Intrauterine viral infection may result in spontaneous abortion, stillbirth, prematurity, growth restriction, and malformations
  - Direct cell injury may result in tissue necrosis and is possibly responsible for congenital malformations
  - Infants often have persistent infection after birth and prolonged viral shedding
  - Infection of placenta may or may not be associated with fetal infection

MACROSCOPIC FINDINGS

General Features

- Villitis is rarely gross diagnosis
  - Placenta may have a pale granular or coarse appearance
  - Small yellow-white areas of agglutinated villi or regions of villous atrophy may be present
  - Thickened layer of fibrinoid is frequently noted at maternal surface associated with villitis
- Hydrops may be present with pale, spongy, thickened placental parenchyma

Villitis and Intervillositis

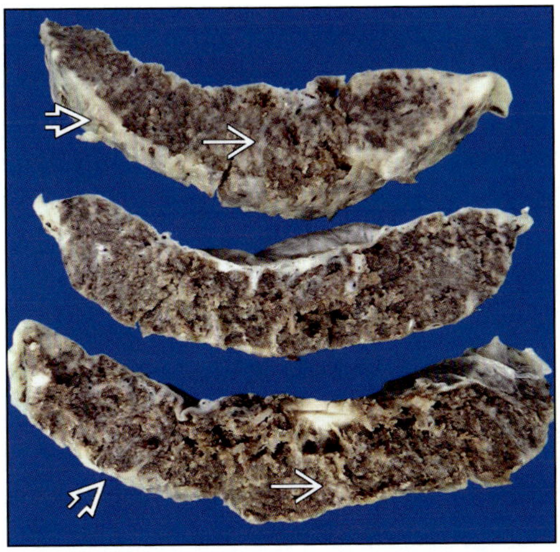

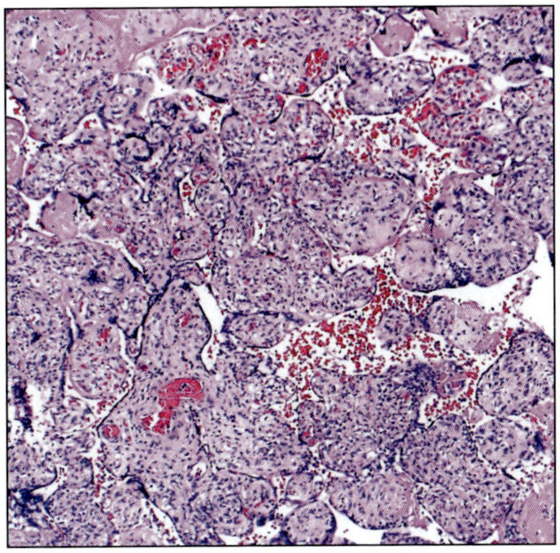

(Left) *Diffuse chronic villitis may be associated with a granular cut surface. There is increased fibrin deposition with the parenchyma* ➔ *and on the maternal surface* ➔*.* ***(Right)*** *Most viral infections are spread to the placenta during maternal viremia. The villi may have neutrophilic, lymphocytic, histiocytic, granulomatous, or plasmacytic inflammation. This case of villitis of undetermined etiology (VUE) is similar to infectious villitis but is usually only lymphohistiocytic.*

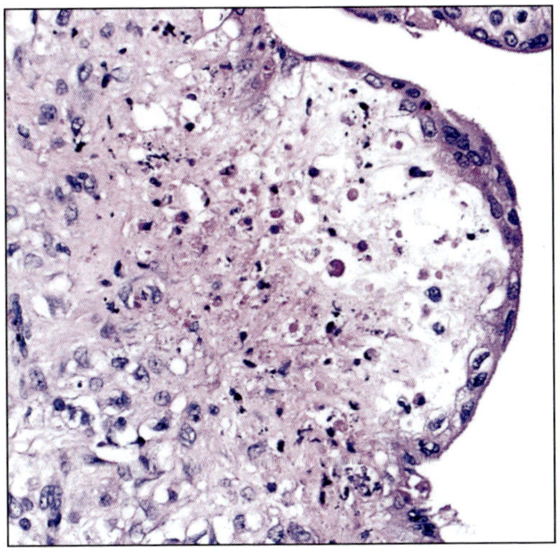

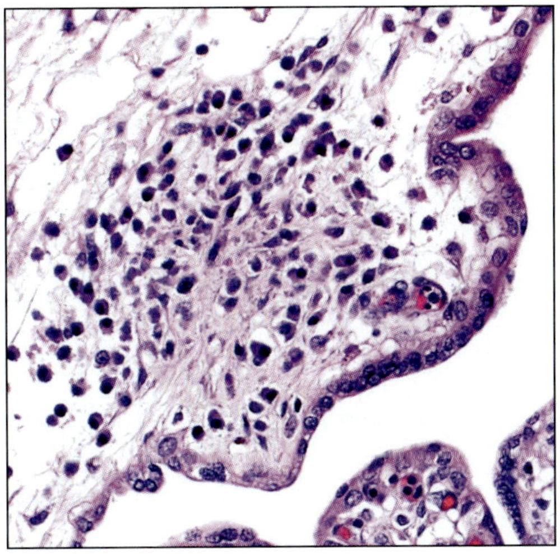

(Left) *Necrotizing villitis is shown here in a case of transplacentally acquired herpes simplex virus.* ***(Right)*** *Lymphoplasmacytic villitis is characteristic of cytomegalovirus (CMV) infection. If no inclusions are identified, an immunohistochemistry stain for CMV or PCR for the virus from formalin-fixed, paraffin-embedded tissue may be useful to confirm the infection.*

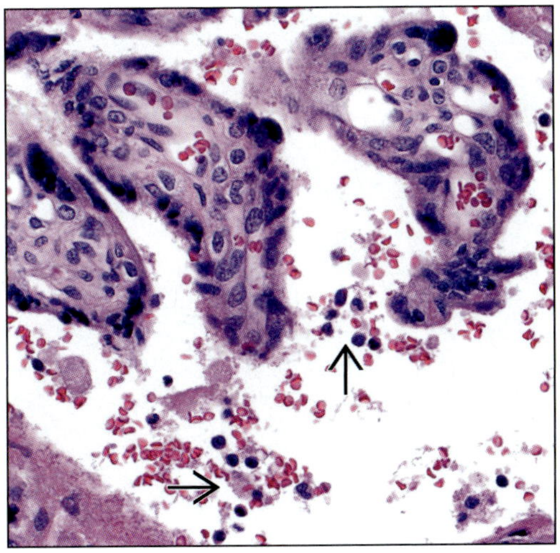

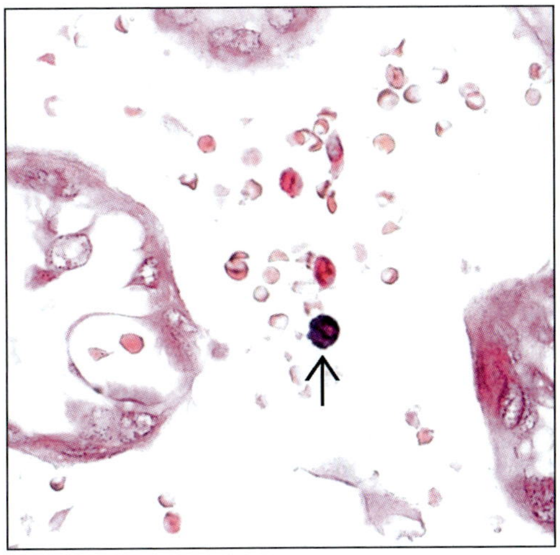

(Left) *The placenta from a case wherein Epstein-Barr virus (EBV) was suspected to have been vertically transmitted to the fetus has an increase in mononuclear cells* ➔ *within the intervillous space.* ***(Right)*** *This in situ hybridization study for EBV (EBV-encoded RNA1 [EBER]) shows a rare positive mononuclear cell* ➔ *in the maternal intervillous space. Finding EBV in the placenta does not necessarily indicate fetal infection.*

OTHER VIRUSES

Varicella-Zoster Virus Infection

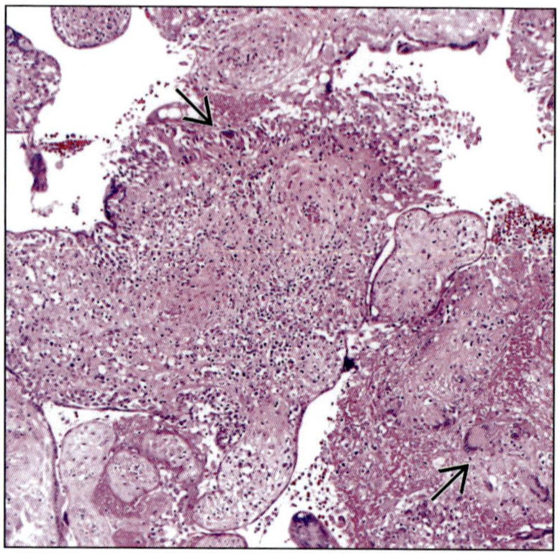

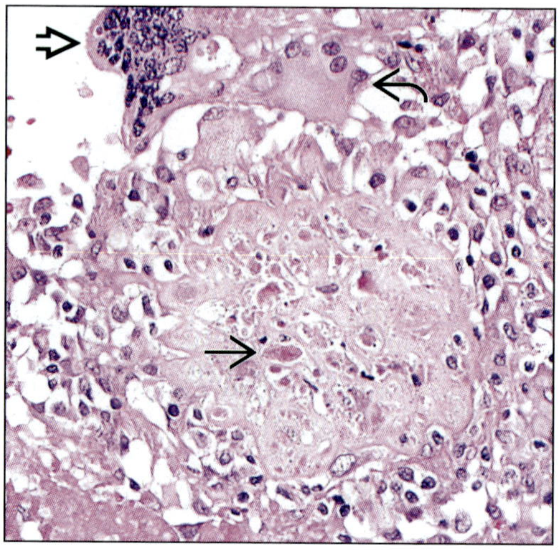

(Left) *In this case, VZV infection is the etiology of fetal demise at 17 weeks gestation. The villi have diffuse granulomatous, necrotizing villitis with Langhans-type multinucleated giant cells* →. ***(Right)*** *H&E shows VZV infection with eosinophilic inclusions* → *in Hofbauer cells. Syncytiotrophoblasts* ⇨ *are usually easily distinguished from Langhans-type multinucleated histiocytic giant cells* ↶.

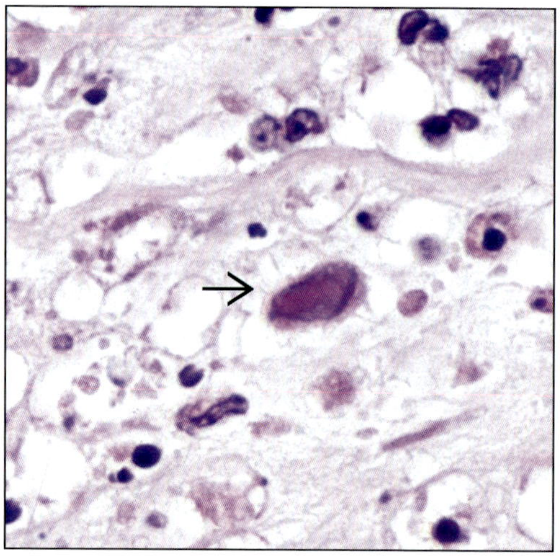

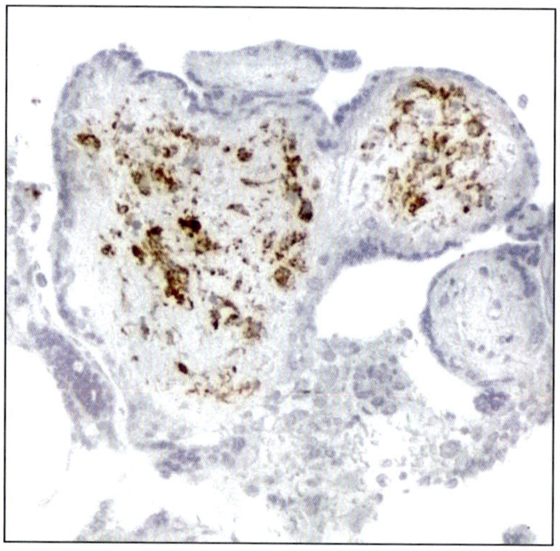

(Left) *H&E of VZV infection shows classic herpes viral inclusion* → *with eosinophilic intranuclear inclusion and peripheral condensed nuclear chromatin.* ***(Right)*** *Immunohistochemistry for VZV is strongly positive within the necrotic villous stromal cells.*

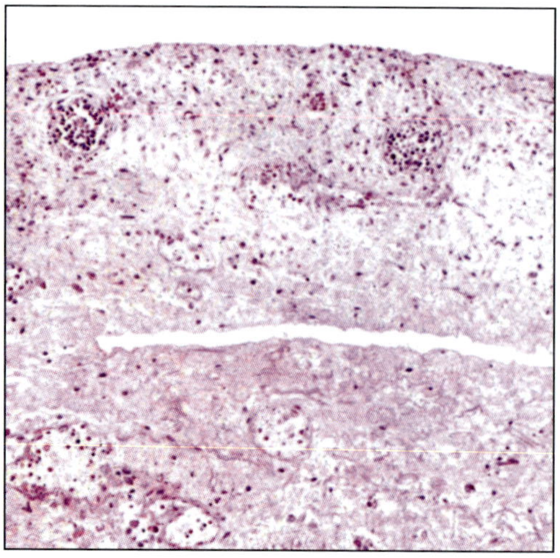

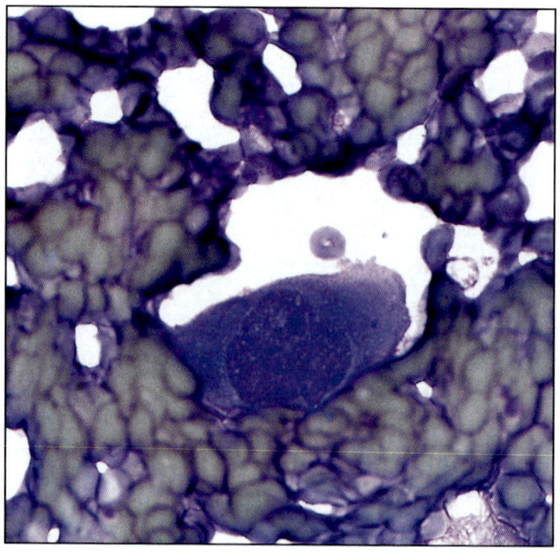

(Left) *In this case, VZV infection in the 1st trimester resulted in fetal demise. Even though markedly macerated, the skin shows cellular changes that are suggestive of herpes infection. This same section was strongly positive with immunohistochemistry.* ***(Right)*** *Tzanck preparation from skin lesions of herpes zoster virus (shingles) has multinucleated viral infected cells indistinguishable from other herpesviruses. The skin lesions of shingles are infectious to those who are not immune.*

Other Viral Infections

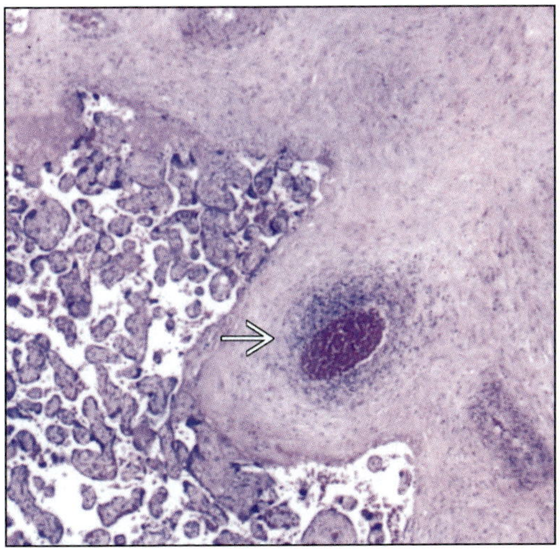
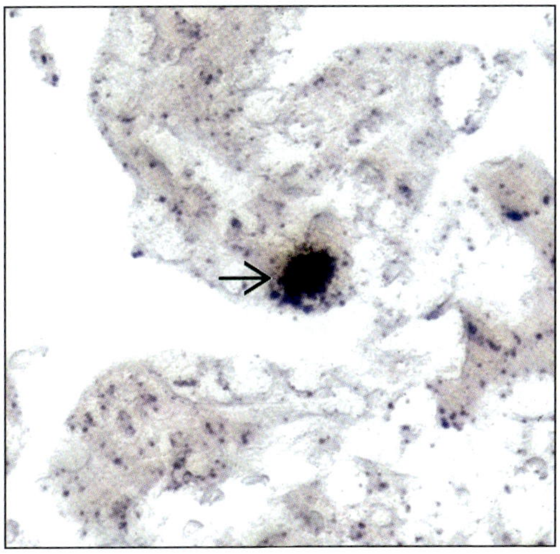

(Left) *Placenta from a case of vertical HIV transmission in utero shows a single focus of chronic vasculitis ➔ noted within a large stem villus.* ***(Right)*** *This image shows an in situ hybridization study for HIV p24 messenger RNA in the placenta from an HIV-infected mother. A placental Hofbauer cell ➔ is positive.*

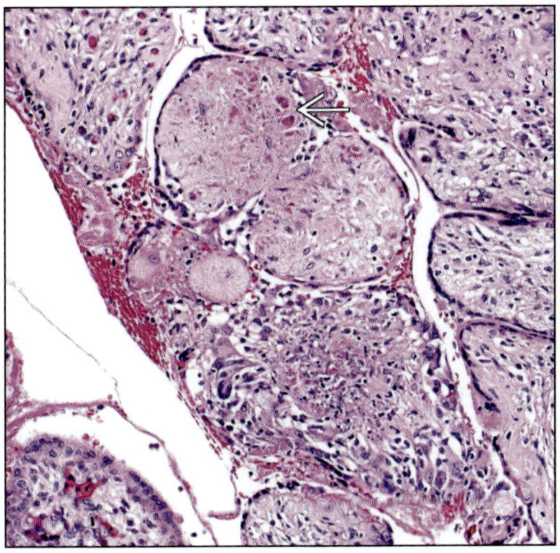
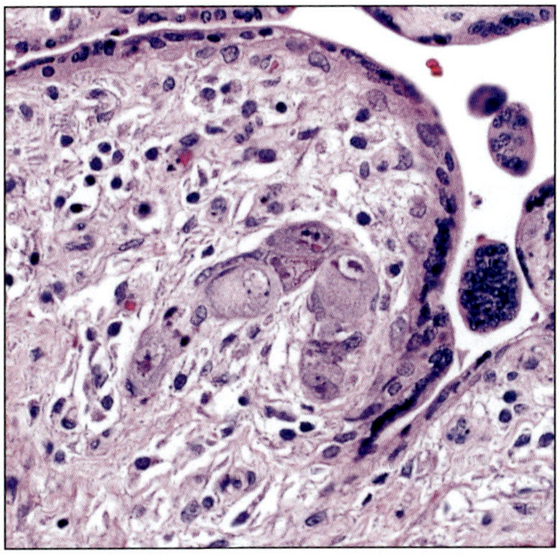

(Left) *Granulomatous and necrotizing villitis is present in this case of reactivation of CMV infection in the presence of HIV coinfection. Multiple eosinophilic cells ➔ suspicious for CMV inclusions are present.* ***(Right)*** *A large number of CMV inclusions are noted in this villus from a patient with coinfection of HIV and CMV.*

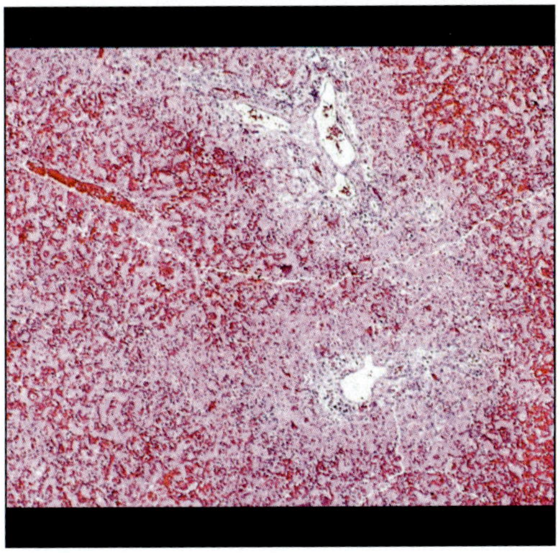
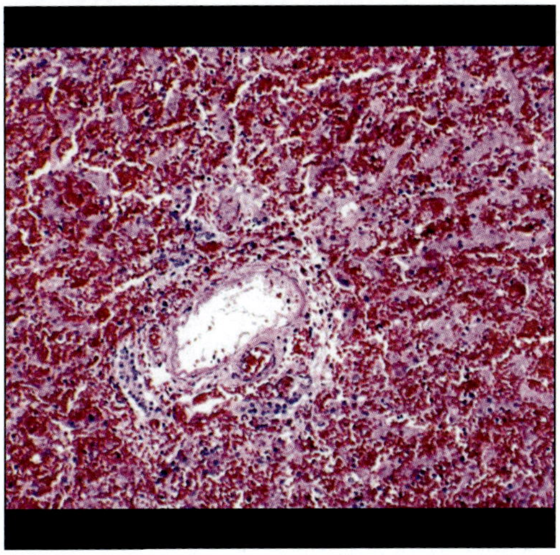

(Left) *Congenital echovirus infection may have massive hepatic necrosis, as shown here.* ***(Right)*** *In massive hemorrhagic hepatic necrosis due to congenital echovirus infection, neither significant inflammation nor viral inclusions are seen.*

SYPHILIS

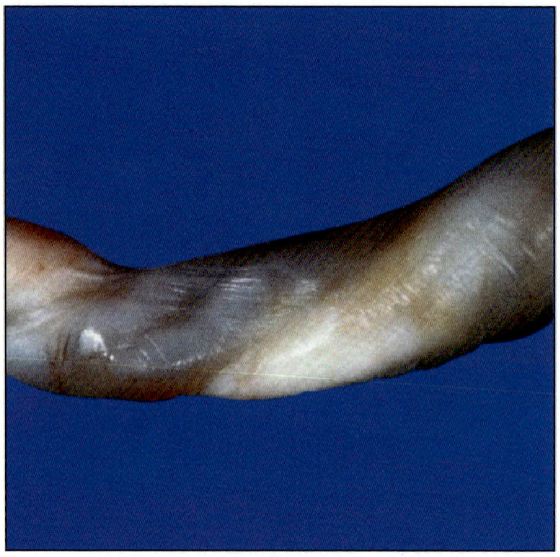

Gross image shows a "barber pole" appearance of the umbilical cord that is due to the accumulation of calcified necrotic debris around the vessels.

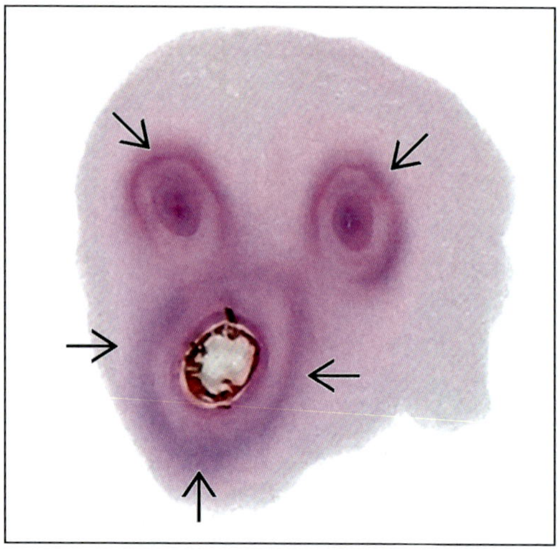

Section of the umbilical cord with necrotizing funisitis shows inflammation that is amniotropic → and oriented toward the amniotic cavity. These changes may be focal, often at the placental end.

TERMINOLOGY

Synonyms

- Treponemal infection

Definitions

- Congenital syphilis is usually acquired in utero during maternal spirochetemia
  - Rarely acquired during delivery through contact with infectious maternal blood or genital lesions

ETIOLOGY/PATHOGENESIS

Infectious Agents

- *Treponema pallidum*

Inadequate Treatment

- Most cases are result of no or inadequate treatment during pregnancy

CLINICAL ISSUES

Epidemiology

- Incidence
  - 10.1 per 100,000 live births
  - Significantly higher in southern United States
- Age
  - More common in young pregnant women (< 19 years of age)
- Ethnicity
  - African Americans more commonly affected

Presentation

- Transmission occurs during all trimesters of pregnancy and at all stages of disease
  - May not see a significant inflammatory response early in gestation
  - Incidence of transmission
    - 50% in primary and secondary syphilis
    - 40-80% in early latent syphilis
    - 30% in late syphilis
- 2/3 of infected infants are asymptomatic at birth
  - Early signs include characteristic vesiculobullous or erythematous maculopapular rash on hands and feet
- 30-40% of infected infants are stillborn
- High incidence of prematurity and intrauterine growth restriction

MACROSCOPIC FEATURES

General Features

- Placenta is thick, friable, and frequently pale
- Umbilical cord has characteristic "barber pole" appearance due to chalky white necrotic debris that partially surrounds vessels in amniotropic fashion

MICROSCOPIC PATHOLOGY

Histologic Features

- Umbilical cord
  - Severe necrotizing funisitis is seen in 50% of cases
    - More common in intrauterine fetal demise (IUFD)
  - Degeneration of inflammatory cells (neutrophils, lymphocytes, plasma cells, and macrophages) in Wharton jelly
  - Spirochetes present in cases that have not received antibiotics during gestation or labor, or in fetuses that are stillborn prior to antibiotic therapy
- Villi
  - Rarely has chronic lymphoplasmacytic villitis
  - Increased fibrosis around fetal stem vessels may be a feature of fetal demise rather than infection
  - Increased nucleated red blood cells
  - Villous edema
  - Increased Hofbauer cells
- Membranes

SYPHILIS

Key Facts

Etiology

- Most cases are result of no or inadequate treatment during pregnancy

Clinical Issues

- High incidence of intrauterine fetal demise (IUFD)
- Transmission occurs during all trimesters of pregnancy and at all stages of disease

Macroscopic Pathology

- Umbilical cord has characteristic "barber pole" appearance due to chalky white necrotic debris that partially surrounds vessels in amniotropic fashion

Microscopic Pathology

- Severe necrotizing funisitis is seen in 50% of cases
  - More common in IUFD
- Spirochetes present in cases that have not received antibiotics during gestation or labor, or in fetuses that are stillborn prior to antibiotic therapy
- Rarely has chronic lymphoplasmacytic villitis
- Increased fibrosis around fetal stem vessels may be a feature of fetal demise rather than infection
- Increased nucleated red blood cells
- Commonly has increased lymphocytes and plasma cells in decidua
- Organisms are disseminated to nearly all organs
- Inflammatory response occurs in perivascular connective tissue rather than parenchyma
- Lung, bone, liver, pancreas, small bowel, kidney, and spleen are most severely affected
- There is diffuse extramedullary hematopoiesis

  - Rarely associated with chorioamnionitis, which is usually due to another organism
- Decidua
  - Commonly has increased lymphocytes and plasma cells
- Congenital syphilis
  - Organisms are disseminated to nearly all organs
  - Inflammatory response occurs in perivascular connective tissue rather than parenchyma
  - Lung, bone, liver, pancreas, small bowel, kidney, and spleen are most severely affected
  - There is diffuse extramedullary hematopoiesis

ANCILLARY TESTS

Histochemistry

- Warthin-Starry stain
  - Difficult stain to interpret due to background staining of necrotic debris
  - Organisms most frequently found in necrotic debris

Immunohistochemistry

- Useful in cases where there are few organisms
- Monoclonal or polyclonal anti-*T. pallidum* antibodies available

DIFFERENTIAL DIAGNOSIS

Other Forms of Villitis

- Cytomegalovirus (CMV)
  - Usually associated with lymphoplasmacytic villitis
    - Rarely has funisitis
- Herpes simplex virus (HSV)
  - May have plasma cell rich infiltrates in membranes, umbilical cord
- Villitis of undetermined etiology (VUE)
  - Usually associated with lymphohistiocytic villitis
    - No funisitis

DIAGNOSTIC CHECKLIST

Clinically Relevant Pathologic Features

- Necrotizing funisitis

Pathologic Interpretation Pearls

- All cases of necrotizing funisitis need to be correlated with maternal syphilis serology

SELECTED REFERENCES

1. Newman L et al: Global estimates of syphilis in pregnancy and associated adverse outcomes: analysis of multinational antenatal surveillance data. PLoS Med. 10(2):e1001396, 2013
2. Kakogawa J et al: Prolonged fetal bradycardia as the presenting clinical sign in congenital syphilis complicated by necrotizing funisitis: a case report. ISRN Obstet Gynecol 2011:320246, 2011
3. Centers for Disease Control and Prevention (CDC): Congenital syphilis - United States, 2003-2008. MMWR Morb Mortal Wkly Rep. 59(14):413-7, 2010
4. Genest DR et al: Diagnosis of congenital syphilis from placental examination: comparison of histopathology, Steiner stain, and polymerase chain reaction for Treponema pallidum DNA. Hum Pathol. 27(4):366-72, 1996
5. Schwartz DA et al: Pathology of the umbilical cord in congenital syphilis: analysis of 25 specimens using histochemistry and immunofluorescent antibody to Treponema pallidum. Hum Pathol. 26(7):784-91, 1995
6. Qureshi F et al: Placental histopathology in syphilis. Hum Pathol. 24(7):779-84, 1993

SYPHILIS

Gross and Microscopic Features

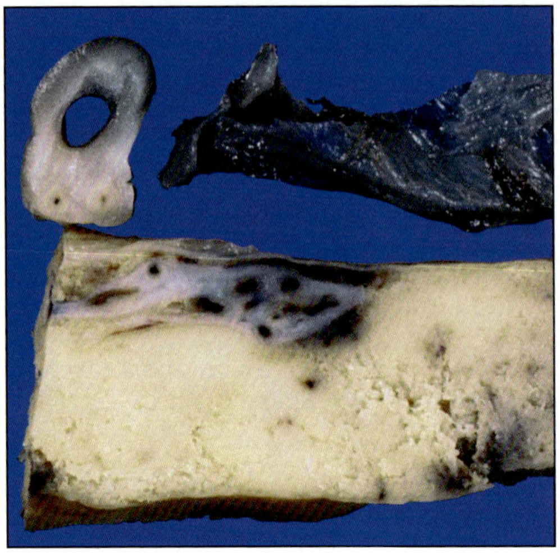
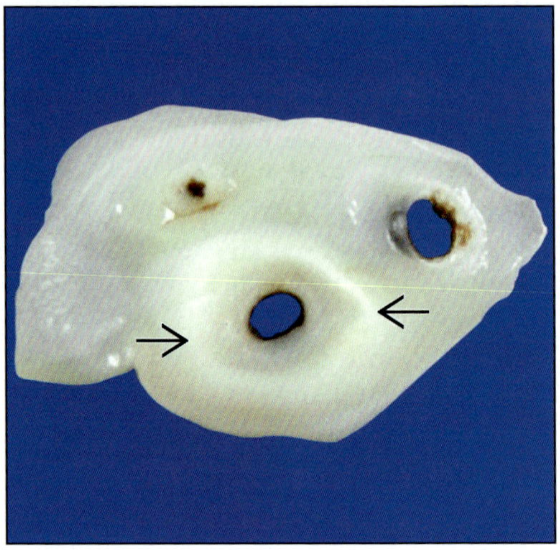

(Left) *Placenta associated with congenital syphilis is very pale. This segment of umbilical cord does not have necrotizing funisitis.* ***(Right)*** *Umbilical cord section with necrotizing funisitis shows that the chalky necrotic debris* ➔ *is most easily seen around the umbilical vein.*

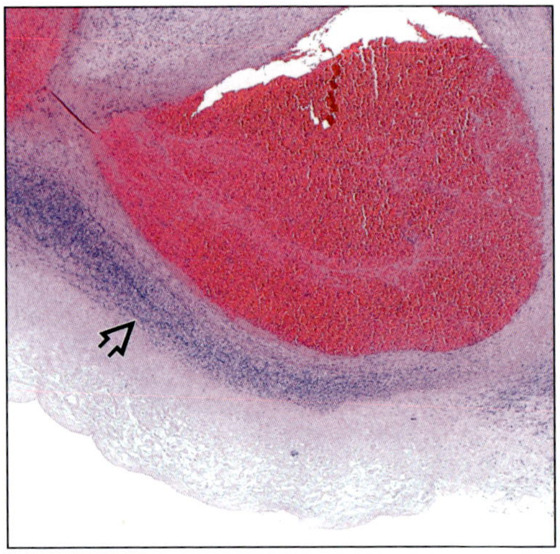
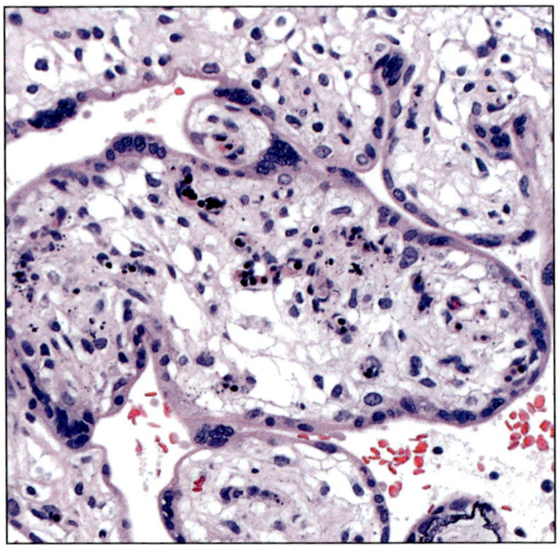

(Left) *The necrotic debris* ⇨ *is seen outside the vessel wall in Wharton jelly. The vessel may thrombose due to the severe inflammation and become devitalized.* ***(Right)*** *There may be a marked increase in nucleated red blood cells within the fetal circulation in congenital syphilis.*

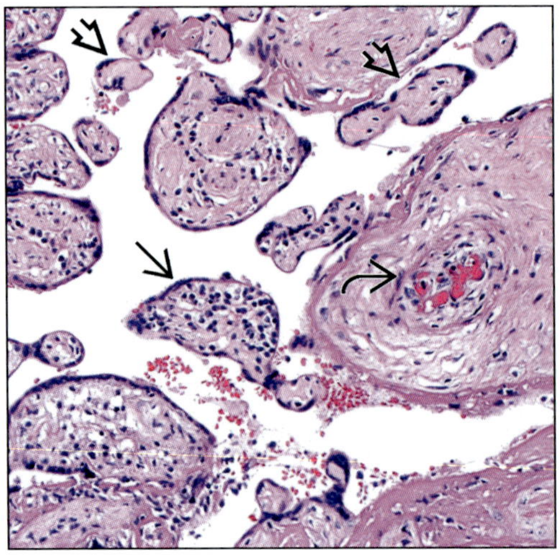
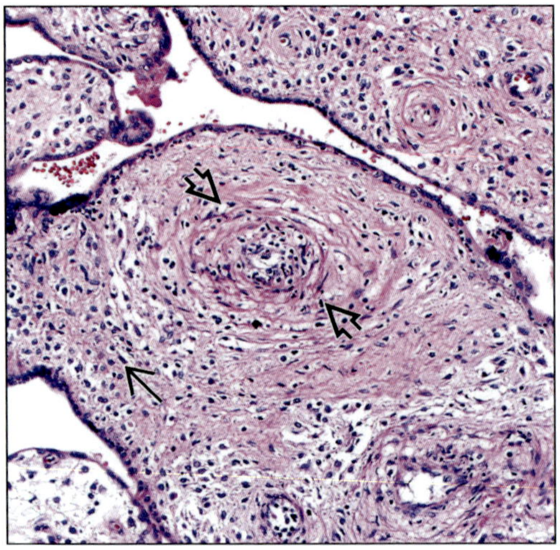

(Left) *Lymphoplasmacytic villitis* ➔ *is an uncommon finding in syphilis. There are also avascular villi* ⇨ *that may be secondary to fibroblast proliferation within the adjacent stem vessel* ↷*.* ***(Right)*** *This stem villus has lymphocytic villitis* ➔ *and is associated with chronic inflammation of the stem vessel, which also shows concentric fibroblast proliferation* ⇨*.*

Features of Congenital Syphilis

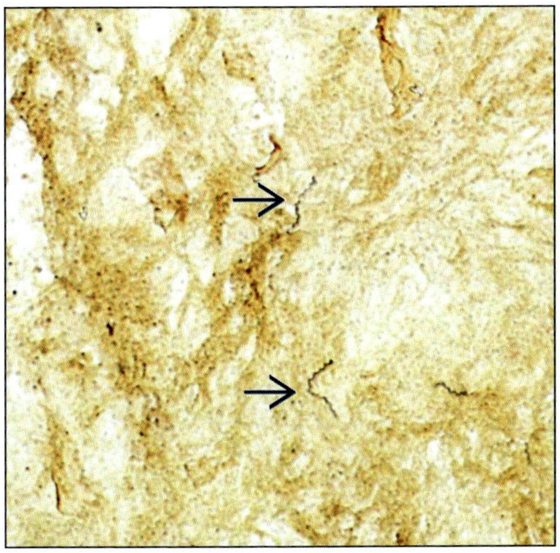

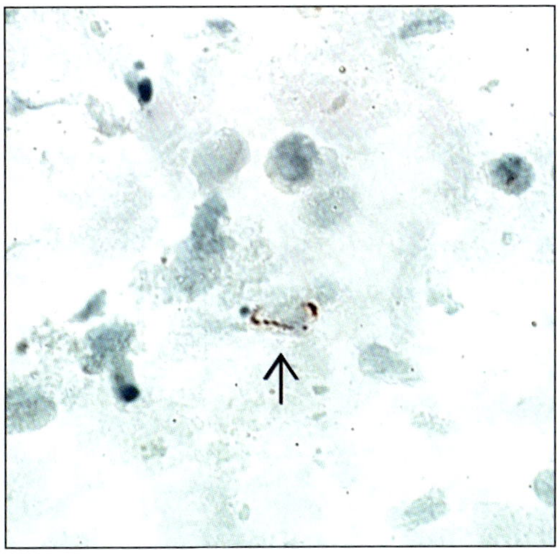

(Left) *Warthin-Starry staining shows several spirochetes* → *from the umbilical cord of a stillborn.* ***(Right)*** *Immunohistochemistry for Treponema pallidum may be useful in identifying rare organisms* →*.*

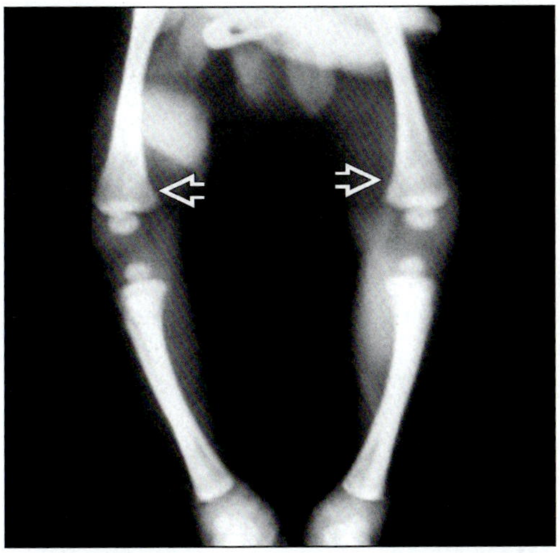

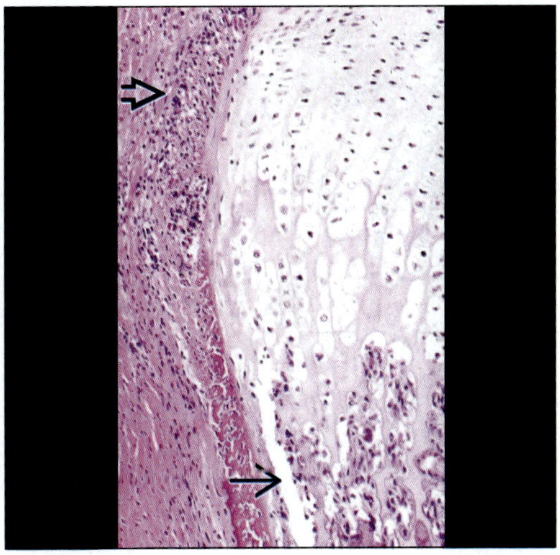

(Left) *Marked flaring of the epiphyses* ➡ *is noted in the case of congenital syphilis. Osteochondritis is a common complication of untreated congenital syphilis and may present with symptoms of osteomyelitis.* ***(Right)*** *A decalcified section from the femoral epiphysis from a fetus with congenital syphilis shows growth disturbance with loss of the marrow free zone* →*. A large number of plasma cells* ⇨ *are seen in the periosteum.*

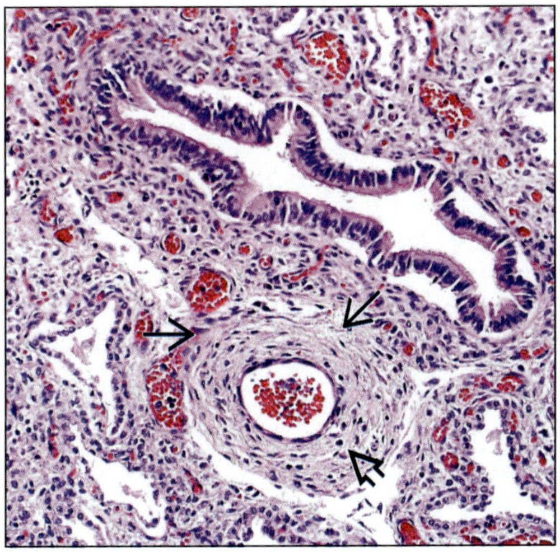

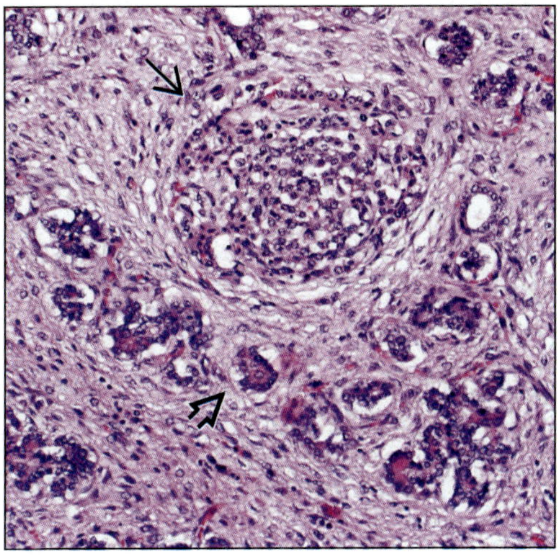

(Left) *Pneumonia alba is characteristic of congenital syphilis. Increased perivascular fibrosis* → *is noted and a rare plasma cell* ⇨ *is present.* ***(Right)*** *Another characteristic feature of congenital syphilis is marked fibrosis within the pancreas involving both islets* → *and acinar* ⇨ *components. Extramedullary hematopoiesis may also be a prominent feature in this location.*

COCCIDIOIDOMYCOSIS

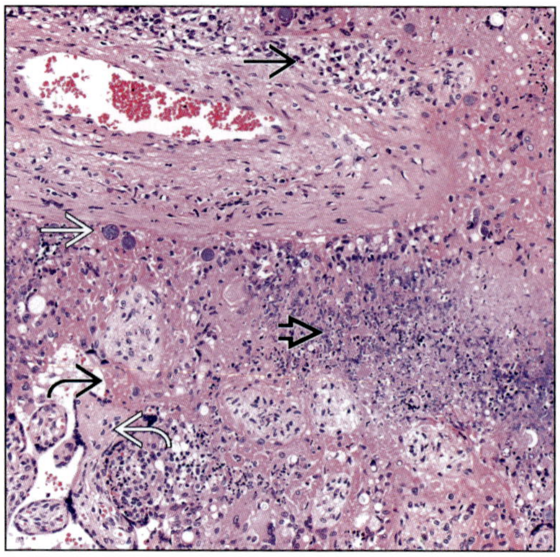

Grossly evident infarcts show a lymphohistiocytic chronic villitis ➡, intervillous organisms ➡, increased fibrin ➡, purulent foci ➡, and adjacent sclerotic villi ➡.

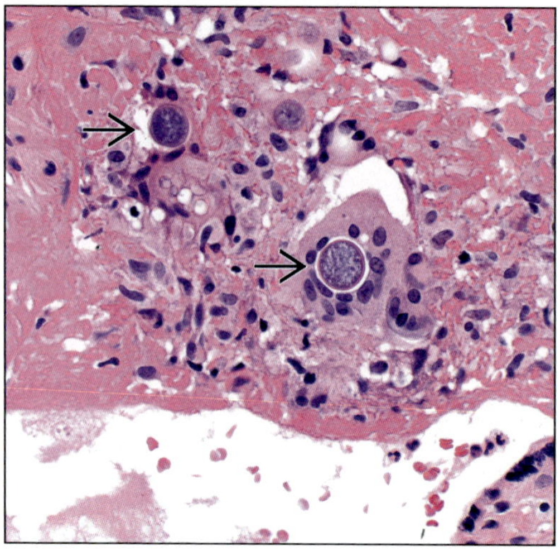

Intervillous fibrin and a maternal foreign body giant cell reaction encases foci with spherules of *Coccidioides immitis* ➡.

TERMINOLOGY

Synonyms

- *Coccidioides immitis*, Valley fever

Definitions

- Soil-borne fungus found mostly in southwestern United States and northern Mexico

CLINICAL ISSUES

Presentation

- Disseminated infection in pregnant mother
- Diagnosis usually clinically obvious in endemic areas

Prognosis

- Despite massive placental burden, transmission to fetus is uncommon

MACROSCOPIC FEATURES

General Features

- Numerous parenchymal tan lesions on cut section
- Variably increased parenchymal fibrin

MICROSCOPIC PATHOLOGY

Histologic Features

- Umbilical cord
  - No fetal inflammatory response
  - Fetal inflammatory response suggests coinfection with ascending chorioamnionitis
- Membranes
  - No significant inflammation of chorion or amnion
  - Chorioamnionitis suggests coinfection with ascending organism
- Villous parenchyma
  - Multiple intervillous and perivillous foci of infection
    - Increased fibrin
    - Abscesses rich in neutrophils and purulent debris
    - Acute villitis is not common
    - Endospore containing spherules (10-100 μm in size) of *C. immitis* visible on H&E stain
    - Foreign body giant cell reaction to spherules
    - Lymphohistiocytic chronic villitis with involution of fetal vasculature in adjacent villi
    - Stainable organisms may be absent if mother treated with antifungal drugs during pregnancy
- Decidua
  - Variable inflammation
  - Abscesses not commonly seen
  - Inhalation of infected decidua postulated as cause of perinatal infection

ANCILLARY TESTS

Histochemistry

- Gomori methenamine silver (GMS), spherules also visible on H&E
  - Reactivity: Positive

DIFFERENTIAL DIAGNOSIS

Other Fungal Infections

- *Candida albicans*
  - Most common fungal infection of placenta
  - Ascending chorioamnionitis pattern with peripheral funisitis
  - Typically does not have villitis or intervillositis component
  - Hyphae visible in affected areas
- *Cryptococcosis neoformans*
  - Rarely seen in placenta
  - Opportunistic infection occurs in severely immunocompromised patients

COCCIDIOIDOMYCOSIS

Key Facts

Macroscopic Pathology
- Tan lesions resembling infarcts on cut section
- Increased fibrin

Microscopic Pathology
- Intervillous and perivillous foci of infection with numerous large fungal spherules
- Adjacent chronic villitis with increased perivillous fibrin, avascular villi
- Foreign body giant cell reaction to spherules
- Intervillous neutrophilic exudate with necrosis

Reporting Considerations
- Despite the heavy placental burden, transmission to fetus is rare
- Fetal inflammatory response is uncommon
  - If present, suggests possible exposure of fetus to *Coccidioides* or concomitant ascending chorioamnionitis

---

  - Yeast buds are 5-10 μm, smaller than spherules of *Coccidioides*
  - Rare reported cases describe intervillous yeasts with minimal inflammation
- *Blastomyces dermatitidis*
  - Rarely seen in placenta
  - Broad-based budding yeasts 10-15 μm in size, smaller than large spherules of *Coccidioides*
  - Reported cases describe chronic villitis and intervillous granulomatous inflammation in a subset of infected mothers
  - Transplacental infection described in ~ 10% of cases, with high infant mortality

Acute Viral Placentitis
- Lymphoplasmacytic villitis, with some villous necrosis and neutrophils in acute cytomegalovirus or HSV infection

Other Infections With Hematogenous Spread
- Tuberculosis
  - Villous and intervillous granulomas, bacilli may be hard to find
- Listeriosis
  - Villous and intervillous abscesses often associated with chorioamnionitis
- Toxoplasmosis
  - Lymphoplasmacytic villitis, with toxoplasma cysts beneath amnion and in cord stroma

DIAGNOSTIC CHECKLIST

Clinically Relevant Pathologic Features
- Fetal inflammatory response (umbilical or chorionic acute vasculitis) is uncommon
  - If present, suggests possible exposure of fetus to *Coccidioides* or concomitant ascending chorioamnionitis

Pathologic Interpretation Pearls
- Large intervillous abscesses with numerous fungal spherules and excess fibrin deposition

SELECTED REFERENCES

1. Youssef D et al: Pulmonary blastomycosis during pregnancy: case report and review of the literature. Tenn Med. 106(3):37-9, 2013
2. Patel M et al: Transplacental transmission of Cryptococcus neoformans to an HIV-exposed premature neonate. J Perinatol. 32(3):235-7, 2012
3. Hooper JE et al: Disseminated coccidioidomycosis in pregnancy. Arch Pathol Lab Med. 131(4):652-5, 2007
4. Crum NF et al: Coccidioidomycosis in pregnancy: case report and review of the literature. Am J Med. 119(11):993, 2006
5. Charlton V et al: Intrauterine transmission of coccidioidomycosis. Pediatr Infect Dis J. 18(6):561-3, 1999
6. Linsangan LC et al: Coccidioides immitis infection of the neonate: two routes of infection. Pediatr Infect Dis J. 18(2):171-3, 1999

MICROSCOPIC FEATURES

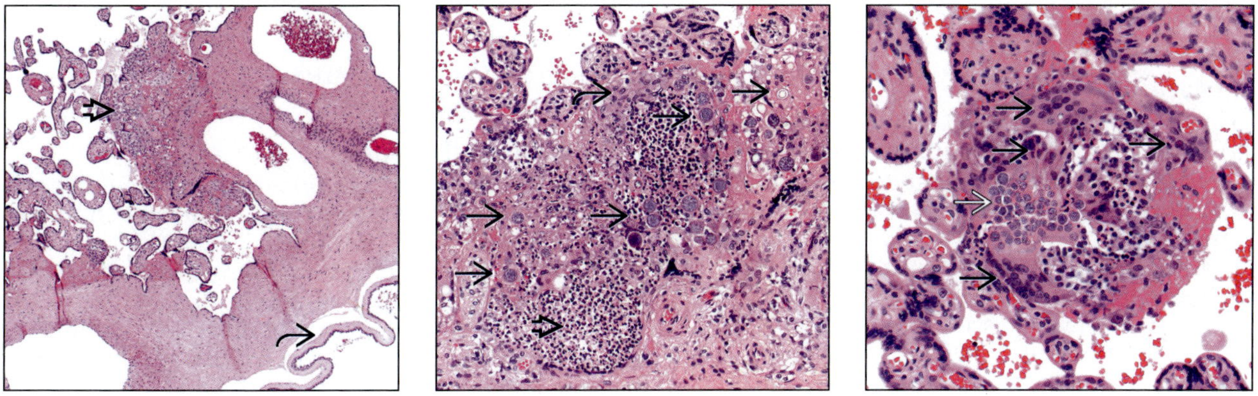

(Left) *Coccidioides immitis is a hematogenously spread infection to the placenta. Infection is confined to the intervillous space accompanied by chronic villitis, with sparing of the membranes and umbilical cord.* ***(Center)*** *Numerous fungal spherules are accompanied by a histiocytic response and neutrophilic exudate.* ***(Right)*** *A prominent foreign body giant cell reaction may be present, surrounding the organism.*

PARASITES

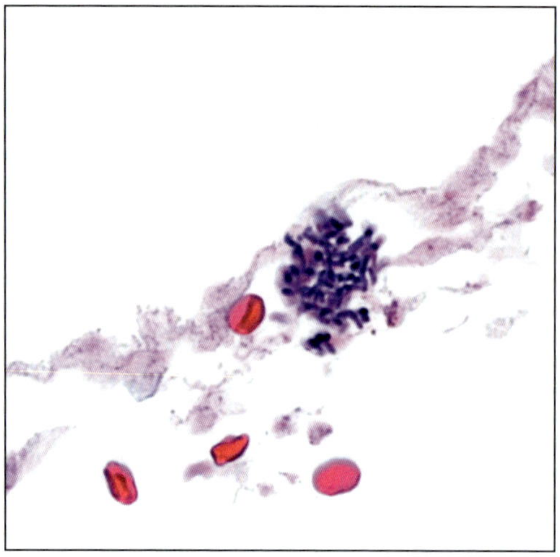

Crescent-shaped toxoplasmosis tachyzoites are present within the connective tissue of the placental membranes.

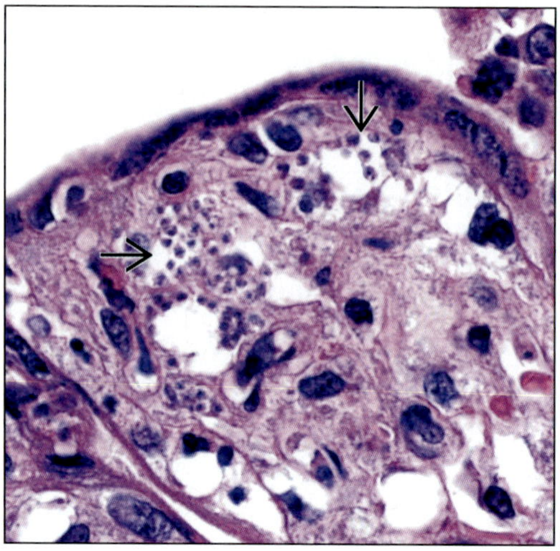

Chagas disease villitis shows numerous intracellular, 3-5 μm amastigotes ⇒ that have a kinetoplast on 1 end of the organism that stains darkly on routine H&E.

TERMINOLOGY

Definitions

- Hematogenous infection: Parasitemia spreads from maternal bloodstream into placental villi
  - Trophoblast epithelium, basal laminae, villous stroma, fetal capillary endothelium are crossed to infect fetal bloodstream
- Vertical transmission: Transmission from mother to child in utero, during delivery from cervical secretions, or postpartum through breast milk

TOXOPLASMOSIS

Toxoplasma gondii

- Ubiquitous obligate intracellular protozoan
  - 3 genotypes: Type II is most common, type I has higher pathogenicity
- Definitive host is cats; cows, pigs, sheep, bird eggs, and humans are intermediate hosts
- Humans usually infected from ingestion of undercooked meat containing cysts and less often from ingesting oocytes from feline feces
- Seroconversion risk is 3-5% per year; immunity is protective against vertical transmission
  - High incidence of false-positive IgM serology

Presentation

- Usually asymptomatic infection in normal host or mild viral-like illness in immunoincompetent host, reactivation possible in immunoincompetent host
- Parasitemic stage occurs 1-2 weeks after ingestion of oocytes or cysts
- Congenital toxoplasmosis occurs in 33-50% of parasitemic pregnant women
  - Risk for transmission varies with gestational age
    - 17% in 1st trimester, 25% in 2nd trimester, and 63% in 3rd trimester
  - Long delay between maternal infection and transmission may occur
  - Most cases are asymptomatic, but increased risk of intrauterine growth restriction (IUGR) and prematurity
  - 5-15% of cases are stillbirths, usually after infection early in pregnancy
  - Symptomatic infants may show hydrops, sepsis, hepatosplenomegaly, jaundice, petechiae, and eye and CNS abnormalities

Treatment

- Spiramycin treatment during pregnancy has questionable impact on outcome, may prevent spread across placenta
- Pyrimethamine, sulfadiazine, and folinic acid during pregnancy for confirmed fetal infection
- Neonatal treatment recommended, even when asymptomatic

Prognosis of Congenital Infection

- Stillbirth in 5-15%
- 85% of survivors have chorioretinitis and may develop unilateral or bilateral blindness
- 10-20% of survivors have hydrocephalus with diffuse intracranial calcifications, learning disorders, or severe intellectual disability

Macroscopic Features

- No specific features

Histologic Features

- Organisms are intracellular in amnion epithelial cells, stromal cells between amnion and chorion, and villous Hofbauer cells
- Pseudocysts contain many tachyzoites, appear round in section, 2 x 6 μm, central nucleus
- True cysts are round to oval in section and may contain hundreds of crescentic bradyzoites that are periodic acid-Schiff (PAS) positive

Malaria

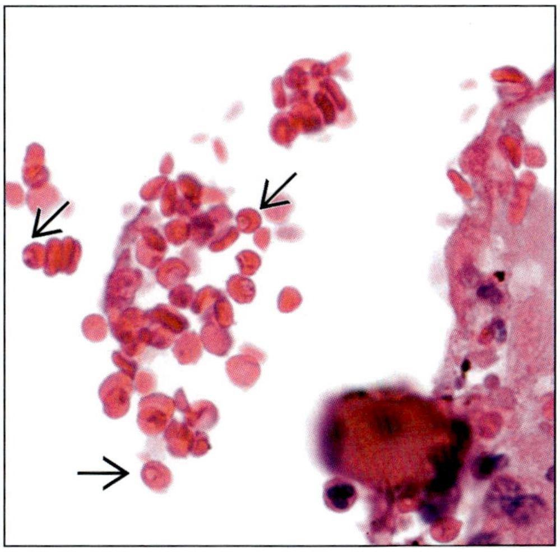
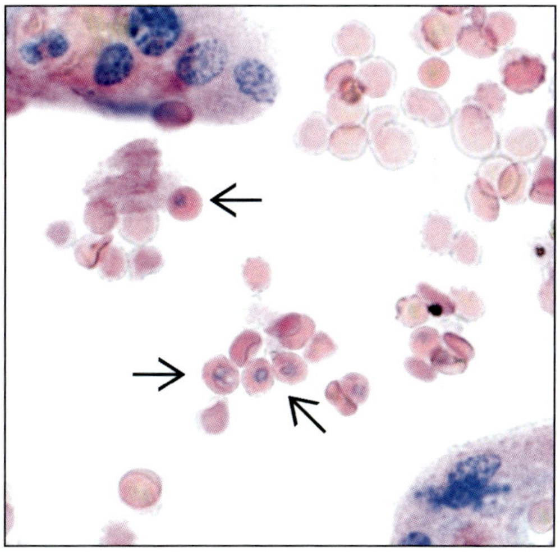

(Left) *Placental intervillous space in acute malaria shows only infected red blood cells. The organisms are difficult to see on an H&E stain and may appear only as vacuoles* →. **(Right)** *Thomas staining of the slide highlights the heavy parasitemia* → *of this case of primary falciparum malaria in a primigravida.*

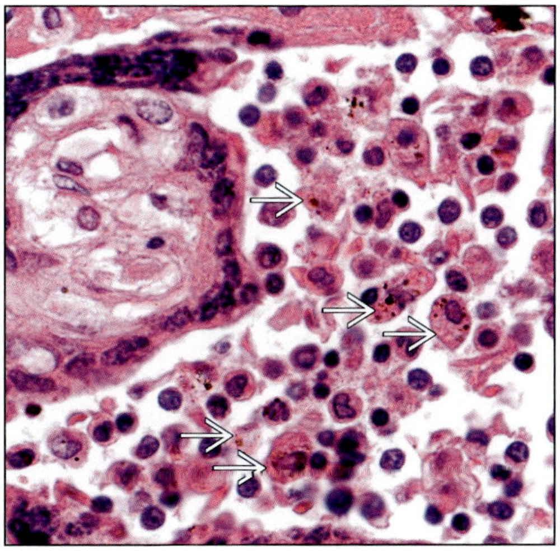
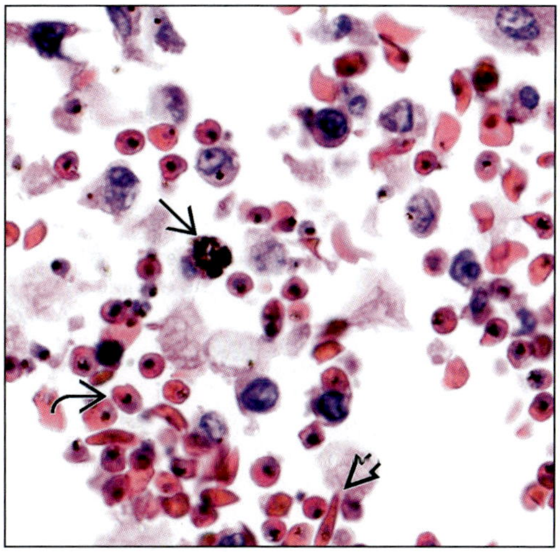

(Left) *Chronic malaria is usually associated with histiocytic intervillositis. The macrophages/histiocytes contain hemozoin pigment* →. **(Right)** *Chronic malaria may show parasites* → *and hemozoin pigment in red blood cells and to a lesser degree within histiocytes* →. *Note that there are sickled red blood cells* → *also present.*

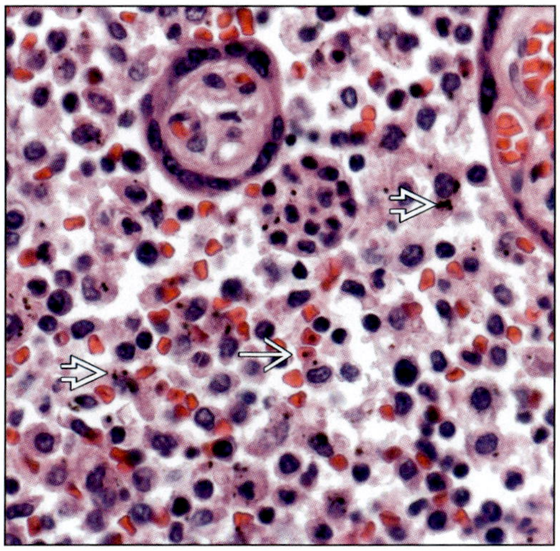
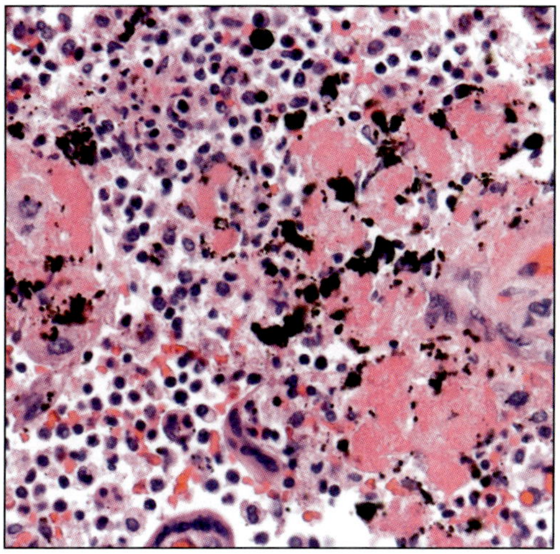

(Left) *Chronic or past infection often displays no parasites in red blood cells, but there may be massive histiocytic intervillositis. Hemozoin pigment is seen within red blood cells* → *and histiocytes* →. **(Right)** *This case of past malarial infection shows massive histiocytic intervillositis and abundant hemozoin pigment, mostly within histiocytes.*

Chronic Inflammatory Lesions

CELLULAR COMPOSITION OF CHRONIC INFLAMMATORY LESIONS

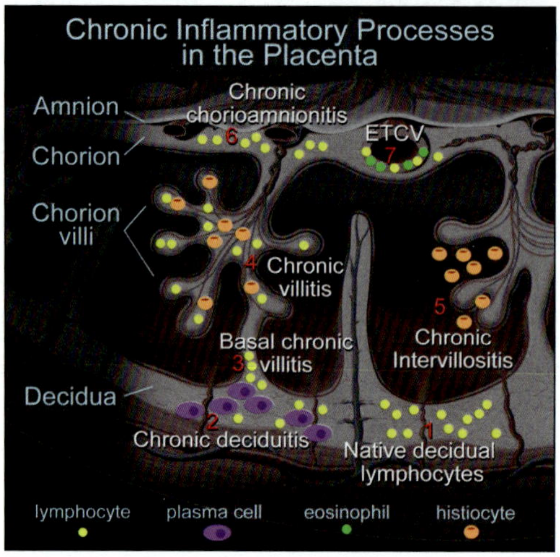

Chronic inflammatory cells occupy compartments of the placenta, including decidua (1 & 2), basal chorionic villi (3), chorionic villi (4), intervillous space (5), chorioamnion (6), and chorionic vessel (7).

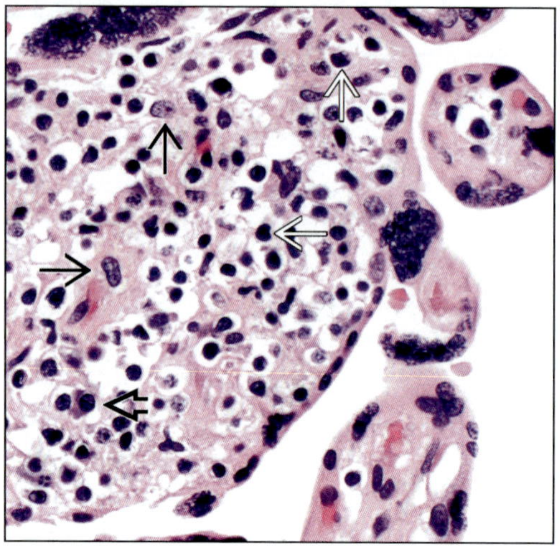

Cytomegaloviral chronic villitis (CV) in a pregnancy with known congenital cytomegalovirus shows 3 types of chronic inflammatory cells: Lymphocytes ➡, histiocytes →, and plasma cells ⇨.

TERMINOLOGY

Definitions

- Chronic inflammation can infiltrate fetal membranes, chorionic surface, and chorionic villi from blood perfusing maternal intervillous space or fetal vasculature
  - Rarely originates from fetal umbilical vessels in cord or chorionic surface

ETIOLOGY/PATHOGENESIS

Infectious Agents

- Chronic inflammatory infiltrates can be a response to infection or autoimmune/alloimmune processes
  - Cytomegalovirus placentitis may have numerous villous plasma cells
  - Herpes simplex virus placentitis may have numerous plasma cells in various locations including umbilical cord

CLINICAL ISSUES

Presentation

- Can correlate with
  - Preterm delivery
  - Intrauterine growth restriction
  - Recurrent abortion
  - Fetal demise in utero

Treatment

- No treatment is recognized for chronic inflammatory lesions of placenta
  - These lesions are not identified until examination of placenta
  - Some infections exhibiting chronic inflammatory lesions of placenta may be clinically evident and treated during pregnancy

Prognosis

- Can recur in subsequent pregnancies

MICROSCOPIC PATHOLOGY

Histologic Features

- Chronic inflammatory cells involved in various lesions include
  - Maternal lymphocytes
  - Fetal histiocytes
  - Eosinophils
  - Plasma cells
- Placental compartments that may contain chronic inflammatory cell infiltrates include
  - Chorionic villi
  - Intervillous space
  - Fetal amniochorion (fetal surface of placenta)
  - Maternal surface decidua
  - Free membranes
  - Fetal vessels of umbilical cord
  - Wharton jelly of umbilical cord

ANCILLARY TESTS

Immunohistochemistry

- CD3 for T lymphocytes
- CD68 for histiocytes

DIFFERENTIAL DIAGNOSIS

Infectious Placentitis

- Cytomegalovirus, herpes simplex virus, *Treponema pallidum*, and toxoplasmosis all may feature similar chronic inflammatory lesions on microscopy

Acute Inflammatory Lesions

- Acute chorioamnionitis

CHRONIC VILLITIS AND INTERVILLOSITIS

Microscopic Features

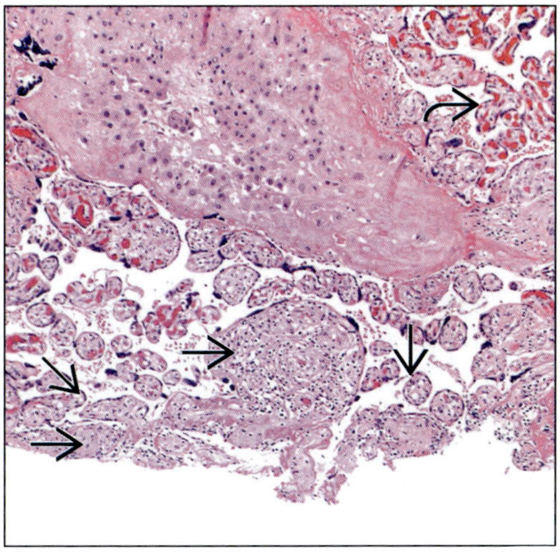
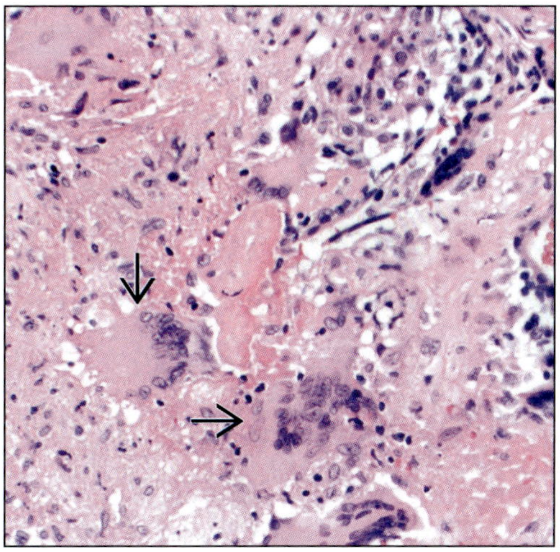

(Left) *Chronic villitis of unknown etiology can affect a placenta focally, multifocally, or extensively. Basal chronic villitis* → *is a common manifestation of focal or multifocal disease. Compared to unaffected villi* ↪*, they appear less vascular and peppered with lymphocytes.* ***(Right)*** *Multinucleated giant cells* → *are variably present in chronic villitis of unknown etiology. They have no known clinical significance within this entity.*

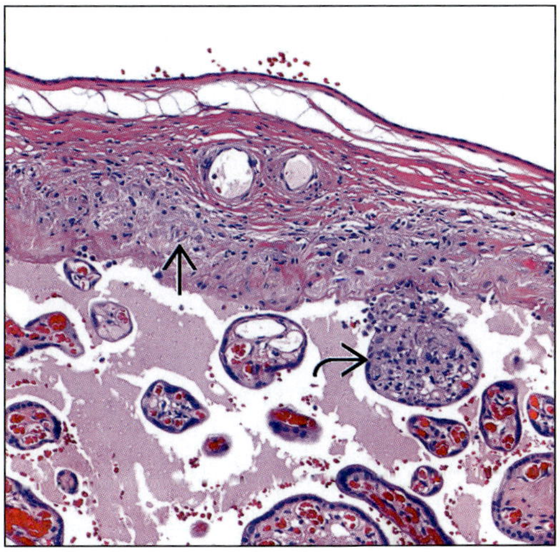
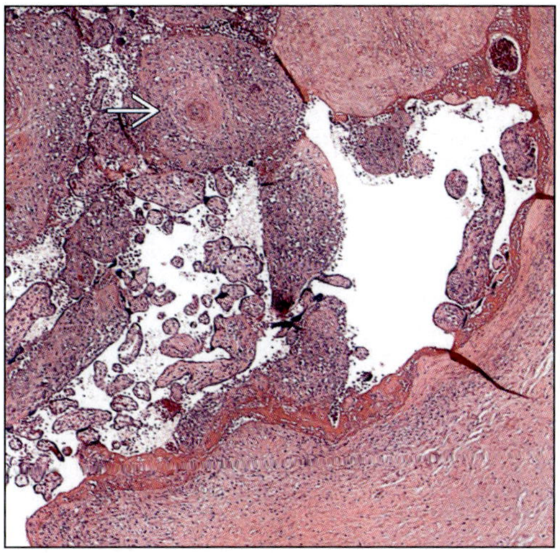

(Left) *In this case, chronic villitis* ↪ *accompanies a lymphohistiocytic infiltrate of the chorionic plate (chronic chorionitis)* →*. The related processes have been likened to a maternal rejection-type immune response against fetal antigens. Involvement of the chorionic plate does not necessarily imply infectious etiology.* ***(Right)*** *Chronic villitis involving the proximal stem villi* ➔ *is termed proximal chronic villitis. The stem villous vasculature may be obliterated.*

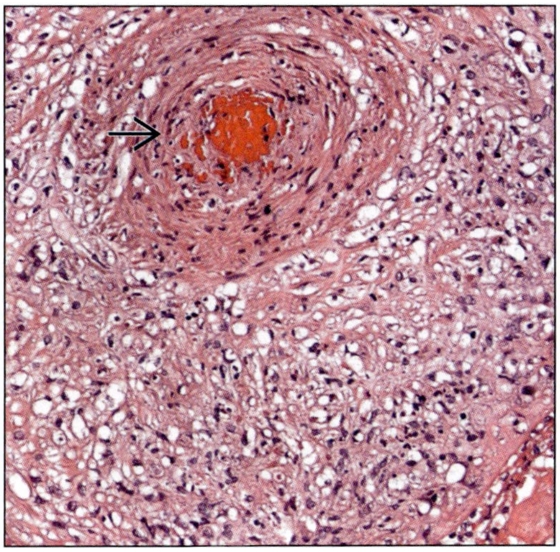
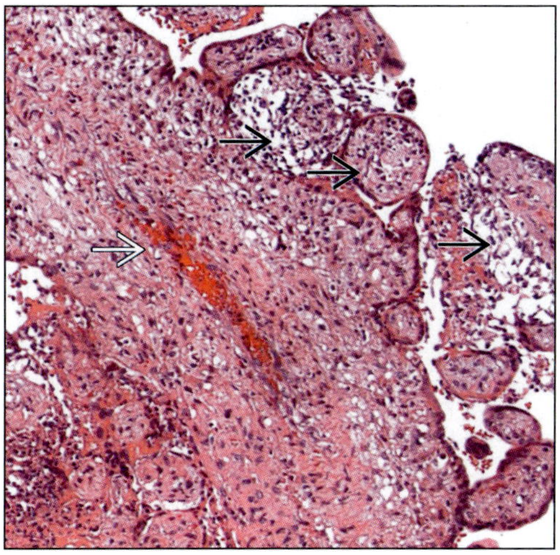

(Left) *Fetal vascular involution occurs in proximal chronic villitis* →*. The changes are similar to those of fetal thrombotic vasculopathy or after fetal demise. The reason for this change is unclear. It may be a mechanism to limit access of hematogenously spread organisms to the fetal vasculature.* ***(Right)*** *Proximal CV with associated fetal vasculopathy is shown. CV involves the terminal villi* → *and stem villus, with vascular involutional changes* ➔ *evidenced by the disrupted endothelium.*

CHRONIC VILLITIS AND INTERVILLOSITIS

Microscopic Features

(Left) *Avascular chorionic villi → are seen in chronic villitis with associated fetal vasculopathy. The presence of true thrombi would be diagnostic of a 2nd unrelated process, concurrent fetal thrombotic vasculopathy.* ***(Right)*** *In some cases of chronic villitis, the inflammation is intense. When admixed neutrophils or significant necrosis are present, lesions are called "active chronic villitis." Infection should be excluded.*

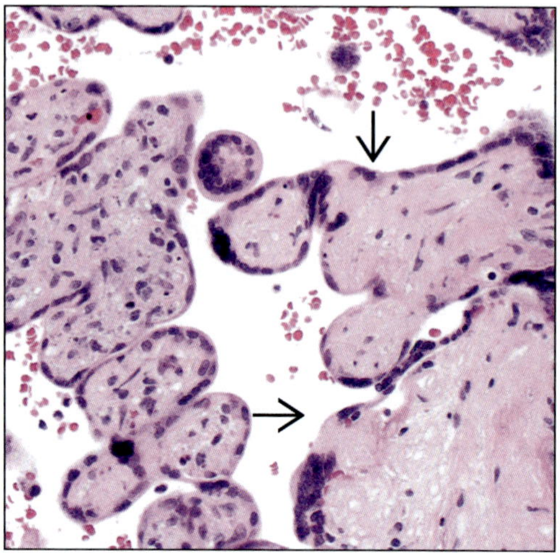

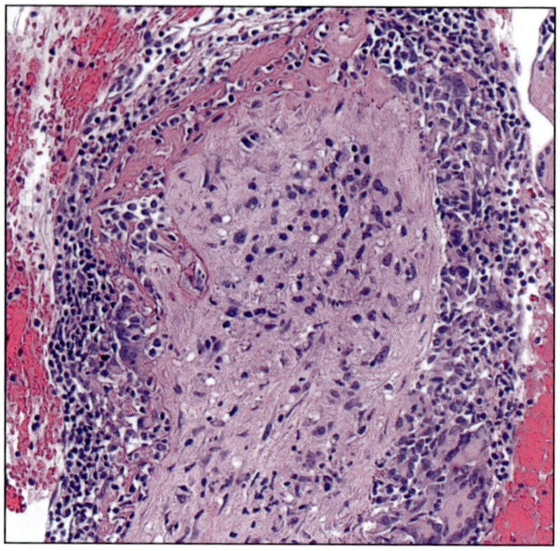

(Left) *This is CV with increased perivillous fibrin. Prolonged damage to the syncytiotrophoblast layer leads to perivillous fibrin deposition. The vessels ⇨ of these stem villi are sclerosed.* ***(Right)*** *The distinction between extensive CV with perivillous fibrin deposition and massive perivillous fibrin deposition (MPFD) can be difficult. These villi → of MPFD are surrounded by fibrin/fibrinoid with prominent extravillous trophoblasts ↶. Compression makes them appear more cellular.*

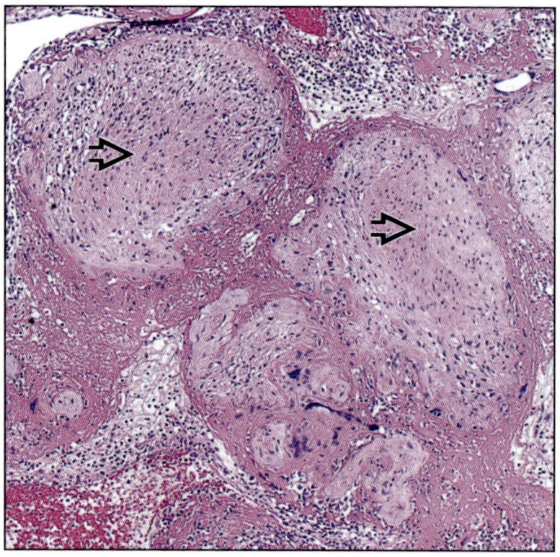

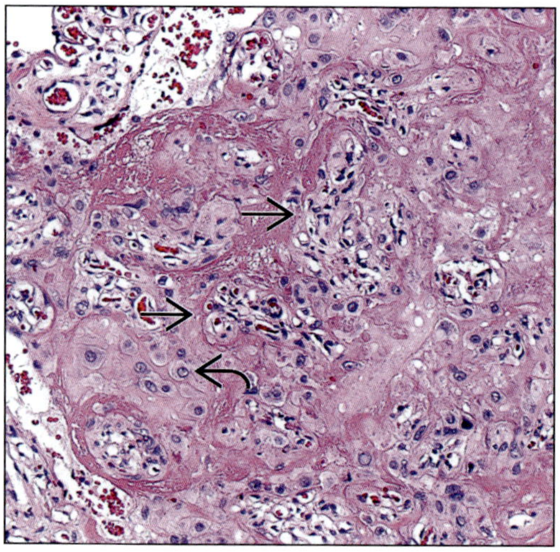

(Left) *Second-trimester chorionic villi have homogeneously cellular stroma that can mimic chronic villitis. Also note that the syncytiotrophoblast layer is intact along the entire villous circumference and no villous agglutination is present.* ***(Right)*** *Chronic villitis seen at higher power contains a nonuniform distribution of inflammatory cells in villi and villous agglutination ⇨ with perivillous fibrinoid deposition →.*

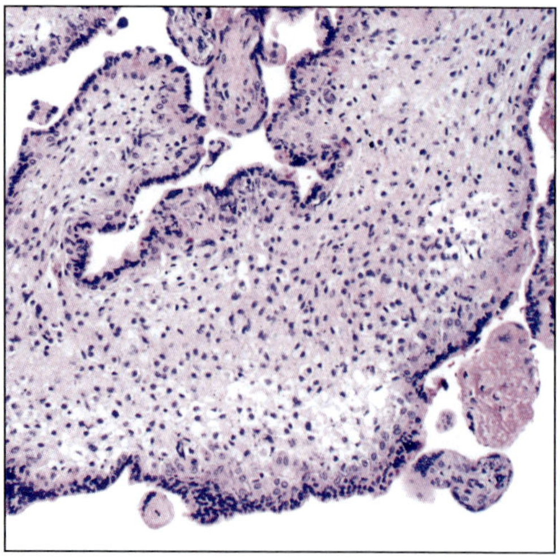

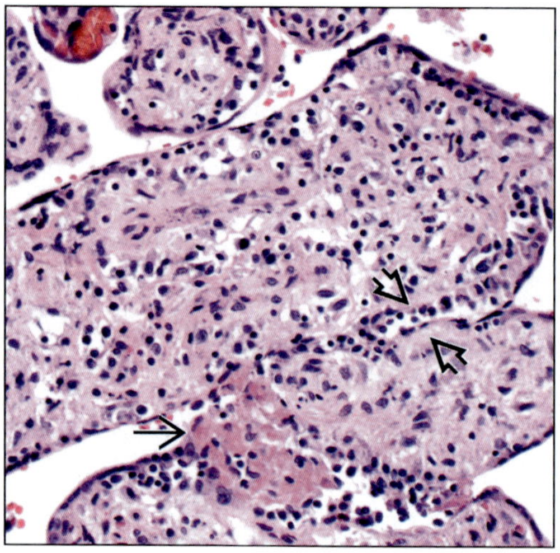

CHRONIC VILLITIS AND INTERVILLOSITIS

Microscopic Features

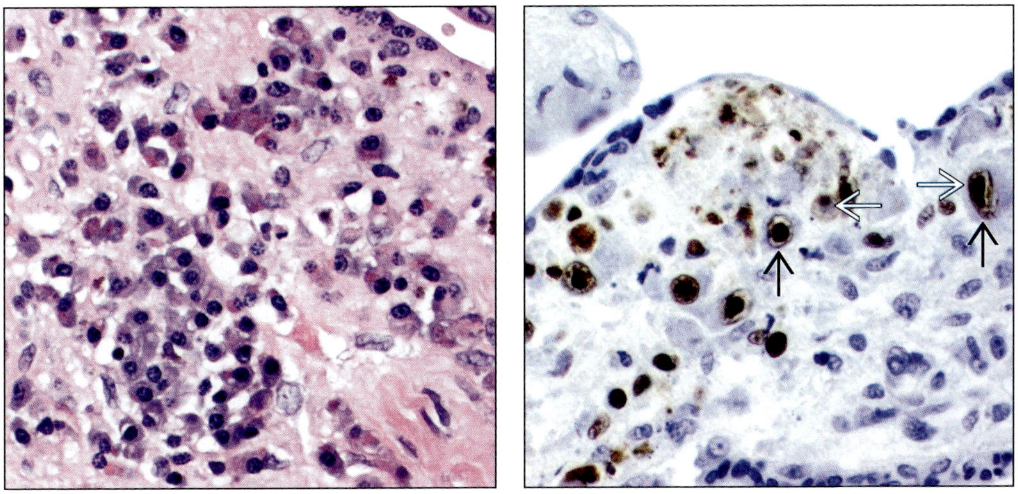

(Left) *Congenital cytomegalovirus can cause plasma cell-predominant chronic villitis in the placenta.* ***(Right)*** *Cytomegalovirus immunostain highlights infected cells in a chorionic villus that includes both nuclear ➡ and cytoplasmic ⇨ inclusions. Viral inclusions may be more difficult to identify on hematoxylin & eosin stains alone.*

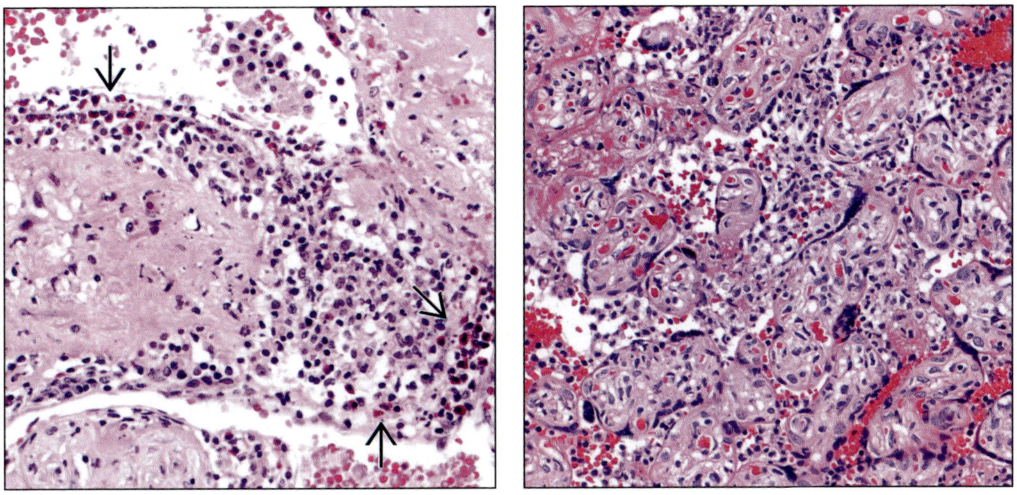

(Left) *Chronic villitis can rarely have unusual cellular infiltration patterns. Here, a mixed lymphocytic and eosinophilic infiltrate ⇨ involves the edges of agglutinated villi while the central portions of the villi are sclerotic.* ***(Right)*** *Chronic histiocytic intervillositis involves the intervillous space. Like chronic villitis, the process can be focal or multifocal. However, even focal lesions appear to have clinical significance, unlike low-grade focal chronic villitis.*

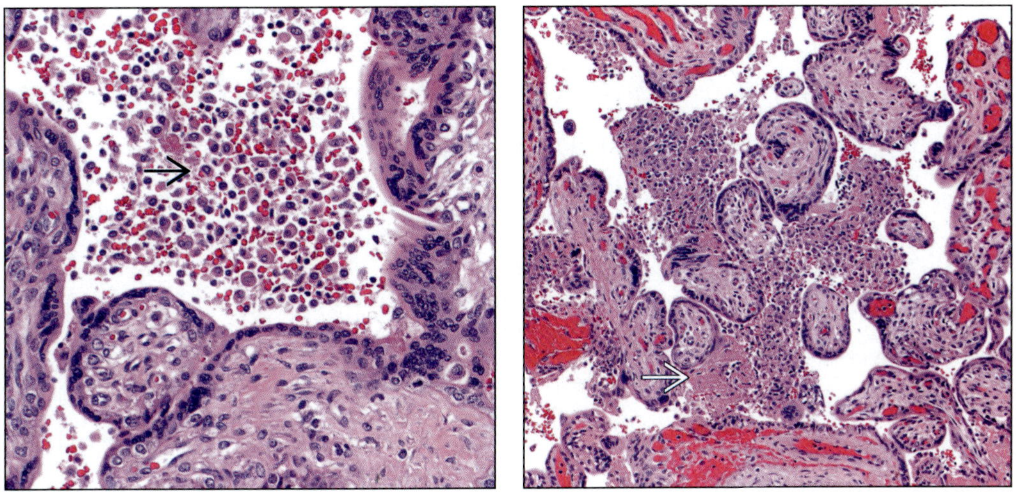

(Left) *Most of the intervillous infiltrate ⇨ is composed of histiocytes, which label with CD68. Unlike chronic villitis, T cells comprise only a minor population (< 5% of cells).* ***(Right)*** *Over time, injury to syncytiotrophoblasts in chronic intervillositis leads to perivillous fibrin accumulation ➡, as in some cases of chronic villitis. The severity of fibrin deposition relates to the degree of fetal growth restriction in a recent study, implying chronicity.*

BASAL CHRONIC VILLITIS AND CHRONIC DECIDUITIS

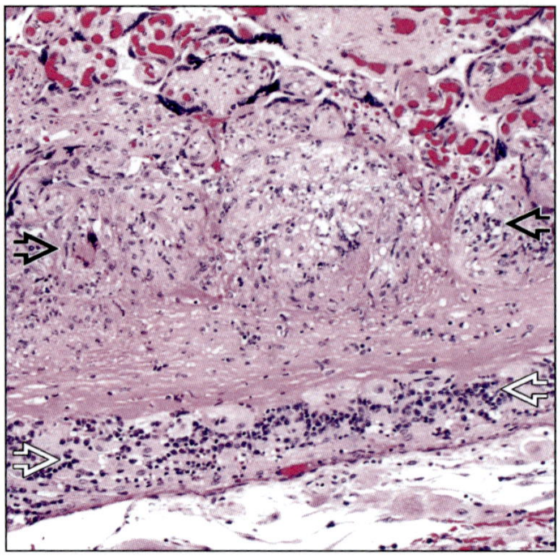

Basal chronic villitis involves villi along the basal floor. Chronic deciduitis is often present concurrently in the subjacent decidua.

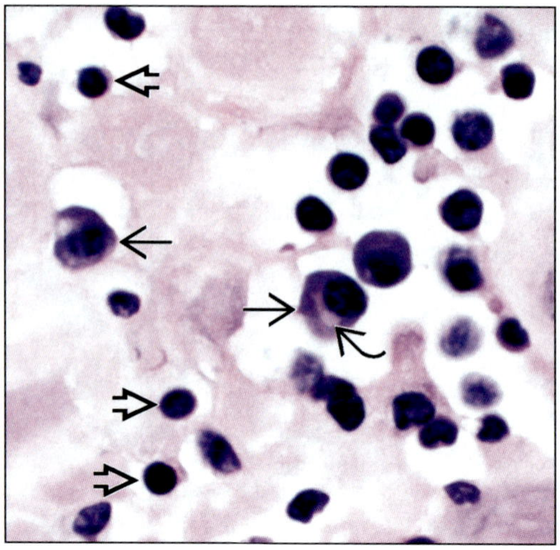

Plasma cells, characterized by their eccentric nucleus and perinuclear hof, are the diagnostic cell for chronic deciduitis. Lymphocytes are usually part of the chronic inflammation in this lesion.

TERMINOLOGY

Definitions

- Basal chronic villitis
  - Restriction of chronic villitis to maternal floor chorionic villi
- Chronic deciduitis
  - Presence of mixed plasma cells and lymphocytes in decidua basalis adjacent to maternal floor

ETIOLOGY/PATHOGENESIS

Infectious Agents

- Less associated with hematogenous infectious etiology than diffuse chronic villitis
- Possible association with subclinical chronic infection of endometrium
  - *Mycoplasma hominis*
  - *Ureaplasma urealyticum*
  - *Streptococcus agalactiae*

Abnormal Immune Response

- Basal plate represents a unique site of maternal and fetal cellular interaction without syncytiotrophoblast
- Basal chronic villitis may be an alloimmune response of maternal lymphocytes to fetal antigens
- Function of plasma cells in chronic deciduitis unknown
- Relationship to chronic endometritis is not defined

CLINICAL ISSUES

Presentation

- Chronic deciduitis
  - Recognized in 1-2% of 3rd-trimester placentas
  - In ~ 10% of placentas from spontaneous abortions and preterm deliveries
  - In ~ 40% of cases of preterm labor without clinical chorioamnionitis
- No reported ultrasonographic findings

Prognosis

- Recurrence
  - Both basal chronic villitis and chronic deciduitis can recur in subsequent pregnancies
  - May be associated with recurrent preterm birth &/or recurrent spontaneous abortion
  - Diffuse chronic capsular deciduitis and capsular decidual plasma cells are associated with periventricular leukomalacia in 1 study

MACROSCOPIC FEATURES

Gross Examination

- Neither basal chronic villitis nor chronic deciduitis are visible on gross examination
- Adequate sampling of maternal surface and membrane roll may identify focal lesions

MICROSCOPIC PATHOLOGY

Histologic Features

- Basal chronic villitis
  - Occurs ± chronic villitis of unknown etiology
  - Chronic deciduitis often present in subjacent decidua
  - Plasma cells occasionally infiltrate into basal chorionic villi
- Chronic deciduitis
  - Plasma cells seen in decidua
    - Can be patchy or focal
    - Decidua of maternal surface or membrane roll can be involved
    - May be underdiagnosed if high-power objective not used

BASAL CHRONIC VILLITIS AND CHRONIC DECIDUITIS

Key Facts

Terminology
- Basal chronic villitis: Restriction of chronic villitis to maternal floor chorionic villi
- Chronic deciduitis: Presence of mixed plasma cells and lymphocytes in decidua basalis adjacent to maternal floor

Clinical Issues
- Prognosis: Basal chronic villitis and chronic deciduitis can recur in subsequent pregnancies
- Chronic deciduitis is more frequent in preterm birth and may be associated with recurrent preterm birth

Microscopic Pathology
- Basal chronic villitis involves anchoring villi and is often seen with adjacent chronic deciduitis
- Chronic deciduitis can include few or many plasma cells that may be seen only focally

Top Differential Diagnoses
- Acute deciduitis
  - More common than chronic deciduitis and involves neutrophils
- 2nd-trimester placenta
  - Increased stromal cellularity in 2nd-trimester chorionic villi can mimic chronic villitis
- Herpes simplex virus

Diagnostic Checklist
- Any plasma cells in basal plate or free membranes consistent with chronic deciduitis
- Lymphoplasmacytic infiltrate in basal chorionic villi may be focal or diffuse

---

- Often seen with chronic villitis and basal chronic villitis
  - Plasma cells of chronic deciduitis can infiltrate basal chorionic villi that are also involved by chronic villitis
- Both entities often seen with chronic chorioamnionitis

ANCILLARY TESTS

Immunohistochemistry
- CD138 positively stains plasma cells
  - Usually not necessary for diagnosis
- Immunostain for herpes simplex virus (HSV) may be useful in cases with extensive plasma cells &/or necrosis

DIFFERENTIAL DIAGNOSIS

Acute Deciduitis
- Mimics chronic deciduitis on low power
- Often associated with decidual necrosis
- Neutrophils are often abundant
- Neutrophils contain multilobated nuclei
- Karyorrhectic debris often associated with neutrophilic infiltrate

2nd-Trimester Placenta
- Large number of stromal cells in 2nd-trimester chorionic villi can mimic chronic villitis
- Stromal cells uniformly increased unlike more patchy involvement by chronic villitis

HSV Infection
- Varied histopathologic findings
- Lymphoplasmacytic deciduitis with numerous plasma cells
- May see necrosis of amnion and chorion with lymphoplasmacytic chorioamnionitis
- May see villous necrosis with viral inclusions

DIAGNOSTIC CHECKLIST

Pathologic Interpretation Pearls
- Basal chronic villitis often occurs with diffuse chronic villitis
  - Basal chronic villitis can occur focally
  - Often has concurrent subjacent chronic deciduitis in basal plate
  - Plasma cells can infiltrate basal chorionic villi
  - Be careful diagnosing basal chronic villitis in 2nd-trimester placentas that have increased villous stromal cellularity
- Chronic deciduitis likely underdiagnosed
  - Decidual plasma cells can be sparse
  - High-power objective examination often required
  - Often accompanies chronic villitis and chronic chorioamnionitis

SELECTED REFERENCES

1. Edmondson N et al: The prevalence of chronic deciduitis in cases of preterm labor without clinical chorioamnionitis. Pediatr Dev Pathol. 12(1):16-21, 2009
2. Maleki Z et al: Periventricular leukomalacia and placental histopathologic abnormalities. Obstet Gynecol. 114(5):1115-20, 2009
3. Khong TY et al: Chronic deciduitis in the placental basal plate: definition and interobserver reliability. Hum Pathol. 31(3):292-5, 2000

BASAL CHRONIC VILLITIS AND CHRONIC DECIDUITIS

Microscopic Features

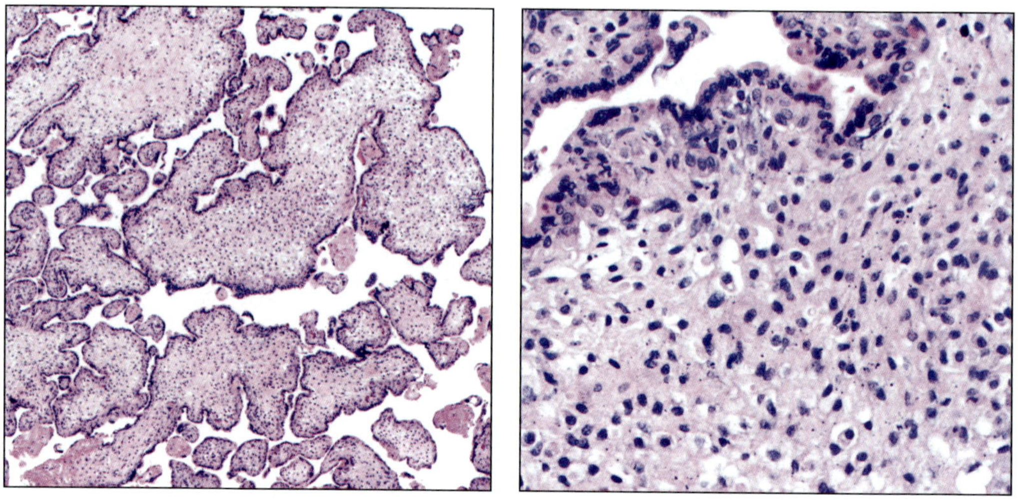

***(Left)** Second-trimester placentas, distinguished by their bulky chorionic villi, also have increased stromal cellularity compared with their 3rd-trimester counterparts. **(Right)** The increased stromal cellularity in 2nd-trimester chorionic villi can be mistaken for chronic villitis on low power. However, as seen here on high power, the stromal cells are uniformly placed within the stroma, and there is no disruption of the surface trophoblast layer.*

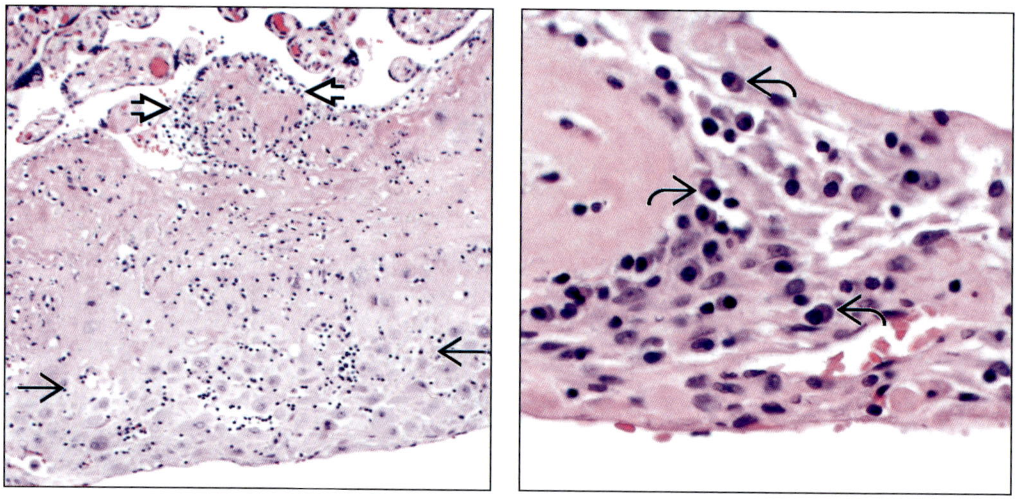

***(Left)** On low power, chronic inflammation is commonly seen in the decidua ➔. Only on high power can the plasma cells of chronic deciduitis be seen. The presence of basal chronic villitis ⇨ should prompt a search for chronic deciduitis. **(Right)** At higher power, plasma cells ↷ become more obvious. They have more cytoplasm than surrounding lymphocytes, and they have eccentric nuclei.*

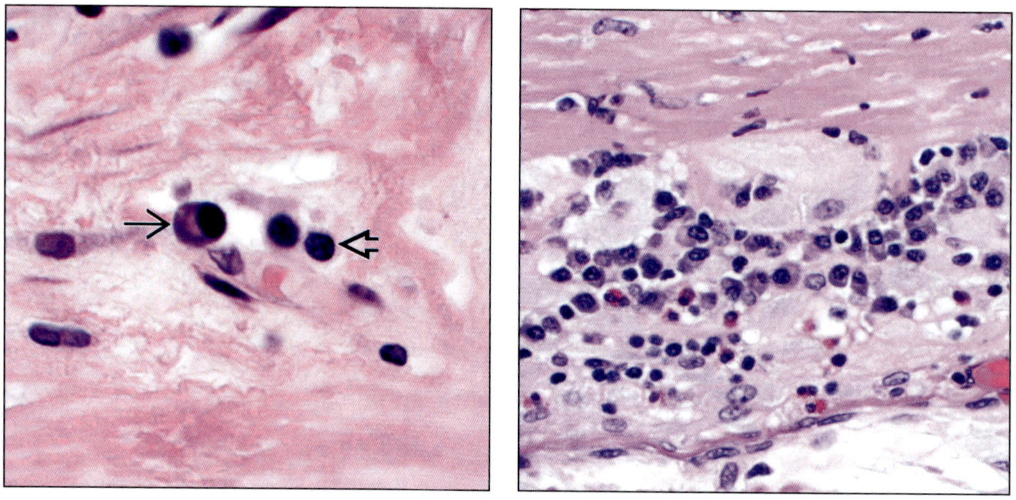

***(Left)** At high power, plasma cells ➔ are easily recognizable when seen next to lymphocytes ⇨. Plasma cells have an eccentric nucleus, abundant cytoplasm, and a perinuclear hof. **(Right)** Occasionally, large numbers of plasma cells are present in chronic deciduitis and can be seen easily at low power.*

Microscopic Features

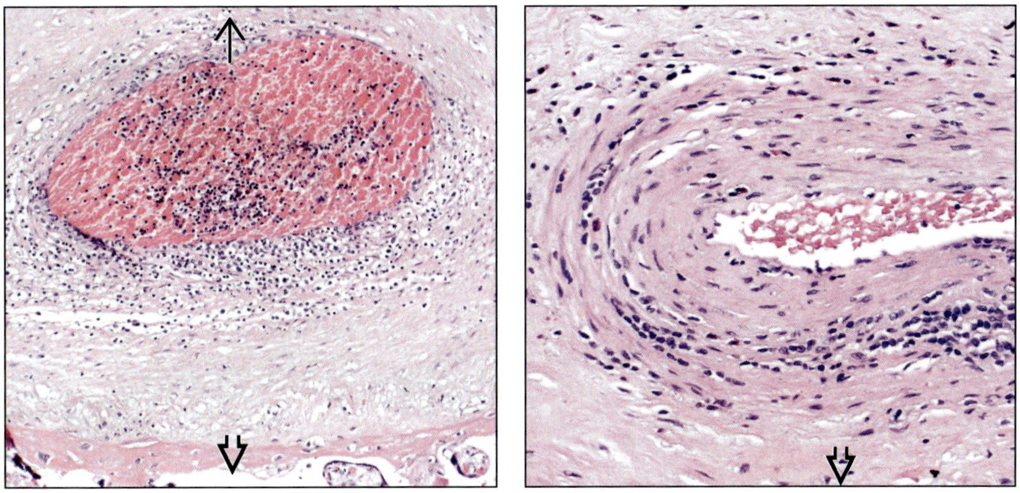

(Left) *In some cases of ETCV, the inflammatory cells appear more circumferential, with perivascular inflammation present in both the vessel wall facing the intervillous space ⇨ and in the vessel wall facing the amnion →, which lies above and is not seen in this image.* ***(Right)*** *Perivascular lymphocytic and eosinophilic inflammation is distributed around this chorionic vessel but is largely concentrated in the vessel wall facing the intervillous space ⇨ (out of view).*

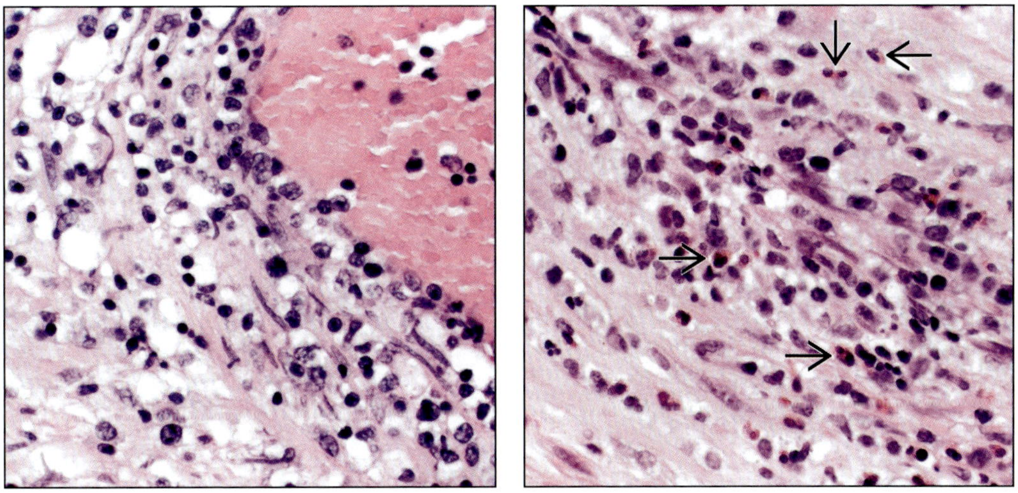

(Left) *Eosinophils may be difficult to find in some cases of ETCV, but often scattered eosinophils can be seen if viewed on high power or on deeper levels of the tissue block. No eosinophils are seen in this image.* ***(Right)*** *In other cases of ETCV, eosinophils → are abundant and intermixed with lymphocytes. Their role in ETCV is not clear, but they are likely attracted by cytokines released by lymphocytes.*

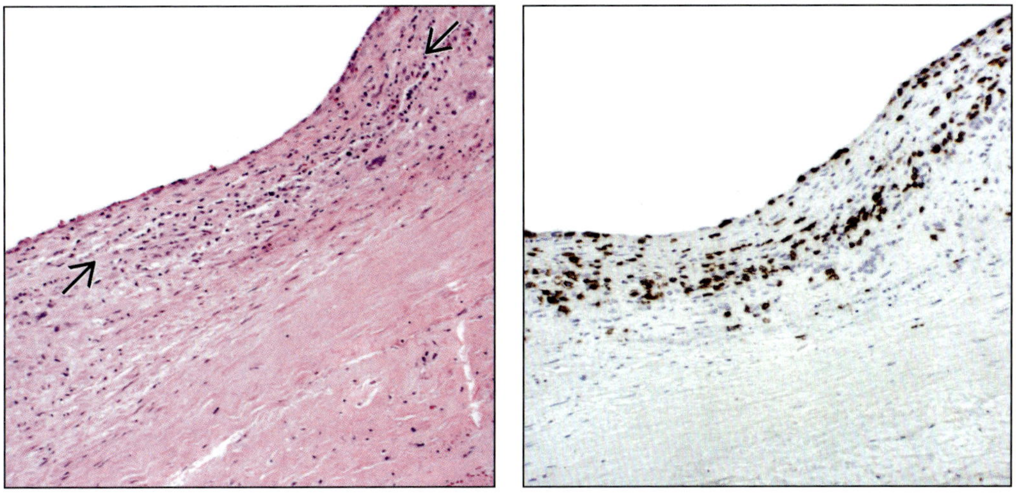

(Left) *Some cases of ETCV have very sparse infiltrates →. A CD3 immunostain can help to highlight them in these cases.* ***(Right)*** *A CD3 immunostain can highlight the presence of T-cell lymphocytes. Eosinophils may be rare and require deeper levels of the block.*

Massive Perivillous Fibrin Deposition and Maternal Floor Infarction

MASSIVE PERIVILLOUS FIBRIN DEPOSITION AND MATERNAL FLOOR INFARCTION

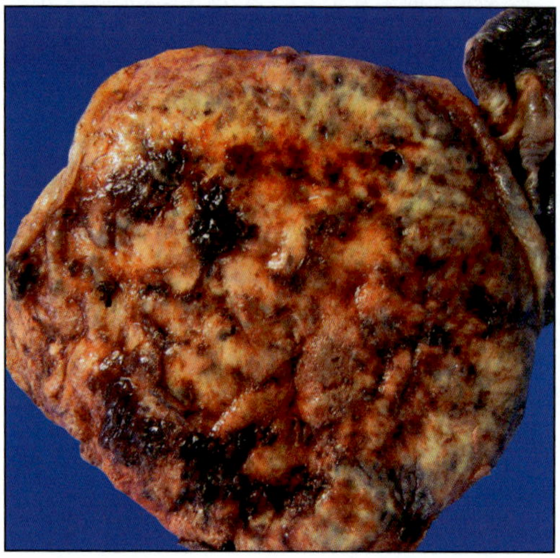

The maternal surface may show diffuse yellow-tan discoloration and thickening in massive perivillous fibrin deposition (MPVFD)/maternal floor infarction (MFI). The individual cotyledons lose their demarcation.

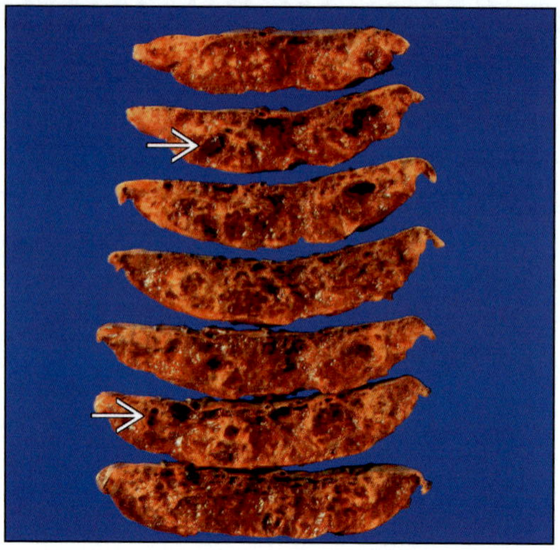

Cut sections of placenta with MPVFD show vertically oriented, firm trabeculae and a lattice-like deposition of fibrin. Intervillous thrombi are also seen ➔.

TERMINOLOGY

Abbreviations

- Massive perivillous fibrin deposition (MPVFD)
- Maternal floor infarction (MFI)

Synonyms

- MPVFD and MFI often used interchangeably
  - May represent a spectrum of the same disease process
- "Gitterinfarkt" is also a term that has been used to describe this entity

Definitions

- MPVFD
  - Excessive fibrin deposition entrapping villi and completely obliterating intervillous space, involving ≥ 30% of parenchyma
  - Involves but is not necessarily confined to basal plate
  - Perivillous fibrin deposition extends vertically toward chorionic plate
- MFI
  - Gross finding of a rind-like, yellow thickening of basal (maternal) placental surface
  - Basal villi are encased in excessive fibrin deposition
  - "Infarct" is a misnomer since deposition of fibrin and villous injury does not display the pattern seen in ischemic injury
- Diagnostic terminology proposed by Katzman (2002)
  - Transmural MPVFD: Perivillous fibrinoid extending from maternal to fetal surface and encasing ≥ 50% of villi on ≥ 1 slide
  - Borderline MPVFD: Involvement of 25-50% of villi on ≥ 1 slide in a transmural or nearly transmural distribution
  - Classic MFI: Basal villi of entire maternal floor encased by fibrinoid ≥ 3 mm on ≥ 1 slide

Fibrin vs. Fibrinoid

- Both terms frequently used interchangeably in literature
  - True fibrin is derived from fibrinogen
  - Fibrinoid
    - Fibrin-like fibrinoid = combination of maternal and fetal serum fibrin with other molecules derived from blood clotting
    - Matrix-type fibrinoid = trophoblast-derived extracellular matrix product
- Nature of perivillous material in MPVFD appears to be a mixture of typical fibrin polymeric formations of probably maternal and fetal origin, with trophoblastic extracellular matrix material

ETIOLOGY/PATHOGENESIS

Etiology

- Currently unknown
- Several mechanisms of formation of abnormal perivillous fibrin have been proposed
  - Stasis of blood in intervillous space
  - Inadequate drainage of intervillous space
  - Abnormal procoagulant properties of intervillous blood or trophoblast
  - Intrinsic abnormality of extravillous cytotrophoblast differentiation leading to excess secretion of extracellular matrix
  - Any mechanism leading to excessive syncytiotrophoblast injury
  - Auto-/alloimmune mechanisms that directly damage syncytiotrophoblast
- Uncertain if MPVFD is a single entity or end stage of several different disorders of pregnancy

Pathogenesis

- Normal perivillous fibrin deposition

MASSIVE PERIVILLOUS FIBRIN DEPOSITION AND MATERNAL FLOOR INFARCTION

Key Facts

Terminology
- Massive perivillous fibrin deposition (MPVFD) and maternal floor infarction (MFI) have often been used interchangeably
- Transmural MPVFD: Perivillous fibrinoid extending from maternal to fetal surface and encasing ≥ 50% of villi on ≥ 1 slide or involving ≥ 30% of parenchyma
- Borderline MPVFD: Involvement of 25-50% of villi on ≥ 1 slide in transmural or nearly transmural distribution
- Classic MFI: Basal villi of entire maternal floor encased by fibrinoid ≥ 3 mm on ≥ 1 slide

Etiology
- Currently unknown
- Several mechanisms of formation of abnormal perivillous fibrin have been proposed including a strong association with auto-/alloimmune disorders

Clinical Issues
- Rare placental lesion with incidence between 0.028% and 0.5% of placentas
- High recurrence rates between 12% and 78%
- Poor obstetrical and neonatal outcomes are common

Top Differential Diagnoses
- Ischemic infarction of chorionic villi
- Fetal thrombotic vasculopathy, longstanding
- Extensive chronic villitis with increased perivillous fibrin deposition

- By-product of turbulence and eddying of intervillous blood flow
- Most prominent in subchorionic area, present at interface between maternal and fetal tissues
- Increases with gestational age
- Typically does not have significant effect on maternofetal exchange
- Response to localized syncytiotrophoblast injury, preventing significant fetal-maternal hemorrhage

- MPVFD
  - Altered (more prominent basally) and increased deposition of perivillous fibrin
    - Fills and obliterates intervillous space
    - Surrounds and chokes off affected chorionic villi
    - Chorionic villi are not devitalized but may become avascular
  - Ultimately leads to impaired exchange of gases and nutrients
    - Can lead to fetal morbidity (growth restriction, prematurity) and mortality

CLINICAL ISSUES

Epidemiology
- Incidence
  - Rare placental lesion with incidence between 0.028% and 0.5% of placentas

Laboratory Tests
- Elevated maternal serum α-fetoprotein is associated with MPVFD

Natural History
- Recurrence rates are reported between 12% and 78%

Treatment
- Low-dose aspirin and Lovenox utilized, theoretically reduces coagulation within intervillous space

Clinical Associations
- Maternal
  - Hypertension, preeclampsia
  - Autoimmune disorders, antiphospholipid antibody syndrome, polymyositis
  - Inherited or acquired coagulopathies
  - Oligohydramnios
  - Poor past reproductive history, with high rates of fetal demise, intrauterine growth restriction, neonatal death
- Fetal/neonatal
  - Kidney disorders, cystic renal dysplasia, renal tubular dysgenesis
  - Long-chain 3-hydroxyacyl-CoA dehydrogenase (LCHAD) deficiency with mutations in *LCHAD* gene
- Placental
  - Discordant presence of MFI in both dichorionic and monochorionic twin placentas has been reported
  - Concurrence of MPVFD with chronic intervillositis has been reported
  - Extensive chronic villitis may have excessive perivillous fibrin deposition
- Infection
  - Villous damage from infection and inflammation can lead to excessive perivillous fibrin deposition

Clinical Outcomes
- Preterm delivery (26-60%)
- Intrauterine growth restriction (24-100%)
- Spontaneous abortion
- Stillbirth (13-50%)
- Long-term neurologic impairment

IMAGE FINDINGS

Ultrasonographic Findings
- Increased placental echogenicity
- Intrauterine growth restriction
- Oligohydramnios: Decreased amniotic fluid index
- Reduced or abnormal blood flow within placenta may also be seen

MASSIVE PERIVILLOUS FIBRIN DEPOSITION AND MATERNAL FLOOR INFARCTION

MACROSCOPIC FEATURES

General Features

- Placenta usually small but may have increased weight due to abundance of fibrinoid and hemorrhages
- Dense, firm placenta with basally located "orange rind" of fibrin (MFI)
- Diffusely distributed pattern of vertically oriented firm trabeculae and lattice-like deposition of fibrin concentrated along basal plate that may extend to chorionic plate (MPVFD)
- Parenchyma has a pale granular appearance
- Cut surface of fibrinoid is homogeneous and shiny
- Chorionic cysts, septal cyst, and intervillous thrombi are commonly seen

Size

- Placenta is typically small for gestational age; however, placenta may be of normal or even increased weight due to presence of abundant fibrin

MICROSCOPIC PATHOLOGY

Histologic Features

- Chorionic villi are encased in amorphous, eosinophilic fibrin/fibrinoid material
- Intervillous space is filled in and obliterated by fibrin/fibrinoid material
- Villi remain separated/individuated without collapse of intervillous space
- Villi show spectrum of changes from villous atrophy to frank avascularity
- Perivillous fibrin may contain cellular proliferation of extravillous cytotrophoblast cells, ± cytotrophoblast cysts
- Intervillous thrombi likely reflect of abnormal blood flow in intervillous space
- Inflammation is not typically seen but may present as secondary component

DIFFERENTIAL DIAGNOSIS

Normal Perivillous Fibrin Deposition

- Typically in scattered foci concentrated in subchorionic zones and around terminal and stem villi and at basal plate (Nitabuch and Rohr fibrinoid)
- MPVFD shows prominent basal distribution as well as more diffuse involvement of intervillous space

Infarction

- True infarcts show collapse of intervillous space **and** coagulative necrosis, features not typically seen in MPVFD
- Decidual vasculopathy is often present in cases with multiple infarcts, a feature not typically seen in MPVFD

Fetal Thrombotic Vasculopathy (FTV), Longstanding

- Typically, avascular villi of FTV show no significant surrounding perivillous fibrin, but with longstanding lesions, fibrin can fill in intervillous space
- In longstanding FTV, avascular villi not encased in fibrin are visible at edges of lesion
- Presence of thrombi in chorionic plate or stem villous vessels can be seen in FTV, features not typically seen in MPVFD

Diffuse Chronic Villitis of Unknown Etiology

- Diffuse chronic inflammatory infiltrates can lead to villous agglutination and perivillous fibrin deposition
- As lesions of chronic villitis age ("burnt out villitis"), villi may become avascular and surrounded by bland fibrin
  - Residual chronic inflammation is usually present
- In MPVFD, chronic inflammation should be minimal

Massive Chronic Intervillositis (MCI)

- While occasional chronic inflammatory infiltrates are present in MPVFD, infiltrates in MCI are much more prominent and diffuse
- Chronic inflammatory infiltrates in MPVFD may represent an overlap between pathologic mechanism in these 2 conditions

DIAGNOSTIC CHECKLIST

Pathologic Interpretation Pearls

- MPVFD is usually a gross diagnosis, villi are surrounded by fibrinoid and not infarcted

SELECTED REFERENCES

1. Faye-Petersen OM et al: Maternal floor infarction and massive perivillous fibrin deposition. In Baergen RN et al: Surgical Pathology Clinics: Placental Pathology. Vol 6:1. Philadelphia: WB Saunders, 2013
2. Linn RL et al: Recurrent massive perivillous fibrin deposition in the placenta associated with fetal renal tubular dysgenesis: case report and literature review. Pediatr Dev Pathol. 16(5):378-86, 2013
3. Romero R et al: Maternal floor infarction/massive perivillous fibrin deposition: a manifestation of maternal antifetal rejection? Am J Reprod Immunol. 70(4):285-98, 2013
4. Griffin AC et al: Mutations in long-chain 3-hydroxyacyl coenzyme a dehydrogenase are associated with placental maternal floor infarction/massive perivillous fibrin deposition. Pediatr Dev Pathol. 15(5):368-74, 2012
5. Taweevisit M et al: Maternal floor infarction associated with oligohydramnios and cystic renal dysplasia: report of 2 cases. Pediatr Dev Pathol. 13(2):116-20, 2010
6. Gogia N et al: Maternal thrombophilias are associated with specific placental lesions. Pediatr Dev Pathol. 11(6):424-9, 2008
7. Katzman PJ et al: Maternal floor infarction and massive perivillous fibrin deposition: histological definitions, association with intrauterine fetal growth restriction, and risk of recurrence. Pediatr Dev Pathol. 2002 Mar-Apr;5(2):159-64. Erratum in: Pediatr Dev Pathol. 6(1):102, 2003

Gross and Microscopic Features

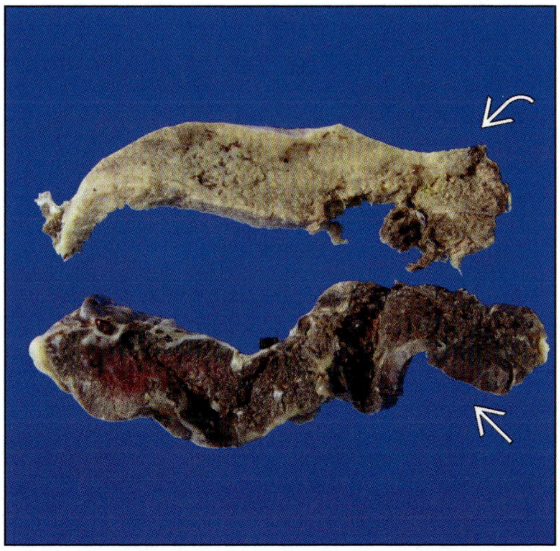
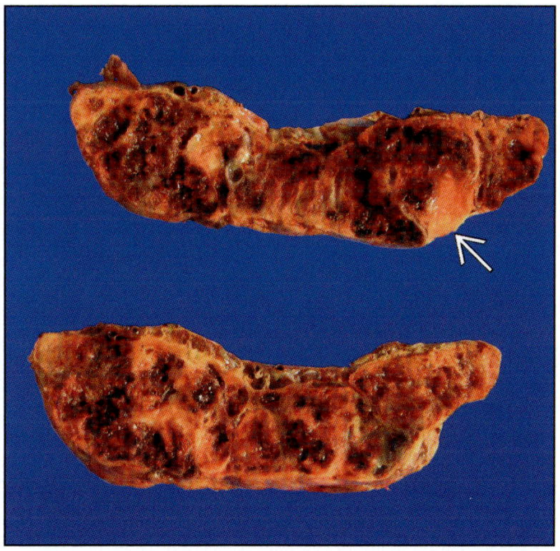

(Left) *This dichorionic twin placenta was discordant for MPVFD. Note the nearly complete involvement of parenchyma of twin A placenta with diffusely pale, tan, firm, and finely granular parenchyma. Twin B has normal spongy, dark-red parenchyma.* ***(Right)*** *Note the diffusely distributed pattern of vertically oriented firm trabeculae and a lattice-like deposition of fibrin in this placenta with MPVFD. Intervillous thrombi are also seen.*

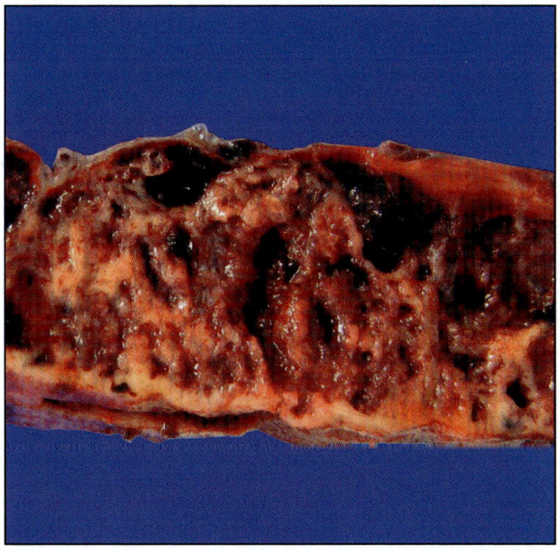
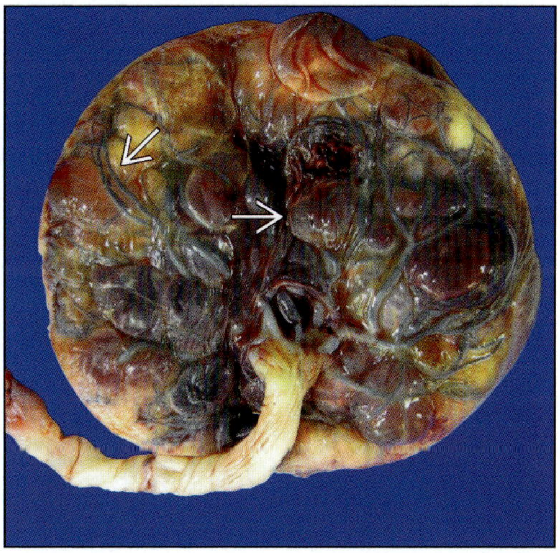

(Left) *Close inspection of the parenchyma in MPVFD shows a granularity that is not typically seen in an ischemic infarct.* ***(Right)*** *Multiple chorionic cysts, some with recent and remote hemorrhage, are frequently seen in association with MPVFD. These cysts are typically lined by extravillous cytotrophoblast, the same cells producing the excessive matrix-type fibrin deposited in MPVFD.*

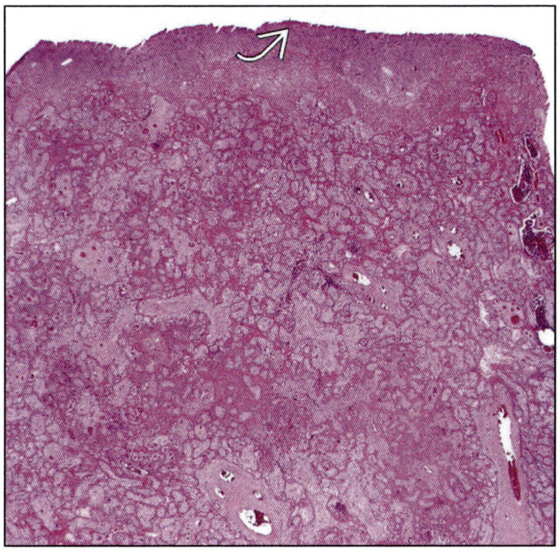
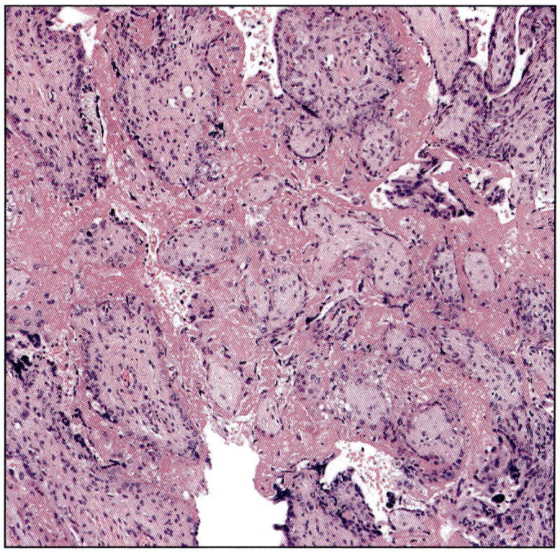

(Left) *Low-power examination in MPVFD shows diffuse, nearly full thickness encasement of the chorionic villi by eosinophilic, bland, noninflamed fibrin. The fibrin typically is most concentrated at the basal surface and extends toward the chorionic plate.* ***(Right)*** *On higher power examination of chorionic villi encased by perivillous fibrin, there is still some preservation of the trophoblast layer and villous stroma, but villous capillaries are sparse.*

Fetal Vasculopathy

LARGE VESSEL FETAL VASCULAR OCCLUSION

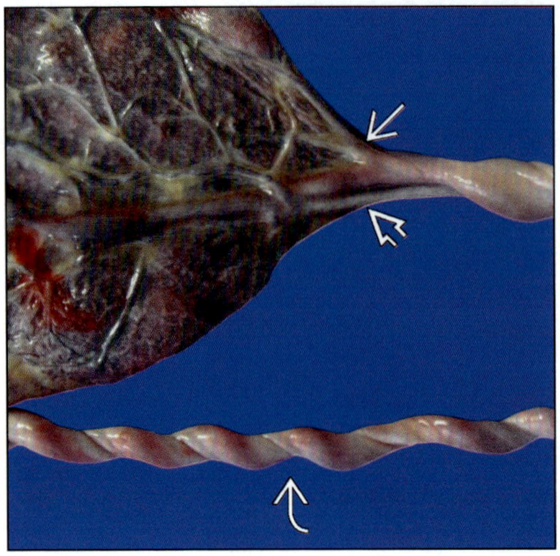

Obstruction or compression of the umbilical cord can lead to vascular flow stasis and thrombosis ⇨. Velamentous insertion ➡ and hypercoiling ➡ are both correlated with thrombosis.

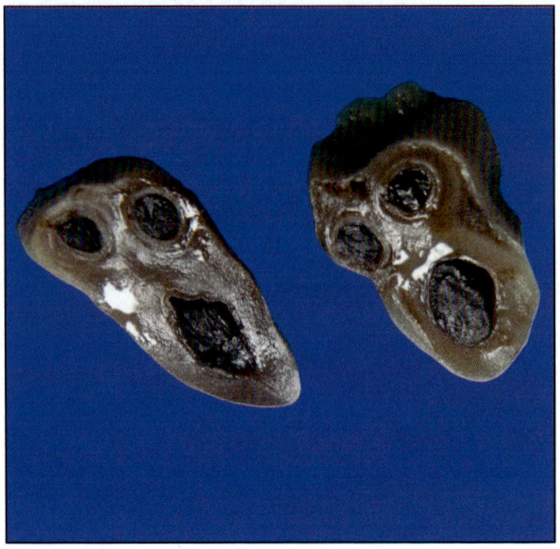

These umbilical vessels are filled with a firm blood clot that appears focally adherent to the wall. Histologic examination is required to distinguish congestion from thrombosis.

TERMINOLOGY

Synonyms

- Similar histologic changes are encompassed by terms
  - Chronic obstructive fetal vasculopathy
  - Chronic fetal vascular obstructive changes
  - Vaso-obliterative fetal vascular changes
  - Fetal vascular involutional changes
  - Fetal thrombotic vasculopathy (FTV)
  - Hemorrhagic endovasculitis (HEV)
  - Villous stromal-vascular karyorrhexis (VSVK)
- Older terminology includes HEV, fibrinous vasculosis, thrombosclerosing placentitis, endarteritis obliterans, and fibromuscular sclerosis

Definitions

- Large fetal vessels of placenta are umbilical vessels, chorionic plate vasculature, and stem villous vessels
- FTV: Characteristic changes in distal villi resulting from cessation of fetal perfusion, often seen in association with large vessel thrombi

ETIOLOGY/PATHOGENESIS

Causes

- Cord compromise from kinking, tight knots, tight nuchal cords or limb/body entanglement, prolapse through cervix, compression of large vessels
- Compression of large fetal vessels not protected by Wharton jelly in velamentous cords, furcate cords, vasa previa
- Thrombosis, occlusive or nonocclusive
- Vasospasm due to meconium or drug effect

Factors That Promote Thrombosis in Fetal Vasculature

- Stasis of fetal blood flow
  - Fetal heart failure, intraabdominal umbilical venous obstruction, polycythemia
  - Interruption of blood flow due to compression or kinking of umbilical or chorionic plate vessels
- Endothelial cell injury
  - Severe acute inflammation of umbilical or chorionic plate vessels in fetal response to amniotic fluid infection
  - Chronic inflammation of proximal stem villi in chronic villitis of unknown etiology, or chronic villitis due to hematogenous infections
- Hypercoagulability of fetal blood
  - Thrombophilia: Genetic or acquired
  - Contribution of genetic thrombophilias is controversial in literature

Thrombotic/Ischemic Complications in Fetus

- Systemic activation of coagulation system
- Emboli from large placental vessels via umbilical vein to central nervous system (CNS) and viscera
- Reduced capacity for maternofetal gas and nutrient exchange due to significant downstream villous compromise (avascular villi)

CLINICAL ISSUES

Epidemiology

- Incidence
  - Thrombosis of umbilical vessels in 1/3,000 deliveries and up to 1/250 high-risk pregnancies
    - Umbilical venous thrombi are more common than umbilical artery thrombi
  - Thrombosis of chorionic plate or stem villous vessel occurs in ~ 4% of placentas submitted for pathologic evaluation; multiple thrombi occur in 3%

Prognosis

- Thrombosis of umbilical vessel is associated with significant fetal morbidity and mortality

LARGE VESSEL FETAL VASCULAR OCCLUSION

Key Facts

Etiology

- Fetal vascular occlusion may be due to thrombi or compression of large fetal vessels

Macroscopic Pathology

- Thrombosis of umbilical, chorionic, and stem villous vessels may be occlusive or mural
- Associated gross umbilical cord abnormalities include abnormal insertion, hypercoiling, excessively long cord, or true knot
- Acute thrombi have vessel ectasia, are rich in red blood cells, and have some adherence to vessel wall
- Subacute to remote thrombi are firm, with white discoloration of vessels and calcification

Microscopic Pathology

- Confirm thrombus with presence of fibrin in lesion and adherence to vessel wall
- Look for associated distal villous changes of fetal thrombotic vasculopathy (FTV) and other associated pathologies

Diagnostic Checklist

- Correlate with clinical history for nuchal cord, limb/body cord entanglement, vasa previa
- Confirm presence or absence of gross umbilical cord abnormality (length, insertion, coiling, knots)
- Look for other associated lesions: Fetal response to amniotic fluid infection, meconium, extensive chronic villitis, eosinophilic T-cell vasculitis, changes of maternal malperfusion/underperfusion

- Significance of chorionic plate or stem villous thrombi is dependent upon other additional placental findings, including
  - Multiple chorionic plate or stem villous thrombi
  - Severe distal villous changes of FTV
  - Extensive chronic villitis
  - Amniotic fluid infection sequence
  - Changes of maternal vascular malperfusion
- Obstetric and neonatal complications associated with FTV

MACROSCOPIC FEATURES

Umbilical Vessels

- Document presence of gross umbilical cord abnormalities, such as abnormal insertion, hypercoiling, excessively long cord, or true knot
- Ectasia without thrombus
  - May indicate obstruction near dilated region; look for compression or maceration of adjacent cord
- Acute thrombosis
  - Distension of vessel by a slightly firm red-tan thrombus
- Subacute to remote thrombosis
  - Firm, variegated, layered, or white

Velamentous Vessels

- Higher risk of injury secondary to lack of protection by Wharton jelly
- Distension, discoloration, or firmness of vessels raises suspicion for thrombosis

Chorionic Vessels

- Ectasia without thrombosis
  - Ectasia = diameter ≥ 4x diameter of an adjacent muscular vessel of similar caliber
- Acute thrombosis
  - Distension of vessel by a slightly firm red-tan thrombus
- Subacute to remote thrombosis
  - Firm
  - Variegated, layered, or white
  - May show chalky calcification

MICROSCOPIC PATHOLOGY

General Features

- Thrombosis, mural or occlusive
  - Thrombi in placental vessels rarely show classic lines of Zahn; vague layering may be present
  - Mural thrombi consist of fibrin and platelets with few red or white cells
  - All thrombi must be adherent to vessel wall
  - Rarely, thrombi of fetal vessels are associated with eosinophilic/T-cell vasculitis
- Chronicity
  - Acute thrombi
    - Vessel is distended
    - Consist mostly of red blood cells, with some fibrin layering
    - Focal attachment to vessel wall
    - Collections of fibrin and cells within vascular lumen are not true thrombi, unless there is definitive attachment to vascular wall
  - Subacute to remote
    - Reduced red cell component; consist mostly of fibrin and platelets
    - Usually nonocclusive
    - May show incorporation into wall ± mural calcification
- Other vaso-obliterative changes of large vessels
  - Loss of endothelial integrity
  - Mural hemorrhage with red cell fragmentation
  - Fibroblastic luminal septation/recanalization
  - Overlap with fetal vascular involutional changes after fetal demise
    - True fibrin or layered thrombus and vascular ectasia of fetal vessels not part of involutional changes after fetal demise
    - Antemortem fetal vascular occlusion is confined to foci; postmortem fetal vascular involution is diffuse in distribution

LARGE VESSEL FETAL VASCULAR OCCLUSION

DIFFERENTIAL DIAGNOSIS

Congestion of Large Fetal Vessels vs. Thrombosis

- Large vessels may appear prominent and filled with abundant blood after fixation
- Congested blood is deeply red and not attached to vascular wall
- Histologic section required to identify fibrin layering, organization, attachment to wall

Endothelial Cushion vs. Mural Thrombus

- Fibrointimal proliferations may protrude into lumen of chorionic plate vessels
  - Termed endothelial cushion defects
  - Unfortunately, some use the term endothelial cushion interchangeably with mural thrombus of chorionic plate vessels
- When deeply eosinophilic fibrin strands &/or calcification are present in lesion, it is a subacute or remote mural thrombus

Refrigeration Artifact

- Endothelial cells degenerate and detach with prolonged refrigeration, resembling loss of endothelial integrity
- Mural hemorrhage, red cell fragmentation, or fibroblastic luminal septation of true vaso-obliterative lesions are not present

DIAGNOSTIC CHECKLIST

General Overview

- Correlate with clinical history for nuchal cord, limb/body cord entanglement, vasa previa
- Confirm presence or absence of gross umbilical cord abnormality (length, insertion, coiling, knots)
- Look for associated findings with thrombus, such as ectasia, or pale parenchymal areas of FTV on gross examination
- Confirm thrombi microscopically, describe as acute or subacute/chronic, occlusive or mural
- Look for additional vaso-obliterative changes and distal villous changes of FTV
- Look for other associated lesions
  - Fetal response to amniotic fluid infection, meconium, extensive chronic villitis, eosinophilic T-cell vasculitis, changes of maternal malperfusion/underperfusion

REPORTING CONSIDERATIONS

Key Elements to Report

- Gross umbilical cord or chorionic plate vascular abnormalities (i.e., velamentous vessels, ectasia)
- Microscopic vascular lesions
  - Number and type of vessels with thrombi
    - Occlusive vs. nonocclusive
    - Acute or subacute to remote
  - Other vascular features associated with thrombus formation: Acute vasculitis, meconium, extensive chronic villitis, eosinophilic T-cell vasculitis, changes of maternal malperfusion/underperfusion
- Microscopic distal villous lesions of FTV
  - Avascular villi
  - VSVK

Society for Pediatric Pathology: Perinatal Section, Fetal Vascular Obstruction Nosology Committee

- Recommends use of header "Changes consistent with chronic fetal vascular obstruction" when thrombi are associated with distal villous changes
  - List findings in fetal umbilical, chorionic plate, and stem villous vasculature (thrombi, vaso-obliterative lesions)
  - List villous findings (avascular villi, VSVK); > 2 foci
- Diagnosis of FTV should be reserved for cases showing
  - Average of ≥ 15 affected villi (avascular villi or VSVK) per slide
    - Fetal vascular thrombi are not required for diagnosis of FTV

SELECTED REFERENCES

1. Ernst LM et al: Gross patterns of umbilical cord coiling: correlations with placental histology and stillbirth. Placenta. 34(7):583-8, 2013
2. Ryan WD et al: Placental histologic criteria for diagnosis of cord accident: sensitivity and specificity. Pediatr Dev Pathol. 15(4):275-80, 2012
3. Pathak S et al: Frequency and clinical significance of placental histological lesions in an unselected population at or near term. Virchows Arch. 459(6):565-72, 2011
4. Rogers BB et al: Avascular villi, increased syncytial knots, and hypervascular villi are associated with pregnancies complicated by factor V Leiden mutation. Pediatr Dev Pathol. 13(5):341-7, 2010
5. Saleemuddin A et al: Obstetric and perinatal complications in placentas with fetal thrombotic vasculopathy. Pediatr Dev Pathol. 13(6):459-64, 2010
6. Taweevisit M et al: Massive fetal thrombotic vasculopathy associated with excessively long umbilical cord and fetal demise: case report and literature review. Pediatr Dev Pathol. 13(2):112-5, 2010
7. Tantbirojn P et al: Gross abnormalities of the umbilical cord: related placental histology and clinical significance. Placenta. 30(12):1083-8, 2009
8. Parast MM et al: Placental histologic criteria for umbilical blood flow restriction in unexplained stillbirth. Hum Pathol. 39(6):948-53, 2008
9. Ariel I et al: Placental pathology in fetal thrombophilia. Hum Pathol. 35(6):729-33, 2004
10. Redline RW et al: Fetal vascular obstructive lesions: nosology and reproducibility of placental reaction patterns. Pediatr Dev Pathol. 7(5):443-52, 2004
11. Genest DR: Estimating the time of death in stillborn fetuses: II. Histologic evaluation of the placenta; a study of 71 stillborns. Obstet Gynecol. 80(4):585-92, 1992

LARGE VESSEL FETAL VASCULAR OCCLUSION

Graphic, Gross, and Microscopic Features

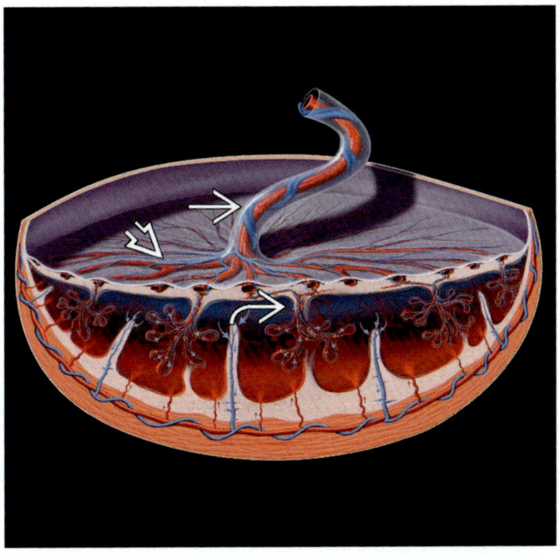

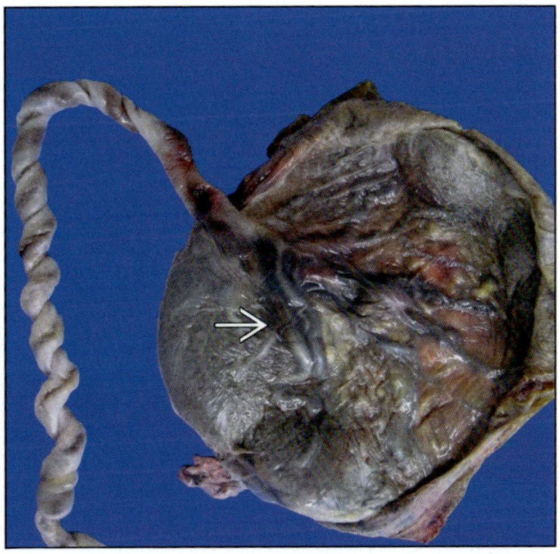

(Left) *Thrombi and other occlusive lesions of the large fetal vessels of the placenta can involve cord vessels, chorionic plate vessels, and stem villous vessels.* ***(Right)*** *Umbilical cord abnormalities, such as hypercoiling and marginal insertion, are associated with large vessel thrombi. These chorionic plate vessels are distended and appear chalky. Histology revealed acute thrombosis.*

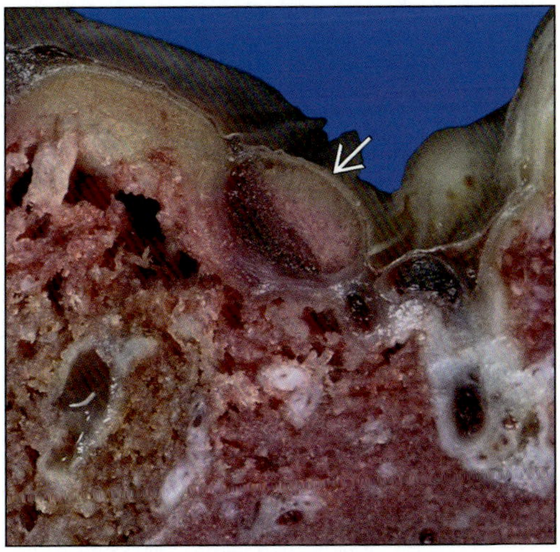

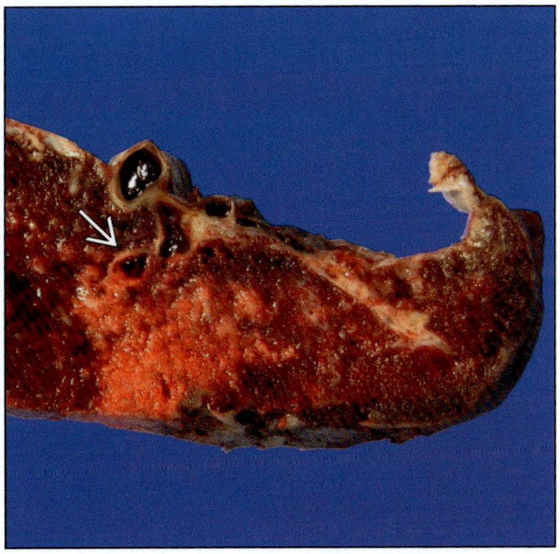

(Left) *This chorionic plate vessel with distension by partly red and partly gray-tan material is highly suspicious for thrombus.* ***(Right)*** *This grossly occluded stem villous vessel is associated with downstream villous pallor, the gross correlate of avascular villi.*

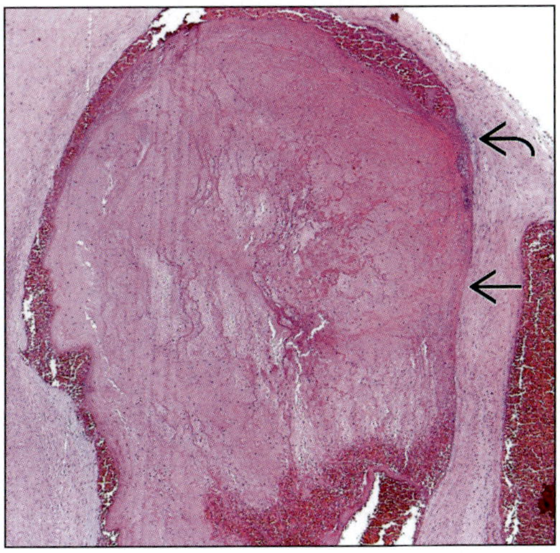

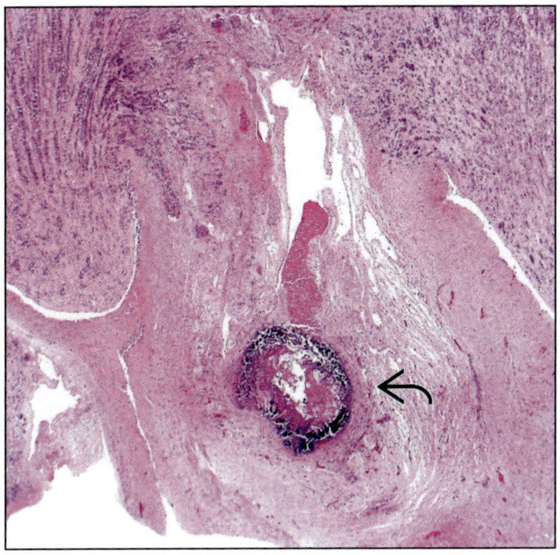

(Left) *This distended chorionic plate vessel has a nearly occlusive thrombus composed mostly of fibrin. Subacute thrombi such as this contain more fibrin than red blood cells (RBC). There is early calcification where the thrombus is attached to the wall.* ***(Right)*** *Thrombi in the placental fetal circulation may embolize to the body. The calcified thrombus in this section of kidney is from a fetus with large fetal vessel occlusion in the placenta.*

LARGE VESSEL FETAL VASCULAR OCCLUSION

Microscopic Features

*(**Left**) Nonocclusive thrombi can be subtle. This chorionic vessel with a myxoid-appearing intimal proliferation has a fibrin thrombus cap ➔, and is therefore a nonocclusive, mural thrombus. (**Right**) This stem villous vessel has no luminal abnormality, but the eosinophilic fibrin strands ⇨ incorporated into the wall suggest a probable organized thrombus. Additional level sections can be useful to identify further features of thrombosis.*

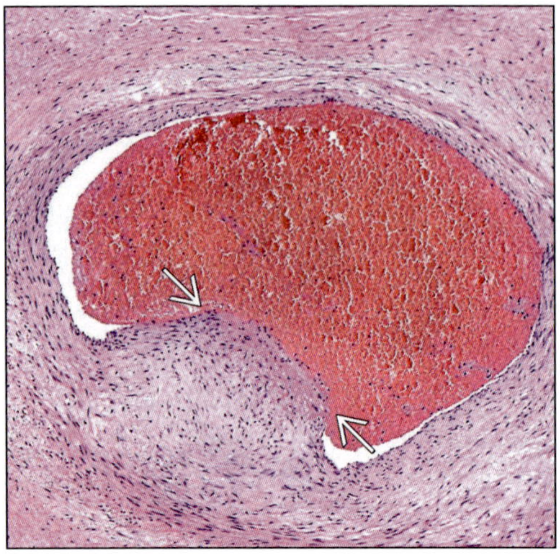

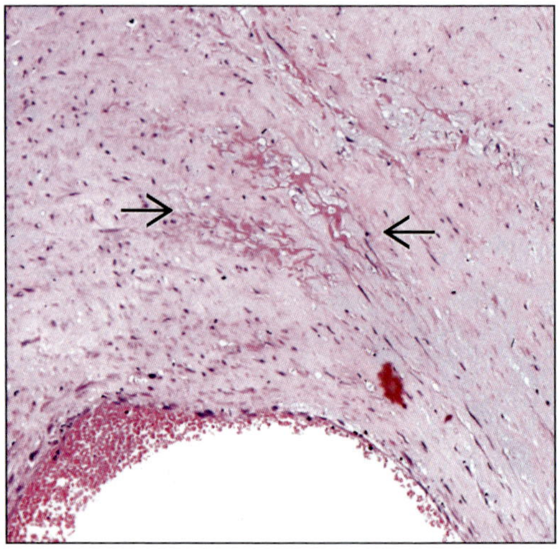

*(**Left**) Isolated luminal aggregates of fibrin alone are not diagnosed as a thrombus; mural attachment must be demonstrated. The rounded appearance of this fibrin nodule ⇨ in a stem villous vessel suggests a thromboembolus. Closer examination is warranted to find additional foci diagnostic of fetal thrombotic vasculopathy (FTV). (**Right**) This stem villous vessel contains an occlusive fibrin thrombus ↗. The vessel also shows septation and endothelial cell fragmentation ⇨.*

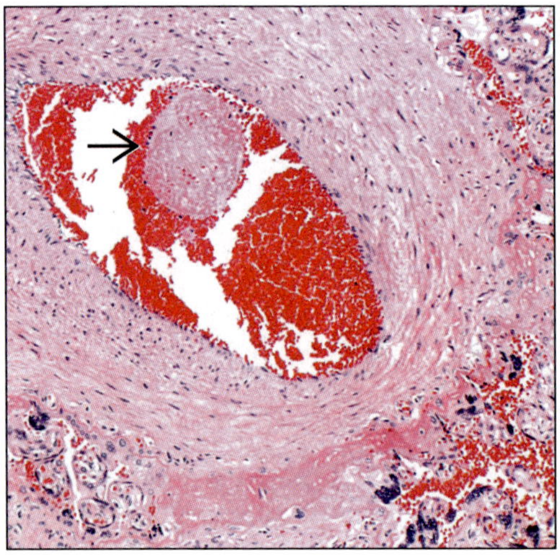

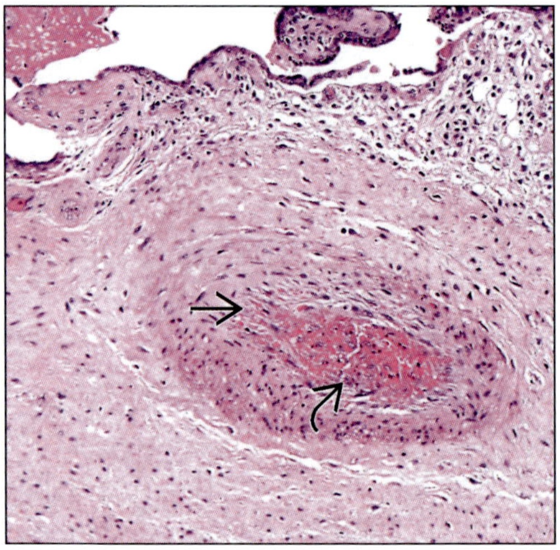

*(**Left**) This nonocclusive, subacute stem villous thrombus ➔ is tightly adherent. (**Right**) Both a large and small stem villous vessel are occluded by a fibrointimal proliferation with red cell fragmentation. Cessation of proximal fetal blood flow due to either fetal death or upstream antemortem vascular occlusion shows similar vaso-obliterative changes.*

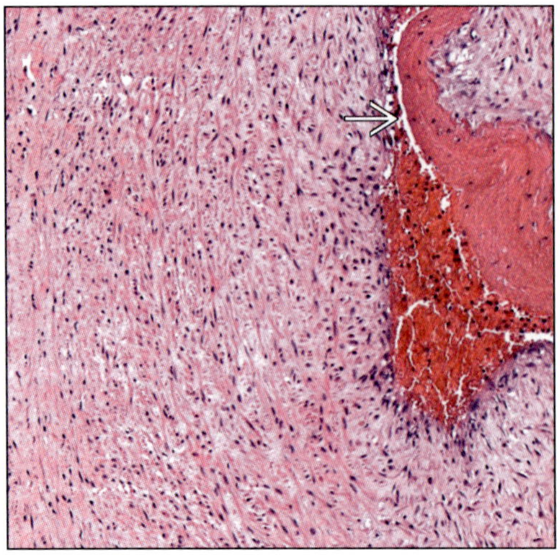

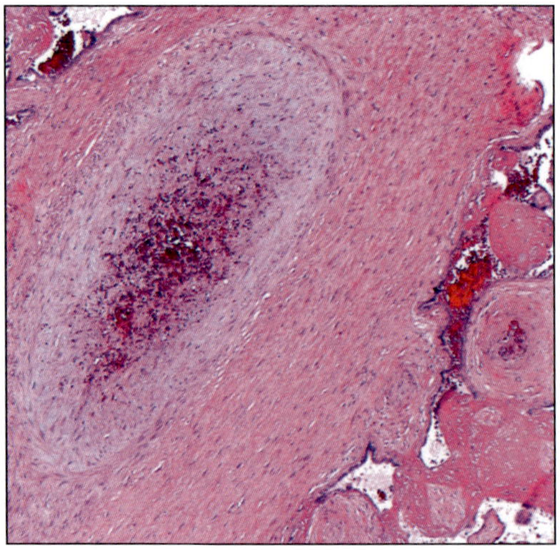

LARGE VESSEL FETAL VASCULAR OCCLUSION

Microscopic Features

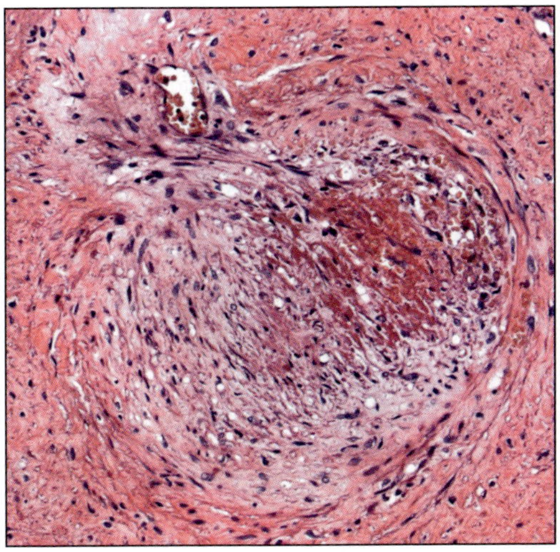
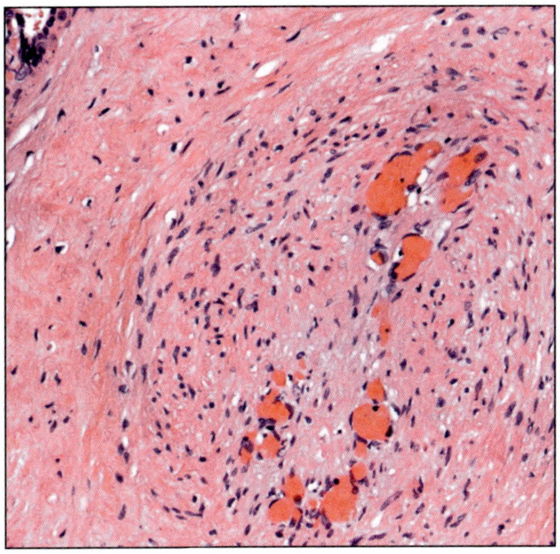

(Left) *The lumen is obliterated by fibrous strands and shows septation resembling recanalization.* ***(Right)*** *Later in the course of these stem villous obliterative changes, only rare fibrous strands or red cell fragments are seen. The lumen is septated into multiple small channels, often forming a ring where the endothelium once lay.*

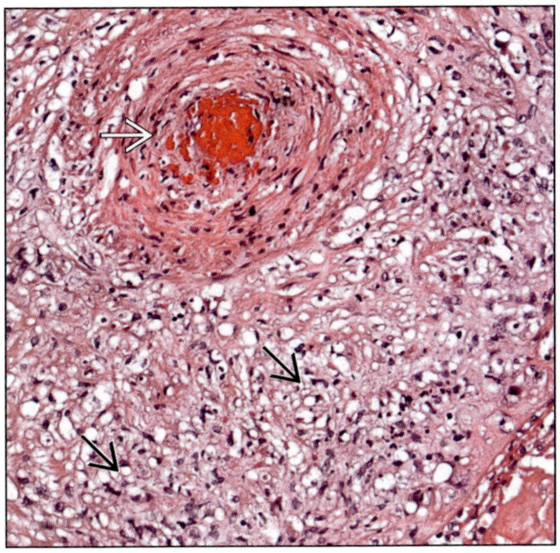
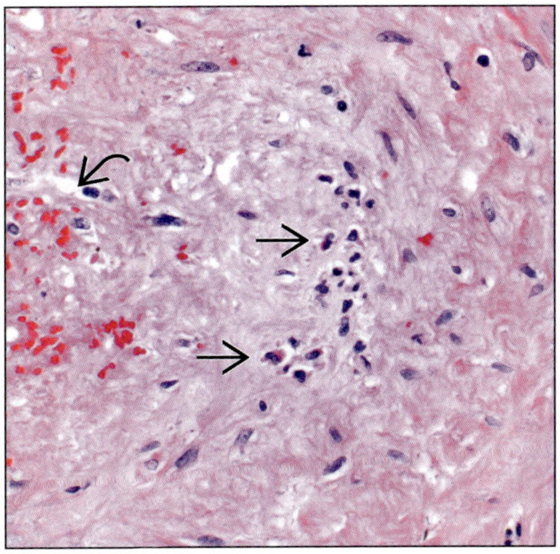

(Left) *The initial injury causing stem villous vessel occlusion may be chronic villitis. This vessel shows loss of endothelial integrity, extravasation, and fragmentation of red blood cells ➔. The villous stroma contains a lymphohistiocytic infiltrate → indicative of chronic villitis.* ***(Right)*** *Rarely, an eosinophilic/T-cell inflammatory infiltrate → accompanies the vaso-obliterative lesions ↪.*

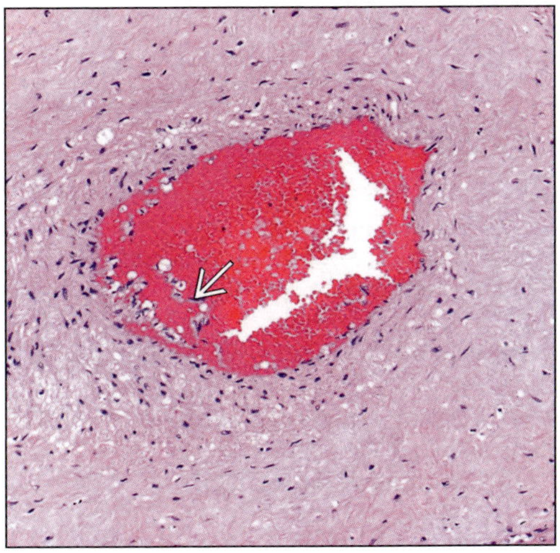
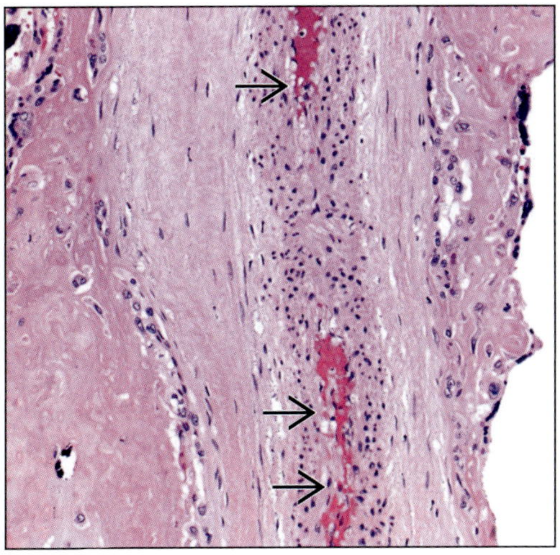

(Left) *Detachment of the endothelium ➔ due to refrigeration artifact, as seen in this chorionic plate vessel, should be distinguished from loss of endothelial integrity or fibrin strands of a vaso-occlusive process.* ***(Right)*** *Refrigeration artifact can also be seen in stem villous vessels → and needs to be distinguished from true lesions of vascular occlusion.*

DISTAL VILLOUS LESIONS ASSOCIATED WITH FETAL VASCULAR OCCLUSION

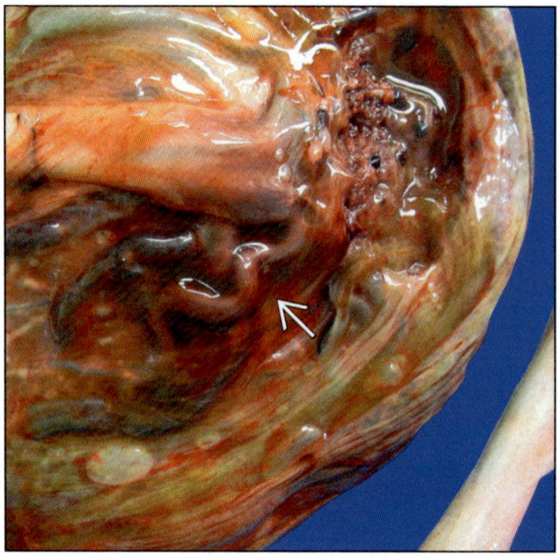

Fetal surface of the placenta of a stillborn term fetus shows a tight nuchal cord. Note the dilated, firm, white, thrombosed vessels on the fetal surface ➡.

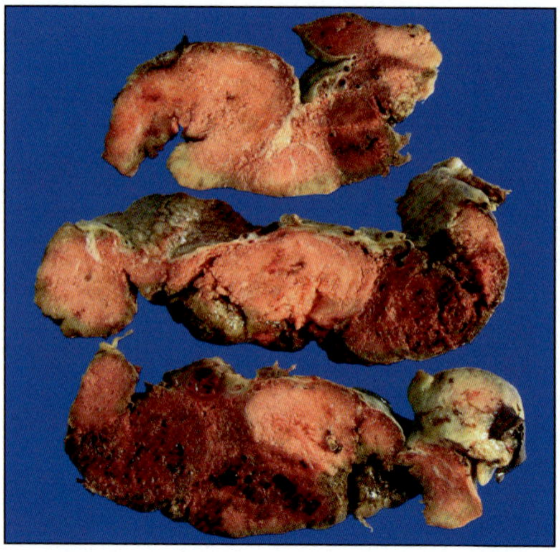

Cut surface of the placenta shows numerous pale areas that appear more granular than typical infarcts. These represent large areas of avascular villi and villous stromal-vascular karyorrhexis.

TERMINOLOGY

Synonyms

- Terms that describe histologically similar changes
  - Fetal thrombotic vasculopathy (FTV)
  - Chronic obstructive fetal vasculopathy
  - Chronic fetal vascular obstructive changes
  - Vaso-obliterative fetal vascular changes
  - Hemorrhagic endovasculitis/hemorrhagic endovasculopathy
  - Fetal vascular involutional changes

Definitions

- FTV
  - Term introduced in 1995 by Redline
  - Encompasses large vessel and distal villous changes of vascular occlusion, but not all may be due to true thrombi
- Villous stromal-vascular karyorrhexis (VSVK)
  - Terminal villi with karyorrhexis of fetal cells, including nucleated red blood cells, leukocytes, endothelial cells, &/or villous stromal cells
  - Important component in diagnosis of FTV
- Avascular villi
  - Terminal villi with total loss of villous capillaries and bland hyaline fibrosis of villous stroma
  - Important component in diagnosis of FTV
- Hemorrhagic endovasculopathy (HEV) (older terminology)
  - Terminal or stem villi with extravasated red blood cells into villous stroma, karyorrhexis of fetal cells, and septation of vessels
  - Controversial entity due to its similarities with changes that occur in stillbirth
  - Difficult to distinguish from VSVK histologically
    - Some consider it to be similar or same lesion
- Chronic villitis of unknown etiology (CVUE) with obliterative fetal vasculopathy
  - VUE of proximal stem vessels occludes fetal perfusion of distal villous tree resulting in VSVK and avascular villi

ETIOLOGY/PATHOGENESIS

Loss of Perfusion From Proximal Fetal Vasculature

- Any condition that ceases perfusion upstream of distal villi can cause VSVK and avascular villi
  - Umbilical cord compromise, arterial thrombi, fetal heart failure, fetal demise
  - Villous capillaries degenerate secondary to lack of fetal perfusion
- VSVK is considered the early stage, and avascular villi is deemed the later stage
  - Supported by progression of in utero demise to delivery interval changes
- VSVK with intravillous hemorrhage or with hemorrhagic appearance similar to HEV may occur secondary to venous obstruction

CLINICAL ISSUES

Epidemiology

- Incidence
  - 5% of placentas from live births submitted for pathologic examination show VSVK or avascular villi
    - ~ 1/2 that number have extensive changes graded as severe
    - Many more placentas from stillbirths have VSVK or avascular villi
  - 1% of placentas from all term births show FTV

Prognosis

- FTV is associated with numerous fetal/neonatal morbidities and mortality

DISTAL VILLOUS LESIONS ASSOCIATED WITH FETAL VASCULAR OCCLUSION

Key Facts

Macroscopic Pathology

- Main gross characteristic of avascular villi is villous pallor on cut sections of placenta
- May also show gross evidence of large upstream vessel occlusion

Microscopic Pathology

- Avascular villi: Terminal villi with total loss of villous capillaries and bland hyaline fibrosis of villous stroma
- Villous stromal-vascular karyorrhexis: Terminal villi with karyorrhexis of fetal cells, including nucleated red blood cells, leukocytes, endothelial cells, &/or villous stromal cells
- Villitis of unknown etiology with obliterative fetal vasculopathy (chronic villitis with associated avascular villi)

Top Differential Diagnoses

- Fetal thrombotic vasculopathy must be distinguished from changes of in utero fetal demise

Diagnostic Checklist

- Recommended use of header: "Changes consistent with chronic fetal vascular obstruction"
  - List findings in fetal vasculature (thrombi, vaso-obliterative lesions)
  - List distal villous findings (avascular villi, villous stromal-vascular karyorrhexis): > 2 foci
- Diagnosis of fetal thrombotic vasculopathy used for most severe cases: Average of ≥ 15 affected villi (avascular or villous stromal-vascular karyorrhexis) per slide

  - Still, most infants born with these lesions in placenta will be healthy

Obstetrical Complications Associated With FTV

- Preeclampsia
- Pregnancy-associated recurrent hemolytic-uremic syndrome
- Intrauterine growth restriction
- Oligohydramnios
- Abnormal umbilical artery Doppler velocimetry
- Decrease in cord blood arterial and venous pH
- Stillbirth
  - Placentas with FTV are associated with 9x increase in rate of stillbirth when compared with control placentas without FTV

Associated Placental Pathologies

- Umbilical cord abnormalities
- Changes of severe maternal vascular malperfusion
- Chronic villitis of unknown etiology with obstructive fetal vasculopathy

Neonatal Morbidity Associated With FTV

- Central nervous system injury: Infarcts, cerebral palsy, neurologic impairment, neonatal encephalopathy
- Visceral ischemic disease: Perinatal liver disease, Budd-Chiari syndrome, renal vein thrombosis, myocardial infarction
- Transverse ischemic limb reduction defects
- Fetal cardiac abnormalities
- Thrombocytopenia
- Thrombophilia
  - Few cases with FTV have thrombophilic mutation identified

MACROSCOPIC FEATURES

General Features

- Avascular villi
  - Small foci are not detectable grossly
  - Larger foci consist of a well-demarcated area of villous pallor on cut surface of placenta
    - Villous beefy-red color is derived predominantly from fetal red blood cells
    - Avascular villi have no fetal capillaries or blood, so they appear pale
    - Pale foci retain fine granularity of villous parenchyma
  - Classically, arterial occlusion is characterized by wedge-shaped area of pallor with apex of wedge pointing to occluded vessel (toward chorionic plate)
- Villous stromal-vascular karyorrhexis
  - Small foci are not detectable grossly
  - Larger foci may show villous pallor or, if there is significant entrapped red cells, foci may appear more hemorrhagic
- Gross abnormalities of umbilical cord should not be overlooked

MICROSCOPIC PATHOLOGY

Histologic Features

- Avascular villi
  - Terminal villi with total loss of villous capillaries and bland hyaline fibrosis of villous stroma
  - Distribution consistent with obstructed flow in large supplying or draining fetal vessel
    - Linear or finger-like pattern, like withered branch(es) of a tree
    - Often clustered together
  - Small amount of karyorrhectic debris is allowable
  - Hemosiderin may be present
  - Surrounding villous trophoblast and intervillous space are preserved
- Villous stromal-vascular karyorrhexis
  - Terminal villi with karyorrhexis of fetal cells, including nucleated red blood cells, leukocytes, endothelial cells, &/or villous stromal cells
  - Stroma may be hypercellular and show mineralization

DISTAL VILLOUS LESIONS ASSOCIATED WITH FETAL VASCULAR OCCLUSION

  - Villi can be hypovascular or show only capillary degenerative changes
  - Entrapped red blood cells and red blood cell fragments are often seen
  - Hemosiderin may be present
  - Surrounding villous trophoblast cells and intervillous space are preserved
- Evidence of large vessel occlusion may or may not also be present

Overlap With Histologic Changes in Stillbirth

- Stasis of fetal blood flow after fetal death leads to involutional changes in fetal vasculature that mimic antemortem changes of fetal vascular obstruction
  - Large fetal vessels of chorionic plate and stem villi can show fibroblast septation with appearance of recanalized thrombus and even total fibrous obliteration
  - Distal villi show intravascular karyorrhexis, stromal debris, and, ultimately, total villous fibrosis (avascular villi)
- True fibrin or layered thrombus and vascular ectasia of fetal vessels are not part of fetal vascular involutional changes after fetal death
- Regionally (as opposed to diffusely) distributed avascular villi also signify antemortem fetal vascular occlusion

DIFFERENTIAL DIAGNOSIS

Parenchymal Infarcts

- Grossly visible foci of avascular villi are often mistaken for infarcts
  - Infarcts are firmer, more homogeneous, and less granular than foci of avascular villi

Chorangioma

- Hemorrhagic foci of VSVK may resemble other hemorrhagic-appearing lesions, such as chorangioma

Chronic Villitis of Unknown Etiology

- VSVK and avascular villi may be found with chronic villitis when stem villi are inflamed
  - The term "CVUE with associated obstructive fetal vasculopathy" is preferred over FTV in this setting

Massive Perivillous Fibrin Deposition

- Avascular villi may be associated with massive perivillous fibrin deposition
  - May be a mechanism of fetal and maternal perfusion matching
- Presence of large vessel occlusive lesions help to distinguish FTV from massive perivillous fibrin deposition

DIAGNOSTIC CHECKLIST

Clinically Relevant Pathologic Features

- FTV must be distinguished from fetal vascular involution due to in utero demise in stillbirth cases
  - Identical villous changes, differ only in focal vs. diffuse distribution

REPORTING CRITERIA

Society for Pediatric Pathology, Perinatal Section, Fetal Vascular Obstruction Nosology Committee

- Recommended use of header: "Changes consistent with chronic fetal vascular obstruction"
  - List findings in fetal vasculature (thrombi, vaso-obliterative lesions)
  - List distal villous findings (avascular villi, VSVK): > 2 foci
- Diagnosis of FTV should be reserved for cases demonstrating
  - Average of ≥ 15 affected villi (avascular or VSVK) per slide
    - Fetal vascular thrombi are not required for diagnosis of FTV, but when identified, they should be reported

SELECTED REFERENCES

1. Ernst LM et al: Gross patterns of umbilical cord coiling: correlations with placental histology and stillbirth. Placenta. 34(7):583-8, 2013
2. Ryan WD et al: Placental histologic criteria for diagnosis of cord accident: sensitivity and specificity. Pediatr Dev Pathol. 15(4):275-80, 2012
3. Saleemuddin A et al: Obstetric and perinatal complications in placentas with fetal thrombotic vasculopathy. Pediatr Dev Pathol. 13(6):459-64, 2010
4. Tantbirojn P et al: Gross abnormalities of the umbilical cord: related placental histology and clinical significance. Placenta. 30(12):1083-8, 2009
5. Parast MM et al: Placental histologic criteria for umbilical blood flow restriction in unexplained stillbirth. Hum Pathol. 39(6):948-53, 2008
6. Ariel I et al: Placental pathology in fetal thrombophilia. Hum Pathol. 35(6):729-33, 2004
7. McDonald DG et al: Placental fetal thrombotic vasculopathy is associated with neonatal encephalopathy. Hum Pathol. 35(7):875-80, 2004
8. Redline RW et al: Fetal vascular obstructive lesions: nosology and reproducibility of placental reaction patterns. Pediatr Dev Pathol. 7(5):443-52, 2004
9. Redline RW: Clinical and pathological umbilical cord abnormalities in fetal thrombotic vasculopathy. Hum Pathol. 35(12):1494-8, 2004
10. Dahms BB et al: Severe perinatal liver disease associated with fetal thrombotic vasculopathy. Pediatr Dev Pathol. 5(1):80-5, 2002
11. Redline RW et al: Placental lesions associated with cerebral palsy and neurologic impairment following term birth. Arch Pathol Lab Med. 124(12):1785-91, 2000
12. Redline RW et al: Fetal thrombotic vasculopathy: the clinical significance of extensive avascular villi. Hum Pathol. 26(1):80-5, 1995
13. Genest DR: Estimating the time of death in stillborn fetuses: II. Histologic evaluation of the placenta; a study of 71 stillborns. Obstet Gynecol. 80(4):585-92, 1992

Microscopic Features

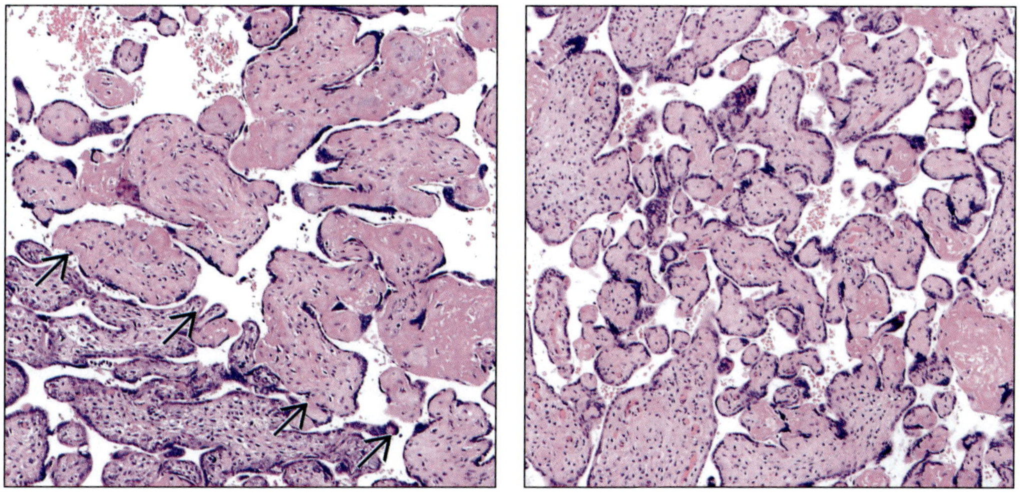

(Left) *Avascular villi* → *show eosinophilic, paucicellular stroma without capillaries. The trophoblast layer is intact. In comparison, the unaffected villi below have more cellular stroma and intact capillaries.* **(Right)** *Avascular villi show eosinophilic, paucicellular stroma without capillaries. On low-power examination, these foci stand out because of their lack of capillaries.*

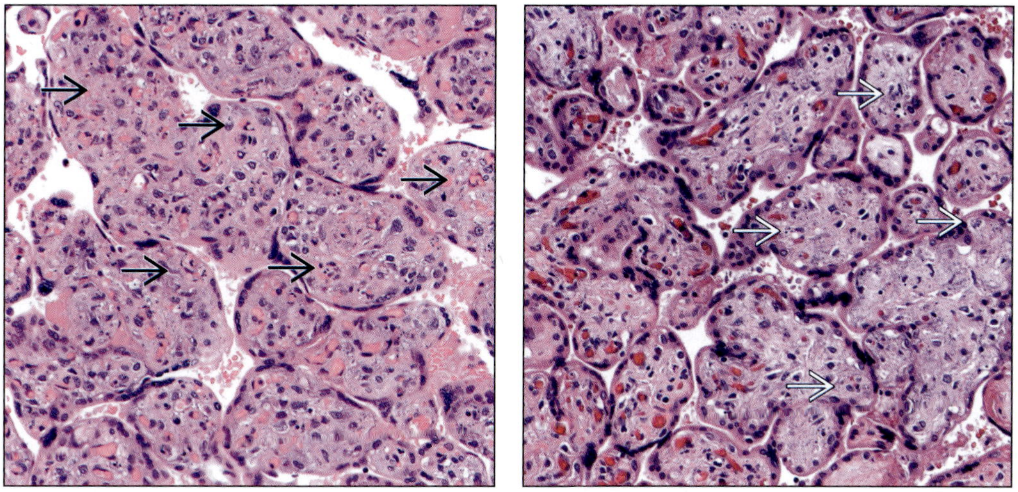

(Left) *In villous stromal-vascular karyorrhexis, some patent capillaries may be visible, but many are showing karyorrhexis* → *of nucleated blood cells, endothelial cells, and stromal cells.* **(Right)** *Villous stromal-vascular karyorrhexis may be more subtle to identify on low power because capillaries may not be completely lost. The eye is directed to paler foci, and high-power examination confirms the presence of karyorrhexis* ➔.

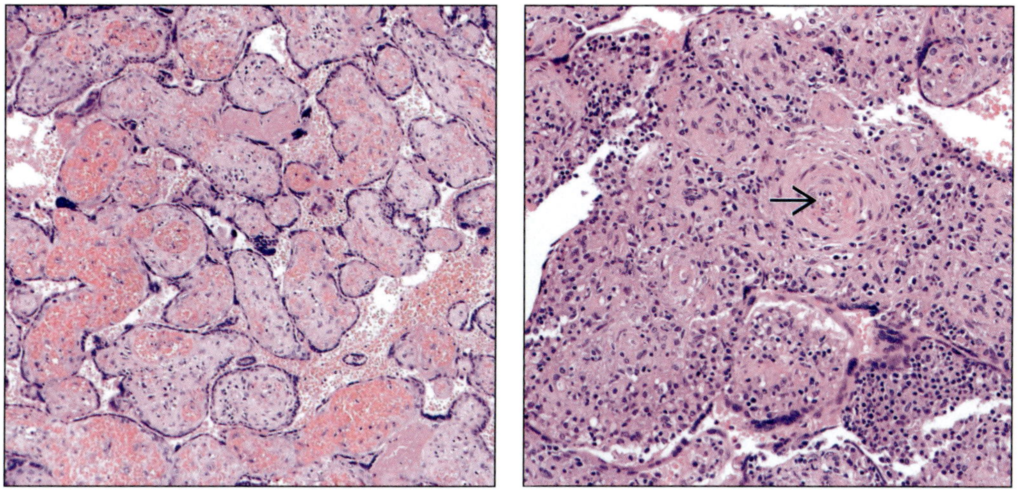

(Left) *In this case, the villi show villous stromal-vascular karyorrhexis in addition to intravillous hemorrhage. The combination of these 2 features suggests obstruction of fetal venous flow in the proximal vasculature. Iron stains may show extensive hemosiderin deposition.* **(Right)** *Proximal chronic villitis involving stem villi causes obliteration of the stem vessels* →*. This focus is associated with downstream avascular villi.*

Features of Lesions of Variable Age

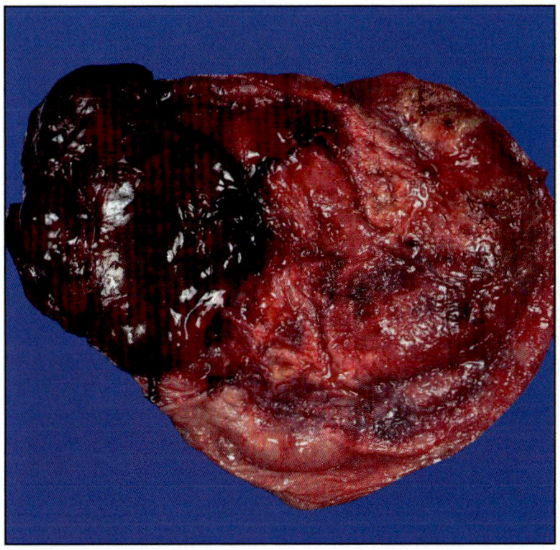

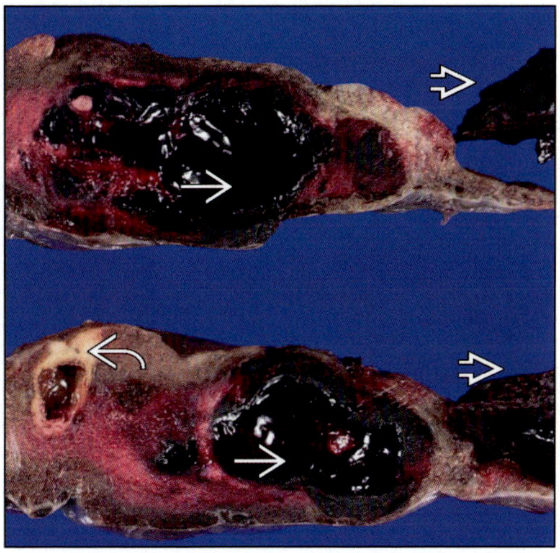

(Left) *A marginal hematoma is present on the maternal surface of a placenta delivered at 31 weeks gestation following intrauterine fetal demise in the setting of maternal preeclampsia.* ***(Right)*** *Cut sections of the same placenta demonstrate multiple lesions of varying age. Acute marginal hematoma compresses the underlying parenchyma. There is a large central infarction hematoma and a smaller, remote one.*

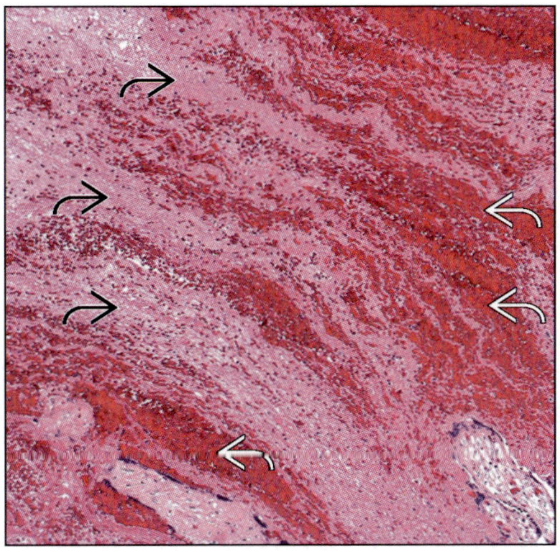

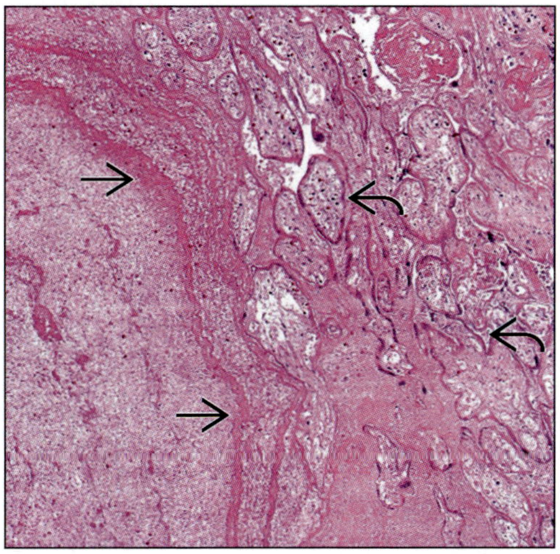

(Left) *The central infarction hematoma an intermediate-aged lesion demonstrating layering of fibrin and red blood cells.* ***(Right)*** *An older lesion consists of laminated fibrin clot with dissolution of red blood cells and an adjacent rim of infarcted villi.*

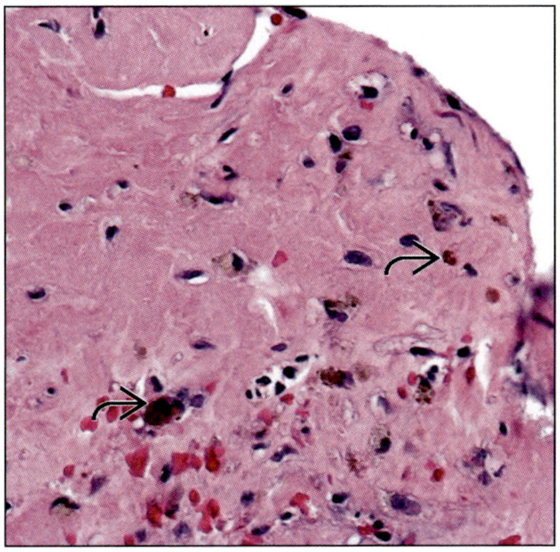

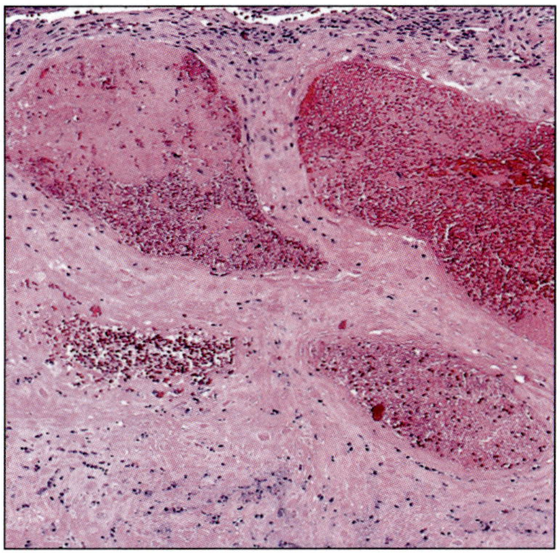

(Left) *This section of the maternal surface contains abundant hemosiderin pigment and macrophages, consistent with remote episodes of retroplacental hemorrhage.* ***(Right)*** *The maternal vessels in the placenta with the marginal hematoma demonstrate focal acute thrombosis and changes of decidual vasculopathy.*

CHRONIC ABRUPTION

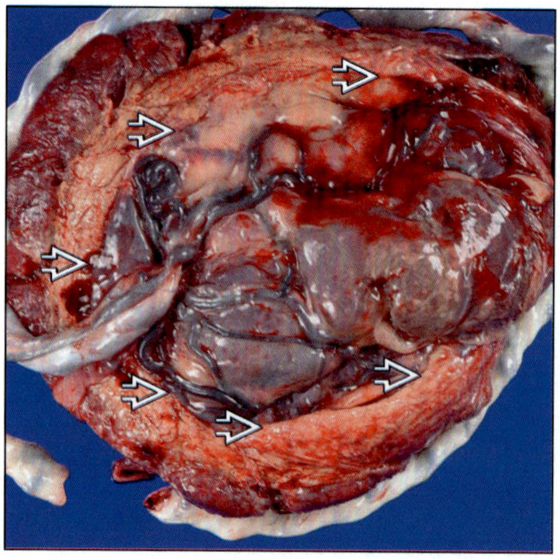

A 496 g placenta with circumvallate membrane insertion ➲ associated with subchorionic to marginal blood clot was seen on prenatal imaging. Delivery was induced due to oligohydramnios.

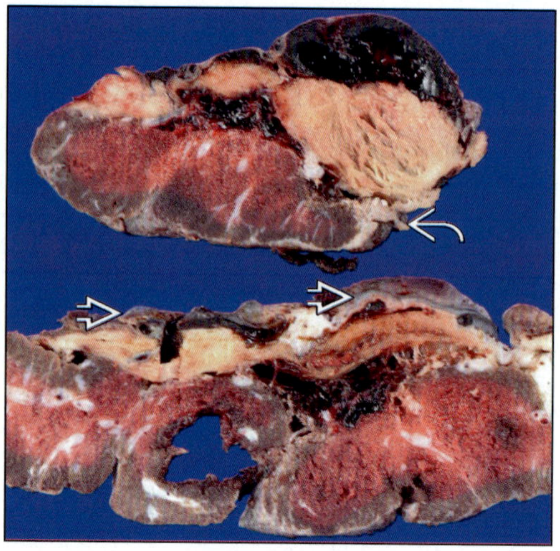

Cross sections of the same placenta demonstrate remote, dissolving clot admixed with fresh clot extending from the margin ➲ under the chorionic plate ➲.

TERMINOLOGY

Synonyms

- Variable usage of language
  - Chronic peripheral separation
  - Retroplacental hemorrhage with delay in delivery > 7 days
  - Marginal placental bleeding
  - Marginal sinus thrombosis or rupture
  - Venous hemorrhage/abruption

Definitions

- Repetitive or persistent hemorrhage with associated placental separation involving peripheral plate or membranes not associated with imminent delivery

CLINICAL ISSUES

Presentation

- May be asymptomatic
- Vaginal bleeding
- Loss of fluid per vagina
- Abdominal pain
- False/threatened preterm labor
- Evolving oligohydramnios
- Premature rupture of membranes
- Intrauterine fetal growth restriction
- Intrauterine fetal death

Treatment

- Increased fetal monitoring
- Surveillance of amniotic fluid levels
- Serial imaging for detection of resolution vs. extension of lesion
- Tocolytics and corticosteroids as appropriate for gestational age and clinical parameters
- Elective delivery in cases of poor fetal growth or fetal distress

Prognosis

- Larger volume of hematoma related to less favorable outcomes
- Related to gestational age and fetal well-being
  - Complications of prematurity, including chronic lung disease
  - Risk of adverse neurodevelopmental outcome
- ~ 60% develop chronic abruption-oligohydramnios sequence (CAOS)

IMAGE FINDINGS

Ultrasonographic Findings

- Sonolucency at site of hematoma/clot
- Decreased amniotic fluid/oligohydramnios

MACROSCOPIC FEATURES

General Features

- Degenerating blood clot ± more recent hemorrhage
- Circumvallate membrane insertion with associated degenerating marginal blood clot
- Subchorionic clot

Less Common Features

- Brown-green discoloration of fetal surface and membranes
- Associated parenchymal lesions, including infarcts

MICROSCOPIC PATHOLOGY

Histologic Features

- Marginal or peripheral subchorionic hematomas
  - Expansion of peripheral corner of placental disc with displacement of chorionic plate, peripheral membranes, or basal decidua by hematoma

CHRONIC ABRUPTION

Key Facts

Etiology

- Hemorrhage, often repetitive or persistent, most likely of venous origin or peripheral in location

Clinical Issues

- Alternative causes of vaginal bleeding, such as placenta previa, should be excluded
- Obstetric management based on volume of hematoma and fetal well-being, including surveillance of amniotic fluid level

Macroscopic Pathology

- Hematomas often located at disc margin with extension into subchorionic region
- Circumvallation with associated marginal blood clot
- Hemosiderotic discoloration of membranes

Microscopic Pathology

- Blood clots of variable age
- Hemosiderin deposition due to chronic hemorrhage

    - Intermediate hematomas consist of laminated fibrin
    - Remote hematomas may be dissolved, appearing as lightly eosinophilic granular or fibrillary material
  - Adjacent parenchyma is variably affected by increased perivillous fibrinoid or villous infarction
- Diffuse chorioamniotic hemosiderosis
  - Increased chorionic macrophages
  - Accumulation of hemosiderin pigment in chorionic plate and extraplacental membranes
- Associated lesions
  - Villous infarcts
  - Regions of decidual necrosis
  - Inflammatory infiltrate associated with hematoma
  - Necrotizing chorioamnionitis

DIAGNOSTIC CHECKLIST

Clinically Relevant Pathologic Features

- Volume of hematoma or affected parenchyma should be estimated and reported

Pathologic Interpretation Pearls

- Chronic abruption is variably defined and accepted as a clinicopathologic entity
- CAOS is a specifically defined entity
  - Clinical hemorrhage with delay of delivery > 7 days
  - Lack of predisposing factor, such as placenta previa
  - Ensuing oligohydramnios without rupture of membranes
  - Increased preterm delivery and increased incidence of chorioamnionitis
- Conflicting evidence of significance of hemosiderosis is present in literature

SELECTED REFERENCES

1. Khong TY et al: Haemosiderosis in the placenta does not appear to be related to chronic placental separation or adverse neonatal outcome. Pathology. 42(2):119-24, 2010
2. Norman SM et al: Ultrasound-detected subchorionic hemorrhage and the obstetric implications. Obstet Gynecol. 116(2 Pt 1):311-5, 2010
3. Walker M et al: Sonographic diagnosis of chronic abruption. J Obstet Gynaecol Can. 32(11):1056-8, 2010
4. Ohyama M et al: Maternal, neonatal, and placental features associated with diffuse chorioamniotic hemosiderosis, with special reference to neonatal morbidity and mortality. Pediatrics. 113(4):800-5, 2004
5. Redline RW et al: Chronic peripheral separation of placenta. The significance of diffuse chorioamnionic hemosiderosis. Am J Clin Pathol. 111(6):804-10, 1999
6. Elliott JP et al: Chronic abruption-oligohydramnios sequence. J Reprod Med. 43(5):418-22, 1998
7. Harris BA Jr: Peripheral placental separation: a review. Obstet Gynecol Surv. 43(10):577-81, 1988
8. Sauerbrei EE et al: Placental abruption and subchorionic hemorrhage in the first half of pregnancy: US appearance and clinical outcome. Radiology. 160(1):109-12, 1986
9. Naftolin F et al: The syndrome of chronic abruptio placentae, hydrorrhea, and circumvallate placenta. Am J Obstet Gynecol. 116(3):347-50, 1973

IMAGE GALLERY

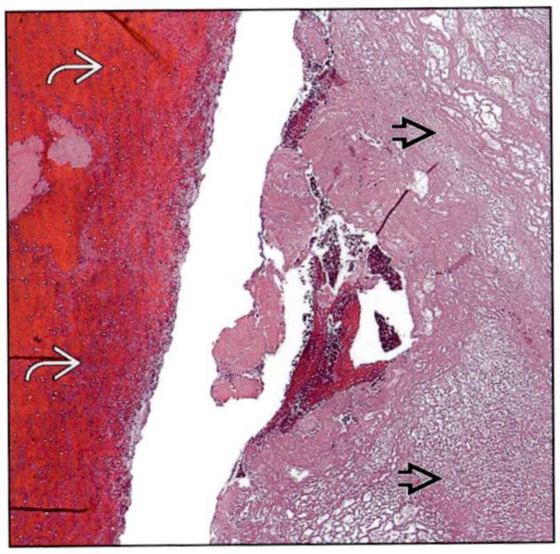
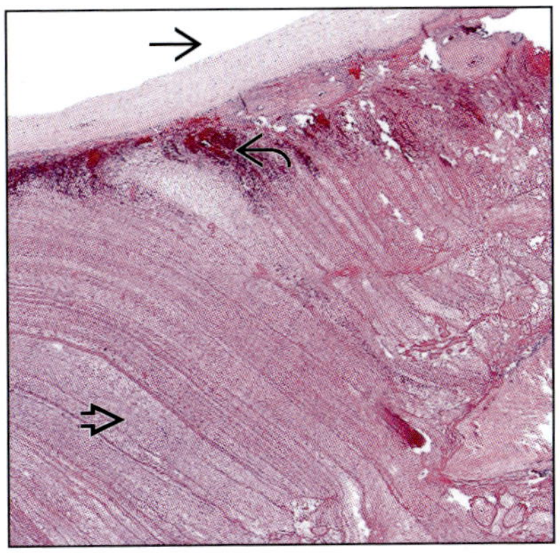
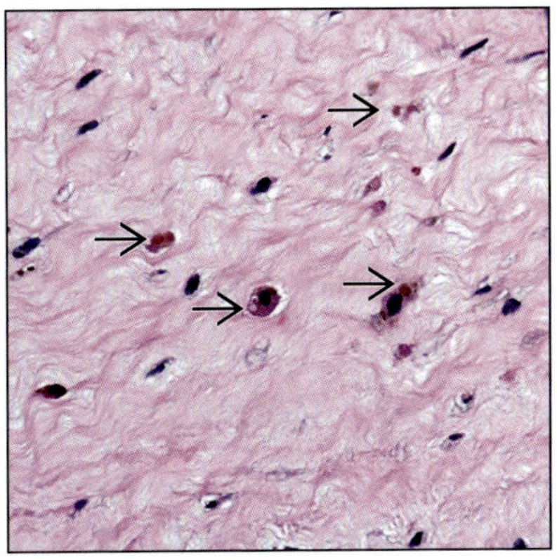

(Left) *The marginal hematoma has juxtaposed layers of new clot ➡ and remote, dissolving clot ⇨.* ***(Center)*** *A remote peripheral thrombohematoma extends beneath the chorionic plate →; the thrombohematoma is composed of fine layers of fibrin ⇨ and is surrounded by small amounts of fresh blood ↶.* ***(Right)*** *Remote hemorrhage adjacent to the chorionic plate or placental membranes can result in accumulation of hemosiderin pigment →.*

Villous Hypervascular Lesions

CHORANGIOSIS

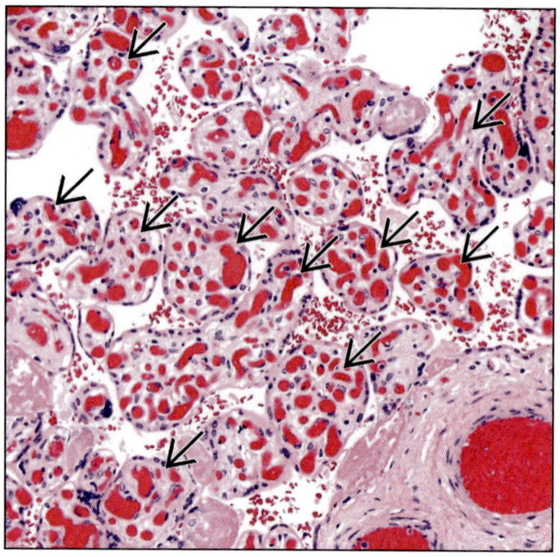

A representative field of a placenta with chorangiosis shows ≥ 10 terminal villi ➔ that contain ≥ 10 capillaries. If 9 other fields in other areas meet these criteria, a diagnosis of chorangiosis is merited.

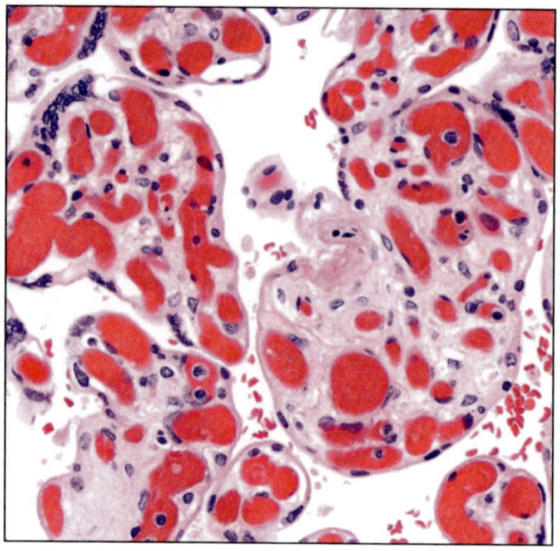

High-power view helps confirm the absence of a continuous pericyte layer around the capillaries.

TERMINOLOGY

Synonyms

- Villous chorangiosis
- Hypercapillarization

Definitions

- ≥ 10 areas of placental parenchyma with ≥ 10 terminal villi, each containing ≥ 10 capillaries

ETIOLOGY/PATHOGENESIS

Environmental Exposure

- Thought to be adaptive response to chronic placental underperfusion
- Cytotrophoblast proliferates more rapidly under hypoxic conditions and induces capillary endothelial proliferation
- Vascular proliferation exceeds stromal growth
  - Increased capillary:villus area ratio
- Stimulated by cytokines, growth factors, &/or increased vascular pressure

Incidence

- 5-10% of all placentas
- Typically only diagnosed in placentas after 37 weeks gestation

Associations

- More frequent in diabetic pregnancies
- More frequent in severely anemic mothers
- More frequent in setting of preeclampsia
- More frequent at higher elevations
- Associated with Beckwith-Wiedemann syndrome
- Variably associated with chronic villitis, villous hypomaturity, cord abnormalities, congenital malformations, and stillbirth

CLINICAL ISSUES

Prognosis

- Clinical significance remains disputed
- Has been associated with poor fetal outcome in some studies, but not in others

MACROSCOPIC FEATURES

General Features

- Lesion(s) not usually visible grossly
- Placentas with chorangiosis are often large for gestational age

MICROSCOPIC PATHOLOGY

Histologic Features

- ≥ 10 medium-powered fields of placental parenchyma with ≥ 10 terminal villi, each containing ≥ 10 capillaries
  - Normal: 2-6 capillaries/villus
- Capillaries are **not** surrounded by a continuous layer of pericytes

ANCILLARY TESTS

Immunohistochemistry

- Muscle-specific actin marks pericytes in chorangioma and chorangiomatosis
  - Absent in chorangiosis
- Endothelial markers, such as CD31 and CD34, should **not** be used
  - Not part of diagnostic criteria; will lead to overdiagnosis

CHORANGIOSIS

Key Facts

Terminology

- ≥ 10 fields of placental parenchyma with ≥ 10 terminal villi, each containing ≥ 10 capillaries

Etiology

- Thought to be an adaptive response to chronic placental underperfusion
- More frequent in diabetic and preeclamptic pregnancies
- Variably associated with chronic villitis, villous hypomaturity, cord abnormalities, congenital malformations, and stillbirth

Clinical Issues

- Clinical significance remains disputed

Macroscopic Pathology

- Placentas with chorangiosis are often large for gestational age

DIFFERENTIAL DIAGNOSIS

Congestion of Normal Terminal Villi

- Fetal capillary bed is normally only ~ 50% filled
  - Congestion will appear hypervascular
- True chorangiosis may have nearly 20 capillaries per villus, which are many more capillaries than would be apparent with vascular congestion

Chorangioma

- Single expansile nodule
- Capillaries have a continuous layer of pericytes

Chorangiomatosis

- Involves intermediate villi, stem villi
- Capillaries have a continuous layer of pericytes

DIAGNOSTIC CHECKLIST

Pathologic Interpretation Pearls

- Diagnosis should be made on H&E-stained slides
- Examine ≥ 10 fields in ≥ 3 areas of the sampled parenchyma
- Can be mimicked by vascular congestion

SELECTED REFERENCES

1. Gupta R et al: Clinico-pathological profile of 12 cases of chorangiosis. Arch Gynecol Obstet. 274(1):50-3, 2006
2. Evers IM et al: Placental pathology in women with type 1 diabetes and in a control group with normal and large-for-gestational-age infants. Placenta. 24(8-9):819-25, 2003
3. Ogino S et al: Villous capillary lesions of the placenta: distinctions between chorangioma, chorangiomatosis, and chorangiosis. Hum Pathol. 31(8):945-54, 2000
4. Kadyrov M et al: Increased fetoplacental angiogenesis during first trimester in anaemic women. Lancet. 352(9142):1747-9, 1998
5. Benirschke K: Obstetrically important lesions of the umbilical cord. J Reprod Med. 39(4):262-72, 1994
6. Benirschke K: Placenta pathology questions to the perinatologist. J Perinatol. 14(5):371-5, 1994
7. Reshetnikova OS et al: Effects of hypobaric hypoxia on the fetoplacental unit: the morphometric diffusing capacity of the villous membrane at high altitude. Am J Obstet Gynecol. 171(6):1560-5, 1994
8. Kaufmann P et al: [Correlations between placental morphology and fetal oxygen supply. Attempt at a cellular biological interpretation of pathohistologic and experimental findings.] Gynakologe. 26(1):16-23, 1993
9. Scheffen I et al: Alterations of the fetal capillary bed in the guinea pig placenta following long-term hypoxia. Adv Exp Med Biol. 277:779-90, 1990
10. Altshuler G: Chorangiosis. An important placental sign of neonatal morbidity and mortality. Arch Pathol Lab Med. 108(1):71-4, 1984

IMAGE GALLERY

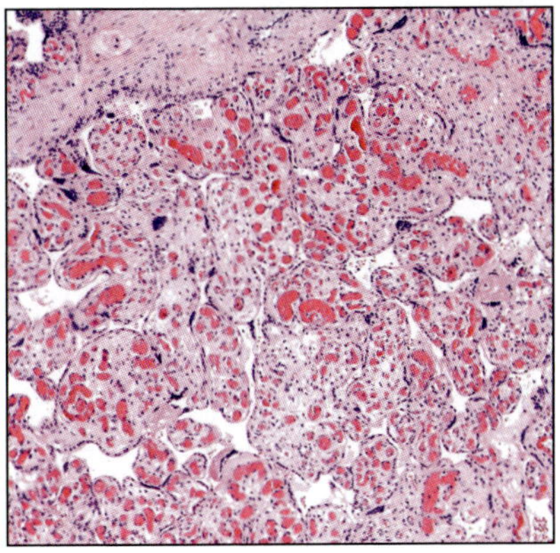

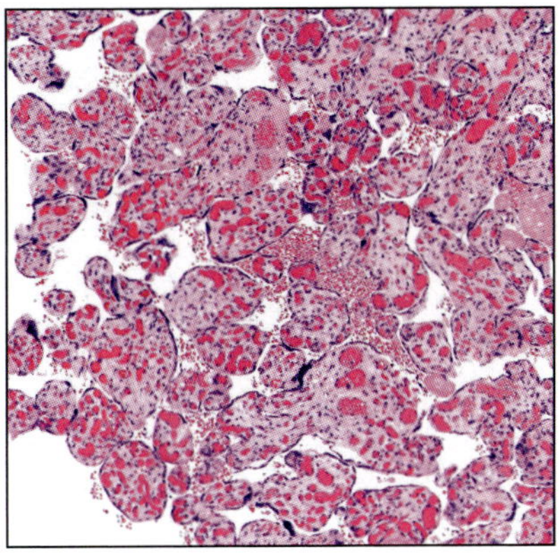

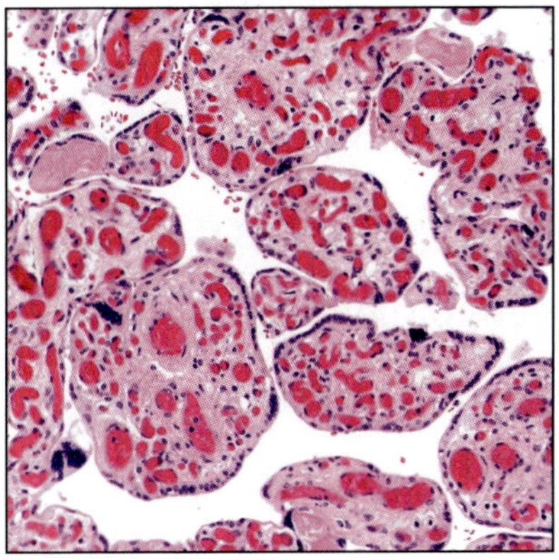

(Left) *Even under low power, the impression of hypervascularity raises suspicion for chorangiosis.* ***(Center)*** *At least 10 villi in each of the 10 areas should contain ≥ 10 capillaries in order to meet the recommended diagnostic criteria.* ***(Right)*** *Higher power view shows excess numbers of villous capillaries lacking a surrounding layer of pericytes.*

CHORANGIOMATOSIS

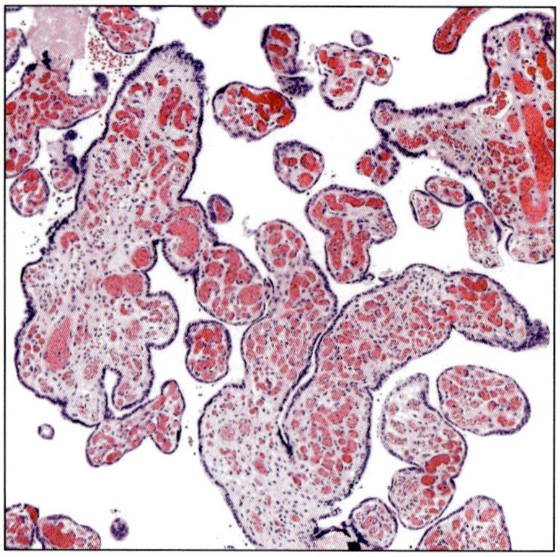

Localized chorangiomatosis shows expansion of multiple, adjacent intermediate villi by proliferating capillaries that are similar to those seen in chorangioma.

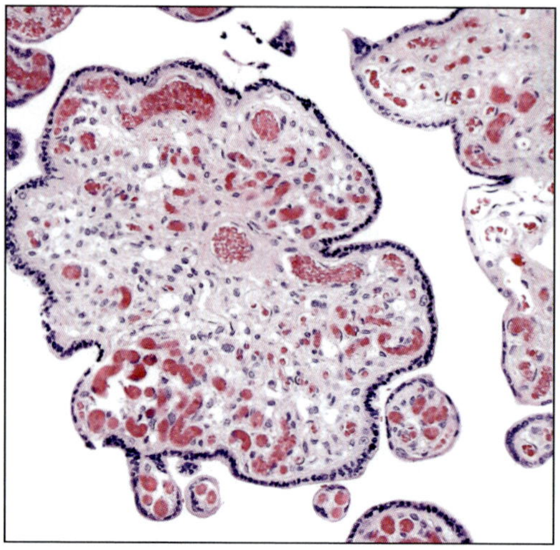

The lesional capillaries are surrounded by pericytes and involve intermediate villi, unlike those seen in chorangiosis.

TERMINOLOGY

Synonyms

- Localized chorangiomatosis
  - Focal chorangiomatosis
  - Segmental chorangiomatosis
- Multifocal chorangiomatosis
  - Diffuse chorangiomatosis
  - Diffuse multifocal chorangiomatosis
  - Multiple chorangiomas

Definitions

- Localized chorangiomatosis
  - Chorangioma-like lesion that extends into and permeates adjacent stem villi in a single area rather than forming a single nodule
- Multifocal chorangiomatosis
  - Chorangioma-like vascular proliferation in multiple adjacent villi in multiple areas of placenta
  - Multiple chorangioma-like lesions scattered throughout placenta

ETIOLOGY/PATHOGENESIS

Developmental Anomaly

- May arise from aberrant overgrowth of peripheral capillary net seen in immature intermediate villi maturing to early stem villi

CLINICAL ISSUES

Epidemiology

- Incidence
  - < 1% of all placentas

Presentation

- Localized chorangiomatosis is associated with maternal preeclampsia and multiple gestation pregnancies
- Multifocal chorangiomatosis is associated with placentomegaly, advanced maternal age, avascular villi, preterm delivery, intrauterine growth restriction, and congenital malformations
- Both forms are associated with other vascular abnormalities, including chorangiosis and chorangiomas
- Platelet sequestration in lesional vessels can lead to thrombocytopenia or disseminated intravascular coagulation in neonates

MACROSCOPIC FEATURES

General Features

- Localized and multifocal chorangiomatosis are not usually grossly identifiable
- Multiple chorangiomas may be evident as scattered small tan or red nodules

MICROSCOPIC PATHOLOGY

Histologic Features

- Localized chorangiomatosis
  - Similar to chorangioma, but rather than forming a single nodule, it involves multiple adjacent stem villi
  - Capillary vessel proliferation throughout the involved stem villi
  - Lesional vessels are surrounded by pericytes and lattice-like reticulin fibers
  - Increased stromal collagenization, sometimes with a central fibrotic core
- Multifocal chorangiomatosis

CHORANGIOMATOSIS

Key Facts

Clinical Issues

- < 1% of all placentas
- Localized chorangiomatosis is associated with maternal preeclampsia and multiple gestation pregnancies
- Multifocal chorangiomatosis is associated with placentomegaly, advanced maternal age, avascular villi, preterm delivery, intrauterine growth restriction, and congenital malformations

Microscopic Pathology

- Localized chorangiomatosis has capillary proliferation within multiple adjacent stem villi
- Multifocal chorangiomatosis has small anastomosing capillaries at periphery of stem villi surrounding a central vessel in multiple areas of placenta
- Pericytes and stromal collagenization are present in localized and multifocal variants

  - Involves multiple foci of multiple stem villi or intermediate villi
  - Small anastomosing capillaries at periphery of stem villi surrounding a central vessel
  - Lesional vessels surrounded by pericytes and increased stromal collagen

ANCILLARY TESTS

Histochemistry

- Reticulin highlights stromal matrix surrounding capillaries
  - Reactivity:
  - Staining pattern
    -

Immunohistochemistry

- Pericytes surrounding capillaries are positive for muscle-specific actin
- Vimentin highlights stromal hypercellularity

DIFFERENTIAL DIAGNOSIS

Congestion of Normal Terminal Villi

- Capillaries should be counted to avoid overcalling prominent, distended vessels

Chorangioma

- Single (or, rarely, multiple) nodule expanding a single stem villus

Chorangiosis

- > 10 terminal villi with > 10 capillaries each in each of the 10 fields
- Lesional vessels lack surrounding pericytes
- Hypervascularity confined to terminal villi

SELECTED REFERENCES

1. Bagby C et al: Multifocal chorangiomatosis. Pediatr Dev Pathol. 14(1):38-44, 2011
2. Amer HZ et al: Chorangioma and related vascular lesions of the placenta--a review. Fetal Pediatr Pathol. 29(4):199-206, 2010
3. Chopra A et al: Diffuse multifocal chorangiomatosis of the placenta with multiple intestinal stenosis of the fetus: combination of rare causes for nonimmune hydrops fetalis. Indian J Pathol Microbiol. 49(4):600-2, 2006
4. Saltzman M et al: Luteinized cystic ovarian hyperplasia associated with placentomegaly due to chorangiomatosis. Fetal Pediatr Pathol. 24(1):31-7, 2005
5. Caldarella A et al: Chorangiosis: report of three cases and review of the literature. Pathol Res Pract. 199(12):847-50, 2003
6. Ogino S et al: Villous capillary lesions of the placenta: distinctions between chorangioma, chorangiomatosis, and chorangiosis. Hum Pathol. 31(8):945-54, 2000

IMAGE GALLERY

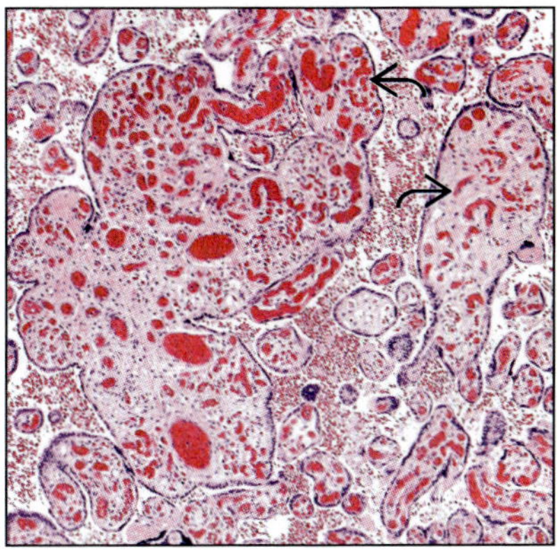

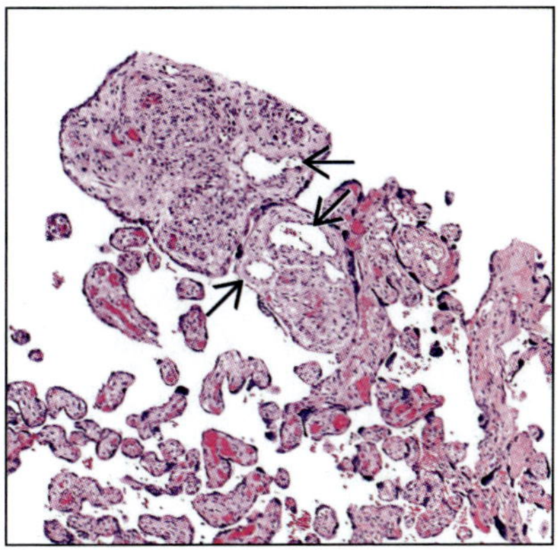

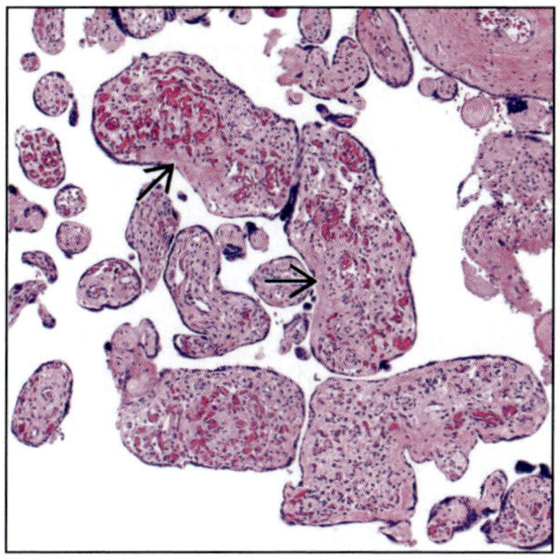

(Left) *Multifocal chorangiomatosis involves several areas ⇨ throughout the parenchyma in this case.* ***(Center)*** *The vessels in multifocal chorangiomatosis often consist of small capillaries at the periphery of the intermediate/stem villus surrounding a larger central vessel(s) ⇨.* ***(Right)*** *The villi have increased stromal cellularity and matrix with areas of collagenization ⇨ and a lattice-like pattern on reticulin stain.*

CHORANGIOMA

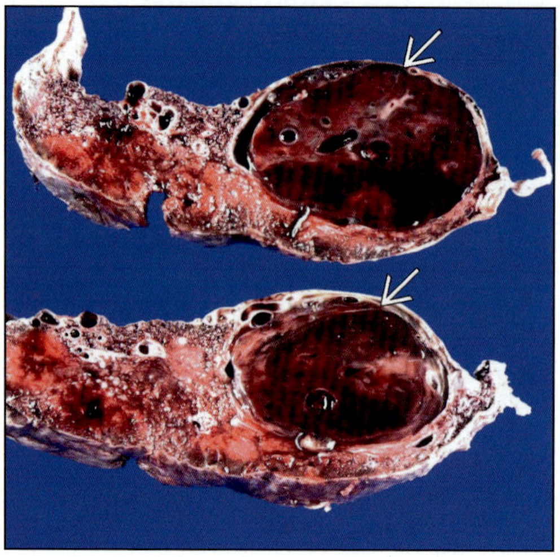

A medium-sized chorangioma ➡ bulges from the underside of the chorionic plate in sections of a placenta. The circumscribed, red, firm appearance is characteristic of these highly vascular lesions.

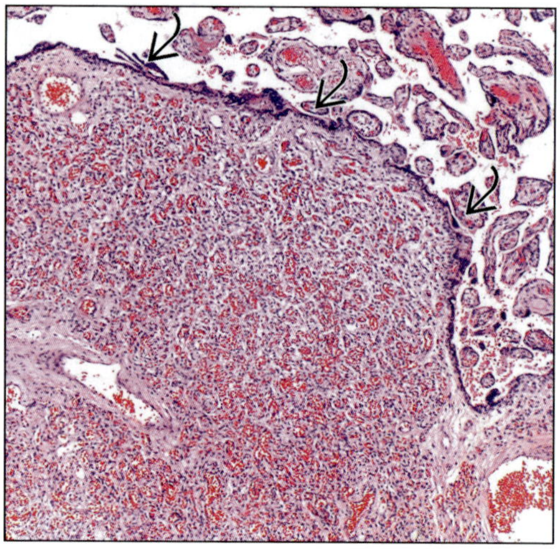

Chorangiomas are composed of capillary proliferations expanding stem villi. The capillaries are surrounded by stromal cells, and the nodule is surfaced by trophoblast ➡ that may be hyperplastic.

TERMINOLOGY

Synonyms

- Chorangioma and placental hemangioma and fibroangiomyxoma

Definitions

- Intraparenchymal nodule composed of capillaries, stromal cells, and trophoblast

ETIOLOGY/PATHOGENESIS

Environmental Exposure

- A reactive proliferation, not a neoplasm
- Placental hypoxia triggers angiogenesis and excessive capillary proliferation

Associations

- More common in preeclamptic pregnancies
- More common in multiple gestation pregnancies
- More common at high altitudes
- May recur in subsequent pregnancies
- Fetal hemangiomas/vascular lesions may occur concurrently

CLINICAL ISSUES

Epidemiology

- Incidence
  - ~ 0.5-1.0% of all placentas

Presentation

- Usually develops during 32-37 weeks gestation
- Small chorangioma is usually asymptomatic
- Medium-sized/large chorangioma is associated with fetal growth restriction
- Large chorangioma can cause
  - Preterm delivery
  - Arteriovenous shunting (with fetal hydrops, high-output heart failure, polyhydramnios, &/or fetal death)
  - Platelet trapping (with fetal thrombocytopenia, hemorrhage, &/or disseminated intravascular coagulation)
  - Maternal "mirror" syndrome (with maternal edema or preeclampsia in association with fetal hydrops)
- Spontaneous involution/regression of large chorangioma is associated with improvement of clinical symptoms

Treatment

- Usually not treated; if fetal distress occurs, delivery can often be induced
- Symptomatic fetal therapy
  - Amnioreduction, blood transfusion
  - Surgical ligation of placental vessels feeding chorangioma
  - Alcohol injection of lesion to induce vascular sclerosis
  - Laser ablation of lesion

MACROSCOPIC FEATURES

General Features

- Single or multiple nodules
- Usually subchorionic or marginal (sites of lower oxygen levels)
- Can be dark and soft (vascular) or firm and tan (fibrotic)

Size

- Range: 1 mm to > 10 cm

CHORANGIOMA

Key Facts

Terminology
- Intraparenchymal nodule composed of capillaries, stromal cells, and surrounding trophoblast layers

Etiology
- Excessive capillary proliferation in response to hypoxia

Macroscopic Pathology
- Single or multiple nodules, 1 mm to > 10 cm
- Usually subchorionic or marginal

Microscopic Pathology
- Vascular proliferation expanding a villus
- May have associated trophoblastic hyperplasia with pleomorphism and atypia

Top Differential Diagnoses
- Localized chorangiosis
- Multifocal chorangiomatosis

MICROSCOPIC PATHOLOGY

Histologic Features
- Capillary vessels set within a variably cellular and collagenous stroma, surrounded by trophoblast layers
- Stroma contains fibroblasts, macrophages, and collagen
- Vascular proliferation expanding a mature stem villus
- May have associated trophoblastic hyperplasia with pleomorphism and atypia, very rarely associated with choriocarcinoma (chorangiocarcinoma)
- Older lesions may have degenerative changes: Calcifications, infarcts, hemosiderin-laden macrophages
- Different subtypes (capillary, cavernous, endotheliomatous, fibrosing, fibromatous) have been described, but all have identical clinical behavior
- Never malignant despite variable mitotic activity, occasional atypical cytology, and variable cellularity

ANCILLARY TESTS

Immunohistochemistry
- Not required, but CD31 and CD34 stain endothelial lining, and muscle-specific actin stains pericytes
- GLUT1 negative (unlike infantile hemangioma)

Cytogenetics
- Not required but shows normal karyotype

Electron Microscopy
- Not required but shows features of normal capillaries and endothelial cells

DIFFERENTIAL DIAGNOSIS

Gross Mimics
- Villous infarcts

Histologic Mimics
- Localized chorangiosis (capillary proliferation limited to distal chorionic villi)
- Multifocal chorangiomatosis

SELECTED REFERENCES

1. Saksiriwuttho P et al: Prenatal three dimensional ultrasonography and expectant management of placental chorioangioma: a case report. J Med Assoc Thai. 96(4):496-500, 2013
2. García-Díaz L et al: Prenatal management and perinatal outcome in giant placental chorioangioma complicated with hydrops fetalis, fetal anemia and maternal mirror syndrome. BMC Pregnancy Childbirth. 12:72, 2012
3. Amer HZ et al: Chorangioma and related vascular lesions of the placenta--a review. Fetal Pediatr Pathol. 29(4):199-206, 2010
4. Taori K et al: Chorioangioma of placenta: sonographic features. J Clin Ultrasound. 36(2):113-5, 2008
5. Quarello E et al: Prenatal laser treatment of a placental chorioangioma. Ultrasound Obstet Gynecol. 25(3):299-301, 2005

IMAGE GALLERY

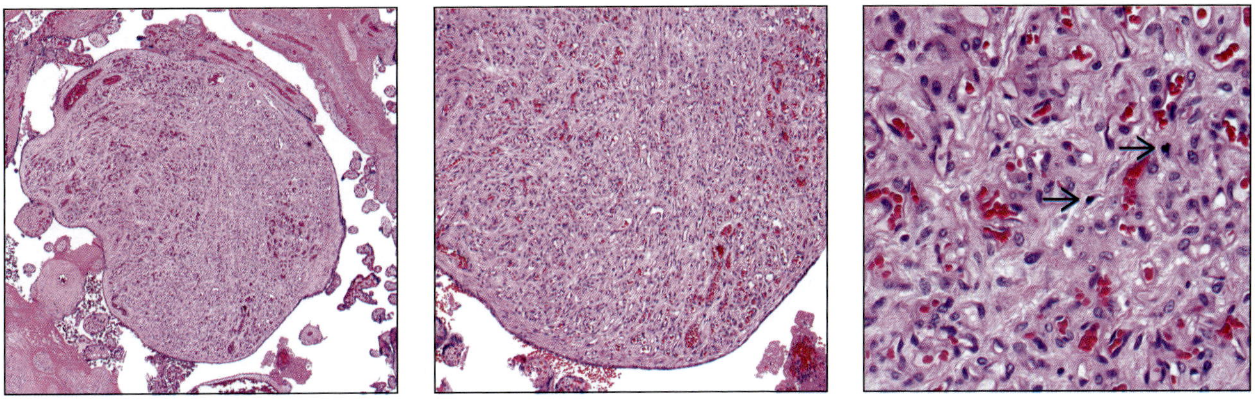

(Left) *Chorangioma is always well circumscribed. It expands the stem villus by a proliferation of capillaries and stroma.* ***(Center)*** *Capillaries are round, elongate, or irregularly shaped.* ***(Right)*** *Stromal mitoses ⇒ are a common finding and do not indicate malignant potential.*

Gestational Trophoblastic Disease and Metastatic Tumors

HYDROPIC DEGENERATION AND HYDATIDIFORM MOLE

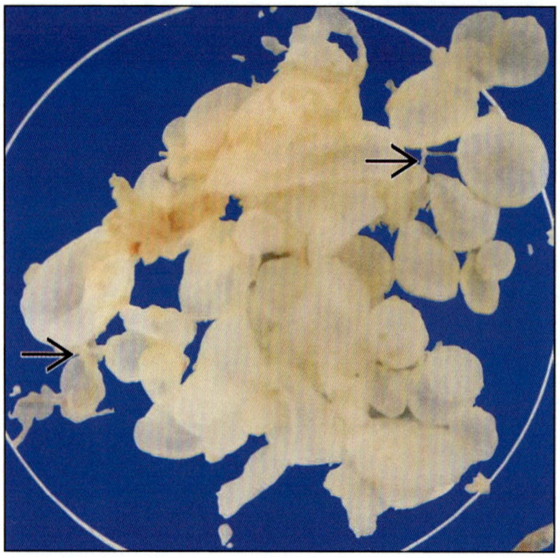

These complete hydatidiform molar villi have been rinsed to remove blood, then rehydrated in water. All villi are vesicular and connected by thin fibrous strands ➔.

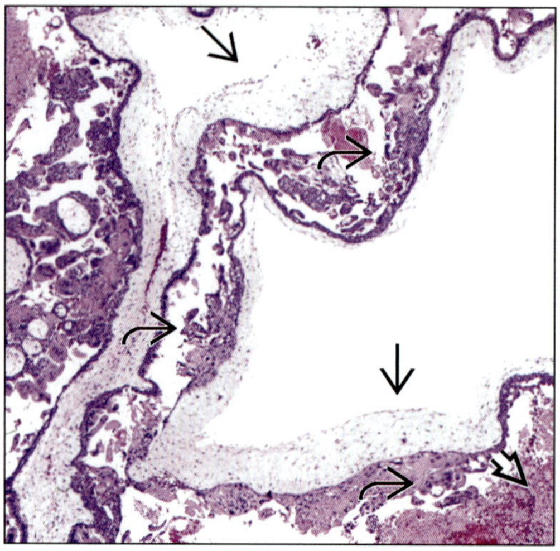

Microscopically, complete hydatidiform moles (CHMs) show well-developed central cisterns ➔, mixed circumferential trophoblast hyperplasia ➔, and focal remote hemorrhage ➔.

TERMINOLOGY

Abbreviations

- Hydropic degeneration (HD)
- Partial hydatidiform mole (PHM)
- Complete hydatidiform mole (CHM)
- Very early complete hydatidiform mole (VECHM)
- Human chorionic gonadotropin (hCG) generally refers to B subunit
- Gestational trophoblastic disease (GTD)

Definitions

- HD
  - Pathologic term referring to edematous microscopic appearance of nonmolar villi

ETIOLOGY/PATHOGENESIS

HD

- 50-75% are secondary to chromosomal abnormalities

PHM

- Triploid, diandrogenetic in origin, with 1 maternal genome and 2 paternal genomes
  - Normal ovum fertilized by 1 sperm that replicates (monospermy) or by 2 sperm (dispermy)
  - 58% are 69,XXY; 38% are 69,XXX; 4% are 69,XYY
  - Rarely tetraploid with 3 paternal components
  - Fetus may be present but usually dies as embryo
    - Live births are rare
  - Excess paternal (but not excess maternal) genomes drive placental overgrowth
  - Digynic triploidy is not associated with molar placenta
    - Very small placenta and severe intrauterine growth restriction (IUGR)
    - 69,XXX usually results in embryonic death, but 32% are liveborn

CHM

- Diandrogenetic, empty ovum fertilized by 1 sperm that replicates (monospermy) or by 2 sperm (dispermy)
- Because it is an abnormal ovum, occurs more commonly at early and late reproductive ages
- Most are diploid, but 6-40% are tetraploid
  - 93% are 46,XX and 4-12% are 46,XY
  - Dispermic in 2% of 46,XX and all 46,XY
  - All tetraploid cases studied have been 92,XXXX
- Biparental complete hydatidiform moles (BiCHM) are a rare autosomal recessive condition
  - Increased risk for recurrent moles and persistent trophoblastic disease
  - Maternal imprinted ovum, genetic defect of *NLRP7* or *KHDC3L* (*C6orf221*)
- By comparison, placental mesenchymal dysplasia (a.k.a. pseudopartial mole) is a mosaic of diandrogenetic cells in placental villous stroma and normal cells
  - Distinct from CHM, in which all cells are diandrogenetic

Invasive Mole

- Molar villi invade into myometrium without intervening decidua and into venous channels
- Theoretically, molar villi themselves can metastasize

Mole and Twin

- Fertilization of 2 ova, with 1 normal ovum and 1 empty ovum
- Rising incidence with induced ovulation

CLINICAL ISSUES

Epidemiology

- Incidence
  - PHM
    - True incidence unknown; may be underdiagnosed

HYDROPIC DEGENERATION AND HYDATIDIFORM MOLE

Key Facts

Microscopic Pathology

- Hydropic degeneration (HD), nonmolar specimens
  - Direct or indirect evidence of fetus
  - Round to oval villi with edematous, amphophilic stroma
  - Syncytiotrophoblast atrophy
  - Normal polar proliferation of anchoring villi
- Partial hydatidiform mole (PHM)
  - Direct or indirect evidence of fetus
  - 2 villous populations
  - 20% of villi may have central cisterns
  - Scalloping with trophoblast pseudoinclusion
  - Central cisterns without karyorrhectic stroma
  - Syncytiotrophoblast proliferation only
- Complete hydatidiform mole (CHM)
  - No direct or indirect evidence of fetus
  - All villi are enlarged
  - Central cisterns with karyorrhectic stroma
  - Mixed trophoblast proliferation is circumferential but may be discontinuous
  - Implantation site with markedly abnormal invasive trophoblasts
- Very early complete hydatidiform mole
  - Variation in villous size
  - Subtle scalloping with bulbus projections
  - Marked stromal cellularity and rare cisterns

Ancillary Tests

- p57
  - Positive in cytotrophoblasts and villous stroma in HD and PHM
  - Negative in cytotrophoblasts and villous stroma in CHM

- CHM
  - ~ 1 in 1,000 pregnancies
  - Invasive mole complicates 2-8% of CHM
  - Mole and twin occurs in 1 per 22,000-100,000 pregnancies

Presentation

- HD
  - Most present as missed abortion
  - Uterus small for dates
  - Decreasing or low hCG
    - In normal early gestation, serum hCG increases 66% every 48 hours
- PHM
  - Present as missed abortion or with vaginal bleeding
  - Uterus usually small for dates
  - Rarely has mildly increased hCG
  - Has been diagnosed in ectopic pregnancy
- CHM
  - Usually present as spontaneous abortion with dark brown vaginal bleeding
  - Uterus usually large for dates
  - More frequent at extremes of reproductive age
  - hCG often elevated > 100,000 mIU/mL
    - High hCG associated with hyperemesis, thecal lutein ovarian cysts, hyperthyroidism, early-onset preeclampsia
    - Tetraploid CHM may have higher hCG
  - May be associated with significant bleeding at time of uterine curettage
  - Has been diagnosed in ectopic pregnancy
- Invasive mole
  - Persistent elevation of hCG
  - Uterine bleeding after evacuation of CHM
  - May have mass in endometrial cavity or in myometrium
  - 15% of cases present with lung or vaginal metastases

Treatment

- Options, risks, complications
  - Follow-up for CHM is serum hCG levels, weekly or biweekly until 3 consecutive negatives, then monthly for 6 months
    - Half-life of hCG is 24 hours
    - hCG should return to negative within 6-8 weeks post evacuation
    - Patients with CHM are advised not to get pregnant for 1 year to allow for adequate follow up
  - Follow-up for PHM is similar to that for CHM, follow serum hCG levels until return to 0
- Surgical approaches
  - Uterine evacuation of products of conception is usually sufficient in PHM, CHM
  - Hysterectomy may be performed for CHM in women > 40 years of age due to increased risk for choriocarcinoma
  - Hysterectomy may be performed for invasive CHM

Prognosis

- GTD clinical risk stratification
  - Low risk
    - Serum hCG < 40,000 mIU/mL
    - Symptoms for < 4 months
    - No liver or brain metastases
    - No prior chemotherapy
    - GTD following a mole, ectopic pregnancy, or spontaneous abortion
  - High risk
    - Serum hCG > 40,000 mIU/mL
    - Symptoms for > 4 months
    - Liver or brain metastases
    - GTD following a term pregnancy
    - Higher hCG does not increase risk in tetraploidy CHM
- PHM
  - Persistent GTD in 0.5-4%
  - Exceedingly rare progression to choriocarcinoma
- CHM
  - Persistent GTD in 15-25%
    - Invasive mole occurs in 15%
    - Uterine choriocarcinoma in 2-8%

HYDROPIC DEGENERATION AND HYDATIDIFORM MOLE

- Metastatic GTD in 3%
  - Sites are lung (80%), vagina (30%), brain (10%), liver (10%)
- Dispermic CHM has nearly 100% persistent GTD; 20% incidence of metastatic disease
- Recurrence risk for developing a subsequent molar pregnancy is 1/100
  - 10x normal risk
- Mole and twin
  - CHM and twin: 55% incidence of persistent trophoblastic disease, 22% metastatic disease
    - Diagnosed later in gestation
    - Present with higher hCG, most likely due to multiple gestation

IMAGE FINDINGS

Ultrasonographic Findings

- HD
  - Gestational sac is smaller than expected for gestational age; no fetal pole or small embryo/fetus without cardiac activity
- PHM
  - Rarely diagnosed prior to pathologic examination
  - Empty gestational sac, or may have an embryo/fetus, usually significantly growth restricted
  - Rare vesicles, best seen on transvaginal ultrasound
- CHM
  - Classic appearance is "snow storm" due to multiple echogenic interfaces
  - No gestational sac or fetal pole
  - Very early complete mole may have small gestational sac, but no fetus
- Invasive mole
  - May have mass in endometrium or myometrium

MACROSCOPIC FEATURES

General Features

- HD
  - Varying amount of villous tissue, dependent on gestational age, but generally not increased
  - Gestational sac, chorionic plate usually present, rarely umbilical cord
  - Rarely identify embryonic or fetal tissues
    - Cartilage and bone will be firm to palpation
  - Hydropic villi rarely measure > 0.28 cm
- PHM
  - May have slightly increased amount of villous tissue
  - Gestational sac and chorionic plate are usually present
  - Gross vesicles, measuring 0.53 cm, are present in only 20% of villi
  - Diandric triploid fetus shows severe symmetric growth restriction, syndactyly of 3rd and 4th fingers &/or toes
    - By comparison, digynic triploid fetus shows asymmetric growth restriction with preservation of head growth, syndactyly of 3rd and 4th fingers &/or toes, not associated with molar villi
- CHM
  - Increased amount of tissue for gestational age
  - Majority of villi are vesicular, 1-2 cm in diameter, attached to one another by thin fibrous strands
  - Increased amount of old hemorrhage with well-formed clot is almost always present
- Very early hydatidiform mole
  - Usually scant tissue
  - Villi may have bulbous appearance but are usually not vesicular, may measure up to 0.7 cm
- Invasive hydatidiform mole
  - Hemorrhagic mass invasive into uterine tissues
- Mole and coexistent twin
  - Both complete and partial moles may be associated with a normal co-twin
  - Molar and nonmolar tissues may be intermixed in curettage specimens

Sections to Be Submitted

- If there is a clinical diagnosis of mole or grossly identified vesicles, submit all of the villous tissue or 10 cassettes
- Implantation site is characterized by increased firmness and yellow color due to fibrinoid deposition
  - Implantation site confirms an intrauterine pregnancy, even in absence of villi
  - Implantation site may identify abnormalities responsible for pregnancy loss
  - CHM has an atypical implantation site that is especially useful in identification of VECHM

MICROSCOPIC PATHOLOGY

Histologic Features

- HD, nonmolar specimens
  - Direct evidence of fetus
    - Embryonic or fetal tissues
  - Indirect evidence of fetus
    - Chorionic plate, amnion, umbilical cord, nucleated red blood cells, yolk sac
  - Villi are round to oval
    - Villous stroma is edematous, frequently amphophilic
    - Residual vessels are often present, sometimes containing nucleated red blood cells or karyorrhectic debris
    - Villous stromal cells may be necrotic with karyorrhexis
    - Variably increased number of Hofbauer cells
    - Syncytiotrophoblast atrophy, corresponds to decreasing hCG
  - No significant trophoblast proliferation
    - Anchoring villi with polar orientation of cytotrophoblast columns will be present
  - Normal invasive trophoblast at implantation site
- PHM
  - Direct or indirect evidence of fetus
  - 2 villus populations: Large hydropic and small fibrotic
    - Hydropic villi ≥ 2.5 mm

- Irregular villous shape (scalloping) resulting in formation of round or oval trophoblast pseudoinclusion
- Central cisterns without karyorrhectic stromal cells
- After 16 weeks, villi may have maze-like cisterns, that are actually dilated vascular structures
- Syncytiotrophoblast proliferation only; circumferential, discontinuous, lacy appearance
  - Normal anchoring villi with polar orientation of cytotrophoblast columns
  - Normal invasive trophoblast at implantation site
- Very early PHM
  - Direct or indirect evidence of fetus
  - Villi vary in size, but no distinct dual population
    - Scattered hydropic villi with rare cisterns, scattered fibrotic villi
    - Rare irregularly shaped villi with trophoblast pseudoinclusion
    - Abnormal but focal trophoblast hyperplasia, usually lacy syncytiotrophoblast
  - Normal invasive trophoblast at implantation site
- CHM
  - Enlarged, round villi, involving all villi
    - Vessels may persist until 10 weeks but will usually not contain nucleated red blood cells
    - Central cisterns with abundant karyorrhectic villous stromal cells, decreased Hofbauer cells
    - Trophoblastic proliferation is circumferential, but may be discontinuous
    - Syncytiotrophoblast proliferation may have a lacy appearance, often necrotic
    - Villous trophoblast proliferation is mixed, containing syncytiotrophoblast, cytotrophoblast, and intermediate trophoblasts
  - Anchoring villi with normal polar proliferations of trophoblast are usually not found
  - Implantation site trophoblast atypia
    - Invasive extravillous trophoblasts are enlarged with nucleomegaly, nuclear pleomorphism, and hyperchromasia and increased mitotic activity
    - May see multiple nucleoli or nuclear pseudoinclusion
    - Trophoblast invasion of maternal vessels for remodeling is diminished
  - Excessive remote hemorrhage
- Tetraploid CHM
  - Associated with larger villi and persistence of villous vessels
- Biparental CHM
  - Most are indistinguishable from androgenetic CHM, but subtle, less pronounced molar features have been reported
- VECHM
  - Variation in villous size
  - Villi have subtle scalloping with bulbus, cauliflower-like projections
    - Few residual villous vessels, rare or absent nucleated red blood cells
    - Abundantly cellular stroma, stromal mucin
    - Mixed trophoblast proliferation, but frequently syncytiotrophoblasts predominate
  - Implantation site changes similar to CHM
- Mole and twin
  - May have totally separate populations of normal and molar villi
  - Curetted samples are usually extensively intermixed and can be confusing
- Invasive mole
  - Villi that are invasive into myometrium generally lose their molar characteristics
    - May be smaller than intracavitary villi
    - Rarely have central cisterns
  - Trophoblastic proliferation is more pronounced and deep into myometrium

ANCILLARY TESTS

Immunohistochemistry

- Cyclin-dependent kinase inhibitor 1C (CDK1C, p57, KIP2)
  - Extravillous trophoblast at tips of columns and some decidual cells are positive in HD, PHM, and CHM
  - Positive nuclear staining in > 10% of villous cytotrophoblasts and stromal cells in HD and PHM
  - < 10% nuclear staining of villous cytotrophoblast and stromal cells in CHM
    - Tetraploid CHM may have absent or low p57 staining
    - Biparental CHM may have positive staining (retained maternal chromosome 11) or absent staining

Flow Cytometry

- Useful to assess ploidy
  - Diploid lesions may be HD or CHM
  - Triploid lesions may or may not be PHM
    - Diandric triploid conceptions are molar, digynic are not

Cytogenetics

- Identifies ploidy and other karyotypic abnormalities
  - Triploid lesions may be partial mole (if diandric)
  - Hydropic degeneration may have chromosomal abnormalities on routine karyotype

Molecular Genetics

- Considered "gold standard" in diagnosis, but cost may limit practical utility
- PCR for short tandem repeats identifies maternal and paternal contributions in a specimen
  - Only method to tell if a diploid result is normal, diandric, or digynic
  - Can determine if triploid result is diandric (PHM) or digynic (nonmolar)

Algorithm for Use in HD Diagnosis

- Morphology alone is effective for most cases of HD vs. mole
- Supplementation with p57 (KIP2) immunostain useful to exclude complete mole
  - Will not distinguish partial mole from HD
    - If clinically necessary, flow, cytogenetics, or FISH can identify triploid DNA of PHM

Serum β-hCG Levels During Normal Pregnancy

Weeks	5th Percentile	Mean	95th Percentile
4	318	719	1,065
6	16,451	41,642	81,650
8	81,313	133,885	232,315
10	50,155	95,670	151,440
12	37,990	79,236	129,005
14	30,500	67,630	136,900
16	15,942	32,889	87,115
18	7,400	26,560	50,000
20	8,963	19,920	37,217
22	12,600	23,855	40,800
24	9,328	19,560	33,130
26	6,800	24,707	57,200
28	13,030	31,584	72,970
30	12,071	21,690	46,650
32	9,160	28,860	77,100
34	5,198	26,374	93,405
36	8,120	30,290	96,700
38	10,360	34,763	10,360
40	5,943	23,138	71,556

β-hCG Values in Pregnancy, Clinical Assays, 1982.

- For research purposes or where clinically necessary, molecular genotyping provides most complete characterization
- Always check hCG and compare to expected normal levels for gestational age

DIAGNOSTIC CHECKLIST

Pathologic Interpretation Pearls

- Most important part of grossing specimen is to rinse out blood and float/rehydrate villi in water
  - This technique can be used even after formalin fixation
- Implantation site shows invasive extravillous trophoblast with marked atypia, helpful in morphologic diagnosis of VECHM
- Villous trophoblast proliferation in CHM is mixed (syncytiotrophoblast, cytotrophoblast, extravillous trophoblast) and is circumferential
- Villous trophoblast proliferation in PHM consists of syncytiotrophoblasts only

SELECTED REFERENCES

1. Banet N et al: Characteristics of hydatidiform moles: analysis of a prospective series with p57 immunohistochemistry and molecular genotyping. Mod Pathol. 27(2):238-54, 2014
2. Buza N et al: Partial hydatidiform mole: histologic parameters in correlation with DNA genotyping. Int J Gynecol Pathol. 32(3):307-15, 2013
3. Sebire NJ et al: Histopathological features of biparental complete hydatidiform moles in women with NLRP7 mutations. Placenta. 34(1):50-6, 2013
4. Sundvall L et al: Tetraploidy in hydatidiform moles. Hum Reprod. 28(7):2010-20, 2013
5. Gupta M et al: Diagnostic reproducibility of hydatidiform moles: ancillary techniques (p57 immunohistochemistry and molecular genotyping) improve morphologic diagnosis for both recently trained and experienced gynecologic pathologists. Am J Surg Pathol. 36(12):1747-60, 2012
6. Baasanjav B et al: The risk of post-molar gestational trophoblastic neoplasia is higher in heterozygous than in homozygous complete hydatidiform moles. Hum Reprod. 25(5):1183-91, 2010
7. Kim KR et al: The villous stromal constituents of complete hydatidiform mole differ histologically in very early pregnancy from the normally developing placenta. Am J Surg Pathol. 33(2):176-85, 2009
8. Vaisbuch E et al: Twin pregnancy consisting of a complete hydatidiform mole and co-existent fetus: report of two cases and review of literature. Gynecol Oncol. 98(1):19-23, 2005
9. Sebire NJ et al: Histopathological diagnosis of partial and complete hydatidiform mole in the first trimester of pregnancy. Pediatr Dev Pathol. 6(1):69-77, 2003

Hydropic Degeneration

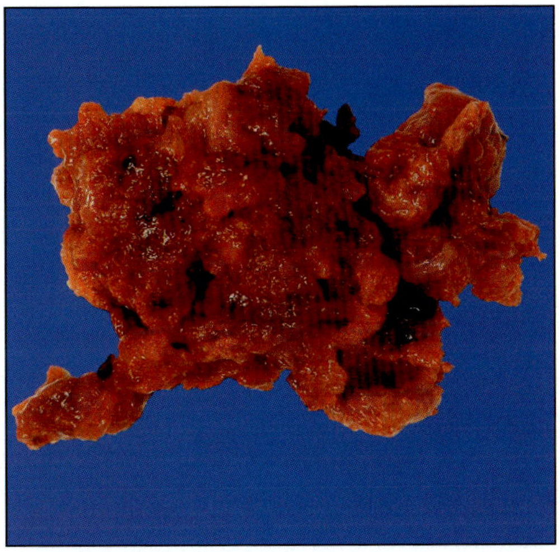

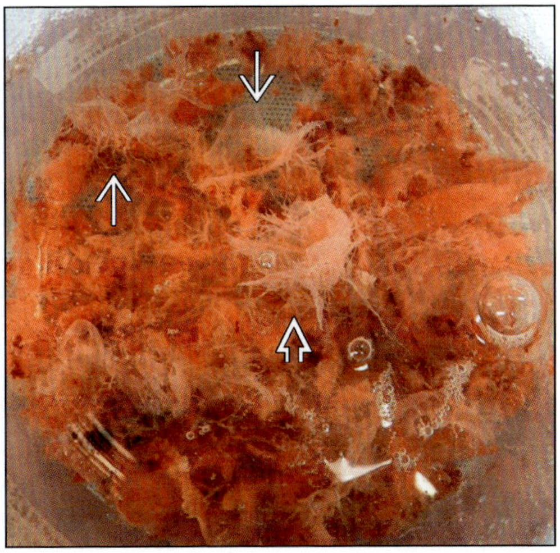

(Left) *Fresh tissue removed from a suction evacuation device without any additional manipulation does not show distinct villous tissue.* ***(Right)*** *This is the same specimen after rinsing through a fine mesh sieve and floating the tissue in water. The placental membranes → and villous tissue ⇨ are easily identified.*

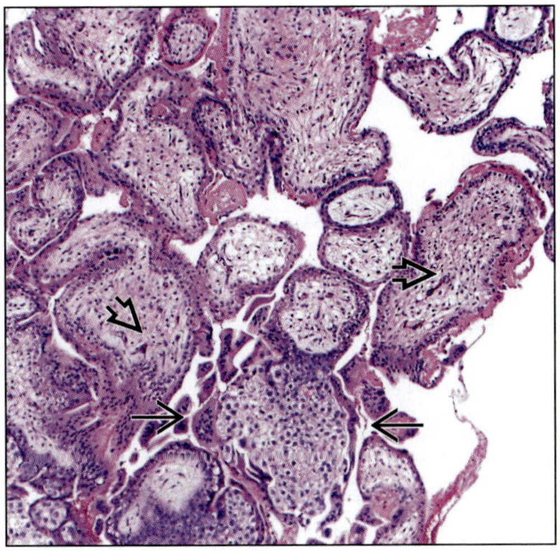

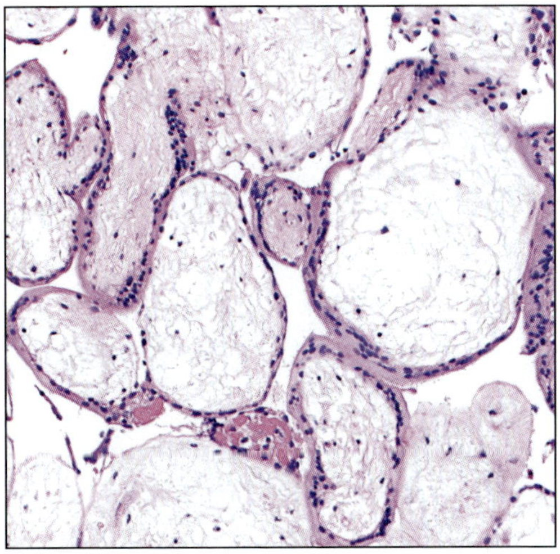

(Left) *First-trimester villi show normal polar trophoblast proliferation of an anchoring villus → with a column of cytotrophoblasts, covered by a layer of syncytiotrophoblasts. Many of the villi have vessels containing red blood cells ⇨.* ***(Right)*** *Hydropic degeneration (HD) shows an amphophilic, hypocellular stroma with no residual vessels. There is atrophy of surrounding trophoblasts. The findings usually indicate embryo loss significantly before evacuation of the uterine contents.*

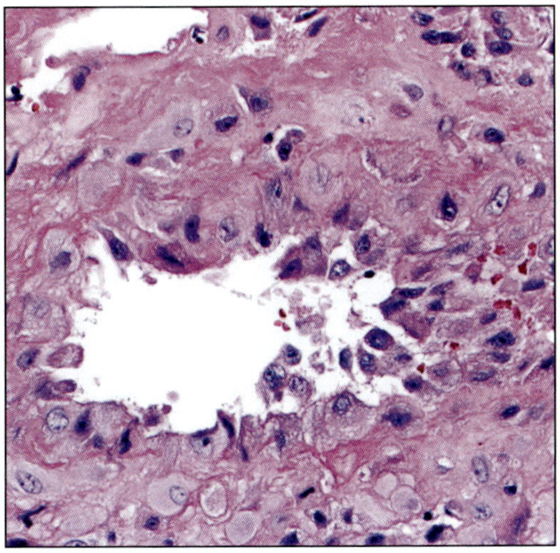

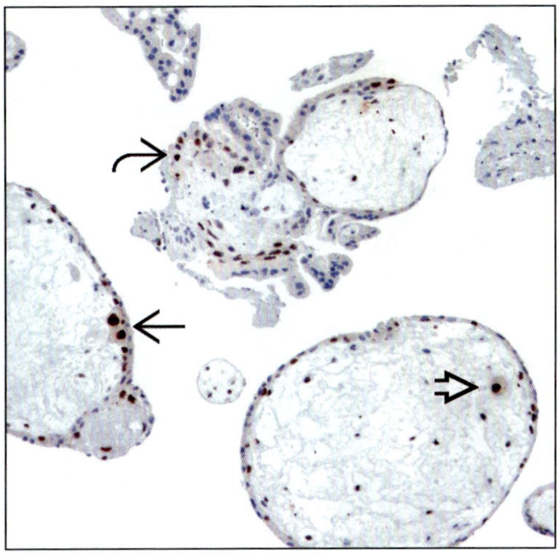

(Left) *This maternal vessel at the implantation site is undergoing normal vascular remodeling. The invasive trophoblast is in the wall and lumen; the muscularis is gone. Vascular remodeling is less common in gestational trophoblastic disease (GTD).* ***(Right)*** *In this case of HD, p57 is differentially expressed in the nuclei of villous cytotrophoblasts → and stromal cells ⇨. p57 is not differentially expressed in invasive trophoblasts ↪; HD, PHM, and CHM would all have nuclear staining in invasive trophoblasts.*

HYDROPIC DEGENERATION AND HYDATIDIFORM MOLE

Implantation Site

*(**Left**) Implantation decidua grossly has a yellow hyalinized appearance due to the deposition of fibrinoid. It is thinner and also has increased resistance. (**Right**) Implantation decidua shows the thick layer of fibrinoid ➔ with invasive trophoblasts ➩ in the decidua. On the surface of the fibrinoid, there are multinucleated syncytiotrophoblasts ↗. If necessary, a cytokeratin can be performed to confirm the presence of invasive trophoblasts.*

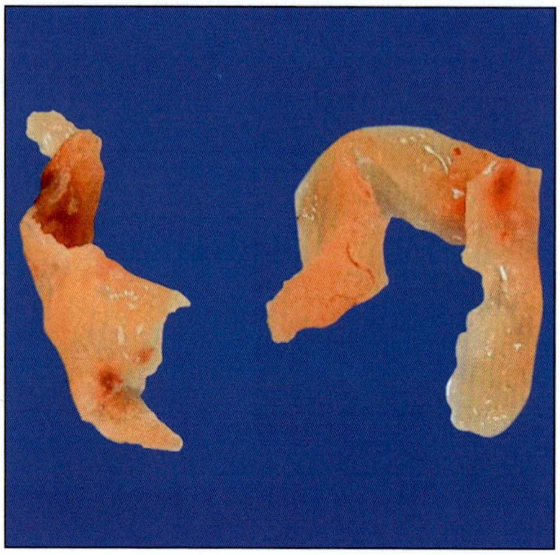

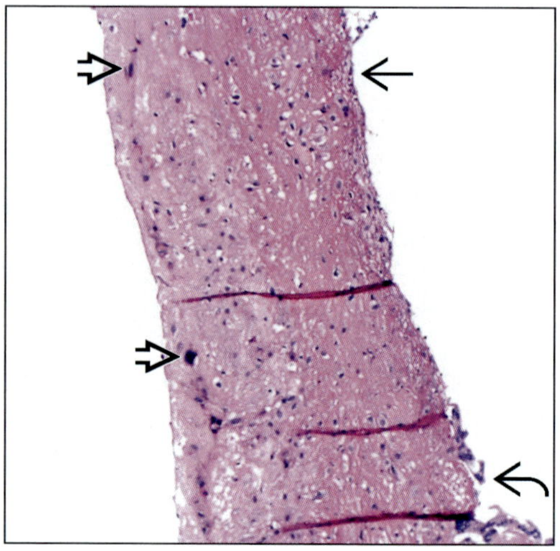

*(**Left**) The basal implantation site should also have maternal vessels that are undergoing adaptation to pregnancy. The vessel lumina normally contain, and may be completely plugged by, intermediate trophoblasts ➔ in the 1st trimester. Nitabuch fibrinoid ➩ is also noted focally. (**Right**) Villi within the chorion laeve frequently have significant hydropic degeneration ➔ and even show central cisterns. This is due to devitalization, as the free membranes are forming.*

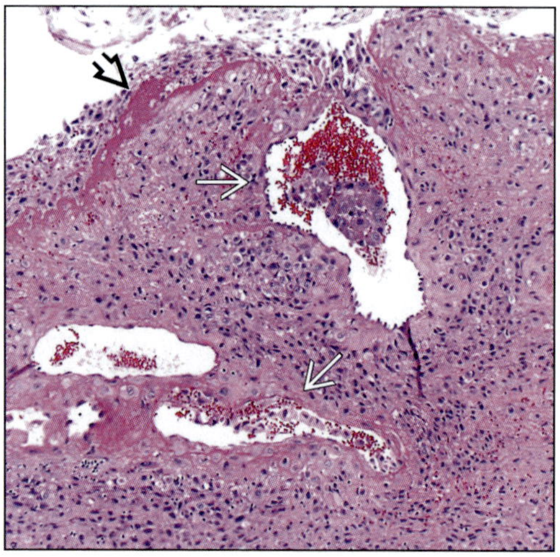

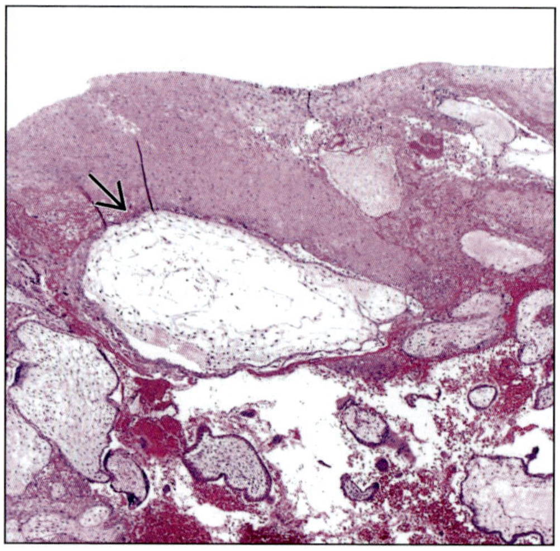

*(**Left**) The nonimplantation site decidua may represent the majority of tissue in early gestation. It is tan-pink, spongy, and usually present in sheets. There may be focal acute hemorrhage. (**Right**) Nonimplantation decidua shows changes of pregnancy hormones on the endometrium, but these changes are not diagnostic of an intrauterine pregnancy. Ectopic pregnancy would show the same decidualization. There is usually minimal acute decidual inflammation in spontaneous abortion.*

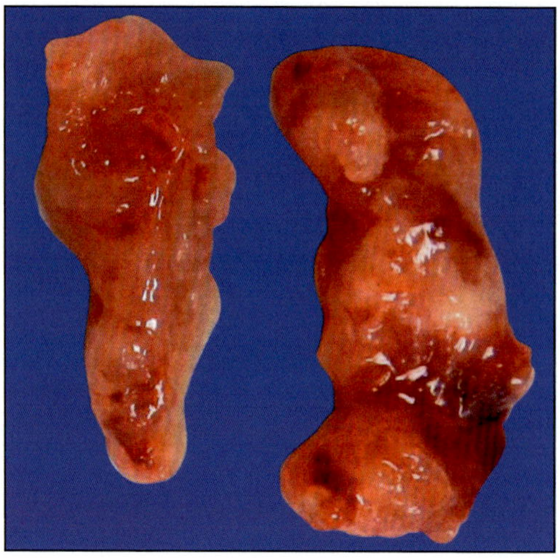

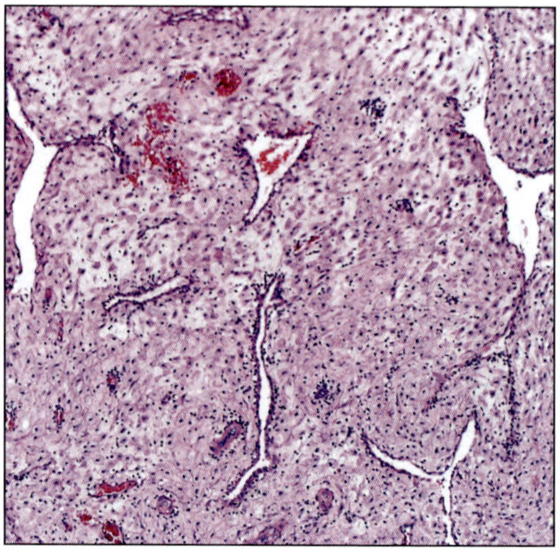

Partial Hydatidiform Mole

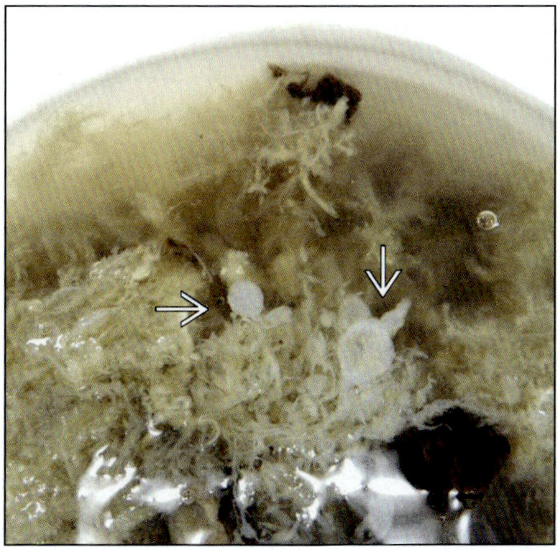

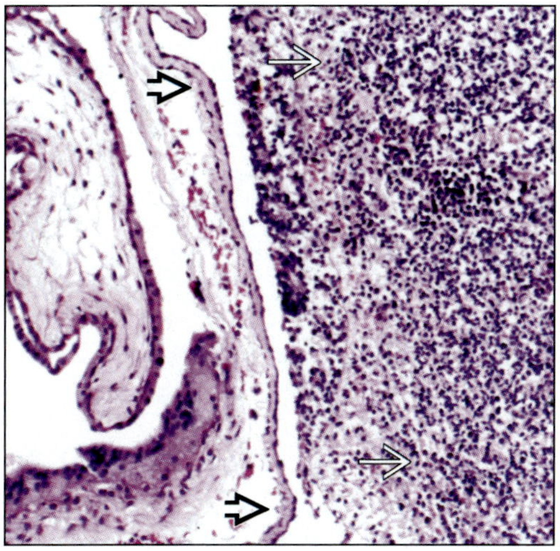

(Left) *This is a partial hydatidiform mole (PHM) that has been rinsed and immersed in water. Most villi are normal in appearance, with only a few grossly evident vesicles* ➡. ***(Right)*** *Embryonic tissue in this section of a PHM shows direct evidence of an embryo/fetus* ➡. *Placental membranes* ⇨ *provide indirect evidence of an embryo/fetus.*

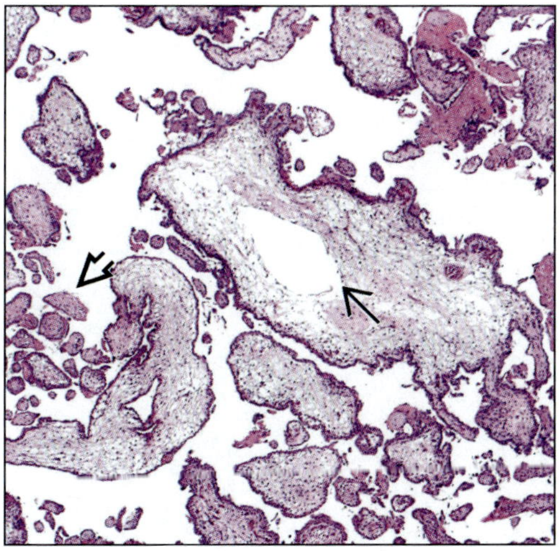

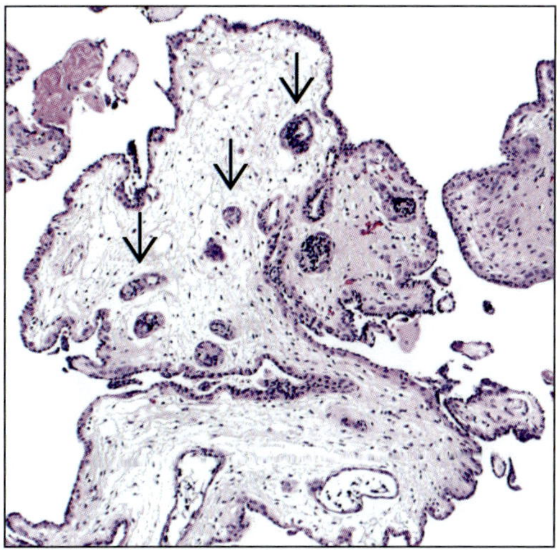

(Left) *This section of PHM shows a dual population of large hydropic villi, including 1 with a central cistern* →, *and smaller fibrotic villi* ⇨. *The villi are irregular in shape, resulting in a jigsaw puzzle piece appearance.* ***(Right)*** *Exuberant trophoblast pseudoinclusions* → *are seen in PHM. They are the result of sectioning of irregular villous contours.*

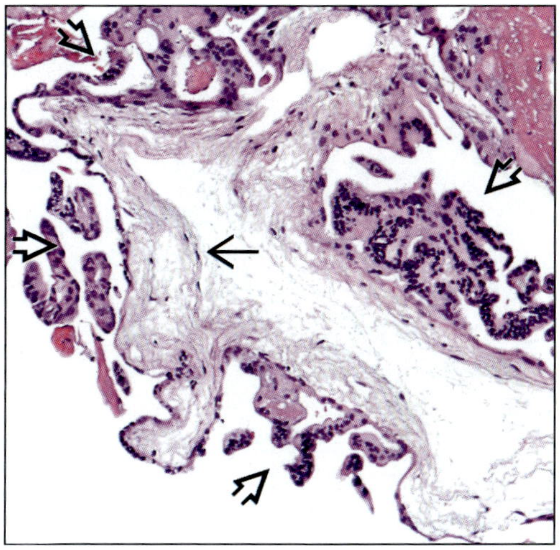

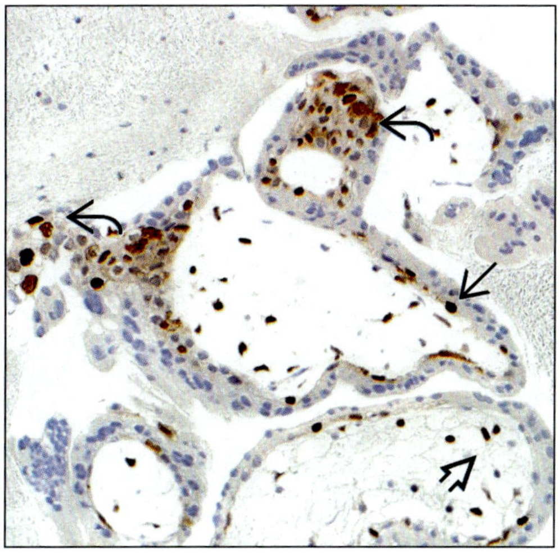

(Left) *This PHM villus contains a central cistern* →. *There is also syncytiotrophoblast proliferation that is circumferential but discontinuous* ⇨. ***(Right)*** *p57 staining of a PHM shows positive nuclear staining in > 10% of cytotrophoblasts* → *and villous stromal cells* ⇨. *Invasive trophoblast* ↷ *staining serves as a positive internal control, as the gene is not differentially expressed in these cells. The p57 staining results rule out CHM but do not distinguish PHM from HD.*

HYDROPIC DEGENERATION AND HYDATIDIFORM MOLE

Complete Hydatidiform Mole

*(**Left**) This transvaginal ultrasound image shows the classic "snow storm" appearance of a CHM. (**Right**) This CHM has previously been formalin fixed. Immersion in water will rehydrate the vesicles. All of the tissue is vesicular with fibrous strands → connecting the vesicles together. There is usually a moderate amount of remote hemorrhage, which was removed for this photograph.*

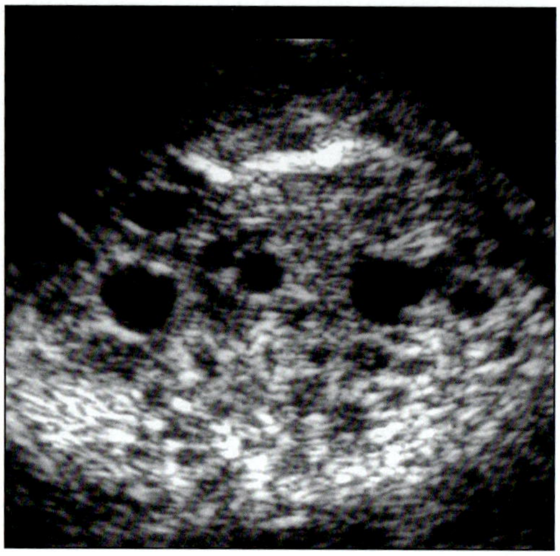

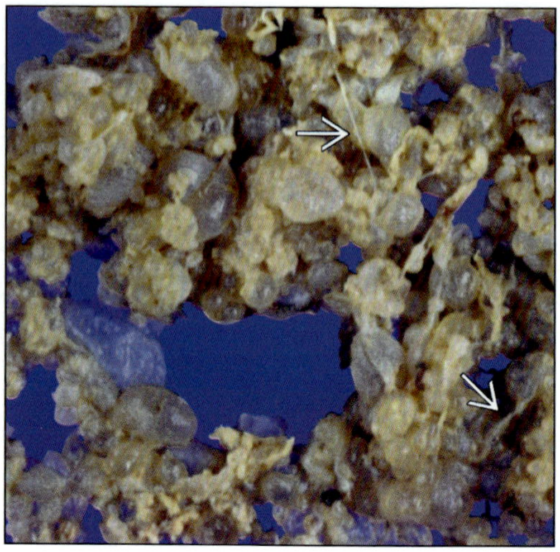

*(**Left**) CHM typically shows huge villi with central cisterns → and mixed trophoblast proliferation that is focally necrotic ⇨. (**Right**) CHM has a mixed trophoblast proliferation that is not as well organized as the normal anchoring villus. Syncytiotrophoblasts may have a lacy appearance →. The invasive trophoblast nuclei are atypical ⇨ and often multinucleate. The small, more regular cytotrophoblasts ↪ are inconspicuous in this section.*

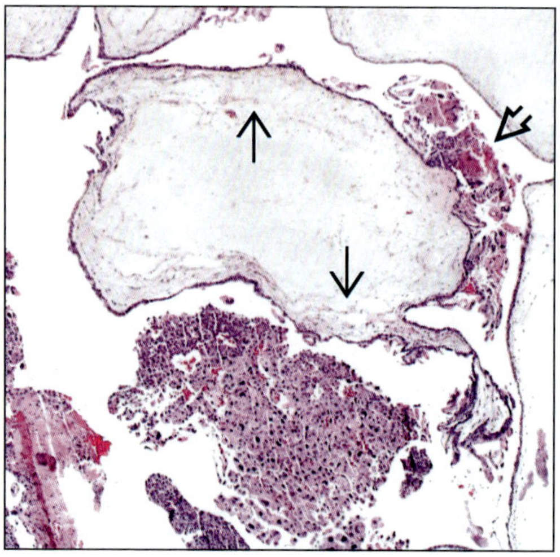

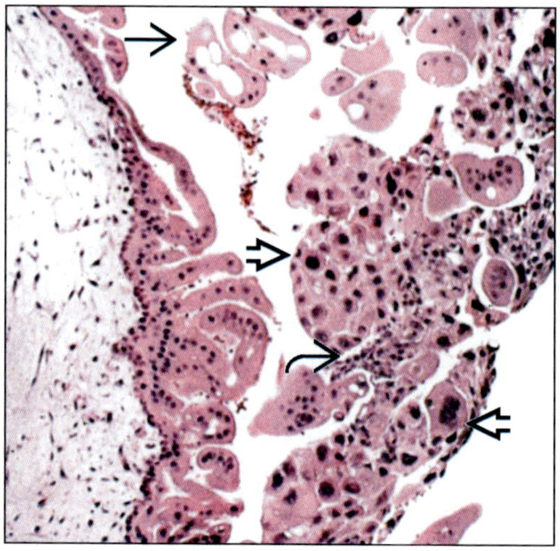

*(**Left**) This is a section from the implantation site of a CHM, showing the marked nuclear enlargement, pleomorphism, and hyperchromasia of the invasive trophoblasts. (**Right**) CHM stained with p57 shows only rare nuclear positivity of the invasive trophoblast →. < 10% of villous stromal cells or cytotrophoblasts are positive. Also note the lacy appearance of the syncytiotrophoblast ⇨ proliferation.*

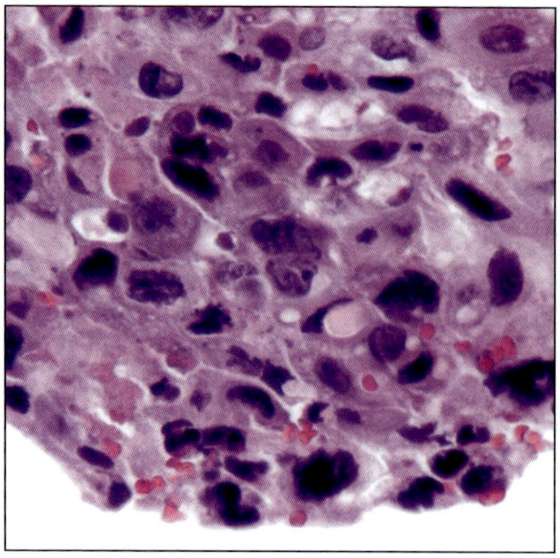

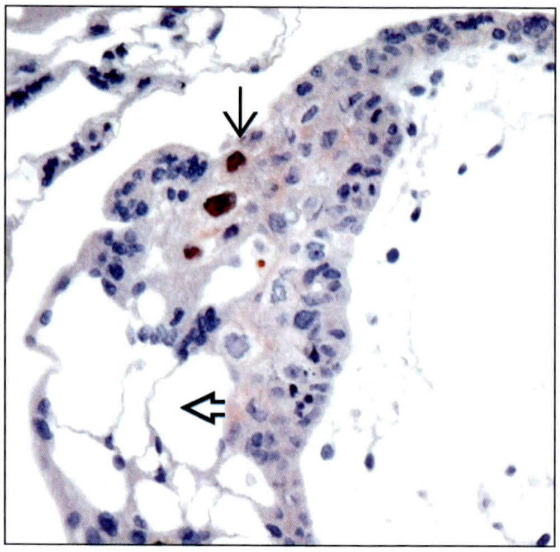

Very Early Complete Hydatidiform Mole

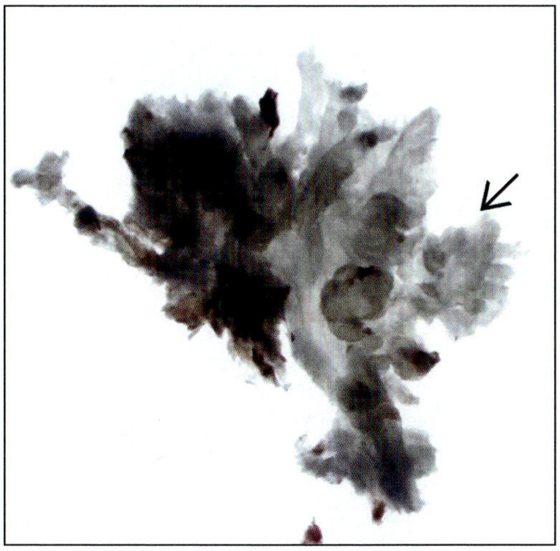

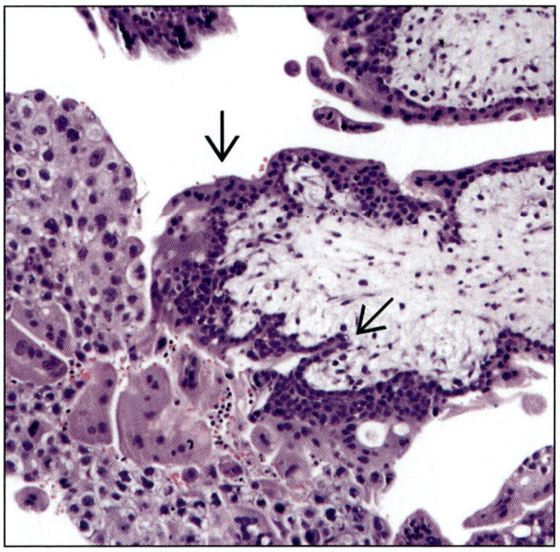

(Left) *This very early complete hydatidiform mole (VECHM) is visualized under a dissecting scope after it has been rinsed and floated in water. Note the uniformly dilated and bulbous appearance of the villi* →. ***(Right)*** *The grossly bulbous villi of VECHM have a gently scalloped, cauliflower-like appearance* →. *There is marked mixed trophoblast proliferation.*

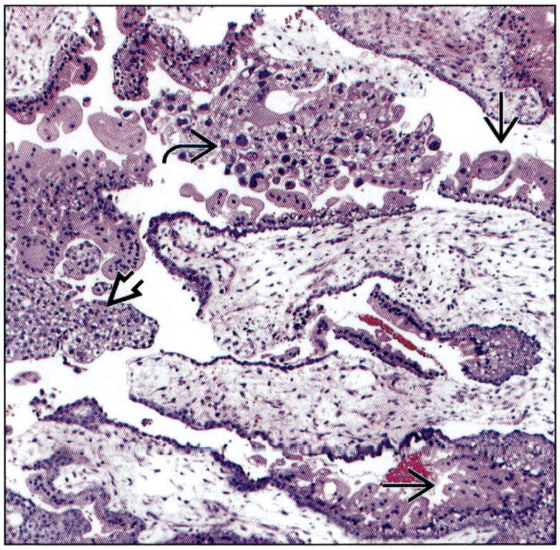

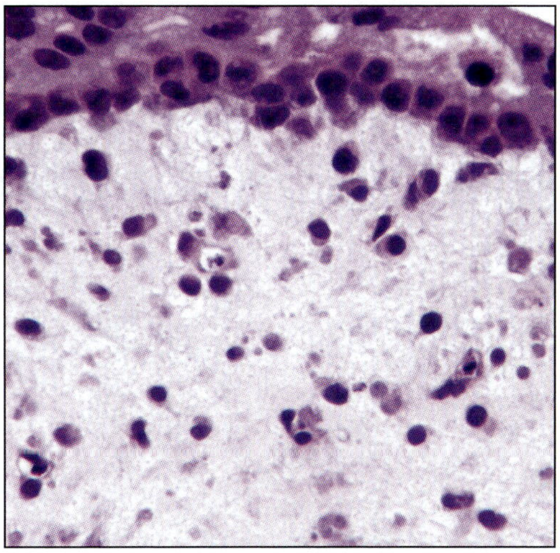

(Left) *This VECHM shows marked mixed syncytiotrophoblast* →, *cytotrophoblast* ⇨, *and intermediate trophoblast* ↷ *proliferation. The villous stroma is highly cellular without central cisterns.* ***(Right)*** *This VECHM villus shows moderate karyorrhexis of the stromal cells.*

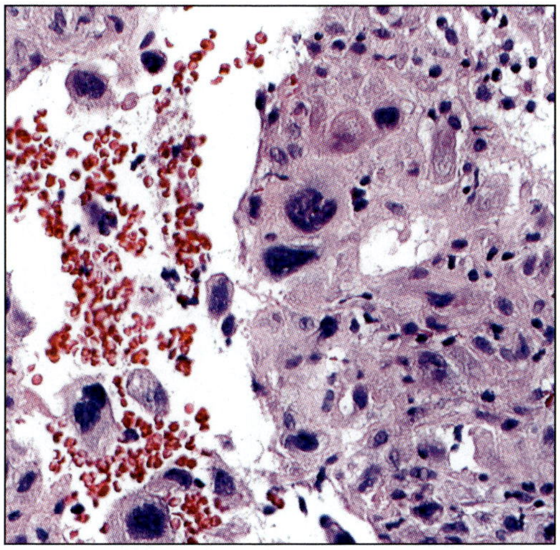

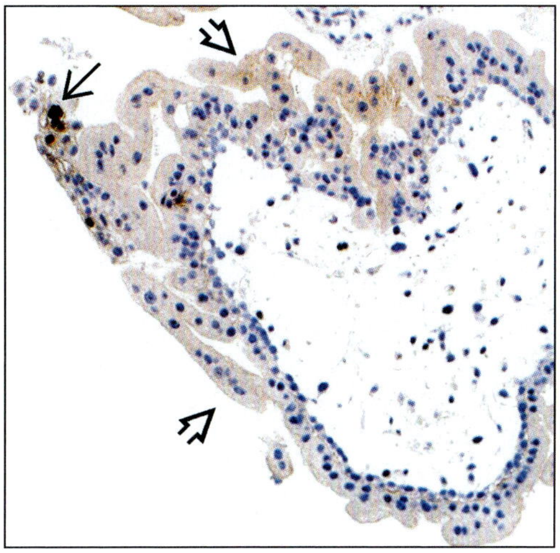

(Left) *The markedly atypical intermediate trophoblast at the implantation site of a VECHM can be very useful in diagnosis. Submission of implantation site decidua is strongly recommended.* ***(Right)*** *p57 immunohistochemistry staining in VECHM shows < 10% nuclear staining of villous cytotrophoblasts and stroma. There is nuclear staining of the invasive trophoblast* →. *There is circumferential syncytiotrophoblast* ⇨ *proliferation.*

HYDROPIC DEGENERATION AND HYDATIDIFORM MOLE

Invasive Mole

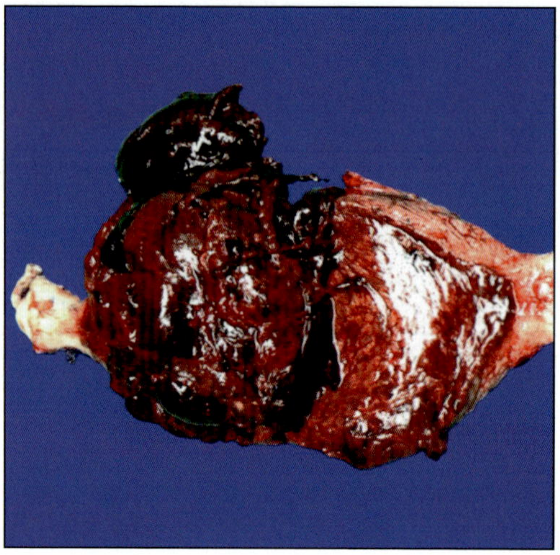

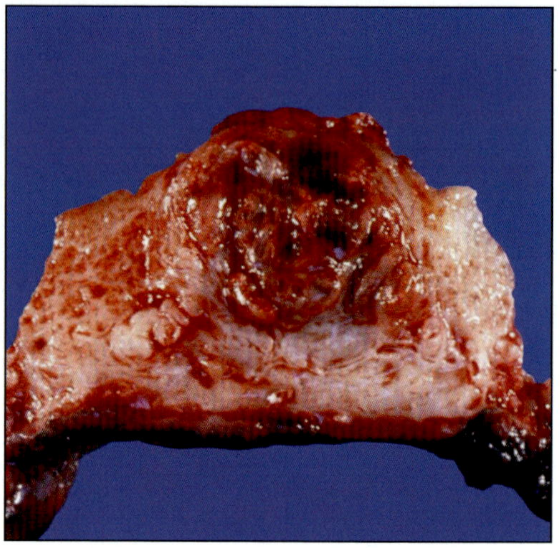

__(Left)__ A hemorrhagic intracavitary mass is grossly noted in this hysterectomy specimen. The patient had a previous diagnosis of CHM but with persistent elevation of serum hCG and uterine bleeding. __(Right)__ Cross section of the uterus shows the deeply invasive friable mass of an invasive mole.

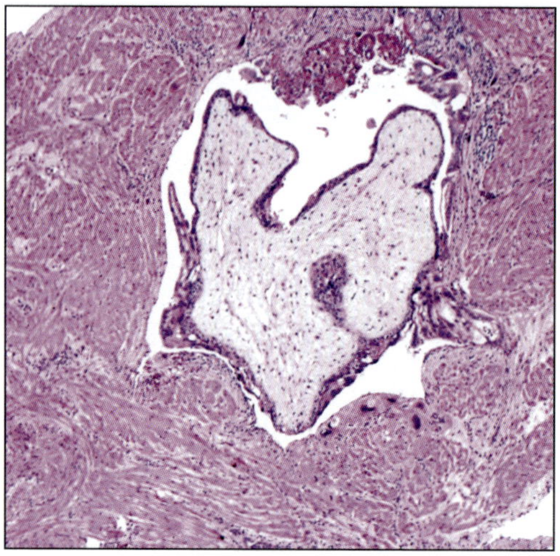

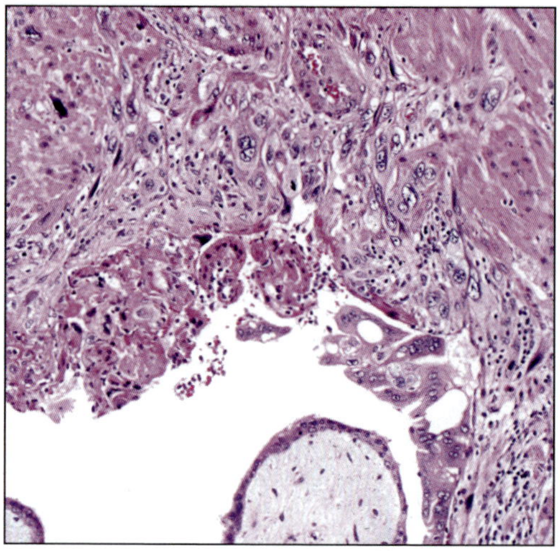

__(Left)__ The villi in an invasive mole are less molar in appearance. Similar to placenta accreta, they are found in the myometrium, often in venous channels. __(Right)__ The trophoblastic proliferation in CHM may become even more pronounced in an invasive mole.

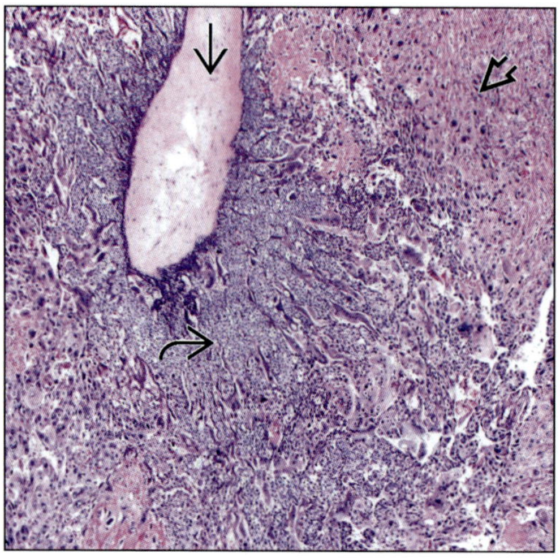

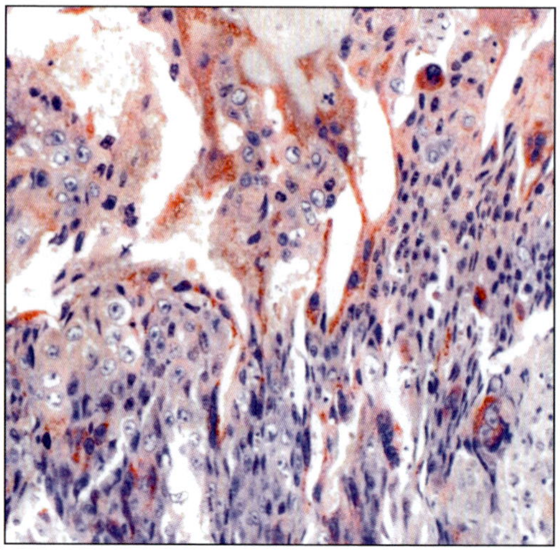

__(Left)__ This invasive CHM could be easily misinterpreted as a choriocarcinoma if the residual villus → were not recognized. The trophoblastic proliferation shows prominent cytotrophoblast columns →, partially covered by syncytiotrophoblast. The invasive trophoblasts → are less conspicuous in this section. __(Right)__ The syncytiotrophoblasts of invasive CHM are HCG positive. This high-power field is indistinguishable from choriocarcinoma.

Key Facts

Terminology

- Placental site nodule (PSN): Small residua of chorionic-type intermediate trophoblast and extracellular matrix persisting long after pregnancy
- Exaggerated placental site (EPS)
  - Implantation site from products of conception where invasive trophoblasts appear increased
  - Atypical invasive trophoblasts are associated with complete hydatidiform mole

Microscopic Pathology

- PSN
  - Round to oval with central hyalinized core and scattered trophoblast arranged singly, in clusters, or in cords
- EPS
  - No specific features distinguish EPS from normal implantation site decidua; may be associated with complete hydatidiform mole

    - Increased trophoblast cellularity; intermediate Ki-67 index (5-8%)
- EPS
  - No specific features useful to distinguish EPS from normal implantation site decidua in products of conception
  - Implantation site of complete hydatidiform mole described as EPS
    - Pleomorphic, mitotically active invasive trophoblast of CHM useful in that diagnosis; should not be confused with atypical PSN or PSTT

ANCILLARY TESTS

Immunohistochemistry

- HPL: Focal staining in PSN, diffuse staining in EPS
- PLAP: Diffuse staining in PSN, focal staining in EPS
- Inhibin-α: Focal positive staining in trophoblast of PSN and EPS
- MEL-CAM (CD146): Focal positive staining in trophoblast of PSN and EPS
- Ki-67: Staining in ~ 5% of PSN trophoblast nuclei, < 1% staining in EPS trophoblast nuclei

DIFFERENTIAL DIAGNOSIS

PSN vs. PSTT

- Microscopic size, circumscription, abundant hyalin matrix, and paucity of trophoblast favor PSN
- Focal staining for MEL-CAM and HPL in PSN, compared to diffuse staining of PSTT

PSN vs. Squamous Cell Carcinoma (SCC) of Cervix

- Circumscription, abundant extracellular matrix, and lack of mitotic activity favor PSN
- Both are cytokeratin, EMA positive; PSN is inhibin-α positive, SCC is not

EPS vs. PSTT

- PSTT forms a tumor mass and is never associated with villi
- Increased trophoblast in PSTT; Ki-67 index is near 0 in EPS but elevated in PSTT (7-21%)

DIAGNOSTIC CHECKLIST

Pathologic Interpretation Pearls

- Only count trophoblast nuclei for Ki-67 index; lymphocytes may have high mitotic activity that is not relevant to differential

SELECTED REFERENCES

1. Shih IM et al: The pathology of intermediate trophoblastic tumors and tumor-like lesions. Int J Gynecol Pathol. 20(1):31-47, 2001
2. Shih IM et al: Placental site nodule and characterization of distinctive types of intermediate trophoblast. Hum Pathol. 30(6):687-94, 1999

EXAGGERATED PLACENTAL SITE

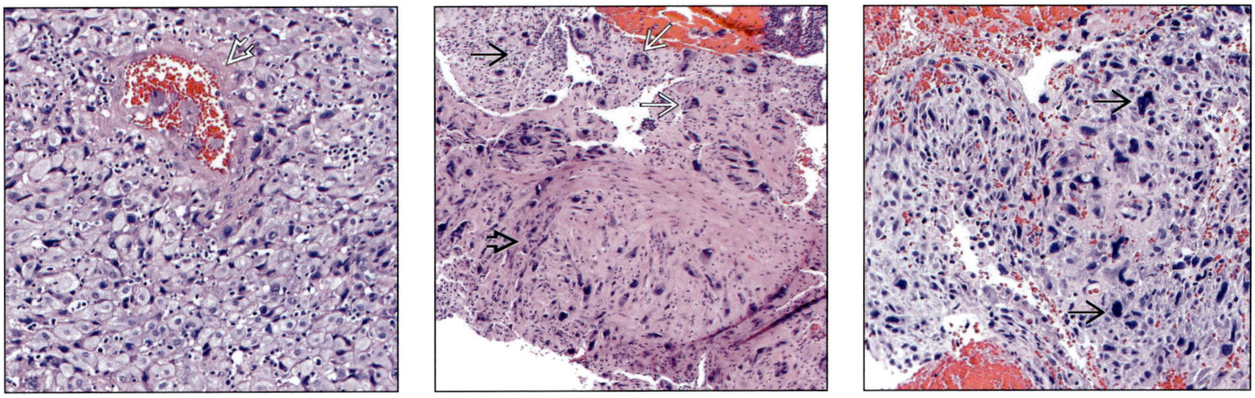

(Left) Large numbers of mononuclear trophoblasts normally invade into the endometrium and uterine spiral arteries ⮕ in early pregnancy. (Center) During normal implantation, trophoblasts invade through the endometrium ⇒ into the inner 1/3 of the myometrium ⇒. Most of the large trophoblasts that are noted are multinucleated ⮕. (Right) Atypical mononuclear invasive trophoblasts ⇒ are characteristic of the implantation site noted with complete hydatidiform mole.

PLACENTAL SITE TROPHOBLASTIC TUMOR AND EPITHELIOID TROPHOBLASTIC TUMOR

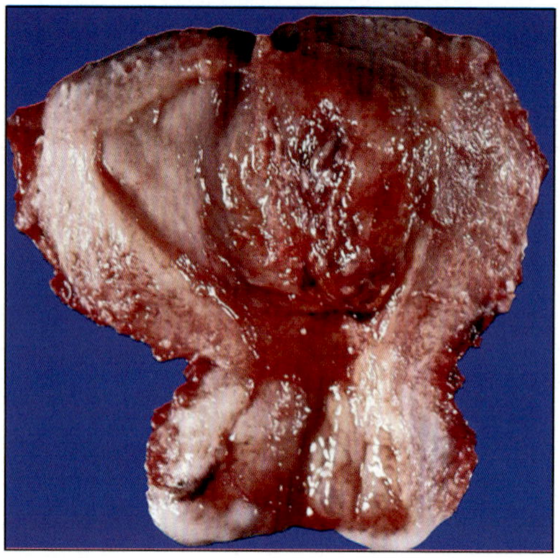

This hysterectomy specimen shows an exophytic placental site trophoblastic tumor (PSTT).

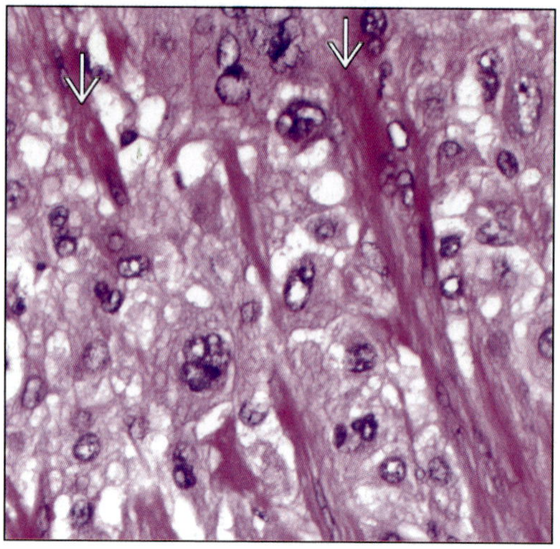

PSTT has polygonal implantation site-type intermediate trophoblasts that invade between myometrial fibers ➡.

ETIOLOGY/PATHOGENESIS

Placental Site Trophoblastic Tumor (PSTT)

- Thought to arise from invasive extravillous trophoblast of implantation site
- Most are diploid, occurring after normal pregnancy or spontaneous abortion

Epithelioid Trophoblastic Tumor (ETT)

- Thought to arise from extravillous trophoblast of chorionic plate or membranous chorion
- Genetics are not well characterized

CLINICAL ISSUES

Presentation

- PSTT
  - Most cases follow term delivery or spontaneous abortion; an antecedent hydatidiform mole is uncommon (5-8%)
  - Most patients present with abnormal menstrual cycles (amenorrhea, menorrhagia, irregular bleeding)
  - Slight uterine enlargement in 25% of patients, may suggest missed abortion
  - Serum β-hCG only mildly elevated
  - May present with erythrocytosis, which resolves after removal of tumor
- ETT
  - Antecedent term delivery in 67% of cases; spontaneous abortion in 16% of cases; hydatidiform mole in 16% of cases
  - Abnormal uterine bleeding, which may occur many years following last pregnancy
  - Usually with low level of hCG (< 2,500 mIU/mL) compared to choriocarcinoma

Treatment

- Surgical approaches
  - Hysterectomy is treatment of choice in PSTT and ETT
- Drugs
  - Chemotherapy is used only in metastatic disease

Prognosis

- PSTT
  - 10-23% metastasize to brain, lungs, liver, lower genital tract, and abdomen
  - Increased mitoses and antecedent pregnancy of > 2 years associated with recurrence
- ETT
  - 20% of patients have metastatic disease; 10% of cases may be fatal

MACROSCOPIC FEATURES

General Features

- PSTT
  - Soft, tan-yellow, usually endophytic mass in uterine wall, may protrude into endometrial cavity
  - Often poorly circumscribed; variable size
  - May extend to serosa, perforate serosa, or extend into broad ligament or adnexa
  - Minimal necrosis or hemorrhage on cut section
- ETT
  - Expansile nodule in endomyometrium or lower uterine segment, up to 5 cm in size, may protrude into endometrial cavity
  - May be solid or cystic on cut section, ± hemorrhage and necrosis

MICROSCOPIC PATHOLOGY

Histologic Features

- PSTT
  - Bland sheets of tumor cells with cords and nests at periphery; rare multinucleate cells

PLACENTAL SITE TROPHOBLASTIC TUMOR AND EPITHELIOID TROPHOBLASTIC TUMOR

Key Facts

Terminology
- Placental site trophoblastic tumor (PSTT): Rare tumor of intermediate, invasive trophoblasts
- Epithelioid trophoblastic tumor (ETT): Very rare tumor of chorionic-type intermediate trophoblasts

Microscopic Pathology
- PSTT
  - Bland, polygonal intermediate trophoblasts forming sheets of tumor cells, with cords and nests extending at periphery
  - Cords of cells separate myometrial fibers with minimal necrosis
  - Associated with abundant eosinophilic extracellular matrix
  - Tumor cells remodel uterine blood vessels as in normal implantation site decidua
  - Mitoses 2-5/10 HPF
- ETT
  - Well-circumscribed nests, cords, and masses of intermediate trophoblasts, typically surrounding blood vessels
  - Extensive necrosis surrounds foci of viable cells, termed geographic necrosis
  - Nodular growth pattern and expansile border differentiate ETT from PSTT
  - Cervical ETT can have growth into endocervical epithelium

Top Differential Diagnoses
- Squamous cell carcinoma vs. ETT
- Placental site nodule vs. ETT, PSTT
- Exaggerated placental site vs. PSTT

  - Cords separate myometrial fibers with minimal necrosis
  - Associated with abundant eosinophilic extracellular matrix
  - Trophoblasts remodel uterine blood vessels as in normal implantation
  - Mitoses 2-5/10 HPF
  - Rare tumors have mixed features of PSTT and choriocarcinoma (mixed choriocarcinoma PSTT)
- ETT
  - Well-circumscribed nests, cords, and masses of intermediate trophoblasts, typically surrounding blood vessels
  - Extensive necrosis surrounds foci of viable cells, termed geographic necrosis
  - Eosinophilic extracellular matrix material associated with trophoblast cells; may mimic keratin
  - Cervical ETT can replace endocervical epithelium
  - Mitoses 0-9/10 HPF

ANCILLARY TESTS

Immunohistochemistry
- Ki-67 proliferation marker
  - Staining in 5-15% of nuclei in PSTT and ETT, but near 0 in placental site nodule (PSN)
- Cytokeratin, EMA
  - Positive in all trophoblastic lesions
- Human chorionic gonadotropin (hCG)
  - Weak and focal staining in both PSTT, ETT
- Human placental lactogen (HPL)
  - Diffusely positive in PSTT, focal in ETT, focal in PSN
- Placental alkaline phosphatase (PLAP)
  - Diffuse staining in ETT, focal staining in PSTT, positive in PSN
- MEL-CAM
  - Diffusely positive in PSTT, focal in ETT, focal or negative in PSN

DIFFERENTIAL DIAGNOSIS

PSN vs. ETT, PSTT
- PSNs are microscopic, well-circumscribed and paucicellular with extensive hyalin-like extracellular matrix

Squamous Cell Carcinoma (SCC) vs. ETT
- Eosinophilic extracellular matrix can mimic keratin; ETT growth pattern can mimic SSC
- Both ETT and SSC may express p16 and p63
- ETT expresses inhibin-α and CK18 whereas SSC does not

Exaggerated Placental Site (EPS) vs. PSTT
- Both consist of implantation site intermediate trophoblast cells, similar immunophenotype
- PSTT shows confluent masses of trophoblast cells with mitotic activity (Ki-67 14 ± 7%)
- EPS is usually an incidental finding with normal implantation site features including decidual stromal cells and anchoring villi; trophoblasts are not mitotically active (Ki-67 < 5%)

SELECTED REFERENCES

1. Luiza JW et al: Placental site trophoblastic tumor: Immunohistochemistry algorithm key to diagnosis and review of literature. Gynecol Oncol Case Rep. 7:13-5, 2013
2. Chew I et al: p16 expression in squamous and trophoblastic lesions of the upper female genital tract. Int J Gynecol Pathol. 29(6):513-22, 2010
3. Houghton O et al: The expression and diagnostic utility of p63 in the female genital tract. Adv Anat Pathol. 16(5):316-21, 2009
4. Kim SJ: Placental site trophoblastic tumour. Best Pract Res Clin Obstet Gynaecol. 17(6):969-84, 2003
5. Shih IM et al: The pathology of intermediate trophoblastic tumors and tumor-like lesions. Int J Gynecol Pathol. 20(1):31-47, 2001

PLACENTAL SITE TROPHOBLASTIC TUMOR AND EPITHELIOID TROPHOBLASTIC TUMOR

Placental Site Trophoblastic Tumor

(Left) Invasive, intermediate trophoblasts intimately surround a blood vessel in placental site trophoblastic tumor. Tumor nuclei may have variable chromasia, similar to implantation site trophoblasts. (Courtesy J. McKenney, MD.) *(Right)* A variable amount of hemorrhage can be seen in placental site trophoblastic tumor, with intravascular tumor cells. (Courtesy J. McKenney, MD.)

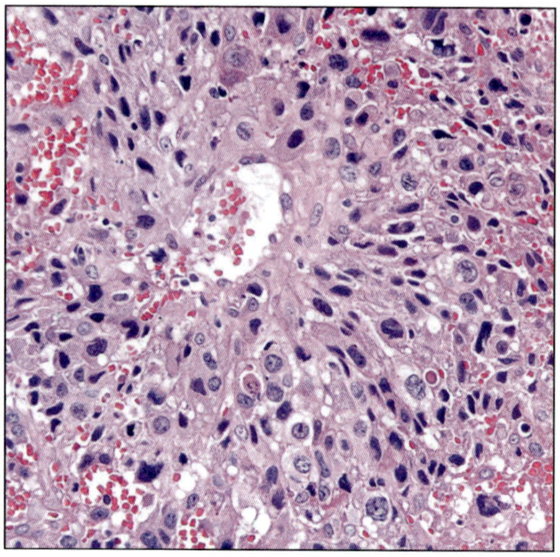

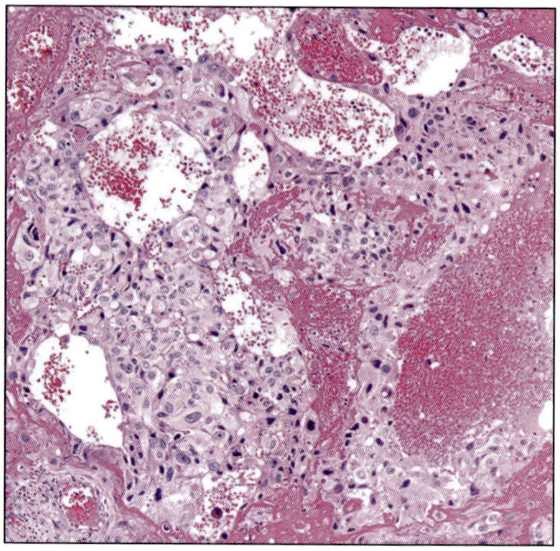

(Left) Hyalin-like eosinophilic extracellular matrix → is seen in both PSTT and ETT. This PSTT shows rare multinucleated trophoblasts ⇨. (Courtesy J. McKenney, MD.) *(Right)* This myometrial vessel shows endovascular trophoblasts → with replacement of vascular smooth muscle by fibrin ⇨. The features are reminiscent of trophoblast-mediated vascular remodeling of pregnancy. (Courtesy J. McKenney, MD.)

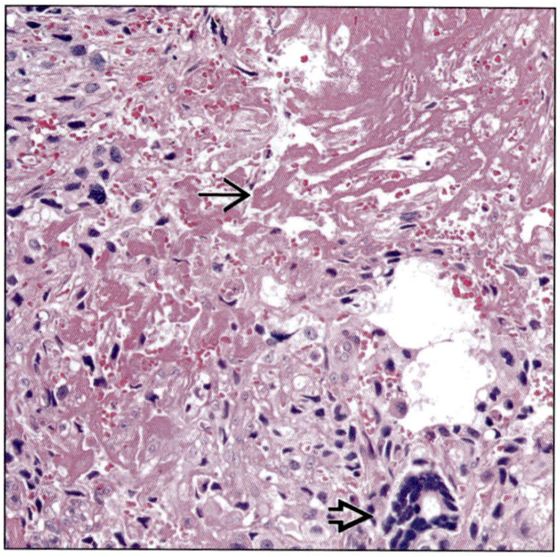

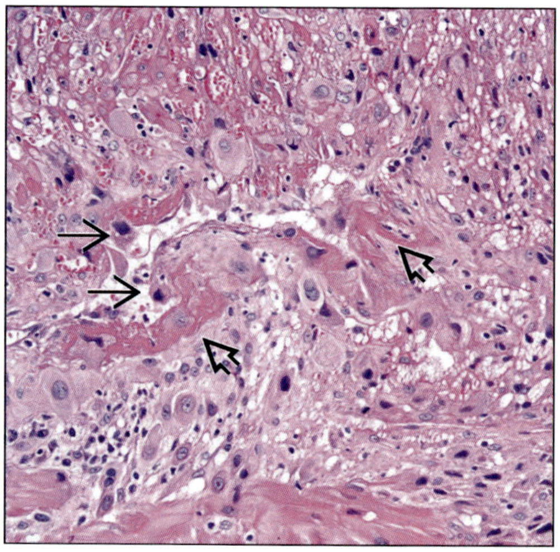

(Left) The tumor cells of PSTT insinuate themselves between myometrial cells → without abundant necrosis. While the cells are much more abundant in PSTT, this feature mimics the normal behavior of invasive intermediate trophoblasts at the placental implantation site. (Courtesy J. McKenney, MD.) *(Right)* Foci of bland necrosis → can be seen in PSTT. (Courtesy J. McKenney, MD.)

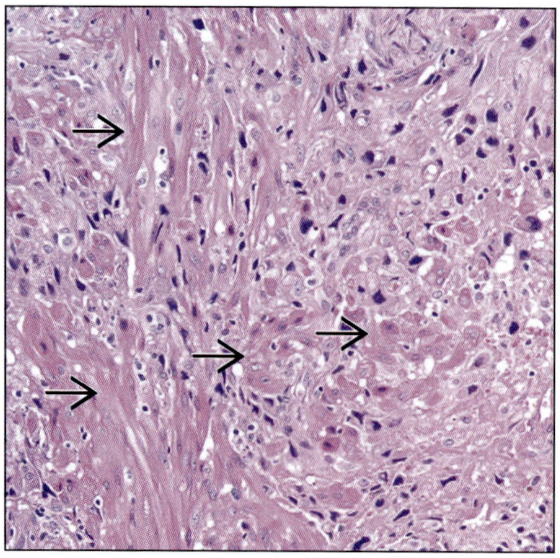

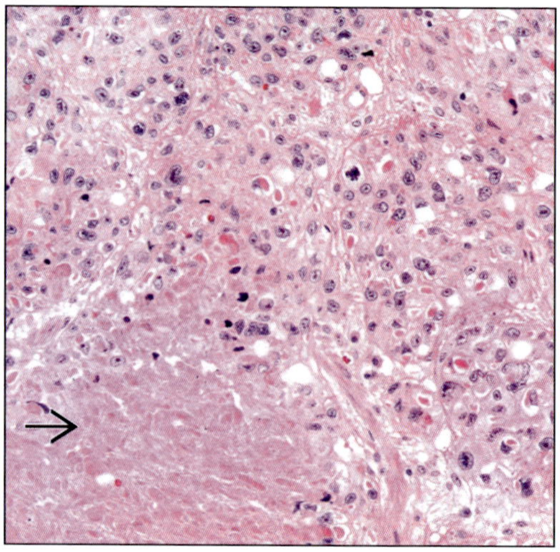

Epithelioid Trophoblastic Tumor

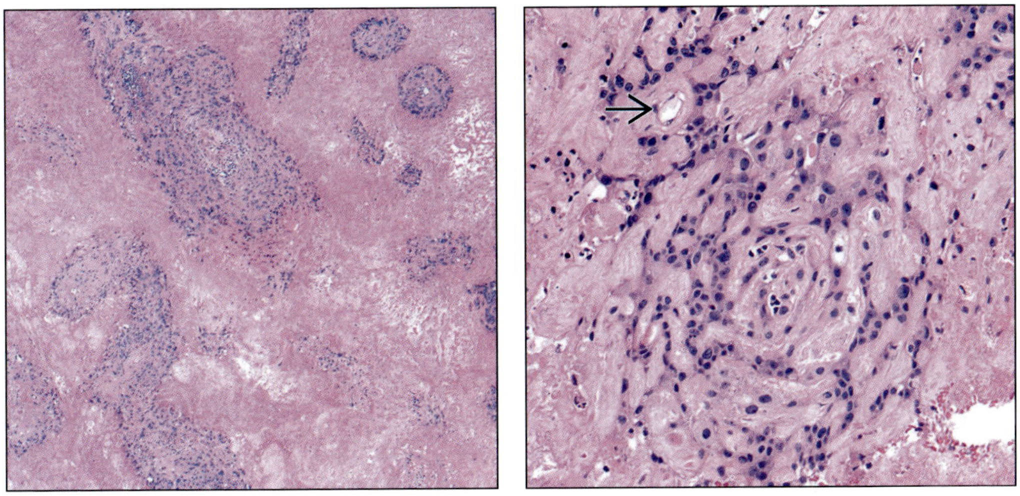

(Left) *Necrosis surrounds nests and islands of tumor cells, forming the characteristic "geographic necrosis" appearance of ETT. (Courtesy J. McKenney, MD.)* **(Right)** *The cords and nests of tumor cells in ETT may surround small blood vessels* →*. (Courtesy J. McKenney, MD.)*

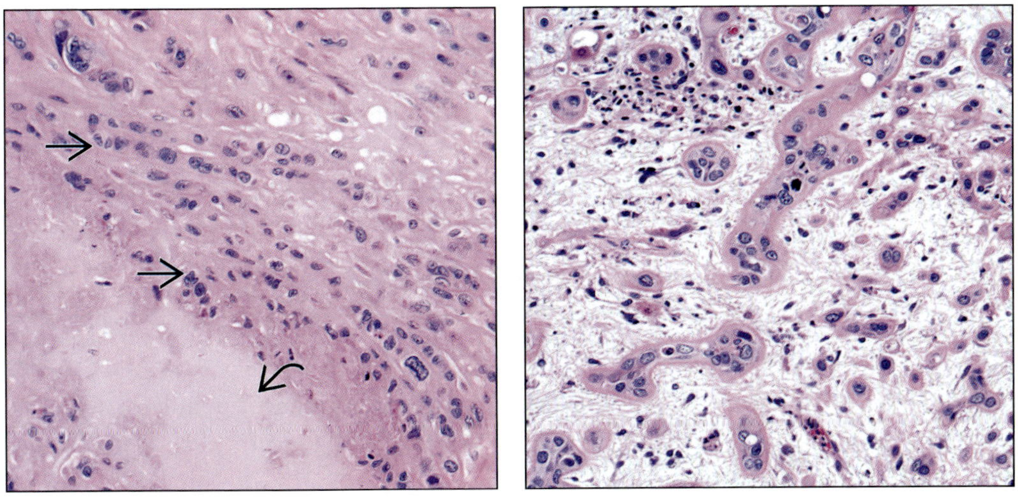

(Left) *ETT has characteristic cords and nests of tumor cells* → *intimately associated with eosinophilic extracellular matrix* ↷*. The matrix resembles the colloid-like material that is produced by extravillous trophoblasts forming septal and subchorionic cysts. (Courtesy J. McKenney, MD.)* **(Right)** *ETT can strongly mimic invasive carcinoma. (Courtesy J. McKenney, MD.)*

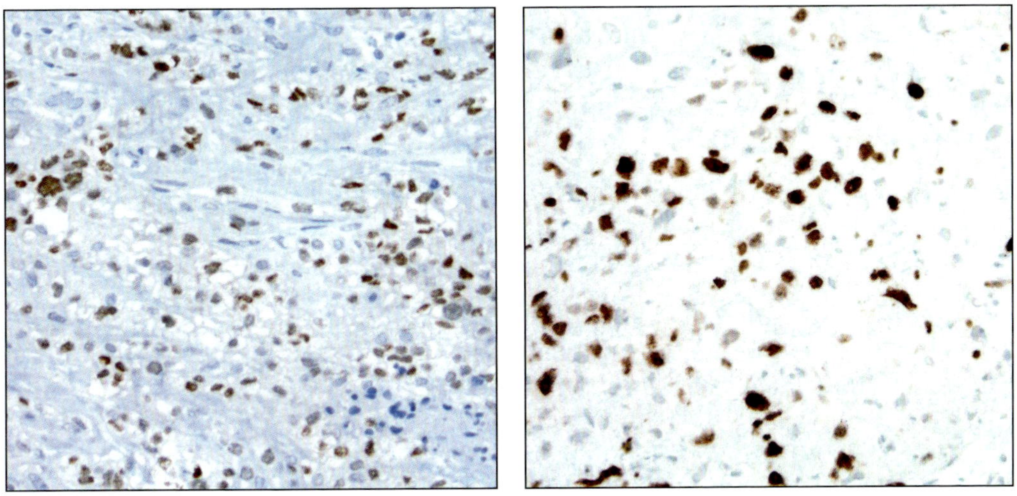

(Left) *ETT can be a difficult mimic of squamous cell carcinoma, particularly in cervical lesions. Both may express p63, as seen here in this image of ETT. (Courtesy J. McKenney, MD.)* **(Right)** *The Ki-67 index of ETT (shown here) and PSTT are both around 5-20%, differentiating these lesions from placental site nodule, which has a very low mitotic index in trophoblast (nearly 0). (Courtesy J. McKenney, MD.)*

METASTATIC TUMORS

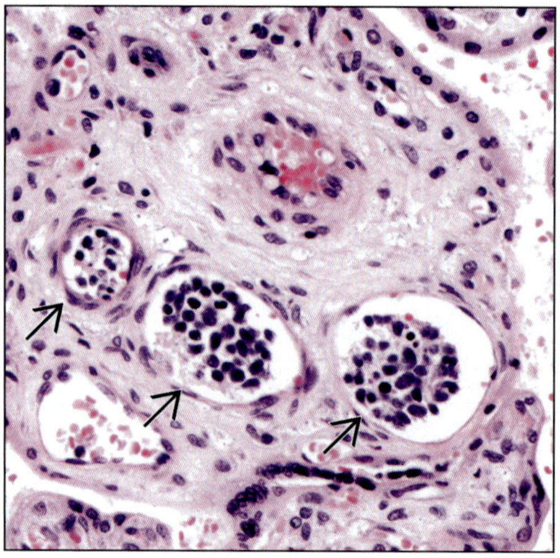

This placenta, from a 36-week-gestation infant with a prenatally diagnosed abdominal mass, weighed 855 g (> 97th percentile). Large clusters of neuroblastoma cells ⇒ are present within the small vessels of intermediate villi.

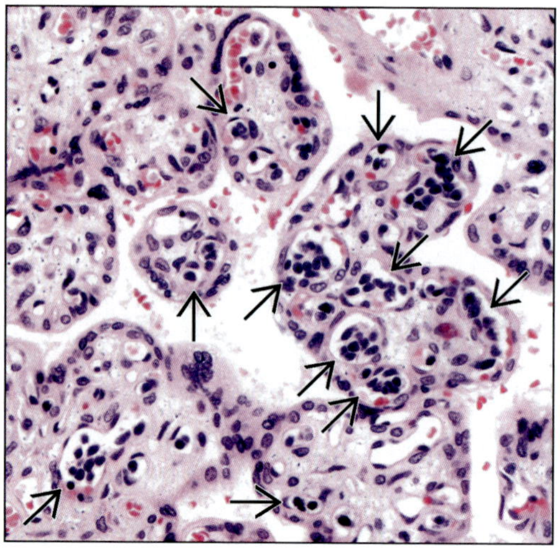

Tumor cells ⇒ are also present in many of the terminal villous capillaries. The cells were positive for synaptophysin by immunohistochemistry; work-up of the resected mass confirmed the diagnosis.

ETIOLOGY/PATHOGENESIS

Maternal Tumors

- Malignant maternal tumor sheds cells into maternal bloodstream, which are carried through decidual arteries and into the blood lake surrounding chorionic villi
- < 0.1% of pregnant women have/develop a malignancy, and only rarely does placental metastasis occur

Fetal Tumors

- Malignant fetal tumor sheds cells into fetal bloodstream, which are carried through umbilical artery and into placental circulatory bed where they lodge in villous capillaries
- Extremely rare event

CLINICAL ISSUES

Presentation

- Most common malignant maternal tumors with placental metastasis (in descending order of frequency)
  - Melanoma
  - Lymphoma/leukemia
  - Breast carcinoma
  - Lung carcinoma
- Most common malignant fetal tumors with placental metastasis (in descending order of frequency)
  - Neuroblastoma
  - Lymphoma/leukemia
  - Hepatoblastoma
  - Melanoma
  - Sarcoma
  - Rhabdoid tumor
- Metastatic fetal tumors often present with nonimmune fetal hydrops; metastatic maternal tumors do not
- Appropriate clinical history (known maternal history of malignancy, fetal tumor seen on ultrasound)

Prognosis

- Fetal hydrops occurring in setting of a malignant fetal tumor is nearly always lethal

MACROSCOPIC FEATURES

General Features

- Metastatic maternal tumors
  - Melanoma may form pigmented nodules
  - Lymphoma (and less often, carcinoma) may form white nodules
- Metastatic fetal tumors
  - Large, pale, hydropic placenta (can exceed 1 kg)
  - Tumor emboli are not usually visible grossly

MICROSCOPIC PATHOLOGY

Histologic Features

- Metastatic maternal tumors
  - Clusters of tumor cells within intervillous space
  - Tumor cells may invade villi (~ 1/2 of melanoma cases)
  - Rarely spread into fetal circulation (melanoma and leukemia/lymphoma)
- Metastatic fetal tumors
  - Clusters of tumor cells within (often distended) fetal vessels within chorionic villi
  - Involved villi usually identifiable within every low-power field
  - In rare cases, tumor cells infiltrate adjacent villous stroma

Placental Mesenchymal Dysplasia

PLACENTAL MESENCHYMAL DYSPLASIA

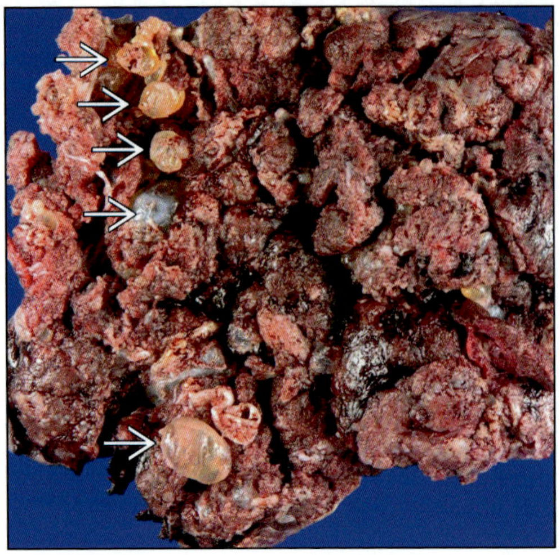

The diagnosis of placental mesenchymal dysplasia (PMD) is suspected on gross exam when presented with an enlarged, bulky placenta containing scattered grape-like cysts ➡ within the parenchyma.

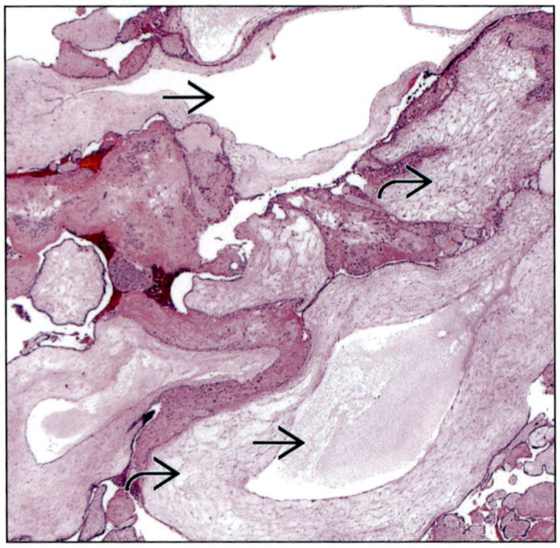

Microscopic exam shows abnormal large villi with cavernous cysts ⇒ and loose, myxoid stroma ⮫. Unlike molar villi, there is no cytotrophoblast proliferation.

TERMINOLOGY

Abbreviations

- Placental mesenchymal dysplasia (PMD)

Synonyms

- Mesenchymal villous dysplasia, pseudopartial mole

Definitions

- Abnormal placental development characterized by placentomegaly, stem-villous hydropic cyst formation, and abnormal villous stroma and fetal vessels
- Androgenetic: Chromosomes of entirely paternal origin, usually from endoreduplication of paternal genes with loss of maternal genome

ETIOLOGY/PATHOGENESIS

Beckwith-Wiedemann Syndrome (BWS)

- 20% of fetuses with PMD have BWS, characterized by macrosomia, organomegaly, hemihypertrophy, macroglossia, omphalocele, and an increased risk of pediatric tumors including hepatoblastoma, Wilms tumor, adrenocortical carcinoma, gonadoblastoma, and brainstem glioma
  - Associated with abnormalities of chromosome 11p15 imprinting with loss of maternal allele expression
- Fetuses with BWS tend to be large for gestational age and have larger PMD placentas

Androgenetic Biparental Mosaicism

- Complete androgenetic development results in a complete hydatidiform mole
  - Complete mole resembles PMD but has trophoblastic hyperplasia and usually no fetus
- At least a subset of PMD cases have androgenetic/ biparental mosaicism
  - Line of cells carrying 2 copies of paternal genome with no maternal component give rise to some of the placental tissues
    - Amount of androgenetic cells is variable, explaining spectrum of changes in PMD, from minimal to severe
  - Probably only a minority of fetal somatic tissues have this abnormal androgenetic cell lineage, if any
    - Could explain association with some features of BWS, or intrauterine growth restriction
    - Could explain preponderance of females as 46,YY fertilized eggs would not be viable
- Most cases are diploid, though rare cases with chromosomal abnormalities confined to placenta or of fetus and placenta are observed

CLINICAL ISSUES

Presentation

- Suspected on ultrasound evaluation when placenta shows molar changes but a fetus is developing
- > 80% of fetuses are female
- Fetus may be normally developed, small for gestational age, hydropic, or show changes of BWS
- Preeclampsia observed in some cases

Prognosis

- Child should be evaluated for possible BWS, given associated risk of malignancy
- Transient anemia and thrombocytopenia described in PMD with chorangioma
- ~ 1/3 of reported cases had fetal demise
- Proportion of parenchyma affected by fetal thrombotic vasculopathy may influence outcome

PLACENTAL MESENCHYMAL DYSPLASIA

Key Facts

Etiology
- ~ 20% of fetuses with placental mesenchymal dysplasia (PMD) have Beckwith-Wiedemann syndrome, at least a subset have androgenetic biparental mosaicism
- Most cases are diploid

Clinical Issues
- Suspected on ultrasound evaluation when placenta shows molar changes but a fetus is developing
- 1/2 of non-BWS fetuses with PMD have intrauterine growth restriction, 1/3 die in utero
- Fetus may be hydropic with anemia and thrombocytopenia associated with chorangioma

Macroscopic Pathology
- Bulky enlarged placenta
- Markedly dilated chorionic plate vessels, varicose-like
- Numerous grape-like cysts in parenchyma

Microscopic Pathology
- Marked dilation of chorionic plate vasculature with mural hemorrhage, thrombi in some cases
- Stem villous cysts, abnormally enlarged villi with stromal and vascular proliferation
- Fetal thrombotic vasculopathy
- Chorangioma and chorangiomatosis

Top Differential Diagnoses
- Partial hydatidiform mole

Diagnostic Checklist
- Absence of trophoblastic proliferation distinguishes PMD from partial mole, partial moles are triploid

MACROSCOPIC FEATURES

General Features
- Bulky enlarged placenta with variably dilated, varicose-like, chorionic plate vessels
- Parenchyma shows grape-like cysts, and regions of tan gelatinous-appearing foci may be found in otherwise spongy red-brown villous parenchyma
- Excessively long, hypercoiled umbilical cord in a subset of cases

MICROSCOPIC PATHOLOGY

Histologic Features
- Chorionic plate vasculature
  - Marked dilation with mural hemorrhage, thrombi in some cases
- Stem villi
  - Cysts, stromal overgrowth, abnormal vasculature
  - Fetal thrombotic vasculopathy with thrombi and changes of fetal vascular involution
  - Chorangioma and chorangiomatosis
- Distal villi
  - Abnormal hypocellular stroma in subpopulation
  - Fetal thrombotic vasculopathy with stromal vascular karyorrhexis and avascular villi

ANCILLARY TESTS

Immunohistochemistry
- Though not necessary for diagnosis, study of p57/KIP2 shows interesting changes
  - Maternally expressed protein; staining is absent in androgenetic cells
    - p57/KIP2 staining is preserved in trophoblast, but lost in villous stroma of dysplastic villi

DIFFERENTIAL DIAGNOSIS

Partial Hydatidiform Mole
- Share cystic villi and presence of normally developed villi
- PMD lacks characteristic trophoblast proliferation around abnormal villi seen in partial mole
- PHM associated with diandric triploidy

DIAGNOSTIC CHECKLIST

Clinically Relevant Pathologic Features
- PMD is an easily recognized cause of fetal and neonatal morbidity and mortality
- ~ 20% of PMD cases associated with BWS in neonate

Pathologic Interpretation Pearls
- Absence of trophoblastic proliferation distinguishes PMD from partial mole

SELECTED REFERENCES

1. Ulker V et al: Placental mesenchymal dysplasia: a rare clinicopathologic entity confused with molar pregnancy. J Obstet Gynaecol. 33(3):246-9, 2013
2. Hoffner L et al: P57KIP2 immunostaining and molecular cytogenetics: combined approach aids in diagnosis of morphologically challenging cases with molar phenotype and in detecting androgenetic cell lines in mosaic/chimeric conceptions. Hum Pathol. 39(1):63-72, 2008
3. Pham T et al: Placental mesenchymal dysplasia is associated with high rates of intrauterine growth restriction and fetal demise: A report of 11 new cases and a review of the literature. Am J Clin Pathol. 126(1):67-78, 2006
4. Jauniaux E et al: Perinatal features associated with placental mesenchymal dysplasia. Placenta. 18(8):701-6, 1997
5. Lage JM: Placentomegaly with massive hydrops of placental stem villi, diploid DNA content, and fetal omphaloceles: possible association with Beckwith-Wiedemann syndrome. Hum Pathol. 22(6):591-7, 1991

PLACENTAL MESENCHYMAL DYSPLASIA

Gross and Microscopic Features

(Left) *Grossly, PMD is characterized by molar-like cysts of stem villi ➡ and a variable degree of chorionic plate vessel dilatation. In this image, a chorionic plate vein is abnormally dilated ➡.* ***(Right)*** *The chorionic plate vasculature ➡ may become cirsoid, or worm-like. In this case, the cord had a furcate insertion ➡ with the abnormal vessels branching before being tethered in the chorionic plate.*

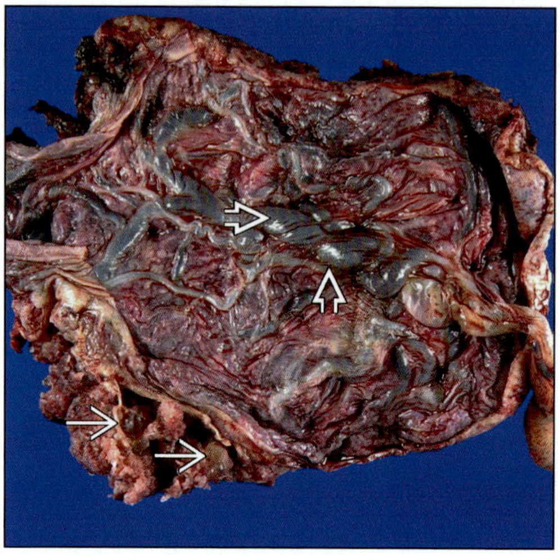

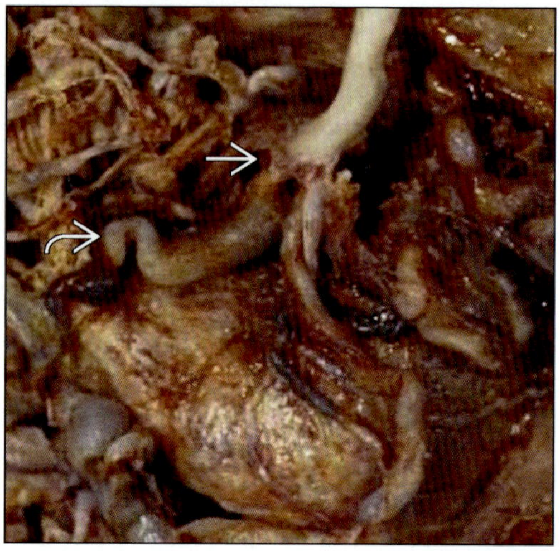

(Left) *This cut section shows glistening cysts ➡. Other placental pathologies, such as fetal thrombotic vasculopathy, infarcts, and increased perivillous fibrin ➡, may also be present.* ***(Right)*** *This PMD placenta shows marked dilation of chorionic plate vasculature ➡ (in this case, veins). (Courtesy S. Kostadinov, MD.)*

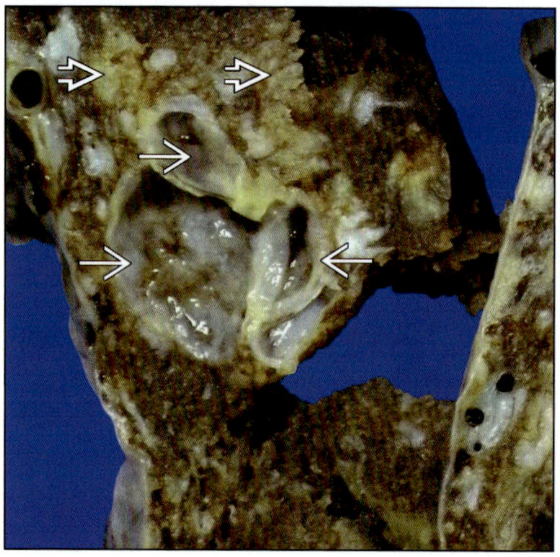

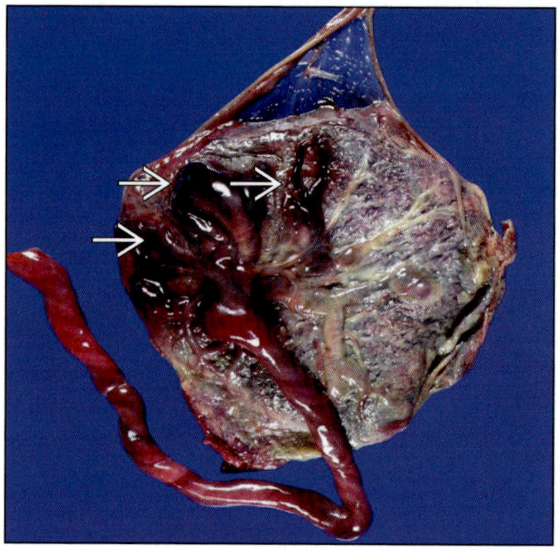

(Left) *Chorangioma histology in PMD differs from that of the usual chorangioma and chorangiomatosis. Capillaries are more loosely arranged and sinusoidal. They are associated with an abnormal stroma with variable cellularity and degenerative changes.* ***(Right)*** *The abnormal vascular proliferation in PMD often shows fetal thrombotic vasculopathy. Thrombus formation ➡ is present in a larger vessel. Neonates with PMD and chorangioma may have a transient but severe coagulopathy.*

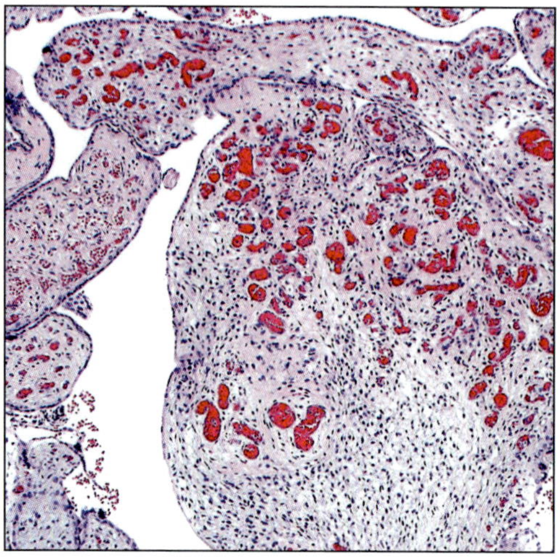

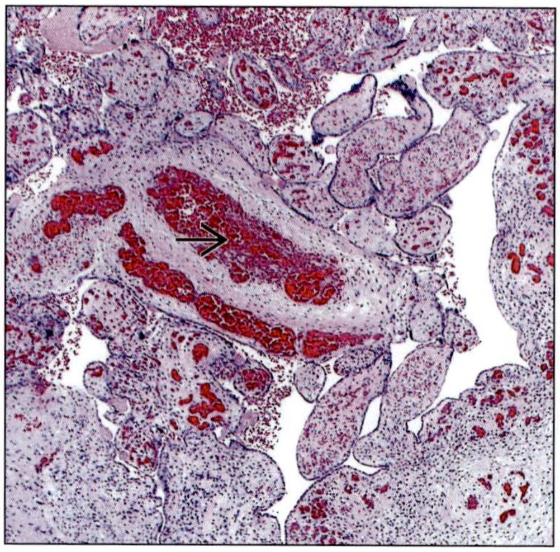

Microscopic Features

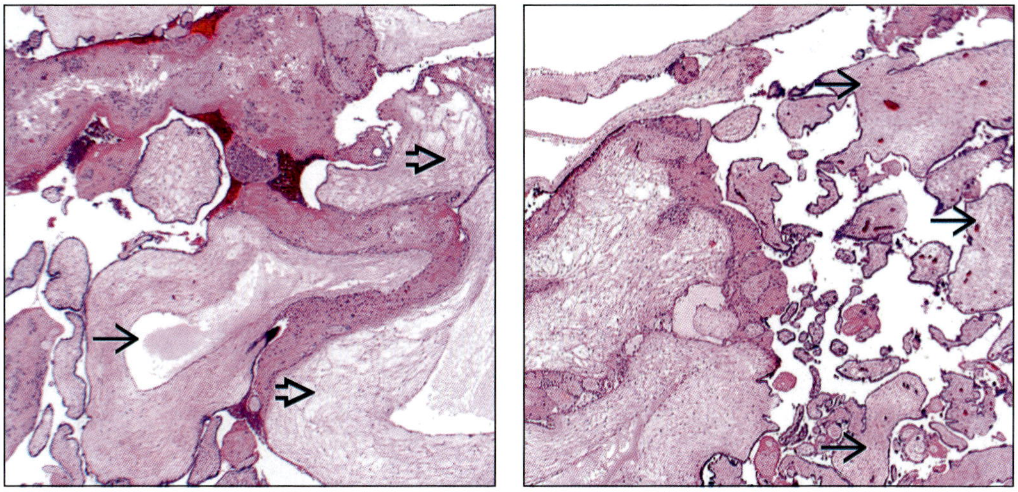

(Left) *On low power, cysts appear as degenerated areas* → *within a loose edematous stroma* ⇨. ***(Right)*** *More normal-sized villi may show stromal overgrowth with abnormal small vessels* →. *Note that there is no trophoblastic proliferation around the abnormal villi.*

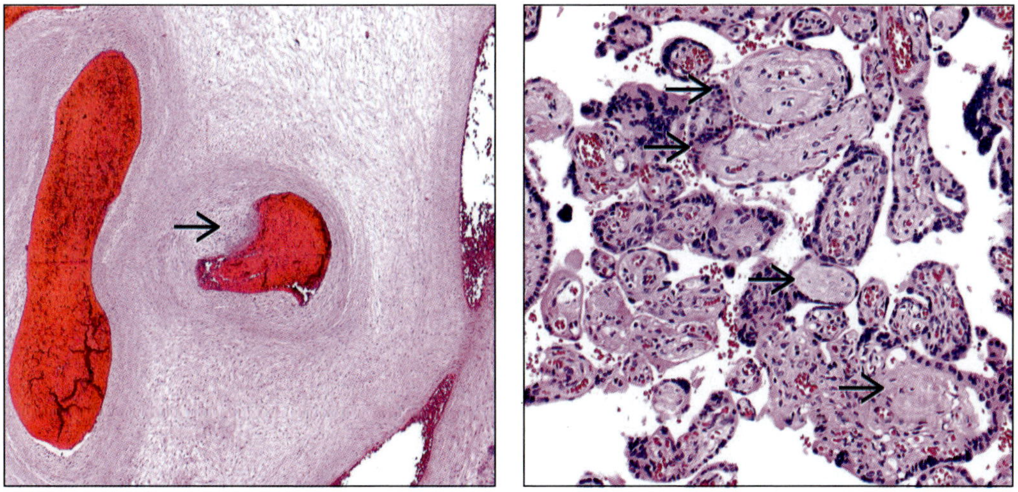

(Left) *This stem villous vessel* → *of a PMD placenta has a mural thrombus. Fetal thrombotic vasculopathy is a common finding in PMD, likely reflecting abnormal hemodynamics through the dysplastic villi. Some cases have umbilical cord abnormalities associated with PMD.* ***(Right)*** *Distal villi may also include abnormal forms* → *with a myxoid hypovascular stroma.*

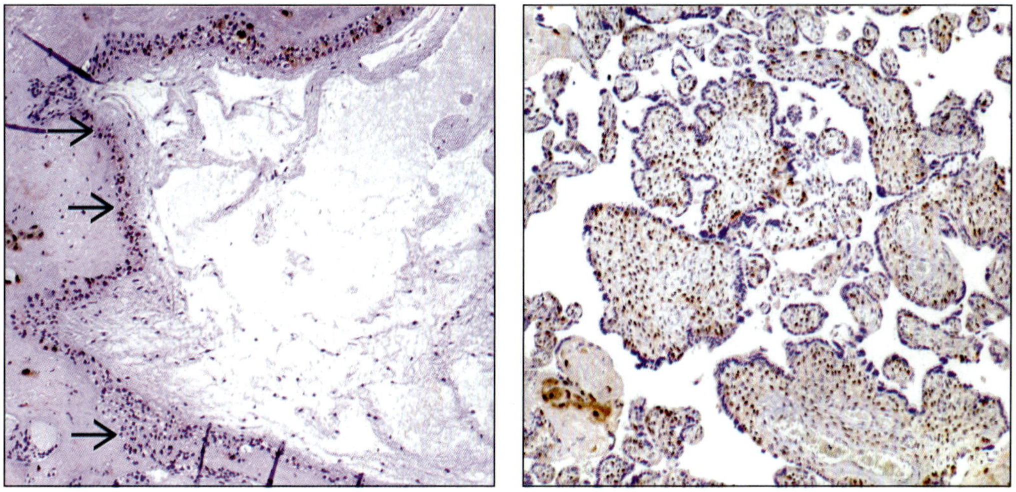

(Left) *p57 immunostaining in PMD suggests androgenetic/biparental mosaicism. The abnormal villi show retention of p57 staining in the cytotrophoblast layer* → *(biparental), derived from the trophoblast embryonic layer, but loss in the stroma (androgenetic) derived from extraembryonic mesoderm.* ***(Right)*** *In contrast, nondysmorphic villi show abundant p57 reactivity in the stroma, consistent with biparental derivation.*

- Normograms for placental weight are based on **trimmed** weight of disc following removal of free membranes, umbilical cord (to within 2 cm of disc insertion), and loosely adherent blood clot
- Multiple sections of villous parenchyma should be examined microscopically to evaluate for potential underlying pathology contributing to increased weight
- Prolonged fresh storage of a placenta can result in decreased weight due to evaporation and leakage of blood/serum
  - Accentuated in hydropic or edematous placentas

Anatomic Features

- Specific macroscopic features of primary pathological processes/diagnoses
  - Villous edema due to any cause including hydrops fetalis, infection, metabolic storage disorders, mass lesions, and fetal anemia
    - Generalized parenchymal pallor
    - Bogginess and increased friability
    - Placental hydrops may also involve umbilical cord, resulting in increased diameter and translucency
  - Maternal diabetes
    - May be pale due to villous edema or plethoric due to fetal hypervolemia
    - Increased friability
  - Placental mesenchymal dysplasia and overgrowth syndromes including Beckwith-Wiedemann syndrome
    - Fetal chorionic vessels with abnormal distribution and aneurysmal dilatation
    - Enlarged stem villi with cyst and vesicle formation
- Placentas from pregnancies affected by maternal anemia and diabetes may have no structural or gross parenchymal abnormalities other than increased weight

MICROSCOPIC FINDINGS

General Features

- Histopathological features relate to parenchymal alterations of the primary process, including
  - Maternal diabetes
    - Distal villous immaturity with increased villous width and prominence of cytotrophoblast layer
    - Villous hypervascularity including chorangiosis
    - Increased fetal nucleated red blood cells
  - Villous edema; changes most evident in gestations < 35 weeks include
    - Increased villous diameters
    - Clearing of villous stroma with "floating" Hofbauer cells
    - Abnormal, scalloped villous contours in cases of extensive edema
  - Placental mesenchymal dysplasia
    - Enlarged stem villi with stromal overgrowth, vascular proliferation, and areas of cystic degeneration or sinusoid formation
    - Distal villi may appear immature and exhibit chorangiosis
  - Metabolic storage disorders
    - Variable vacuolization of trophoblast, stromal cells, or amnion depending on specific disorder
    - Cases involving trophoblast demonstrate diffuse thickening of the trophoblast layer
    - Stromal cells may have distinct foamy appearance as opposed to clear spaces surrounding cells in villous edema

SELECTED REFERENCES

1. Hecht JL et al: Reference weights for placentas delivered before the 28th week of gestation. Placenta. 28(10):987-90, 2007
2. Pinar H et al: Reference values for singleton and twin placental weights. Pediatr Pathol Lab Med. 16(6):901-7, 1996
3. Naeye RL: Do placental weights have clinical significance? Hum Pathol. 18(4):387-91, 1987

IMAGE GALLERY

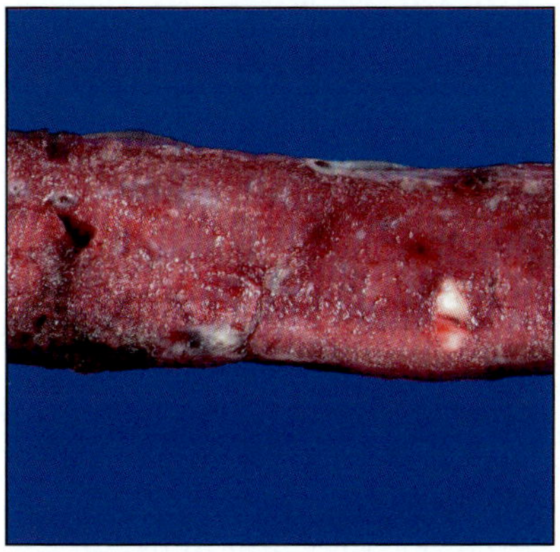

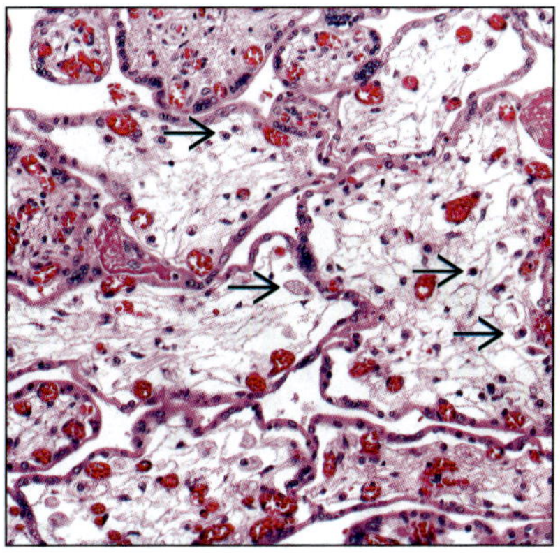

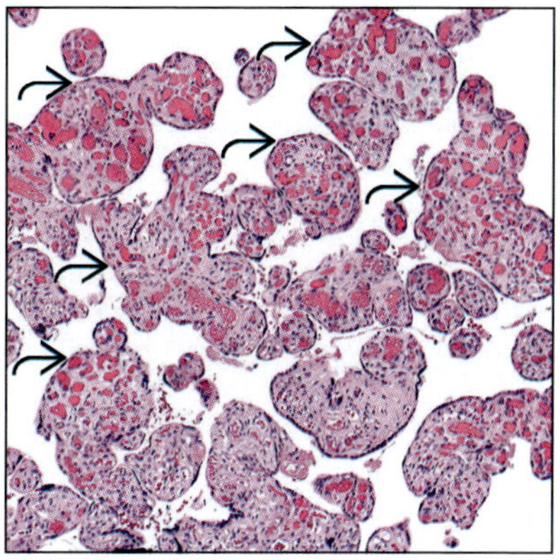

(Left) *This pale, glossy cut surface is due to villous edema and chorangiosis in a 719 g placenta delivered at 36 weeks. The pregnancy was complicated by fetal cardiac defects and polyhydramnios.* ***(Center)*** *H&E shows villous edema with increased width and clear spaces containing "floating" Hofbauer cells ⇨ in a 503 g placenta at 32 weeks from a pregnancy complicated by hydrops and polyhydramnios.* ***(Right)*** *Chorangiosis is seen with > 10 capillaries per villus ⇗ in an 824 g placenta at 38 weeks.*

DISTAL VILLOUS IMMATURITY

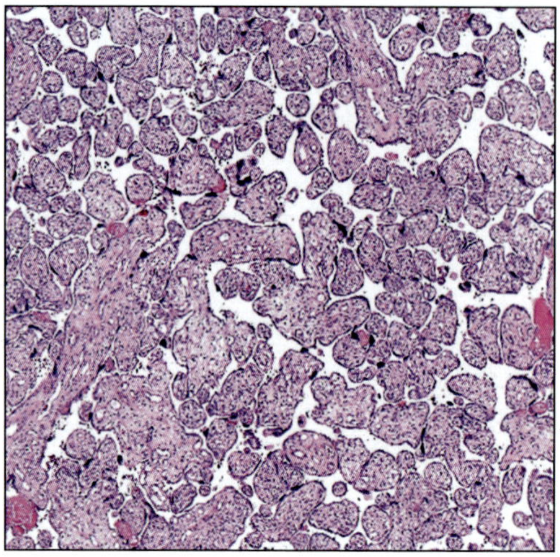

Low-power image demonstrates distal villous immaturity (DVI) in an 800 g placenta at 36 weeks, with increased villous diameter for the gestational age and incomplete terminal villous maturation.

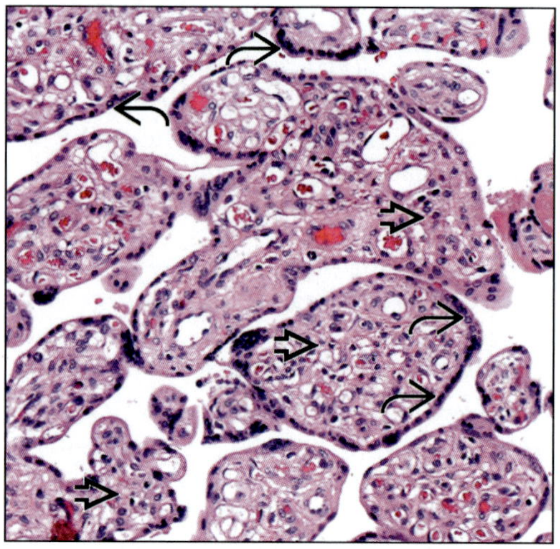

These enlarged distal villi display a continuous trophoblast layer ➩, increased stromal cellularity ➩, and centrally located capillaries with poor vasculosyncytial membrane formation.

TERMINOLOGY

Abbreviations

- Distal villous immaturity (DVI)

Synonyms

- Delayed villous maturation, retarded villous maturation, deficiency of normal terminal villi, absent vasculosyncytial membranes, and placental maturation defect all describe similar changes

Definitions

- Diffuse abnormality of distal villi characterized by poor vasculosyncytial membrane formation, prominent villous cytotrophoblast cellularity, and increased villous stroma

ETIOLOGY/PATHOGENESIS

Potential Etiologic Mechanisms

- Exact mechanism unclear; hypotheses include
  - Excessive growth factors or nutrients (e.g., diabetic pregnancies, maternal obesity) favoring continued growth of tertiary stem villi over maturation of distal villi
  - Alterations in fetal blood flow (stasis, decreased pressure) inducing stromal-vascular remodeling
  - Genetic abnormalities leading to abnormal villous development

Effect on Placental Function

- Paucity of vasculosyncytial membranes leads to inefficient gas and nutrient exchange, decreased fetal tolerance for hypoxia, and other acute stress

CLINICAL ISSUES

Epidemiology

- Incidence
  - Occurs in 1-6% of pregnancies
    - Data from placentas submitted for pathologic examination; population is enriched for conditions such as gestational diabetes or fetal demise

Presentation

- Most commonly associated with maternal diabetes
- Less commonly associated with maternal obesity, excessive weight gain in pregnancy, chronic variable umbilical cord obstruction, fetal chromosomal abnormalities
- May be clinically silent
  - Lack of prenatal and ultrasound markers

Prognosis

- Associated with increased perinatal mortality
  - Increase risk of fetal death at > 35 weeks
    - Up to 5% risk of recurrent stillbirth
  - Mildly increased risk of early neonatal death

Fetal/Neonatal Characteristics

- Altered fetal growth
  - More commonly increased birth weight, large for gestational age
  - Less commonly fetal growth restriction
- Associated with admission to neonatal care units

MACROSCOPIC FEATURES

General Features

- Decreased fetoplacental weight ratio
- Disc may be large for gestational age or normal in shape and size
- Decreased vascularization may result in pallor

DISTAL VILLOUS IMMATURITY

Key Facts

Clinical Issues
- Distal villous immaturity (DVI)
  - Definition: Diffuse abnormality of distal villi with poor vasculosyncytial membrane formation
  - Occurs most commonly with maternal diabetes
  - Clinically silent until late adverse event
  - Risk of recurrent stillbirth

Macroscopic Pathology
- Decreased fetoplacental weight ratio
- Umbilical cord may be thick, hypercoiled

Microscopic Pathology
- Enlarged distal villi with decreased vasculosyncytial membranes, increased villous cellularity and connective tissue

Diagnostic Checklist
- Correlate villous maturation with gestational age
- Assess degree of vasculosyncytial membrane formation

MICROSCOPIC PATHOLOGY

Histologic Features
- Thick cord due to increased Wharton jelly
- Increased ratio of immature intermediate or tertiary stem villi to distal villi
- Distal villi show increased diameter, increased cellularity of cytotrophoblast, variable capillary density with poor vasculosyncytial membrane formation, increased stromal cellularity and connective tissue

Associated Features
- Increased nucleated fetal red blood cells (NRBCs) due to acute hypoxia
- Other villous vascular lesions, such as chorangiosis, chorangiomatosis, edema, or foci of avascular villi

DIFFERENTIAL DIAGNOSIS

Age-Appropriate Villous Immaturity
- Requires familiarity with normal maturation of villi
- Relatively high ratio of proximal:distal villi; prominent immature intermediate villi with loose, reticular stroma
- Distal villous immaturity not diagnosed before 34 weeks gestation

Chorangiosis
- Increased villous size with markedly increased capillary density
- Vasculosyncytial membranes present

DIAGNOSTIC CHECKLIST

Pathologic Interpretation Pearls
- DVI not diagnosed in < 34 weeks
- Assess degree of vasculosyncytial membrane formation
- Villous changes present in majority of tissue sections

SELECTED REFERENCES

1. Treacy A et al: Delayed villous maturation of the placenta: quantitative assessment in different cohorts. Pediatr Dev Pathol. 16(2):63-6, 2013
2. Higgins MF et al: Clinical and ultrasound features of placental maturation in pre-gestational diabetic pregnancy. Early Hum Dev. 88(10):817-21, 2012
3. Redline RW: Distal villous immaturity. In Clarke B et al: Diagnostic Histopathology. Oxford: Elsevier/Medicine Publishing. 18(5): 189-94, 2012
4. Higgins M et al: Clinical associations with a placental diagnosis of delayed villous maturation: a retrospective study. Pediatr Dev Pathol. 14(4):273-9, 2011
5. de Laat MW et al: Hypercoiling of the umbilical cord and placental maturation defect: associated pathology? Pediatr Dev Pathol. 10(4):293-9, 2007
6. Stallmach T et al: Rescue by birth: defective placental maturation and late fetal mortality. Obstet Gynecol. 97(4):505-9, 2001

IMAGE GALLERY

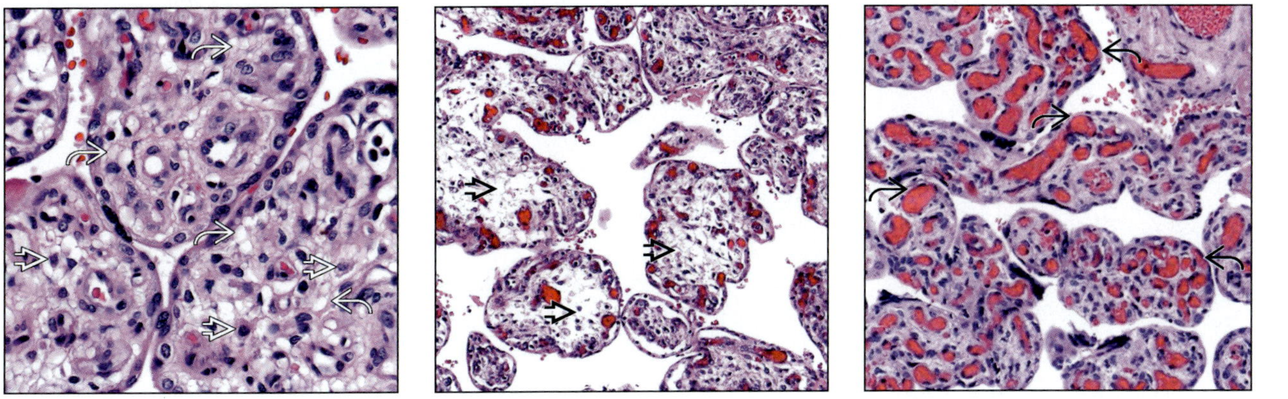

*(**Left**) H&E shows DVI with a complete lack of vasculosyncytial membranes, increased interstitial fluid, and prominent Hofbauer cells. (**Center**) Appropriately immature villi at 23 weeks gestation demonstrate the peripheral location of capillaries with loose mesenchymal stroma and no increase in connective tissue matrix. (**Right**) H&E shows chorangiosis of term villi with hypercapillarization. Vasculosyncytial membranes are present and stromal cellularity is not increased.*

Preeclampsia and Uteroplacental Malperfusion

PREECLAMPSIA AND RELATED HYPERTENSIVE DISORDERS

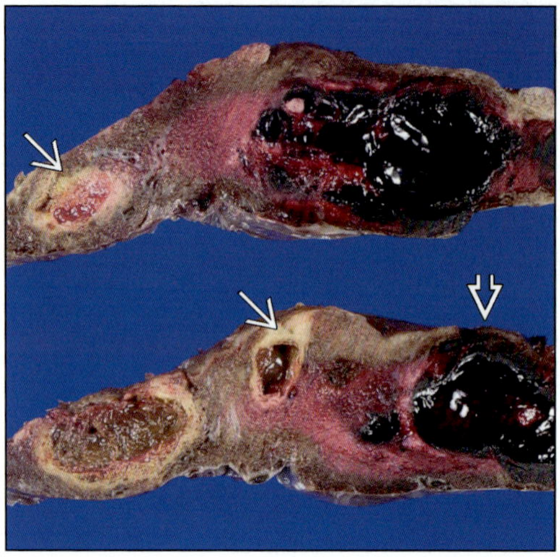

This small placenta has multiple infarcts of variable age, including infarction hematomas, as most commonly seen in preterm PE. White infarcts ➡ are ≥ 7 days old, whereas red infarcts ⇨ are more recent (2-3 days).

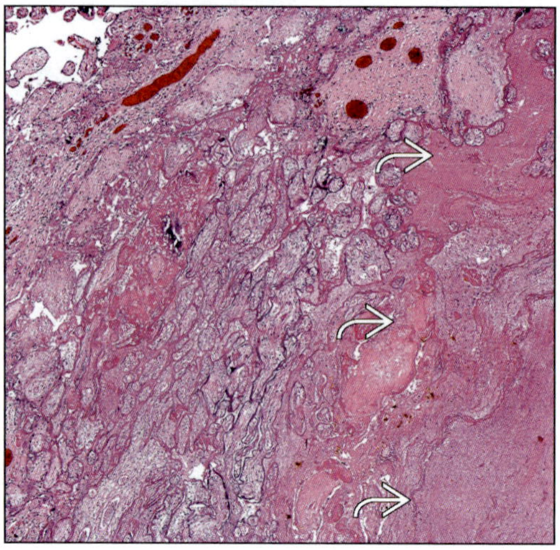

This image from one of the older infarcts in the adjacent placenta demonstrates central hemorrhage ↗, a feature associated with an increased incidence of poor perinatal outcome.

TERMINOLOGY

Abbreviations

- Pregnancy-induced hypertension (PIH)
- Preeclampsia (PE)
- Early-onset or preterm preeclampsia (EOPE)
- Hemolysis, elevated liver enzymes, low platelets (HELLP)

Definitions

- Chronic hypertension: Systolic pressure ≥ 140 mm Hg or diastolic ≥ 90 mm Hg, diagnosed
  - Prior to pregnancy or at < 20 weeks gestation
  - Persisting beyond 12 weeks postpartum
- Gestational or PIH: Blood pressure is ≥ 140/90 mm Hg, diagnosed
  - After 20 weeks gestation
  - Resolves by 12 weeks postpartum
  - Absence of proteinuria or pathologic edema
- PE: Blood pressure is ≥ 140/90 mm Hg with proteinuria and edema
  - Preterm PE (early onset): Development of PE prior to 34 weeks gestation
- PE superimposed on chronic hypertension, onset usually after 24 weeks
  - 15 mm Hg rise in diastolic or 30 mm Hg rise in systolic pressure
- Eclampsia
  - Preeclampsia plus seizures
- HELLP syndrome
  - Severe disease related to preeclampsia with additional, specific clinical features

EPIDEMIOLOGY

Incidence

- Hypertensive disorders affect 5-10% of pregnancies
  - Increased rates in industrialized countries
- PE affects 3-5% of pregnancies
  - 2% progress to eclampsia
- HELLP syndrome affects < 1%
  - Most cases coexist with PE

Age Range

- Increased incidence of chronic hypertension with advancing maternal age
- Increased risk of PE at extremes of reproductive age

Ethnic and Geographical Variation

- Increased rates of PE among African Americans and Hispanics in United States
- Increased prevalence in southern United States
- Filipinas and Samoans with increased risk of PE compared to other Asian subgroups

Mortality

- Hypertensive disorders are leading worldwide cause of maternal mortality
- African Americans have increased risk of mortality

ETIOLOGY/PATHOGENESIS

Genetic Predisposition

- Combined effect of multiple gene variants/ polymorphisms
  - Increased risk of PE in 1st-degree relatives
  - Increased risk of PE with some combinations of paternal HLA and maternal decidual NK cell immunoglobulin receptor genes
  - Increased risk of PE in nonnative populations at high altitudes (e.g., individuals of European descent in Peru)

Immune Mechanisms

- Altered interaction of maternal immune cells and HLA expressed on extravillous trophoblast
  - Decreased tolerance to fetal expressed paternal antigens

Pathogenesis of Maternal Morbidity in Term and Preterm PE

- Angiogenic factors elaborated by trophoblast
  - Altered levels prior to clinical signs/symptoms
  - Correlate with disease severity
  - Release of apoptotic debris into circulation
- Antiangiogenic factor imbalance
  - Increased soluble fms-like tyrosine kinase-1 (sFlt-1), accentuated in trisomy 13, multiple gestation, molar pregnancy
  - Increased soluble endoglin
    - Leads to decreased nitric oxide production
  - Decreased placental growth factor (PIGF)
  - Decreased vascular endothelial growth factor
- Resulting endothelial dysfunction
  - Vasoconstriction with end organ ischemia
  - Endothelial injury with increased thrombosis
  - Glomerular endotheliosis with decreased GFR, decreased renal blood flow and proteinuria

Pathogenesis of Placental Findings

- Preterm PE associated with restricted trophoblastic invasion of decidua, myometrium, and spiral arteries
  - Incomplete conversion of spiral arteries leads to malperfusion of placenta
    - May result from failure of normal trophoblast and uterine NK cell interactions
    - Manifest histologically as maternal decidual vasculopathy
    - Leads to secondary parenchymal ischemic changes such as infarcts, and altered villous growth (distal villous hypoplasia)
  - While these findings are common to preterm PE, they may also be seen in preterm birth or intrauterine growth restriction without PE
- Term PE often lacks reproducible changes in placental morphology

CLINICAL IMPLICATIONS

Clinical Presentation

- PE/eclampsia
  - Maternal hypertension
    - Mild = blood pressure ≥ 140/90 mm Hg
    - Severe = systolic blood pressure ≥ 160 mm Hg or diastolic ≥ 110 mm Hg
    - Mild disease may rapidly progress to severe disease
  - Proteinuria documented on 2 random specimens 6 hours apart
    - Mild = ≥ 100 mg/dL (trace or 1 positive dipstick) urine protein levels or ≥ 300 mg protein in 24-hour collection
    - Severe = ≥ 5,000 mg protein in 24-hour collection
  - Nondependent edema with increased weight gain
  - Epigastric, right upper quadrant pain
  - Neurologic irritation
    - Headache, blurred vision or scotomata
  - Progression to eclampsia with generalized tonic clonic seizures
    - 1/3 cases occur postpartum
    - Younger women are more likely to have seizures with lower blood pressure
  - Fetal growth restriction with EOPE and severe disease
  - Increased risk of preterm labor and delivery
  - May be superimposed on chronic hypertension
  - Symptoms usually resolve within 48 hours postpartum
- HELLP syndrome
  - Hypertension ± other signs of PE
  - Hematological changes
    - Red blood cell hemolysis; abnormal peripheral smear (burr cells, schistocytes), bilirubin ≥ 1.2 mg/dL, LDH > 600 IU/L, decreased haptoglobin
    - Decreased platelet count; < 100,000 uL
  - Elevated liver enzymes; AST (SGOT) ≥ 72 IU/L
- Death can occur due to
  - Hemorrhagic stroke
  - Cardiopulmonary arrest
  - Disseminated intravascular coagulation (DIC) often associated with placental abruption
  - Adult respiratory distress syndrome, severe pulmonary edema
  - Renal failure
  - Intraabdominal hemorrhage due to ruptured hepatic capsule
  - Hypoxic ischemic encephalopathy
  - Findings at autopsy
    - Glomerular endotheliosis
    - Hepatic necrosis in periportal zone 1

Diagnosis

- Primarily based on clinical criteria
  - BP should be repeatedly abnormal
- Potential preclinical markers of PE
  - Decreased β-hCG levels in 1st-trimester maternal serum screening
  - Impaired renal function with
    - Increased serum uric acid
    - Increased creatinine
  - Abnormal uterine artery Doppler velocimetry
    - Persistent early diastolic notch at > 24 weeks
  - Maternal plasma sFlt-1:PIGF
    - Specific diagnostic criteria under investigation

Clinical Risk Factors

- Prior PE or family history
- Obesity
- Primiparity or long interpregnancy interval
- Preexisting maternal disease
  - Chronic hypertension
  - Diabetes mellitus
  - Renal disease
  - Other vascular disease such as lupus
  - Thrombophilia
- Multiple gestations or hydatidiform pregnancy

Prognosis

- 10% worldwide perinatal and neonatal mortality
- Minimal maternal and fetal effects with blood pressure control
- Fetal complications associated with

- Prematurity
  - Necrotizing enterocolitis
  - Hypoxic brain injury
  - Chronic neonatal lung disease
  - Retinopathy of prematurity
- Growth restriction in severe and preterm PE
  - Usually asymmetric with preservation of head/brain growth
- Other effects of placental insufficiency including developmental delay

- Maternal complications
  - Risk of recurrence in future pregnancies
    - Increased risk with severe, early-onset disease
  - Persistent, chronic hypertension
  - Increased lifetime risk of cardiovascular, cerebrovascular, and renal disease
  - Long-term neurologic sequelae including impaired vision
- Maternal mortality increased with severe PE, eclampsia, and HELLP

Treatment

- Published guidelines to decrease blood pressure
- Expectant management to balance risks of prematurity and maternal welfare
  - Steroid administration prior to delivery at < 32-34 weeks
    - Maximizes fetal lung maturity and may protect central nervous system
- Magnesium sulfate for
  - Seizure prophylaxis
  - Maternal neuroprotection
- Prompt delivery with increasing severity

MACROSCOPIC FINDINGS

General Features

- Size
  - Small for gestational age placenta in preterm and severe PE
  - May be within normal range in term PE
  - Rarely, placentas may be large, even hydropic

Common Gross Findings

- Infarcts
  - Extensive (> 5% of placenta) in severe disease
    - Large, central and of variable age, more common in preterm PE
- Retroplacental &/or marginal hematomas (placental abruption)

Specimen Handling

- Routine sectioning with attention to sampling maternal vessels
  - Basal plate biopsies (wedge sections, or enface of maternal surface)
  - 2 membrane rolls
- Additional sections to characterize focal lesions

MICROSCOPIC FINDINGS

Changes Associated With Preterm PE

- Maternal decidual vasculopathy in both decidua parietalis &/or basalis
  - Persistence or mural hypertrophy of smooth muscle, fibrinoid necrosis, acute atheromatous change, perivascular lymphocytes
- Distal villous hypoplasia and accelerated villous maturation
- Increased syncytial knots for age (Tenney-Parker change)
- Villous agglutination and infarcts
- Increased perivillous fibrin

Other Changes Associated With PE

- Uneven villous maturation
- Proliferation of basal extravillous cytotrophoblast cells
- Laminar necrosis of decidua parietalis
- Increased multinucleate trophoblast cells in decidua basalis
- Proliferation and prominence of villous cytotrophoblast cells
- Thickened trophoblast basement membrane (highlighted by PAS stain)
- > 3% of villi with fibrinoid necrosis
- Increased frequency of fetal thrombotic vasculopathy

SELECTED REFERENCES

1. Rana S et al: Angiogenic factors in diagnosis, management, and research in preeclampsia. Hypertension. 63(2):198-202, 2014
2. Abildgaard U et al: Pathogenesis of the syndrome of hemolysis, elevated liver enzymes, and low platelet count (HELLP): a review. Eur J Obstet Gynecol Reprod Biol. 166(2):117-23, 2013
3. Ananth CV et al: Pre-eclampsia rates in the United States, 1980-2010: age-period-cohort analysis. BMJ. 347:f6564, 2013
4. Kovo M et al: Placental vascular pathology as a mechanism of disease in pregnancy complications. Thromb Res. 131 Suppl 1:S18-21, 2013
5. Lo JO et al: Hypertensive disease of pregnancy and maternal mortality. Curr Opin Obstet Gynecol. 25(2):124-32, 2013
6. Naljayan MV et al: New developments in the pathogenesis of preeclampsia. Adv Chronic Kidney Dis. 20(3):265-70, 2013
7. Repke JT: What is new in preeclampsia?: best articles from the past year. Obstet Gynecol. 121(3):682-3, 2013
8. Mustafa R et al: A comprehensive review of hypertension in pregnancy. J Pregnancy. 2012:105918, 2012
9. van Patot MC et al: The hypoxic placenta. High Alt Med Biol. 13(3):176-84, 2012
10. Brosens I et al: The "Great Obstetrical Syndromes" are associated with disorders of deep placentation. Am J Obstet Gynecol. 204(3):193-201, 2011
11. Silasi M et al: Abnormal placentation, angiogenic factors, and the pathogenesis of preeclampsia. Obstet Gynecol Clin North Am. 37(2):239-53, 2010
12. Redline RW et al: Maternal vascular underperfusion: nosology and reproducibility of placental reaction patterns. Pediatr Dev Pathol. 7(3):237-49, 2004

Maternal Vasculopathy

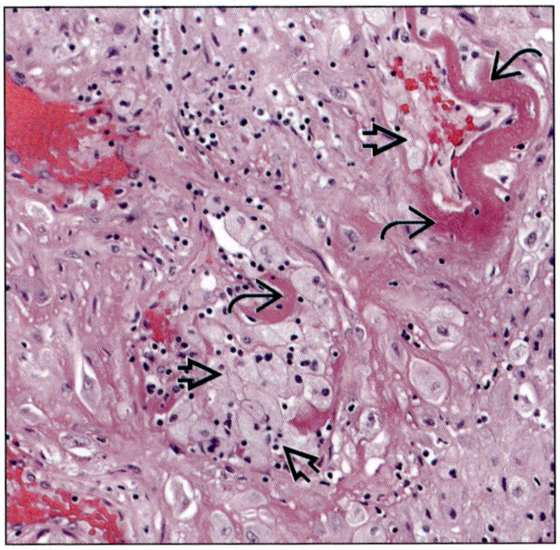

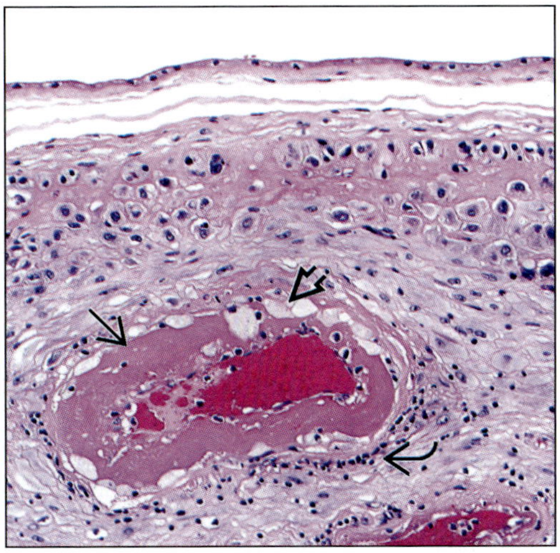

(Left) *Spiral arteries shown here demonstrate fibrinoid necrosis of the vessel walls and marked accumulation of foamy macrophages or atheroma formation.* ***(Right)*** *This section from the free membranes shows an acute atheroma within a maternal vessel of the decidua parietalis. There is fibrinoid necrosis, foamy macrophages, and a cuff of surrounding lymphocytes.*

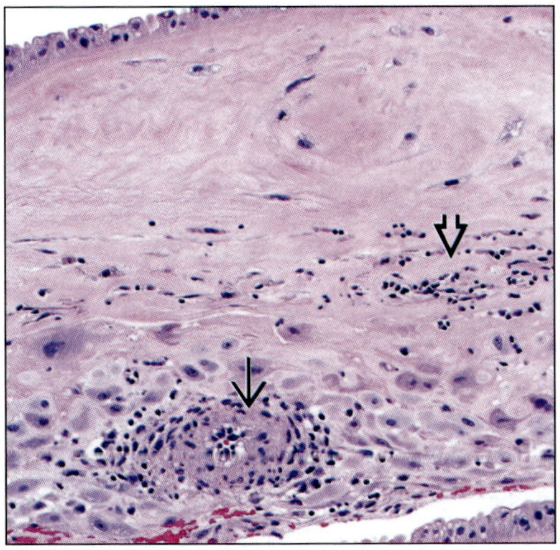

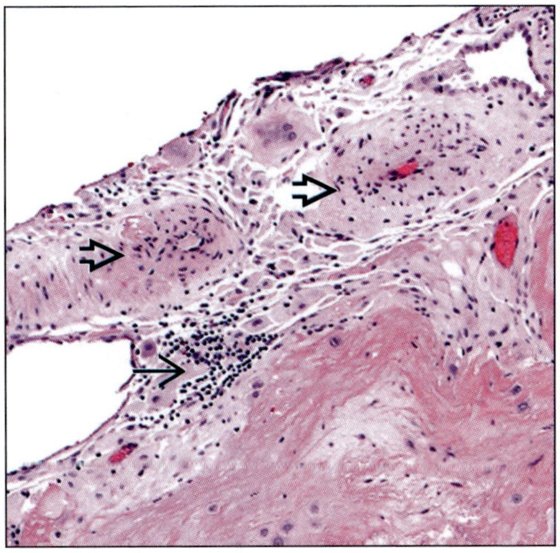

(Left) *This section of the free membranes shows a maternal vessel with medial hypertrophy; the vessel is also surrounded by a cuff of lymphocytes. The lymphocytes are also present in the adjacent chorion.* ***(Right)*** *Maternal vessels in the decidua basalis from the same case demonstrate a lack of physiologic remodeling and a similar degree of mural hypertrophy. There is also an increase in lymphocytes within the decidua.*

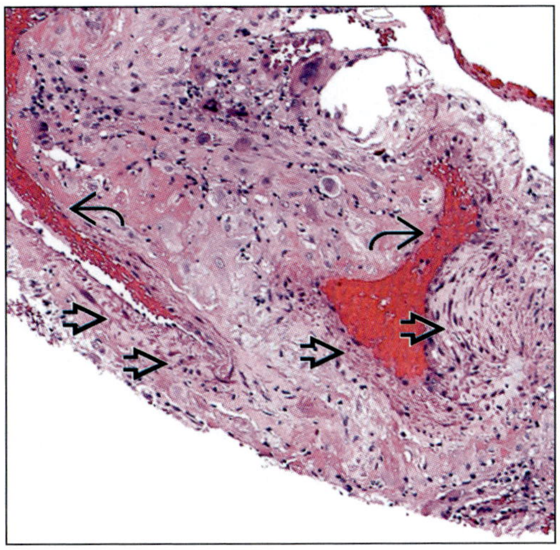

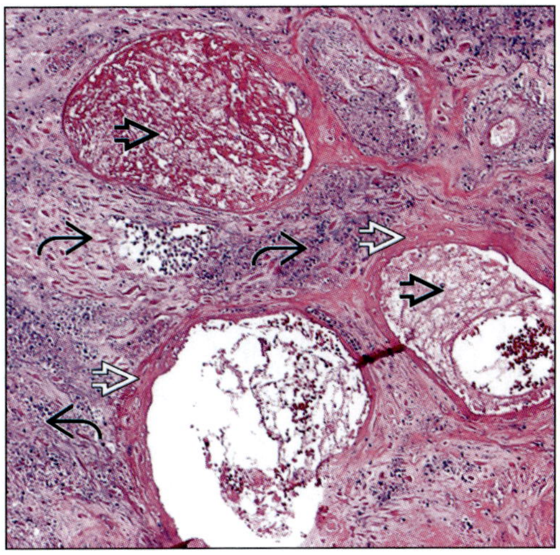

(Left) *This image contains 2 maternal spiral arteries incompletely adapted for pregnancy with persistent mural smooth muscle in a 250 g placenta at 36 weeks gestation with multiple infarcts. The pregnancy was complicated by PE in a woman with a history of deep venous thrombosis.* ***(Right)*** *Recent thrombosis complicates fibrinoid necrosis of a maternal spiral artery in a 290 g placenta at 35 weeks gestation from a pregnancy with PE. The adjacent decidua is necrotic.*

Villi in Preeclampsia

*(**Left**) This preeclamptic placenta shows accelerated villous maturation at 28 weeks gestation with predominantly small villi with vasculosyncytial membranes → and syncytial knots →, rather than large immature intermediate villi. (**Right**) Distal villous hypoplasia, an extreme form of accelerated maturation, is characterized by linear villous profiles →, decreased distal villi, and prominent syncytial knots →. Markedly dilated stem vessels → are associated with abnormal umbilical artery Doppler flow.*

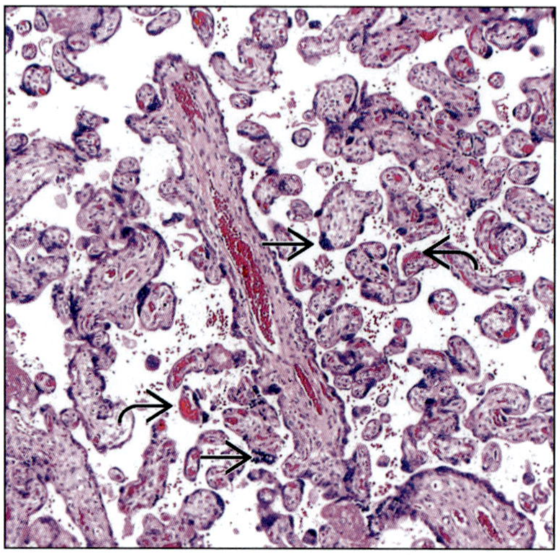

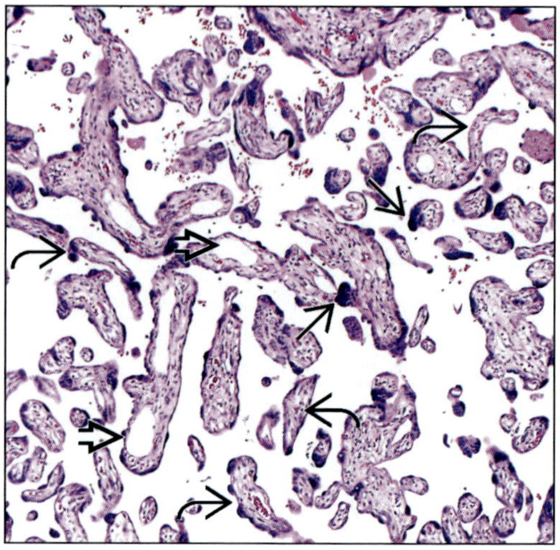

*(**Left**) Markedly exaggerated syncytial knotting, referred to as Tenney-Parker change, is characterized by enlarged knots → containing many syncytiotrophoblast nuclei with condensed nuclear chromatin. Tenney-Parker change is frequently seen in preterm PE and also at the periphery of infarcts. (**Right**) Villous agglutination refers to small areas of villi that appear stuck together; it is frequently seen in placentas with other features of decreased uteroplacental blood flow.*

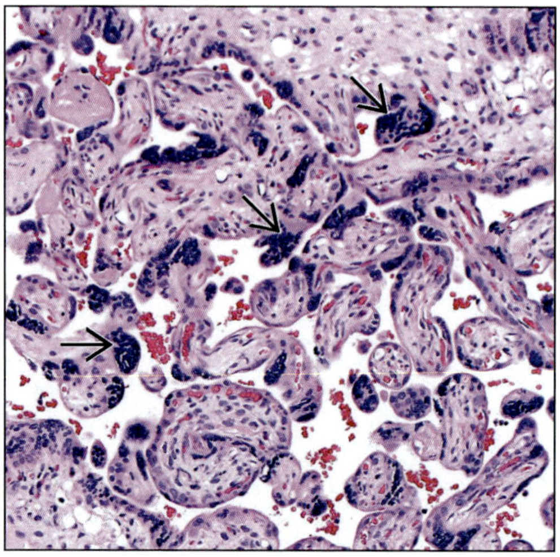

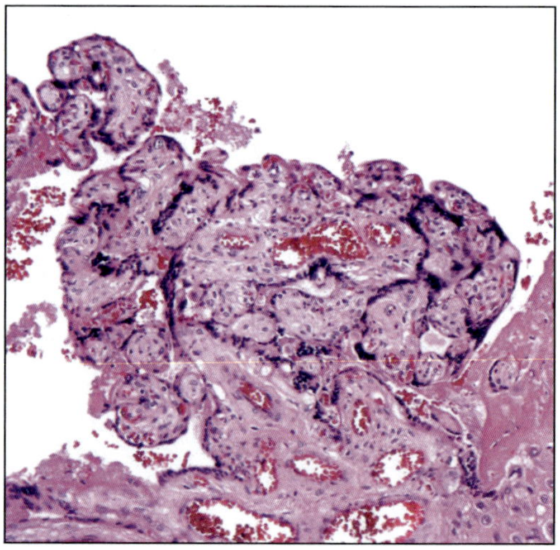

*(**Left**) Preeclampsia is associated with an increased number of villi with fibrinoid necrosis →. The villi are completely or partially replaced by fibrinoid material and maintain a cover of syncytiotrophoblast. (**Right**) Villous changes of PE also include prominence of cytotrophoblast →. This change is considered to be a response to syncytiotrophoblast injury. This image also shows a marked increase in nucleated red blood cells →, a feature of fetal hypoxia.*

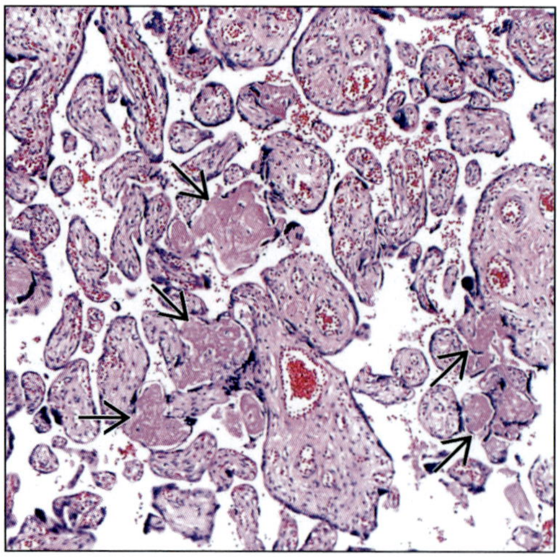

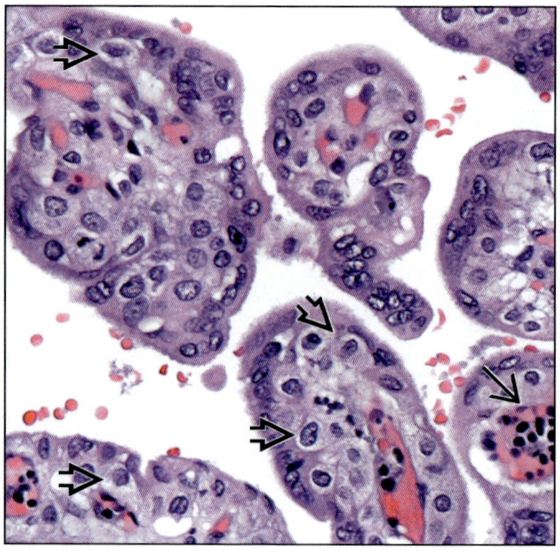

Basal Plate in Preeclampsia

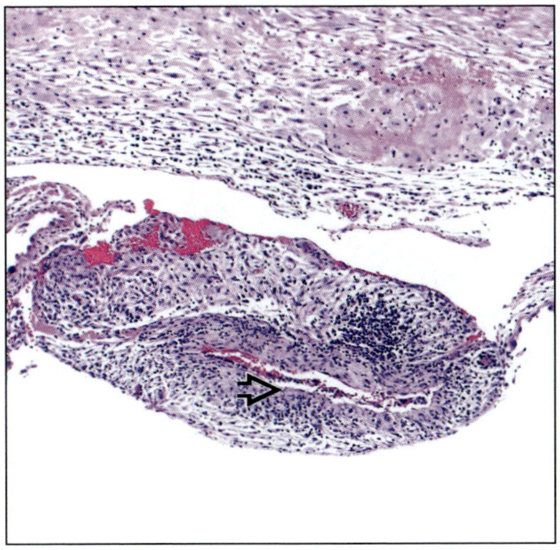

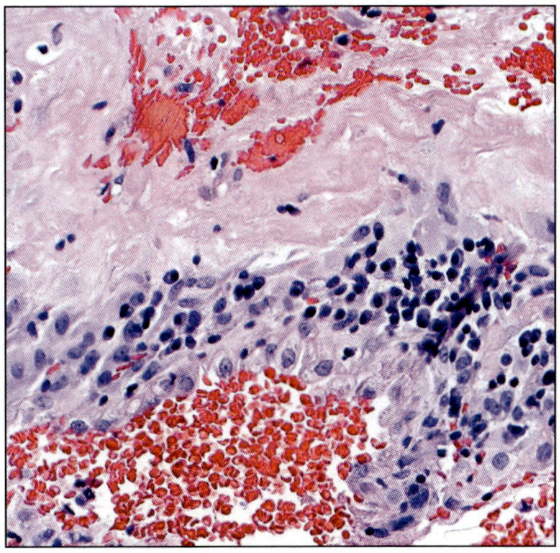

(Left) *Chronic inflammation is frequently increased in the placenta with preeclampsia. This placenta shows marked lymphocytic vasculitis of a maternal spiral artery at the basal plate.* ***(Right)*** *Plasma cells frequently accompany increased lymphocytes at the basal plate in preeclampsia. They are less commonly found within the decidua parietalis of the free membranes.*

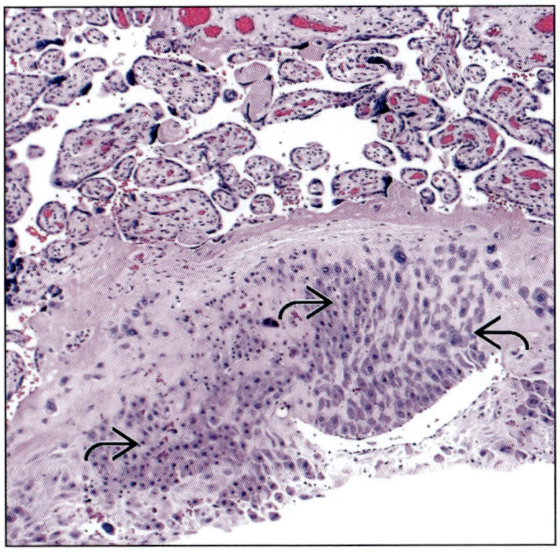

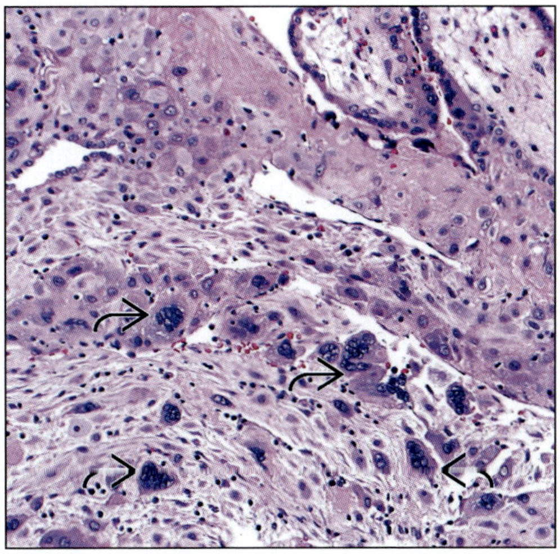

(Left) *PE has been attributed to a failure of trophoblast cells to invade uterine tissues and facilitate vascular remodeling, termed "superficial implantation." This is supported by increased number of extravillous intermediate trophoblast cells remaining at the basal plate.* ***(Right)*** *Fusion of invasive trophoblast to form multinucleate cells generally occurs at the end of migration. Frequent multinucleate trophoblasts in the decidua basalis suggests "superficial implantation."*

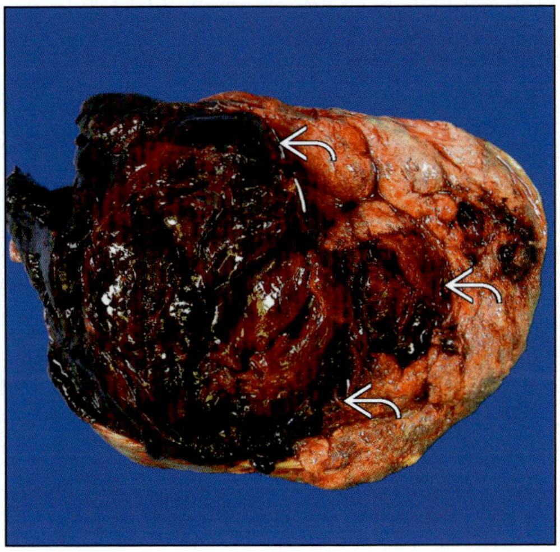

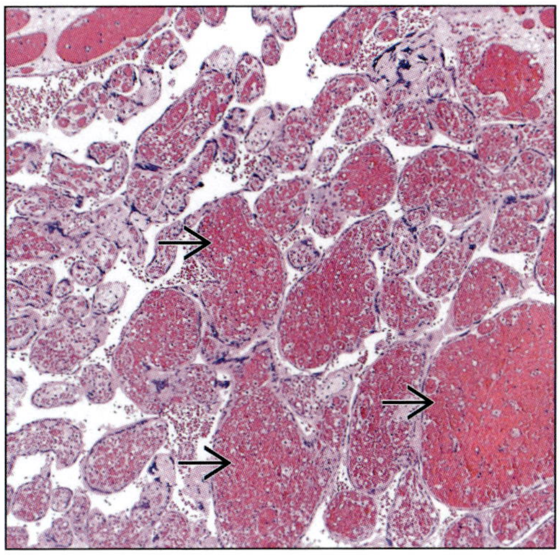

(Left) *Acute retroplacental hematoma occupying at least 50% of the maternal surface, as seen in this image, is usually lethal.* ***(Right)*** *A hyperacute infarct is often associated with recent abruption. The retroplacental hematoma causes a loss of blood flow to the maternal intervillous space, resulting in the loss of maternal blood pressure. A living fetus becomes hyperdynamic and intravillous stromal hemorrhage occurs due to rupture of the villous capillaries.*

SMALL FOR GESTATIONAL AGE PLACENTA

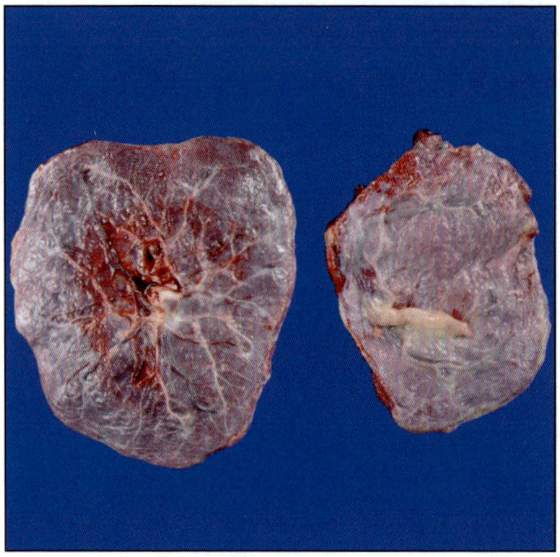

Assessment of placental size is relative to gestational age. These placentas from approximately 37 weeks are visibly discordant in size with the placenta on the right being small for gestational age.

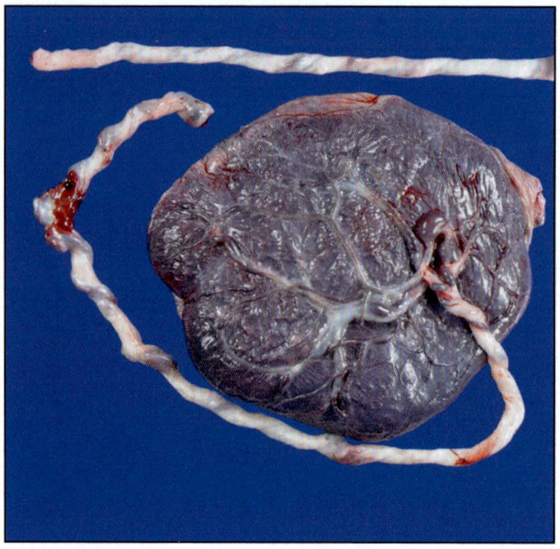

This markedly small placenta weighed only 174 g at 36 weeks, with a maximal diameter of 13 cm, and was composed of dysmorphic villi; the pregnancy was complicated by fetal holoprosencephaly.

TERMINOLOGY

Definitions

- Macroscopic diagnosis based on comparison of placental weight to normative values for given gestational age
  - Variably defined by weight below 10th, 5th, or 3rd percentile
  - Significant pathology more likely in weights below 5th or 3rd percentile

Synonyms

- Placental undergrowth
- Underweight placenta
- Placental growth restriction

ETIOLOGY/PATHOGENESIS

Generalized Growth Impairment With Normal Villous Morphology

- Constitutional small size due to ethnic/genetic variation
- Secondary to maternal disease
- Confined placental mosaicism
  - Discrepant karyotypic, or molecular genetic (e.g., loss of heterozygosity) abnormality present in placenta, absent in fetus
  - Occurs in 1-2% of pregnancies
  - Subcategorized as types 1, 2, or 3
    - Type 1 mosaicism confined to trophoblast
    - Type 2 mosaicism confined to villous stroma
    - Type 3 mosaicism involves trophoblast and stromal cells
  - Type 3 most associated with placental growth impairment

Placental Growth Impairment With Villous Maldevelopment

- Aneuploidy with dysmorphic villi
- Early-onset uteroplacental malperfusion with distal villous hypoplasia

Secondary Pathology Associated With Loss of Functional Parenchyma

- Chronic uteroplacental malperfusion
- Chronic obstructed fetoplacental perfusion
- Parenchymal inflammation, infectious and idiopathic
- Extensive fibrinoid deposition in intervillous space

CLINICAL IMPLICATIONS

Clinical Risk Factors

- Maternal disease associated with fetal growth restriction and small placenta
  - Hypertensive disorders including preeclampsia
  - Autoimmune disorders
  - Thrombophilic disorders
  - Severe malnutrition, poor weight gain during pregnancy
  - Tobacco use during pregnancy
    - Ratio of placental weight to birth weight relatively increased
- Prior pregnancy affected by lesion with known risk of recurrence
  - Early onset, severe preeclampsia
  - Massive perivillous fibrinoid deposition/maternal floor infarct
  - High-grade chronic villitis/villitis of unknown etiology
  - Chronic histiocytic intervillositis of unknown etiology

Clinical Presentation

- Correlates with low fetal weight/growth restriction

DISTAL VILLOUS HYPOPLASIA

Microscopic Features

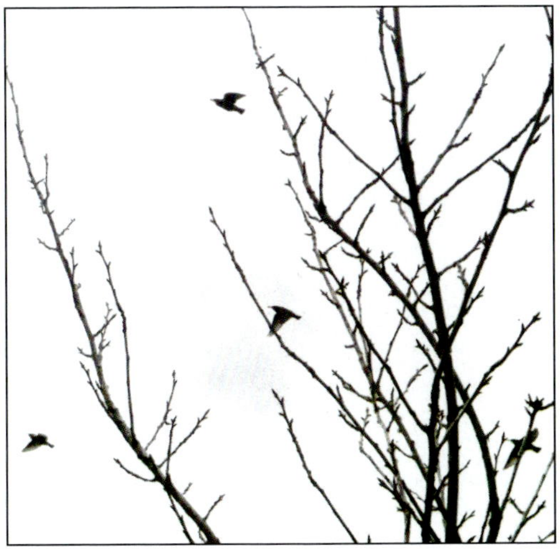

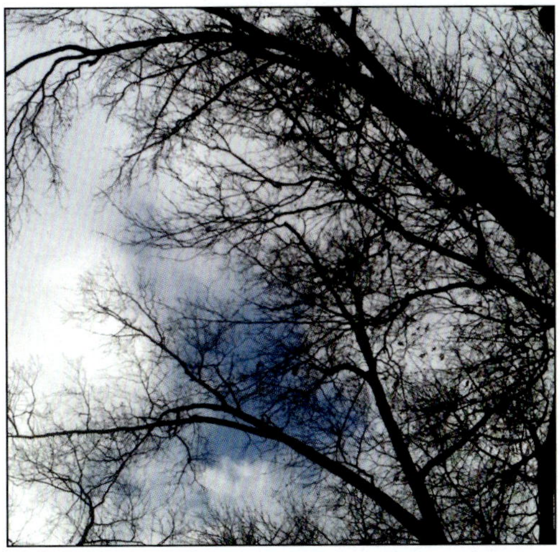

(Left) *Distal villous hypoplasia can be likened to this sparse-appearing tree. Nonbranching angiogenesis alone yields long slender structures. They abruptly give rise to small gas exchange units (mature villi with vasculosyncytial membranes), like leaves.* ***(Right)*** *In comparison, normal placental development includes branching and nonbranching angiogenesis, like the branching pattern of this tree, yielding a greater density and size variation of structures.*

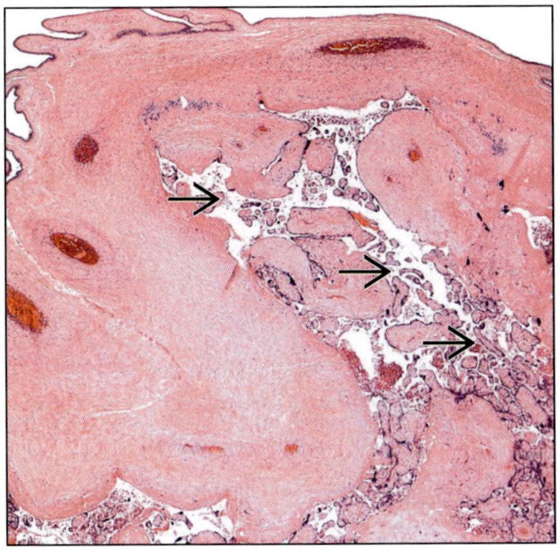

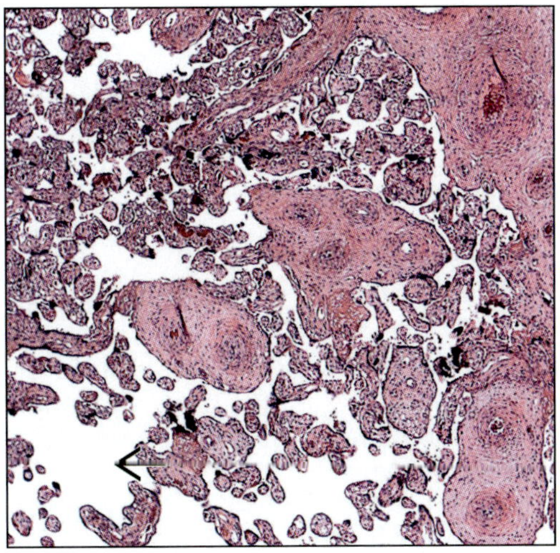

(Left) *Villi beneath the chorionic plate commonly show features of DVH →. This subchorionic region has the most sluggish and inconsistent maternal perfusion, as blood must travel from the basal plate.* ***(Right)*** *A focal region of the mature placenta, often at the periphery of a lobule, can also resemble DVH →. DVH should involve 30% of the parenchyma for diagnosis. This avoids overcalling the feature in the normal variation of villous morphology.*

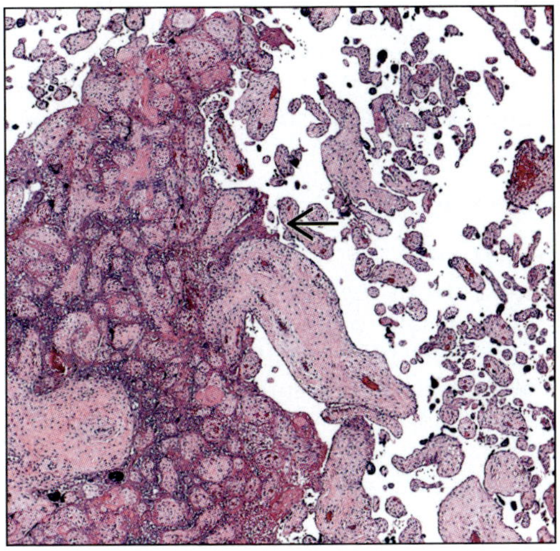

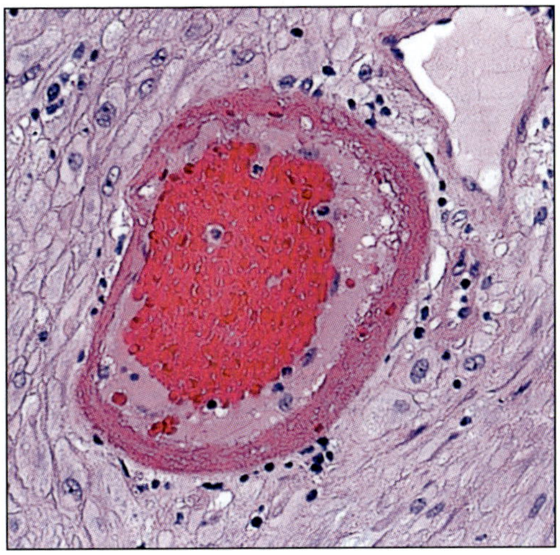

(Left) *Villi adjacent to infarcts → often show DVH. This likely represents the common pathophysiology of poor maternal perfusion and also the location of the villi at the periphery of a lobule.* ***(Right)*** *DVH often accompanies maternal decidual vasculopathy in the preterm placenta from preeclamptic mothers. The failure of the maternal vasculature to appropriately remodel early in pregnancy underlies the chronic malperfusion of the placenta, giving rise to DVH.*

MATERNAL DECIDUAL VASCULOPATHY

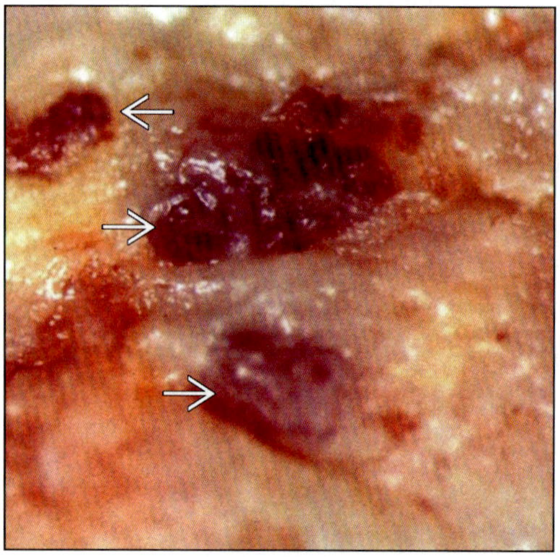

Detection of maternal decidual vasculopathy (MDV) requires sampling of the decidua basalis (spiral arteries ➔) and the membranous decidua on membrane rolls.

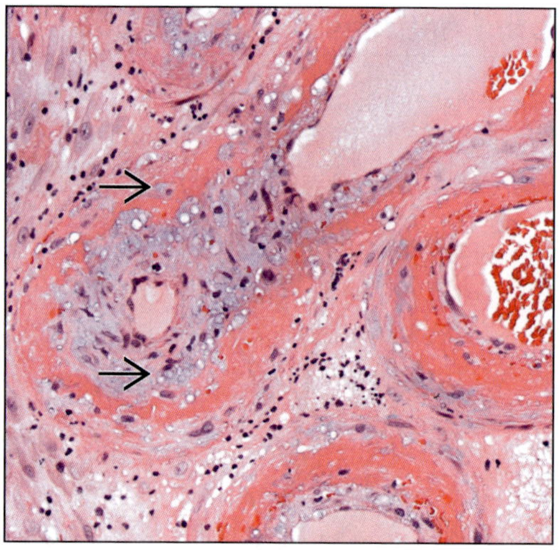

Acute atherosis is unrelated to atherosclerosis. The vessel wall is necrotic and appears replaced by fibrin. Numerous subendothelial and mural foamy macrophages ➔ are seen.

TERMINOLOGY

Abbreviations

- Maternal decidual vasculopathy (MDV)

Synonyms

- Membrane mural hypertrophy and hypertrophic decidual vasculopathy
- Muscular basal plate arteries and incomplete adaptation of spiral artery (SA) for pregnancy

Definitions

- Pathologic changes of maternal decidual vessels, subtypes include
  - Acute atherosis: Glassy pink necrosis of SA walls with subendothelial and intramural foamy macrophages
  - Hypertrophic decidual vasculopathy: SA wall thickness > 1/3 of vessel diameter
  - Incomplete adaptation for pregnancy: Failure of normal physiologic conversion of SA during pregnancy

ETIOLOGY/PATHOGENESIS

Incomplete Adaptation for Pregnancy

- Trophoblast cells normally remodel preplacental SA in decidua basalis and underlying myometrium
  - Failure of early uterine NK-cell/trophoblast interactions that normally facilitate remodeling

Acute Atherosis

- SAs that are not remodeled by trophoblast cells are susceptible to acute atherosis
  - Visible in membranous decidua
  - Visible in decidua basalis when trophoblast remodeling fails to occur
- Cause is unclear
  - May be late effort to remodel vessels, immune-mediated effect, or effect of other soluble factor
- Despite name and appearance, pathogenesis is not related to atherosclerosis

Hypertrophic Decidual Vasculopathy

- SA throughout decidua thin their vascular smooth muscle early in pregnancy
- When SA thinning fails, vessels remain thick
  - Associated with preexisting vascular disease
    - Hypertension
    - Diabetes
- May be evident in cases that otherwise have appropriate trophoblast-mediated remodeling in decidua basalis

CLINICAL ISSUES

Epidemiology

- Incidence
  - Occurs in < 1% of uncomplicated pregnancies
  - More frequent in pregnancies complicated by small for gestational age (SGA), preeclampsia, or pregnancy-induced hypertension

Prognosis

- Associated with recurrent indicated preterm birth

Clinical Implications

- Clinical conditions featuring MDV
  - Preeclampsia, especially preterm with SGA
  - Pregnancy-induced hypertension
  - Indicated preterm birth for poor fetal growth
  - Gestational diabetes

MATERNAL DECIDUAL VASCULOPATHY

Key Facts

Terminology
- Maternal decidual vasculopathy (MDV)
  - Microscopic changes of spiral artery are evident in membranous decidua and decidua basalis
  - Incomplete adaptation for pregnancy
  - Hypertrophic decidual vasculopathy
  - Acute atherosis

Etiology
- Results from failure of normal vascular remodeling for pregnancy

Clinical Issues
- Incidence
  - Occurs in < 1% of uncomplicated pregnancies
  - More frequent in pregnancies complicated by small for gestational age, preeclampsia, or pregnancy-induced hypertension

Microscopic Pathology
- Incomplete adaptation for pregnancy
  - Persistence of smooth muscle in SA of central 2/3 decidua basalis
- Hypertrophic decidual vasculopathy
  - SA wall thickness > 30% of vessel diameter
- Acute atherosis
  - Fibrinoid necrosis of SA wall with subendothelial or mural foamy macrophages, ± thrombus
- MDV associated with infarcts, distal villous hypoplasia

MACROSCOPIC FEATURES

General Features
- MDV is not visible grossly, excepting prominent thrombi

Sections to Be Submitted
- Membranous decidua
  - 2 rolls of membranous decidua with chorioamnionic membranes improves detection of maternal decidual vasculopathy
  - If membranous chorion has separated from decidua, SA may be absent
- Basal plate decidua
  - When placental malperfusion is suspected, submit cassette of multiple wedge sections from central 2/3 of disc basal surface

Associated Gross Features
- Small for gestational age trimmed placenta weight, infarcts, thin umbilical cord

MICROSCOPIC PATHOLOGY

Incomplete Adaptation for Pregnancy
- Muscular SA in central 2/3 of basal decidua
  - Thinned muscular arteries are normal in membranous decidua and peripheral basal plate

Hypertrophic Decidual Vasculopathy
- Abnormally thickened SA in membranous decidua or decidua basalis

Acute Atherosis
- Red-blue glassy fibrinoid necrosis of muscular wall of spiral artery with foamy macrophages in subendothelium or wall
  - Can be seen in any muscular SA of membranous decidua and basal decidua, including margin
- Early stage
  - May show only fibrinoid necrosis of wall
- Late stage
  - May show thrombosis in necrotic vessel

Associated Microscopic Findings
- Distal villous hypoplasia, increased syncytial knots, infarcts

DIFFERENTIAL DIAGNOSIS

Mimics
- Entrapped villi in basal fibrin with muscular fetal vessels mimic muscular maternal vessels in basal plate
- Normal early vascular remodeling in 1st-trimester placenta can resemble acute atherosis
  - Use caution when calling these early processes pathologic
  - Acute atherosis recognized in early spontaneous abortion associated with systemic lupus erythematosus

DIAGNOSTIC CHECKLIST

Pathologic Interpretation Pearls
- Understanding normal vascular remodeling is key to appreciating MDV

SELECTED REFERENCES

1. Stevens DU et al: Decidual vasculopathy in preeclampsia: lesion characteristics relate to disease severity and perinatal outcome. Placenta. 34(9):805-9, 2013
2. Roberts DJ et al: The placenta in pre-eclampsia and intrauterine growth restriction. J Clin Pathol. 61(12):1254-60, 2008
3. Redline RW et al: Maternal vascular underperfusion: nosology and reproducibility of placental reaction patterns. Pediatr Dev Pathol. 7(3):237-49, 2004
4. Robertson WB: Uteroplacental vasculature. J Clin Pathol Suppl (R Coll Pathol). 10:9-17, 1976

MATERNAL DECIDUAL VASCULOPATHY

Vascular Remodeling in Decidua Basalis

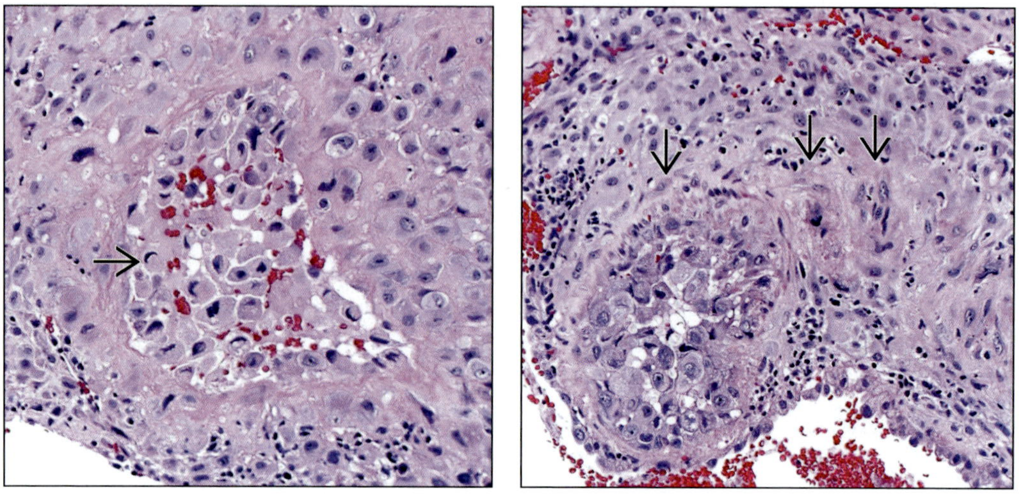

(Left) *This 1st-trimester spiral artery (SA) is filled with invasive cytotrophoblast cells* →*, forming a plug. The occlusion may have a role in protecting the conceptus from the pressure and oxygen tension of arterial blood.* ***(Right)*** *In early transformation, the smooth muscle is attenuated and trophoblast cells plug* → *the lumen. Associated immune cells aid in the transformation.*

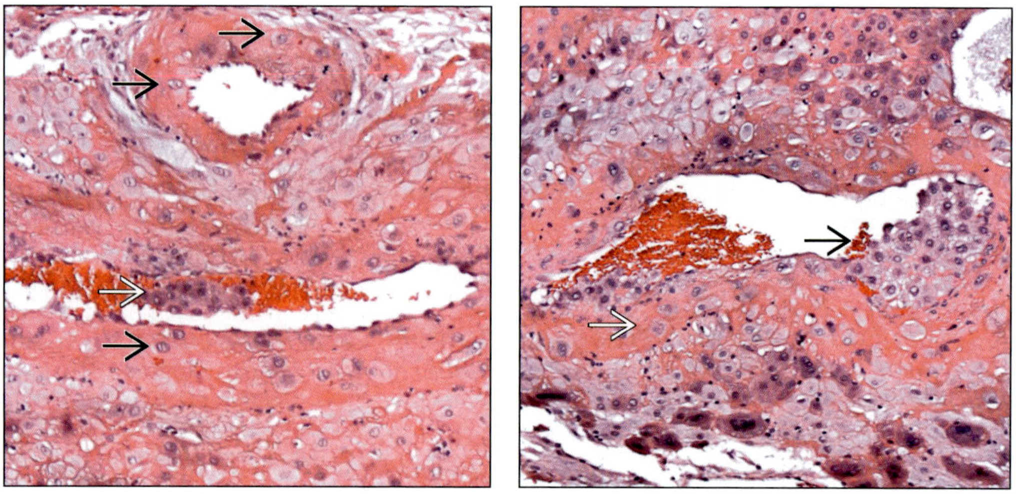

(Left) *In trophoblast-mediated remodeling, vascular smooth muscle is replaced by matrix-type fibrinoid and occasional mural trophoblast cells* →*. Luminal trophoblast cells* ➡ *are expected in the 1st and 2nd trimesters. Near term, they may indicate incomplete remodeling for pregnancy.* ***(Right)*** *This vessel shows ongoing remodeling. Smooth muscle is replaced by matrix-type fibrinoid, and trophoblast cells persist in the lumen* → *and are in the remodeled vessel walls* ➡*.*

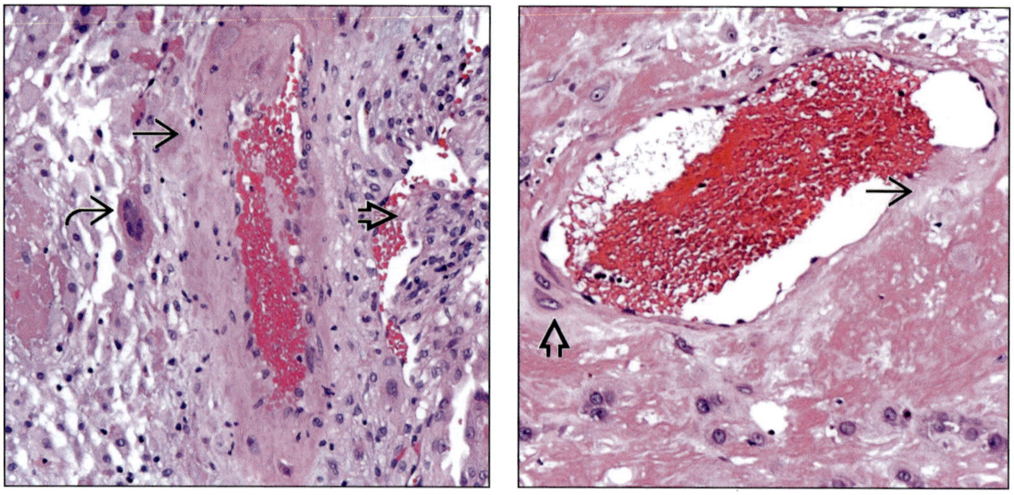

(Left) *In this remodeled vessel, the muscularis is replaced by fibrin* →*. Nearby are extravillous trophoblast cells from an anchoring villus* ⇨ *as well as a multinucleated trophoblast cell* ↪*.* ***(Right)*** *This spiral artery is fully remodeled. The vessel is distinguished from veins by the matrix* → *surrounding the lumen and the mural trophoblast cells* ⇨*.*

Incomplete Adaptation for Pregnancy

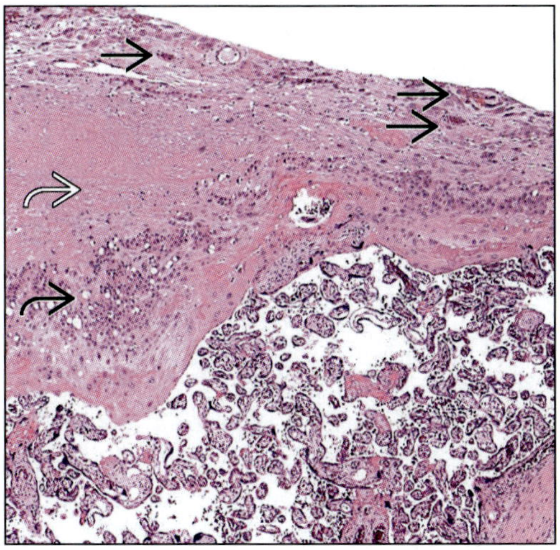
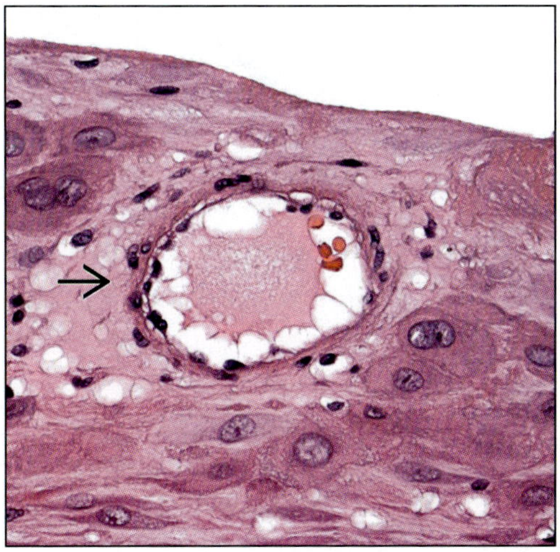

(Left) *SAs ➔ in the decidua basalis are typically deep to the basal trophoblast cell ➔ and fibrin ➔ layers. The small SAs shown have not been adapted for pregnancy.* ***(Right)*** *This muscular SA ➔ shows incomplete adaptation for pregnancy. By the 3rd trimester, SA from the central 2/3 of the decidua basalis should be transformed by trophoblast cells, allowing for free flow of maternal blood unimpeded by changes in muscular tone.*

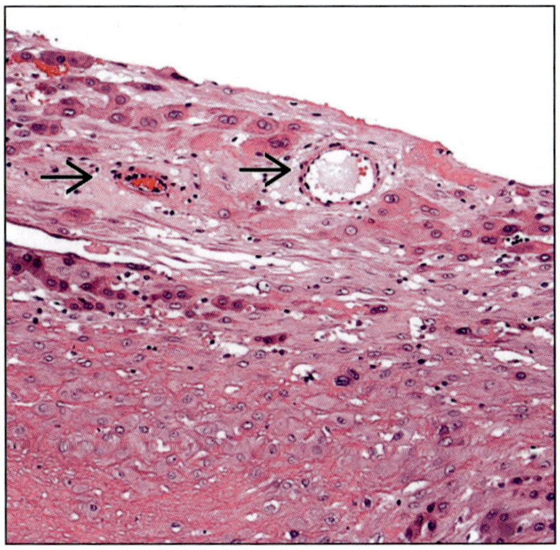
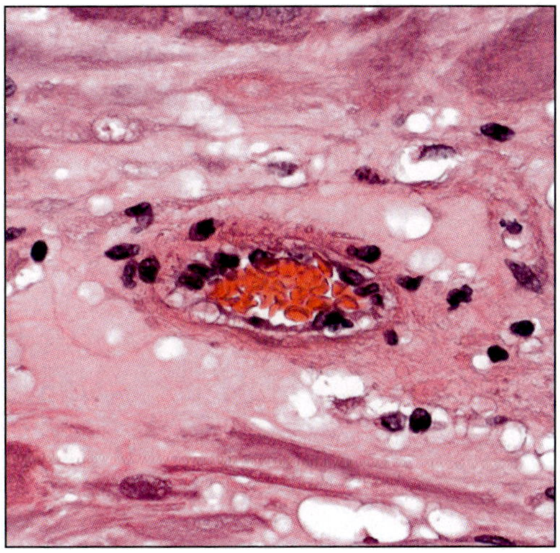

(Left) *Incomplete adaptation for pregnancy ➔ can be easily missed at scanning magnification, especially if one does not realize that these normal-appearing vessels are abnormal in the decidua basalis.* ***(Right)*** *Higher magnification may be needed to see the muscularis. This vessel retains a thin muscular wall and did not undergo the normal widening that results from remodeling. Unremodeled SAs are vulnerable to acute atherosis, whereas remodeled SAs are not susceptible.*

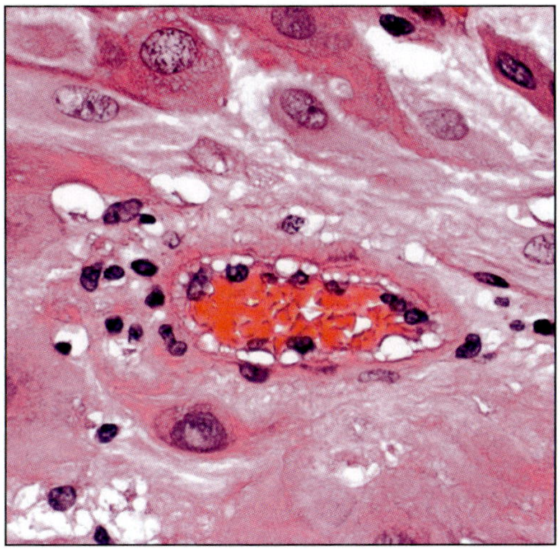
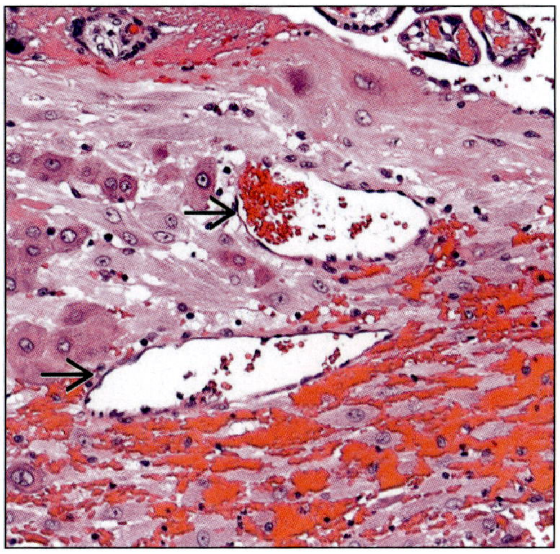

(Left) *Unremodeled SAs limit perfusion to the intervillous space because they remain small and are susceptible to vasoconstriction. The flow dynamics are therefore different. Blood delivered to the intervillous space is of higher pressure and inconstant.* ***(Right)*** *Maternal veins ➔ in the decidua basalis usually have no smooth muscle or incomplete single layers. They are not remodeled by trophoblast.*

MATERNAL DECIDUAL VASCULOPATHY

Hypertrophic Vasculopathy and Acute Atherosis

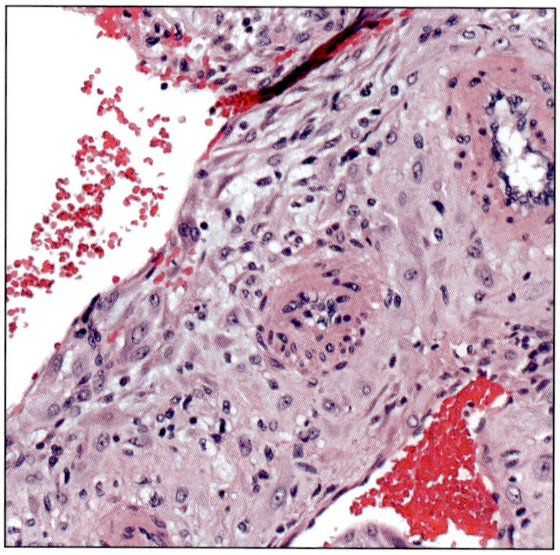

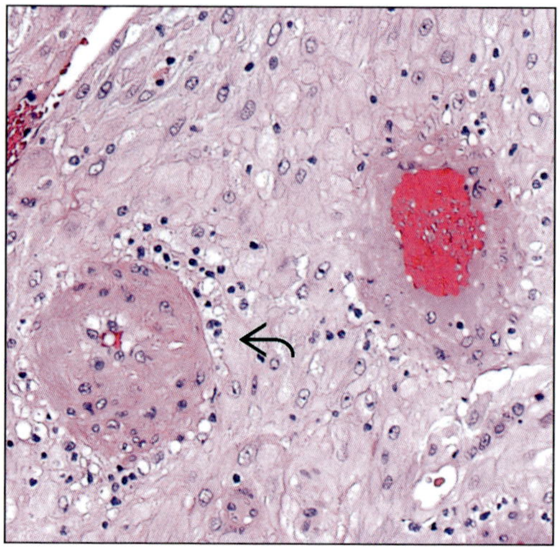

(Left) *The decidual arterial muscularis should thin in response to pregnancy. In hypertrophic decidual vasculopathy, the walls are too thick (wall thickness > 30% of diameter). This feature may be seen in the membranous decidua or in the decidua basalis.* ***(Right)*** *These membranous decidual SAs ↷ not only did not thin out in response to the hormonal milieu of pregnancy, they are also abnormally thickened. The findings are similar to hypertensive changes elsewhere in the body.*

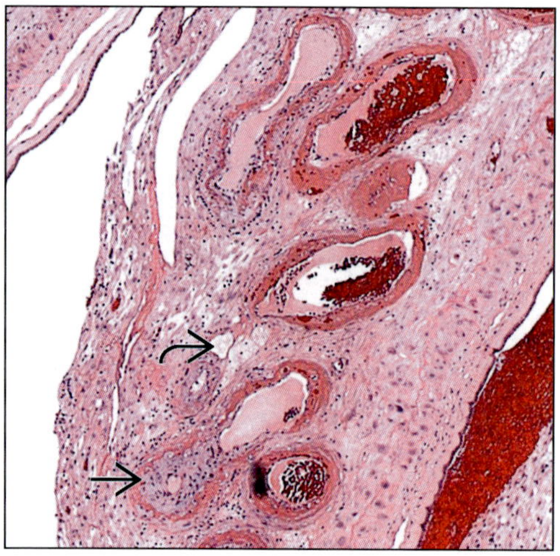

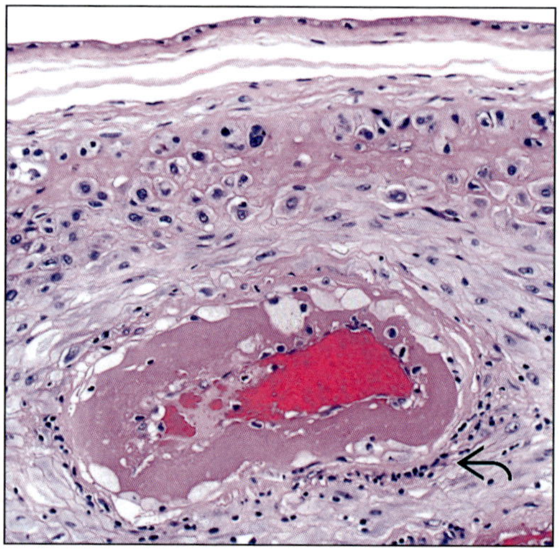

(Left) *In acute atherosis, the vessel walls have the intense eosinophilia of fibrinoid necrosis. Subendothelial foamy cells appear basophilic →. Larger foamy cells are in the necrotic wall ↷. Acute atherosis only occurs in vessels that have not undergone trophoblast-mediated remodeling.* ***(Right)*** *A cuff of lymphocytes ↷ is often found in association with acute atherosis.*

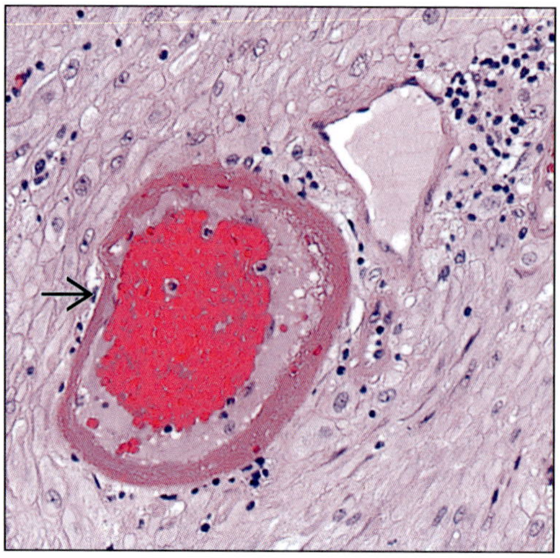

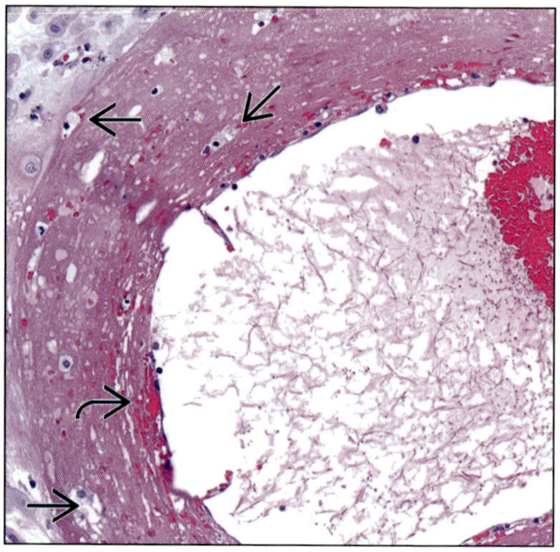

(Left) *Only 1 turn → of this SA appears affected by acute atherosis. MDV can be focal. Submission of 2 membrane rolls may aid in detecting MDV in the membranous decidua.* ***(Right)*** *This vessel shows characteristic intensely eosinophilic fibrinoid necrosis, with scattered foam cells →. There is also early clot formation ↷, evidenced by entrapped red blood cells (RBCs) in the necrotic wall.*

EXTRAVILLOUS CYTOTROPHOBLAST CYSTS

Key Facts

Terminology
- Trophoblast cysts
  - Pools of matrix-type fibrinoid material surrounded by extravillous trophoblast (EVT)
  - Found in sites where EVT proliferate: Cellular chorion of membranes and chorionic plate, placental cell islands, septa, basal plate
- May be macroscopic or microscopic (e.g., microcysts)

Etiology
- Accompany proliferations of EVT
- Contents resemble placental matrix-type fibrinoid

Clinical Issues
- **Membranous trophoblast microcysts**
  - Associated with conditions of uteroplacental hypoxia, including preeclampsia
  - Require ≥ 3 foci to report, include as a supporting finding of maternal malperfusion when accompanied by other features; if an isolated finding, significance is unclear
- **Chorionic plate and septal trophoblast cysts**
  - Associated with delivery at high altitude (preplacental hypoxia)
  - Large cysts on chorionic plate surface (> 4.5 cm) associated with intrauterine growth restriction
  - Associated with massive increased perivillous fibrin (maternal floor infarction)

Microscopic Pathology
- Cysts of homogeneous, colloidal appearing pink fluid lined by EVT cells

  - Associated with massive increased perivillous fibrin deposition (maternal floor infarction)
    - Large (> 4.5 cm) and multiple cysts

MACROSCOPIC FEATURES

General Features
- Membranous trophoblast microcysts are grossly inapparent
- Chorionic trophoblast cysts are frequently large and visible on chorionic plate
  - May have blood-tinged contents when large
- Septal and cell island trophoblast cysts in the parenchyma may be visible on gross cut section

MICROSCOPIC PATHOLOGY

Membranous Trophoblast Microcysts
- Cysts of homogeneous, colloidal appearing pink fluid in cellular chorion of free membranes
- Lined by epithelioid-appearing chorionic trophoblast

Chorionic Plate Trophoblast Cysts
- Cysts appear similar to microcysts in membranous chorion, but are located beneath stroma of chorionic plate
- Can elevate overlying fetal vasculature
- Often have admixed blood of probable fetal origin

Septal and Cell Island Trophoblast Cysts
- Cysts appear similar to membranous chorionic microcysts, but can be larger
- Located in aggregates of extravillous cytotrophoblast within villous parenchyma
- Septal cysts have associated decidual stromal cells of septa
- Cell islands are likely extensions off of septa

DIFFERENTIAL DIAGNOSIS

Regressed Villi
- Remnants of villi that initially covered entire gestational sac in 1st trimester (chorion laeve)
  - Similar size as chorionic microcysts, also often rimmed by chorionic trophoblast
  - Usually have residual polygonal stromal cells
    - Chorionic microcysts may contain macrophages, but no polygonal cells
  - Regressed villi lack the homogeneous appearance of chorionic microcysts

Endometrial Glands
- May have similar proteinaceous fluid as chorionic microcysts
- Located deeper in membranous decidua and are not continuous with chorionic trophoblast

SELECTED REFERENCES

1. Bendon RW et al: Reassessing the clinical significance of chorionic membrane microcysts and linear necrosis. Pediatr Dev Pathol. 15(3):213-6, 2012
2. Stanek J: Membrane microscopic chorionic pseudocysts are associated with increased amount of placental extravillous trophoblasts. Pathology. 42(2):125-30, 2010
3. Stanek J et al: Microscopic chorionic pseudocysts in placental membranes: a histologic lesion of in utero hypoxia. Pediatr Dev Pathol. 10(3):192-8, 2007
4. Soma H et al: Characteristics of histopathological and ultrastructural features of placental villi in pregnant Nepalese women. Med Mol Morphol. 38(2):92-103, 2005
5. Kaufmann P et al: The fibrinoids of the human placenta: origin, composition and functional relevance. Ann Anat. 178(6):485-501, 1996
6. Vernof KK et al: Maternal floor infarction: relationship to X cells, major basic protein, and adverse perinatal outcome. Am J Obstet Gynecol. 167(5):1355-63, 1992
7. Ruckhäberle EK et al: Clinical correlations of morphologic trophoblast findings: a contribution to the pathologic anatomy of placental insufficiency. J Perinat Med. 10(4):185-95, 1982

EXTRAVILLOUS CYTOTROPHOBLAST CYSTS

Microscopic Features

*(**Left**) Trophoblast microcysts in the membranes are shown. Pools of eosinophilic substance ➔ in the membranous chorion are visible at low power. The cyst content resembles colloid in the thyroid. (**Right**) Higher power examination shows the homogeneity of the cysts in the membranous chorion. Occasional trophoblast cells ➔ may appear within the lumen, which reflects the irregular contour of the cysts.*

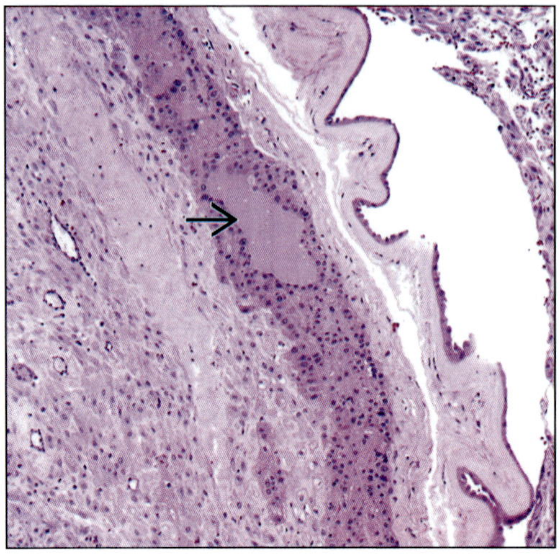

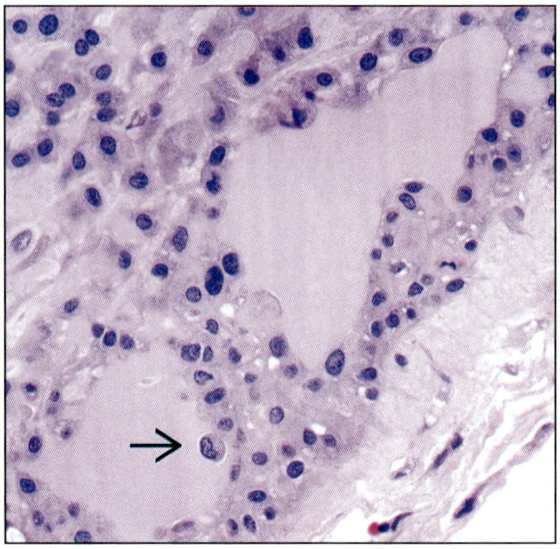

*(**Left**) Trophoblast microcyst in the membranes is shown. The cyst fluid is more dense in the membranes than in other trophoblast cyst locations. (**Right**) The closest mimic of trophoblast cysts in the membranes are regressed villi. These may also be surrounded by trophoblast ➔. Unlike the cysts, they have an internal stroma and are not fluid filled.*

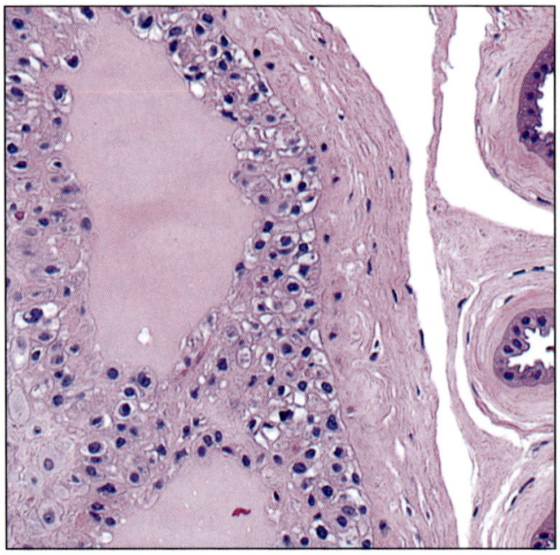

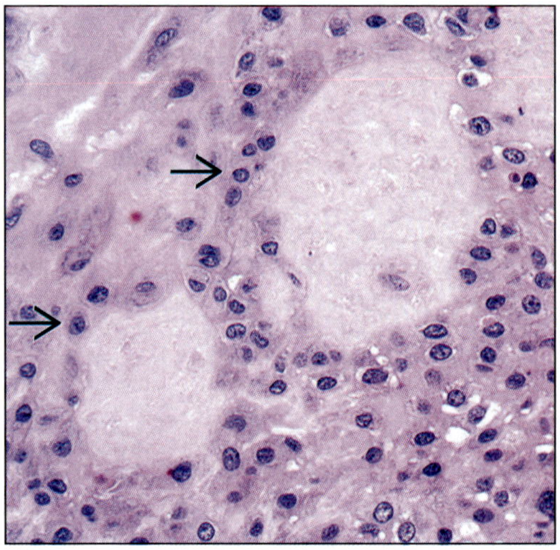

*(**Left**) Endometrial glands in the decidua ➔ may also mimic trophoblast cysts. Their location within the decidua, and not within trophoblast accumulations, are an important clue. (**Right**) Fluid-filled endometrial gland ➔ in membranous decidua is shown. The secreted substance may appear very similar to that of trophoblast microcysts. However, the location is in the decidua, not chorionic trophoblast ⇨.*

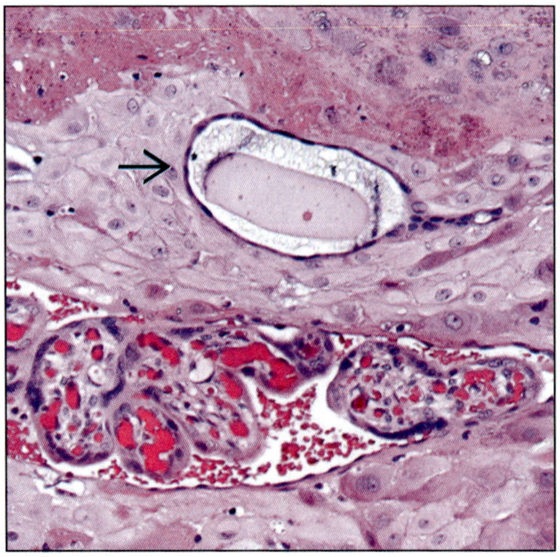

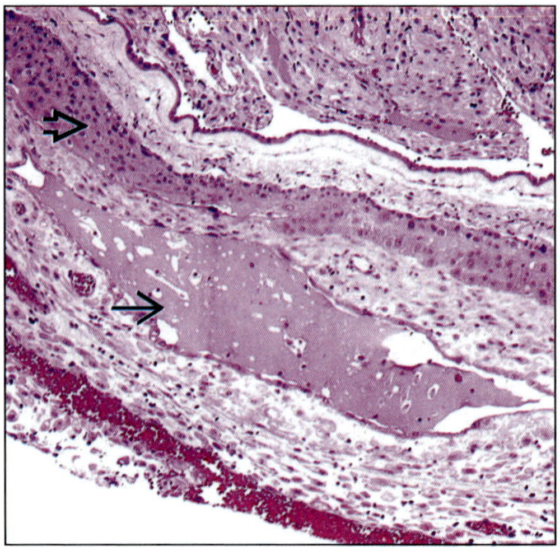

Microscopic Features

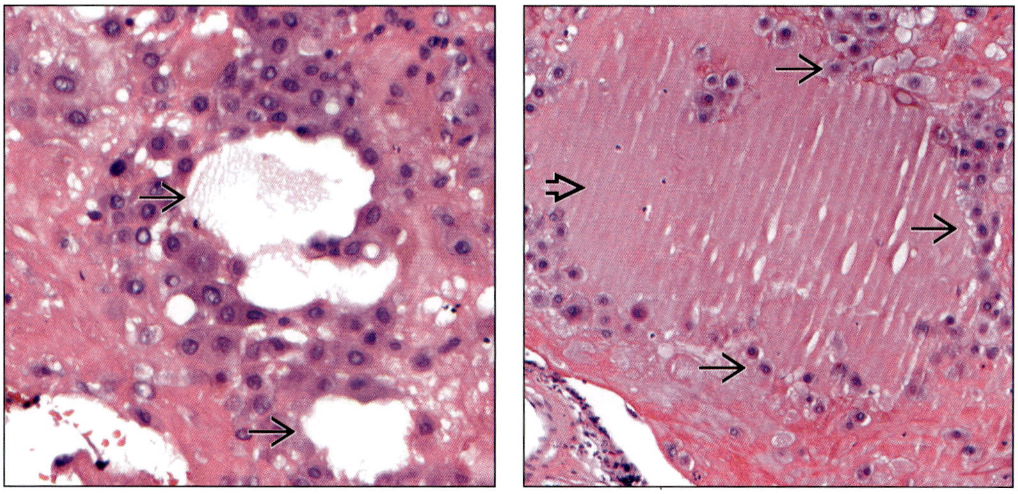

(Left) *In these small trophoblast cysts → in a cell island, the fluid appears less dense than in other locations.* **(Right)** *Larger trophoblast cyst is seen at the tip of a septum, just below the chorionic plate. The eosinophilic matrix product ⇨ appears similar to that of the microcysts of the membranes, but the cyst is less well circumscribed by trophoblast →.*

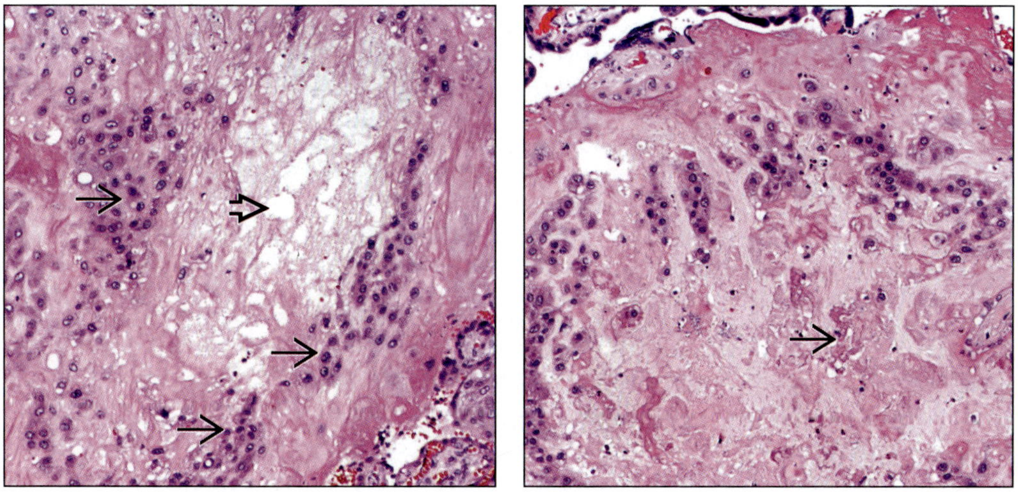

(Left) *Cell island is shown. The loose matrix ⇨ with peripheral trophoblast → resembles a trophoblast microcyst but is not recognized to have the same clinical associations.* **(Right)** *Cell island is shown. Note the dense, matrix-type fibrinoid → in the island core. The trophoblast cells secrete their product usually in a nonpolarized fashion, giving rise to amorphous masses of matrix-type fibrin rather than well-defined cysts.*

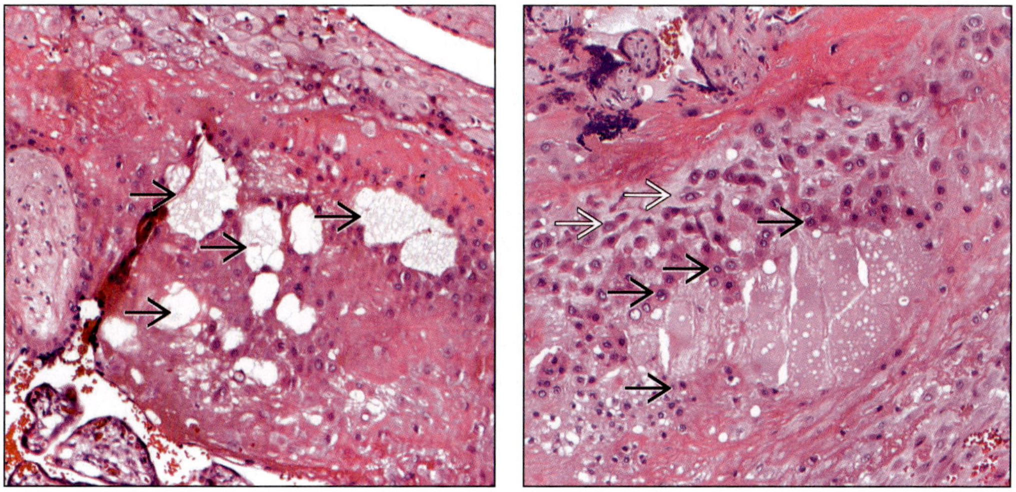

(Left) *Trophoblast cysts → in the basal plate are shown. Abundant matrix-type fibrinoid from these trophoblast cells, together with blood-type fibrin from the maternal circulation, bond together elements of the basal plate and adhere the placenta to the underlying decidua.* **(Right)** *Trophoblast cyst in basal plate is shown. Smaller, epithelioid-appearing trophoblast cells → rim the fluid collection, whereas the trophoblast with larger nuclei ➡ is surrounded by the matrix product.*

LAMINAR DECIDUAL NECROSIS

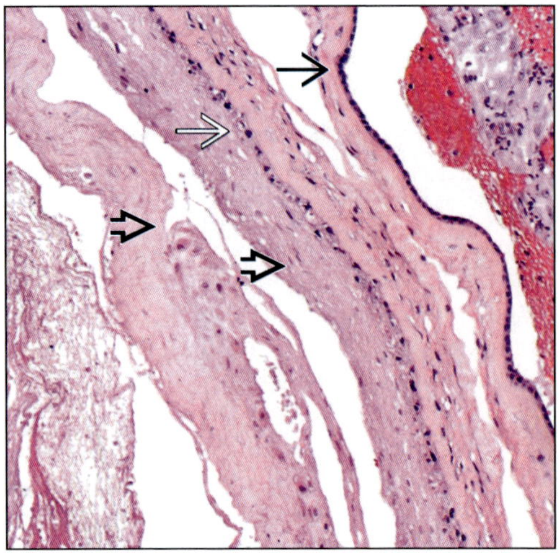

In laminar decidual necrosis (LDN), the amnion → and cellular chorion ➡ are viable with normal nuclear basophilia. The membranous decidua ⇨ shows loss of nuclear basophilia.

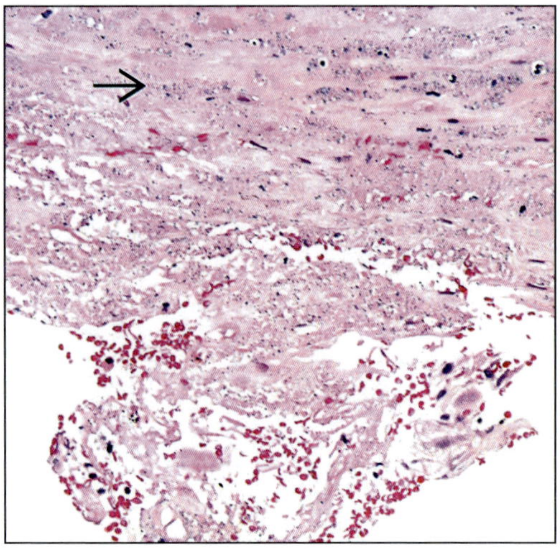

In diffuse decidual leukocytoclastic necrosis (DDLN), decidual stromal cells show loss of nuclear basophilia with karyorrhectic debris →. Neutrophilic karyorrhexis may or may not be discernible.

TERMINOLOGY

Abbreviations

- Laminar decidual necrosis (LDN)
- Diffuse decidual leukocytoclastic necrosis (DDLN)

Synonyms

- Decidual degeneration
- Bland decidual necrosis
- Diffuse decidual leukocytoclastic necrosis

Definitions

- LDN: Coagulative necrosis of membranous decidua
- DDLN: Coagulative necrosis of decidua basalis with residual karyorrhectic nuclear debris

ETIOLOGY/PATHOGENESIS

LDN

- Cause is unclear; hypotheses include
  - Ischemic necrosis in chronic uterine underperfusion
  - Physiologic degeneration of membranous decidua
    - Possibly related to distance from placentally produced hormone
  - Residue of interface between decidua capsularis and decidua parietalis in early gestation
  - Physiologic change of normal term parturition
  - May be more significant preterm
    - May reflect ischemia from maternal malperfusion

DDLN

- Believed to represent an ischemic change
  - Intact or karyorrhectic neutrophils may be present
    - Located on decidual side only
    - Likely reacting to necrotic tissue
    - Not associated with amniotic fluid infection
    - Not associated with spontaneous preterm rupture of membranes

CLINICAL ISSUES

Epidemiology

- Incidence
  - LDN
    - Reported incidence varies greatly
    - 6% of placentas selected for pathologic evaluation in 1 study
    - 18% of unselected placentas (predominantly uncomplicated deliveries at term)
  - DDLN
    - ~ 25% of early preterm births (23-32 weeks gestation)
    - 2% of term placentas

Implications

- **LDN**
  - More common in pregnancies complicated by hypertensive disorders in 1 study
  - Frequent in normal term deliveries in another study
- **DDLN**
  - Association with medically indicated preterm birth (23-32 weeks gestation)
  - Association with recurrent indicated preterm birth
  - Association with preeclampsia and poor fetal growth
  - No association with spontaneous preterm birth and chorioamnionitis
- **Level of evidence is controversial**
  - Newly described entities in literature
  - Data for LDN as isolated finding is less convincing
    - Frequently identified in normal term placentas
    - Unclear if LDN is a normal physiologic process at term
    - May be more significant in preterm placentas
  - Data for DDLN from Alabama Preterm Birth Study suggests stronger association with maternal malperfusion in early preterm births

LAMINAR DECIDUAL NECROSIS

Key Facts

Clinical Issues
- Laminar decidual necrosis
  - More common in pregnancies complicated by hypertensive disorders; suggested association with acute hypoxia
  - Frequent in normal term deliveries in another study
- Diffuse decidual leukocytoclastic necrosis
  - Associated with indicated preterm (23-32 weeks gestation) and recurrent indicated preterm birth
  - Associated with preeclampsia and poor fetal growth
  - Not associated with spontaneous preterm birth and chorioamnionitis

Macroscopic Pathology
- Not usually identified grossly unless extensive or associated with old hemorrhage
- Identified in decidua capsularis of membrane rolls
- Seen in basal plate decidua of full thickness parenchyma sections or basal plate wedge sections

Microscopic Pathology
- Laminar decidual necrosis
  - Loss of nuclear basophilia of decidual stromal cells and vessels in band-like pattern involving at least 10% of membrane roll
- Diffuse decidual leukocytoclastic necrosis
  - Similar to laminar necrosis but with residual karyorrhectic nuclear debris
  - Should involve 30% of represented decidua

Top Differential Diagnoses
- Mimics include excessive matrix-type fibrin in membranes

MACROSCOPIC FEATURES

General Features
- Not usually identified grossly unless extensive or associated with old hemorrhage

Sections to Be Submitted
- Decidua capsularis of membrane rolls
  - 2 submitted
- Basal plate decidua of full thickness parenchyma sections or basal plate wedge sections

MICROSCOPIC PATHOLOGY

LDN
- Loss of nuclear basophilia in decidual stromal cells and vessels in band-like pattern beneath chorion of membranes
  - Quantitative criteria not universally established
  - Suggested: Involvement of at least 10% of membrane
- May accompany recent or remote hemorrhage

DDLN
- Similar to laminar decidual necrosis but with residual karyorrhectic nuclear debris
  - Suggested: Involvement of at least 30% of sampled decidua
- Often with associated microfocal hemorrhages and hemosiderin deposition
- Often present adjacent to infarct or microabruption

DIFFERENTIAL DIAGNOSIS

Excessive Matrix-Type Fibrin in Membranes
- Low power resembles "band of pink" seen in LDN
- Interspersed regressed chorionic villi prove that this is not a decidual lesion
- No ghost decidual stromal cells or nuclear karyorrhexis are seen

DIAGNOSTIC CHECKLIST

Pathologic Interpretation Pearls
- Identification of decidual stromal cells with loss of nuclear basophilia is key to proper recognition of LDN
- Required involvement
  - 10% of membrane decidua for LDN
  - 30% of basal or membranous decidua for DDLN

SELECTED REFERENCES

1. Stanek J: Hypoxic patterns of placental injury: a review. Arch Pathol Lab Med. 137(5):706-20, 2013
2. Bendon RW et al: Reassessing the clinical significance of chorionic membrane microcysts and linear necrosis. Pediatr Dev Pathol. 15(3):213-6, 2012
3. Stanek J: Placental membrane laminar necrosis and chorionic microcysts. Pediatr Dev Pathol. 15(6):514-6, 2012
4. Stanek J: Diagnosing placental membrane hypoxic lesions increases the sensitivity of placental examination. Arch Pathol Lab Med. 134(7):989-95, 2010
5. Stanek J: Acute and chronic placental membrane hypoxic lesions. Virchows Arch. 455(4):315-22, 2009
6. Goldenberg RL et al: The Alabama Preterm Birth Study: diffuse decidual leukocytoclastic necrosis of the decidua basalis, a placental lesion associated with preeclampsia, indicated preterm birth and decreased fetal growth. J Matern Fetal Neonatal Med. 20(5):391-5, 2007
7. Stanek J et al: Laminar necrosis of placental membranes: a histologic sign of uteroplacental hypoxia. Pediatr Dev Pathol. 8(1):34-42, 2005
8. Salafia CM et al: Placental pathologic features of preterm preeclampsia. Am J Obstet Gynecol. 173(4):1097-105, 1995

LAMINAR DECIDUAL NECROSIS

Microscopic Features

*(**Left**) Ghosts of decidual stromal cell nuclei → are barely visible in the membranous decidua of LDN. The overlying chorion and amnion are unaffected. (**Right**) Maternal spiral arterioles → in the membranous decidua undergo a similar bland necrosis.*

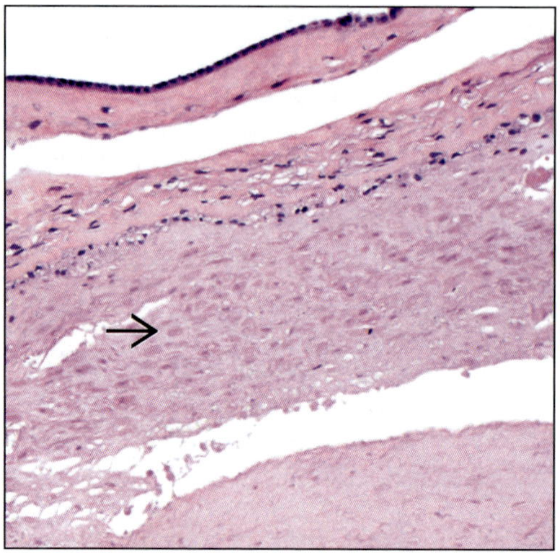

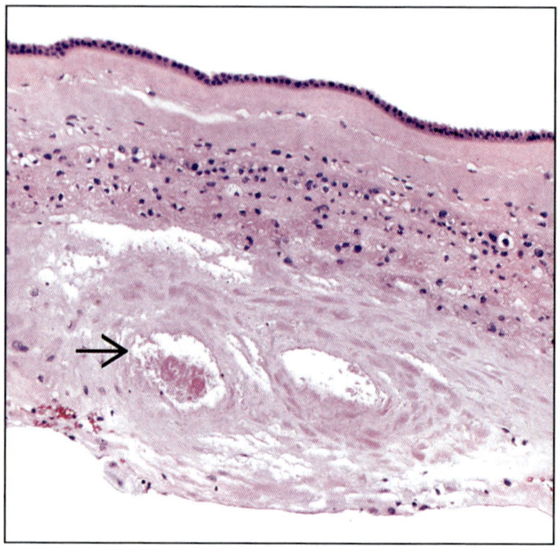

*(**Left**) Viable chorionic trophoblast cells → are distinct from the subjacent necrotic decidua ↪. The histology suggests ischemic necrosis of the decidua, but why it only affects the maternal decidual cells (and not the trophoblast or fetal origin amnion) is unclear. (**Right**) Excessive fibrin → can mimic laminar decidual necrosis. The matrix-type fibrin is a product of chorionic trophoblast. Note that viable decidua ➡ is present, and there are no ghost cells.*

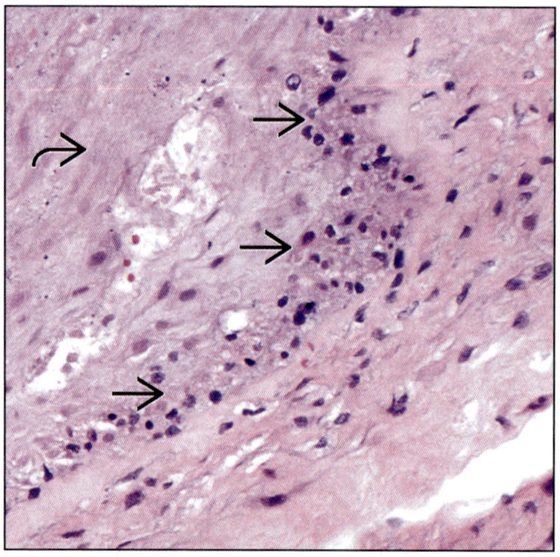

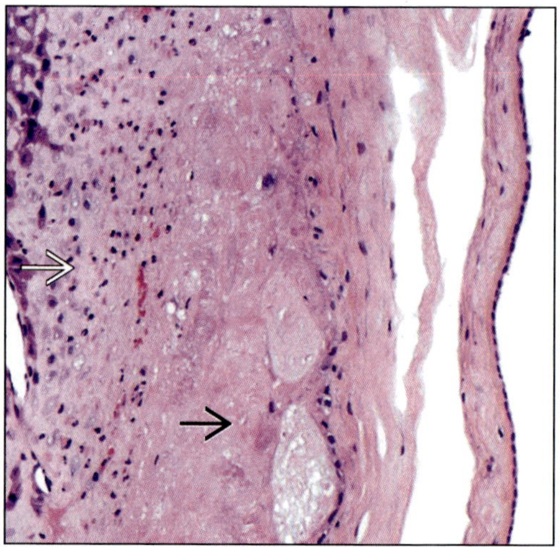

*(**Left**) Excessive matrix-type fibrin and fibrin from previous membranous hemorrhage mimic LDN. Note regressed villi → in the center of the fibrin. True LDN would be deep to this layer. Regressed villi are not present in the membranous decidua layer. (**Right**) Excessive matrix-type fibrin and hemorrhage mimic LDN. Only a small portion of true decidua ↪ is present in this field. Note that regressed villi → of the chorion are present.*

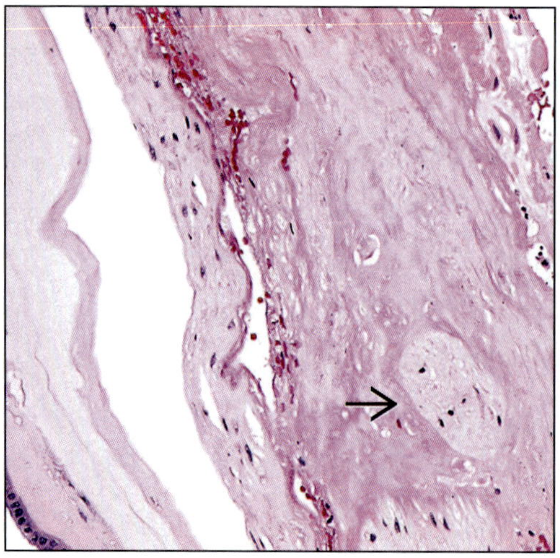

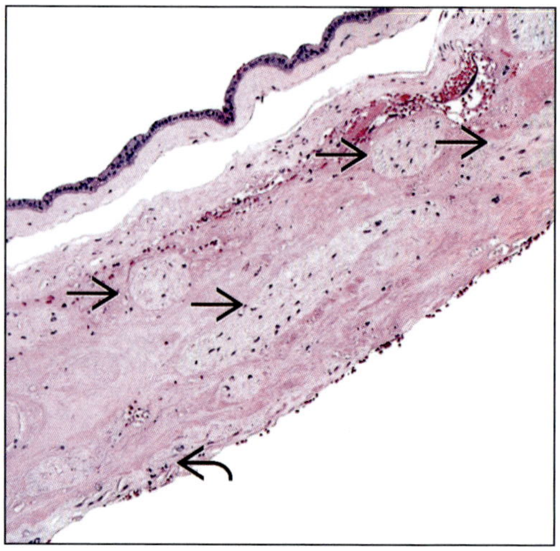

Microscopic Features

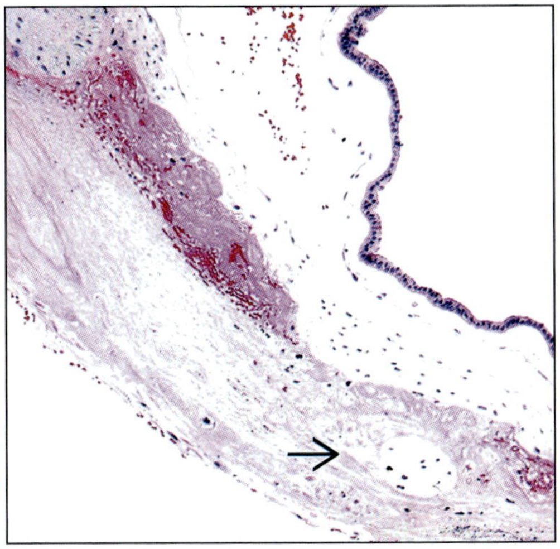

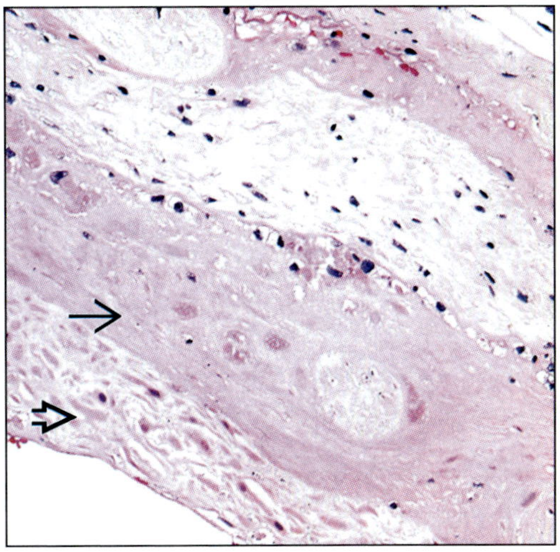

(Left) *Low power suggests laminar decidual necrosis, but higher power examination would be needed to confirm LDN. The presence of regressed villi* ➔ *in the "band of pink" confirms the presence of excessive matrix-type fibrin.* ***(Right)*** *Excessive fibrin* ➔ *is present adjacent to laminar necrosis of the decidua. The fibrin appears more homogeneous, as it is an extracellular product, compared with the individual decidual stromal cells of LDN that have lost nuclear basophilia* ⇨.

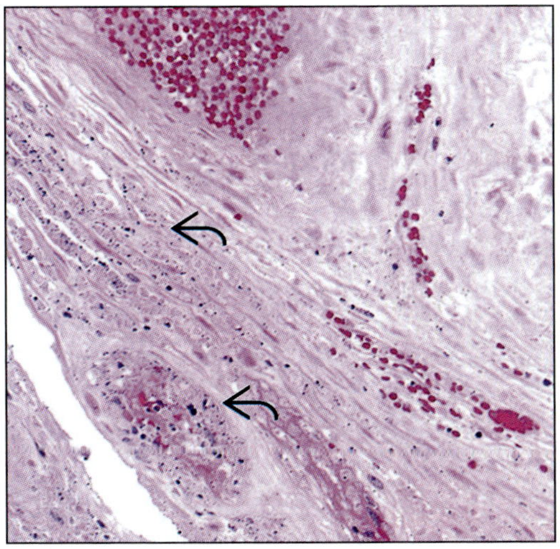

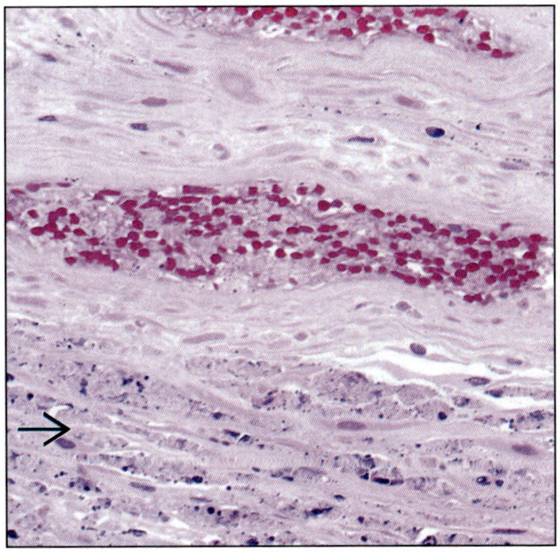

(Left) *Decidual leukocytoclastic necrosis in the decidua basalis is characterized by karyorrhectic nuclear dust* ↶ *along with ghost cells. Karyorrhectic cells often include occasional intact neutrophils, likely reacting to necrotic tissue.* ***(Right)*** *The density of nuclear debris* ➔ *suggests that a leukocytic infiltrate is present. DDLN may coexist with chorioamnionitis. Amniotropic inflammation should be sought elsewhere to diagnose amniotic fluid infection.*

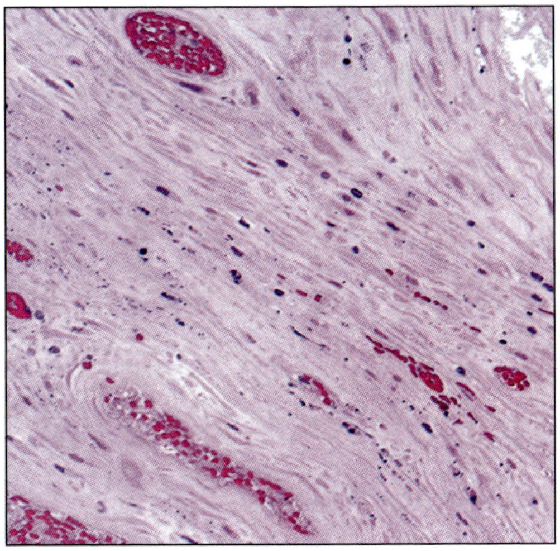

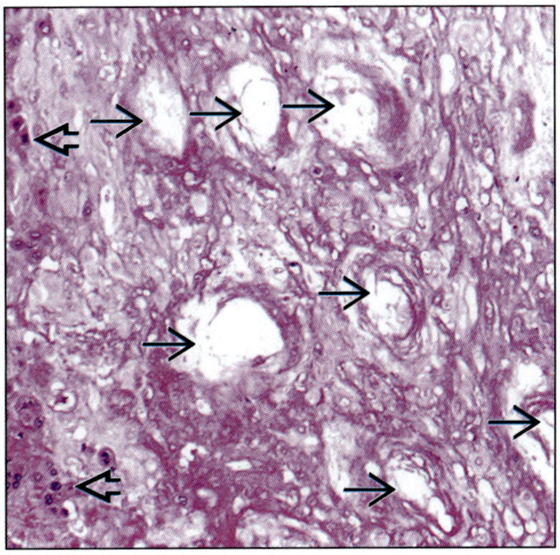

(Left) *In DDLN, microbial studies are usually negative. Other findings suggest that this may be a marker of poor placental perfusion.* ***(Right)*** *Outlines of a maternal spiral artery* ➔ *are seen in this remote infarct of the decidua basalis. Viable trophoblast cells* ⇨ *are present. This finding is more remote than leukocytoclastic decidual necrosis or laminar necrosis and is not pathologic when present at the periphery of the placenta.*

Gross and Microscopic Features

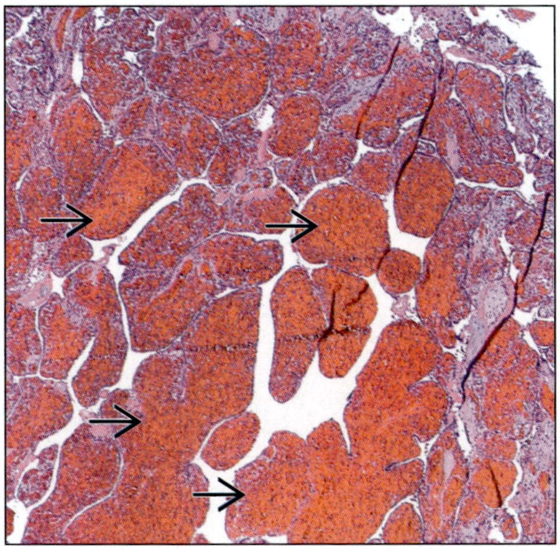
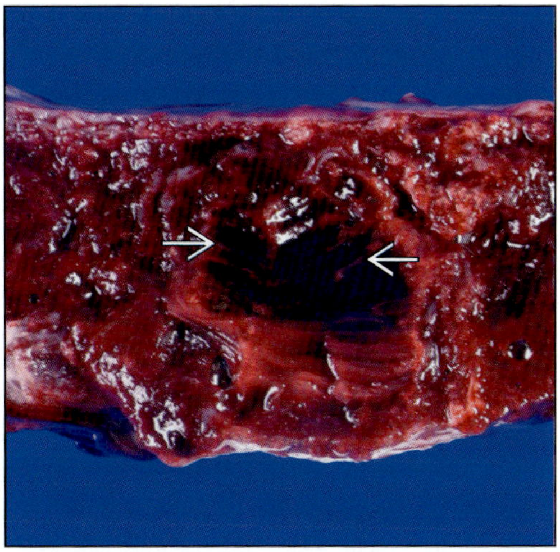

(Left) *Retroplacental hemorrhage (acute abruption) and trauma may cause acute FMH due to massive bruising of the chorionic villi. Extensive intravillous hemorrhage* → *yields fragile sacs of fetal blood ready to burst.* ***(Right)*** *Intervillous thrombi commonly have angular contours. Lines of Zahn* ➔ *identify this as a true thrombus vs. an unclotted collection of maternal blood (i.e., flow void).*

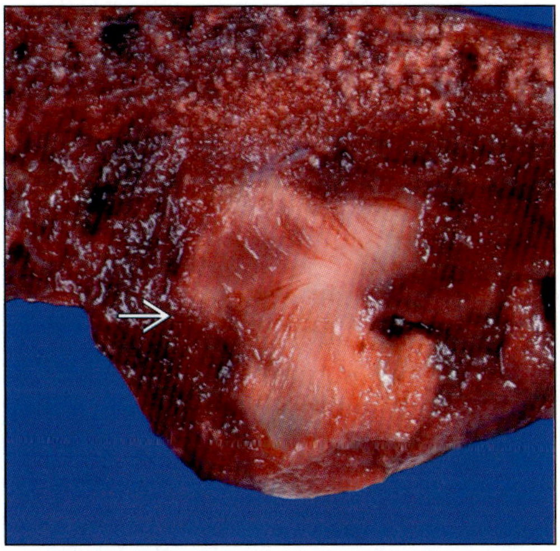
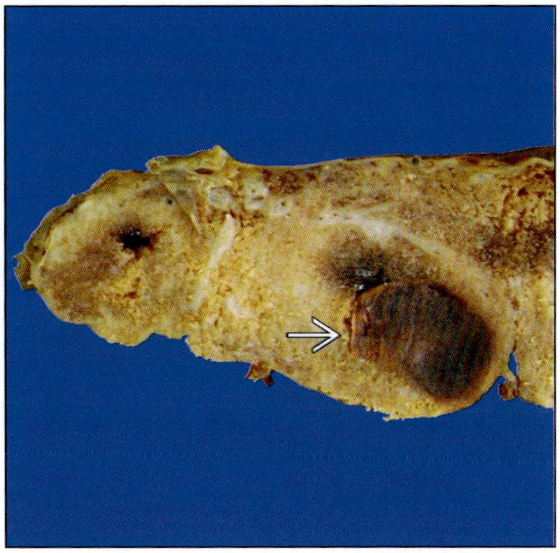

(Left) *This older intervillous thrombus* ➔ *has more fibrin deposition. Intact fetal NRBCs are not likely to be found in older lesions. Immunohistochemistry for fetal HbF may be useful to confirm FMH if the lesion is large or multiple lesions are found.* ***(Right)*** *This recent intervillous thrombus* ➔ *appears dark against the pallor of adjacent parenchyma, suggesting fetal anemia. The differential diagnosis in this location includes microabruption.*

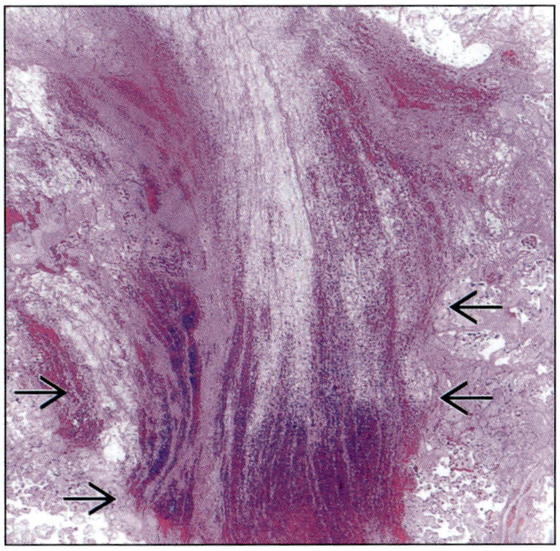
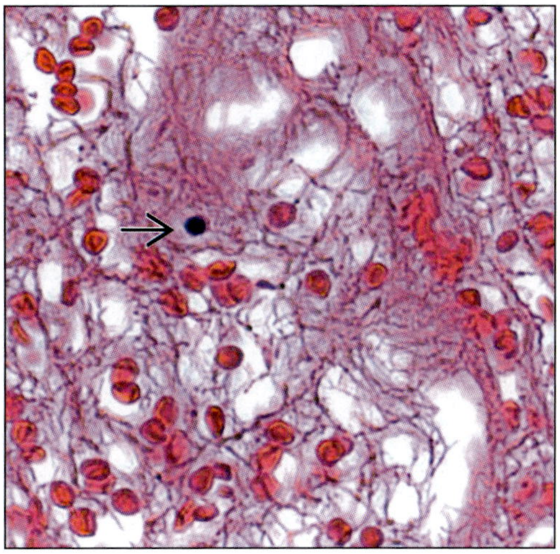

(Left) *The laminated thrombus of an intervillous thrombus laterally displaces chorionic villi* →*. Intervillous thrombi are often due to FMH, but may also represent maternal blood clotting in regions of sluggish flow, or extension of retroplacental hematomas.* ***(Right)*** *A careful search for nucleated RBCs* → *is key to identifying the fetal blood component in an intervillous hematoma. Immunohistochemical stains for fetal hemoglobin are also useful when available.*

FETAL-MATERNAL HEMORRHAGE

Gross and Microscopic Features

*(**Left**) Massive subchorionic thrombohematoma are historically termed Breus mole. The differential for these gross lesions includes hemorrhage into a massive chorionic cyst. Either way, they may represent significant fetal hemorrhage if the lesion is found to contain fetal blood. (**Right**) In contrast to intervillous thrombi, retroplacental hematomas are associated with maternal hemorrhage at the disc margin and from behind the placenta.*

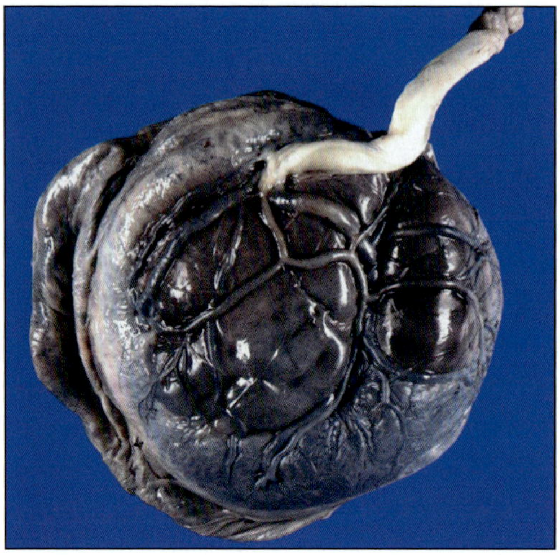

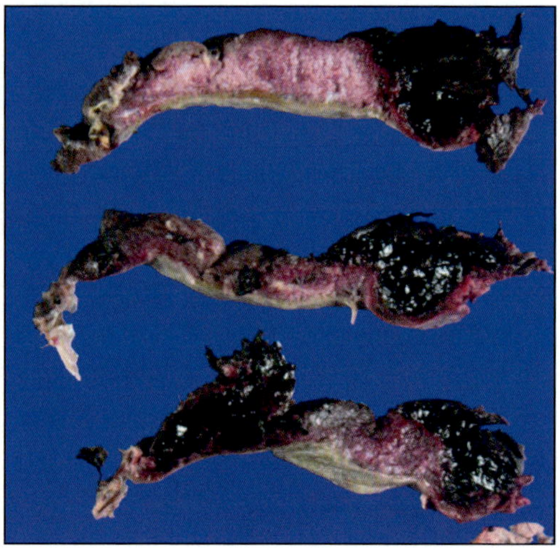

*(**Left**) Microabruption (a.k.a. rounded intraplacental hematoma) pushes up into the placental parenchyma from the underlying decidua basalis. This lesion is composed of maternal blood. The overlying parenchyma is compressed, and continuity with the decidua basalis is present. (**Right**) An immunohistochemical stain for fetal hemoglobin identifies NRBCs → and erythrocytes ⇨ in this focus of fetal hemorrhage into the intervillous space.*

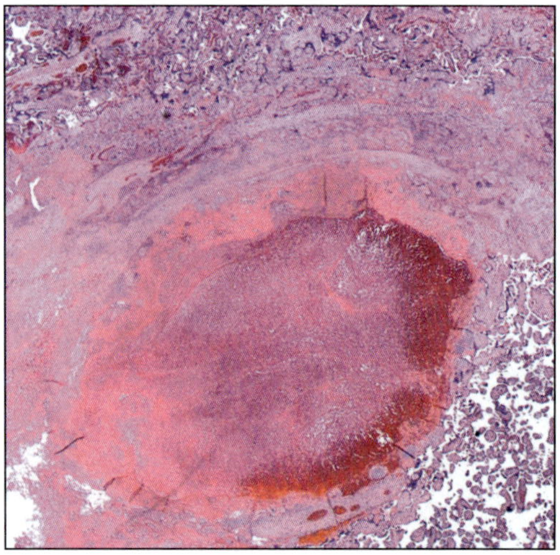

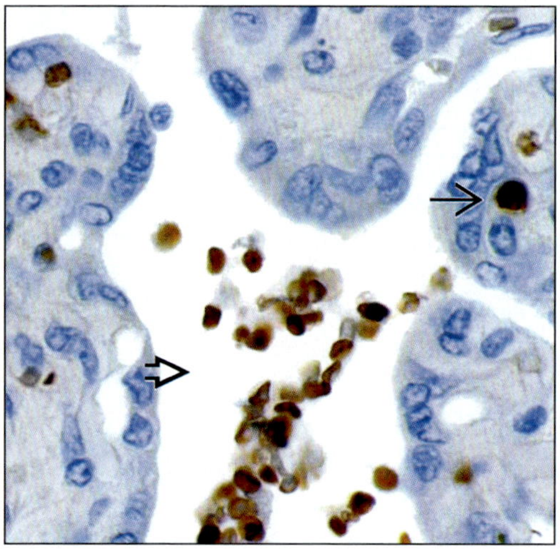

*(**Left**) Fetal nucleated RBCs → are recognized by round, densely dark nuclei against a cytoplasm similar to surrounding erythrocytes. More primitive erythroblasts ⇨ have less dense chromatin and more purple-colored cytoplasm. Lymphocytes ➡ have a higher N:C ratio and less pink cytoplasm. (**Right**) Erythroblastosis in a case of severe fetal anemia due to FMH is shown. Rare NRBCs have irregular nuclei with buds →, a sign of stressed hematopoiesis.*

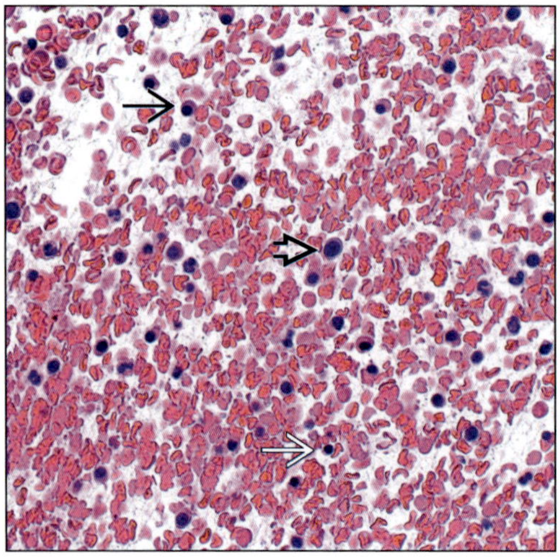

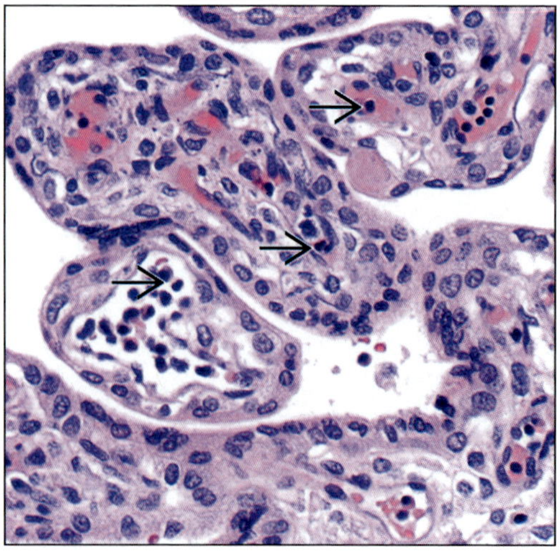

Gross and Microscopic Features

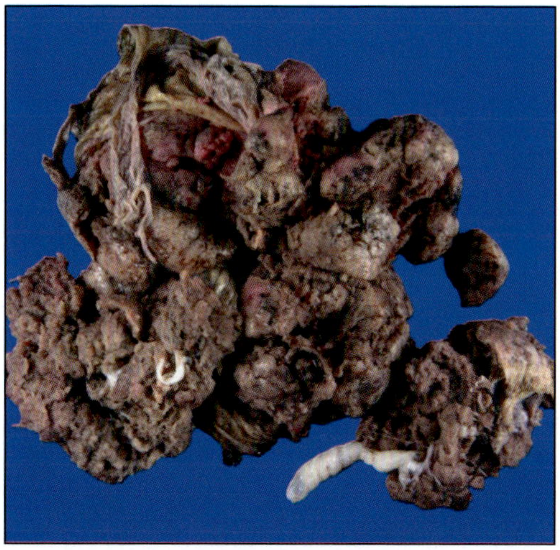
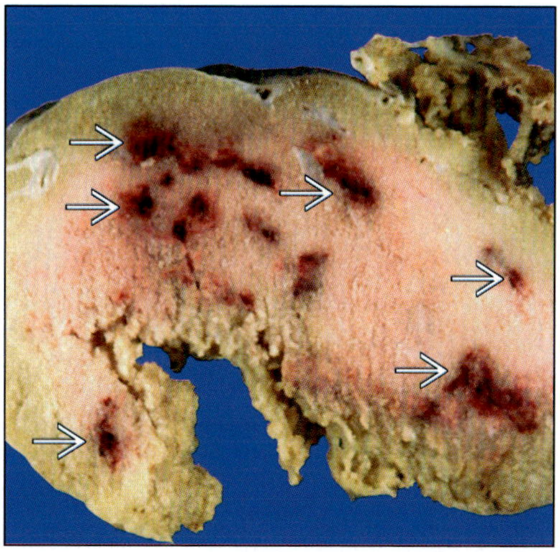

(Left) *This case of chronic fetal-maternal hemorrhage resulted in a bulky and friable placenta due to severe edema.* ***(Right)*** *Note the marked pallor of the parenchyma on cut section from the placenta on the left. Blood appears confined to the Kline hemorrhages ➡. Note also the absence of lamination in the lesions. Poor clotting of FMH lesions is part of the pathogenesis of chronic FMH. Shared maternal and fetal ABO blood types may be associated with worsened FMH.*

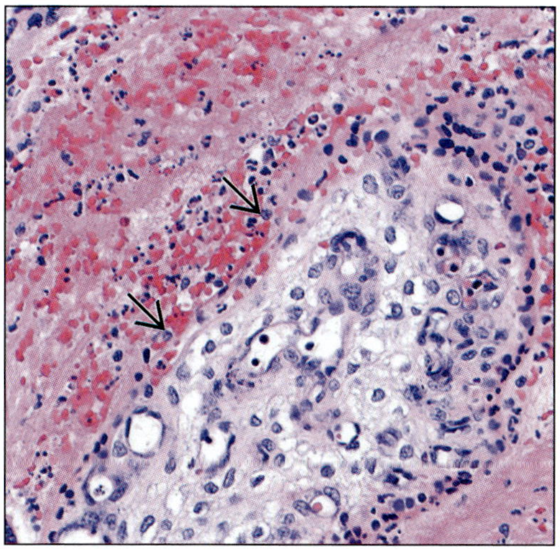
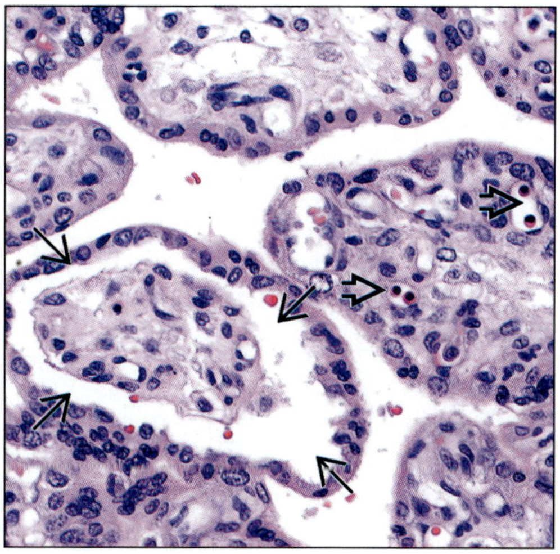

(Left) *Injury to the vasculosyncytial membrane ➡ precipitates FMH.* ***(Right)*** *Chronic FMH shows villous edema ➡ and increased fetal NRBCs ➡ microscopically. The syncytiotrophoblast layer has separated from the parenchyma due to edema. The villous edema likely exacerbates the condition, causing more injury to the villi and more opportunities for FMH.*

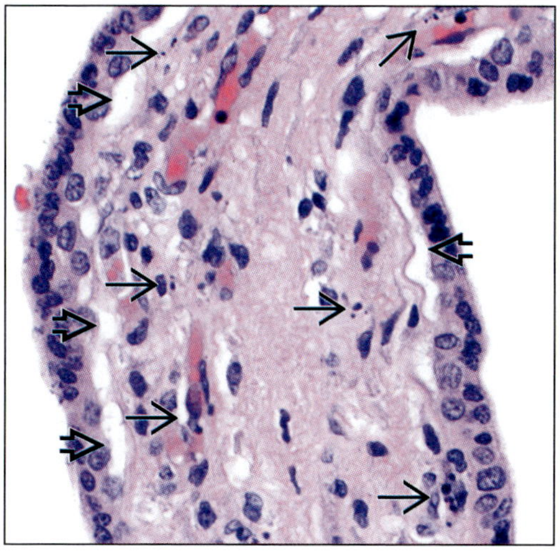
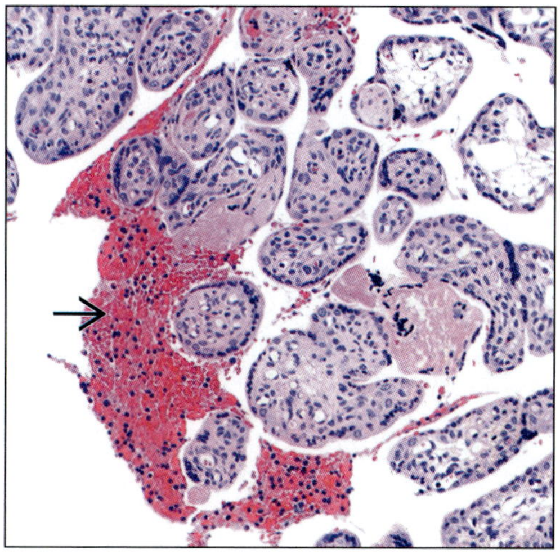

(Left) *Villous edema and stromal vascular karyorrhexis may be seen in chronic FMH. Separation ➡ of the syncytiotrophoblast layer from the villous stroma indicates edema. Fetal vessels are undergoing early involutional changes with karyorrhexis of endothelium and stromal cells ➡, likely from ischemia/hypoxia associated with the severe fetal anemia.* ***(Right)*** *Abundant fetal blood ➡ is seen outside the villi in chronic FMH, proven by the presence of numerous NRBC.*

Intrauterine Growth Restriction

PLACENTAL CAUSES OF POOR FETAL GROWTH

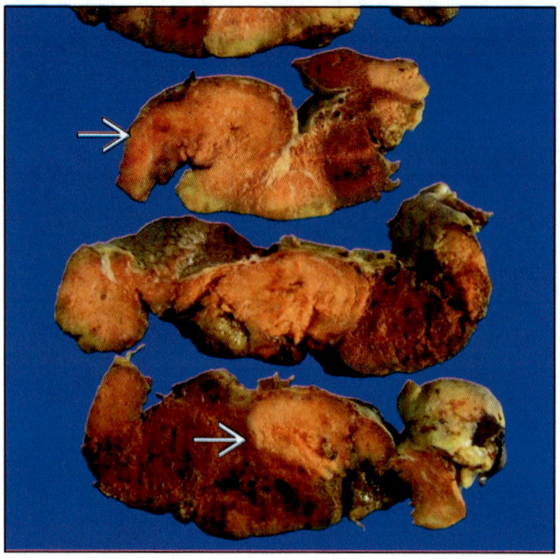

Placental causes of fetal growth restriction affect large areas of the parenchyma. These areas of villous pallor ➔ occupy > 50% of the parenchyma. Histologically, they were avascular villi of fetal thrombotic vasculopathy.

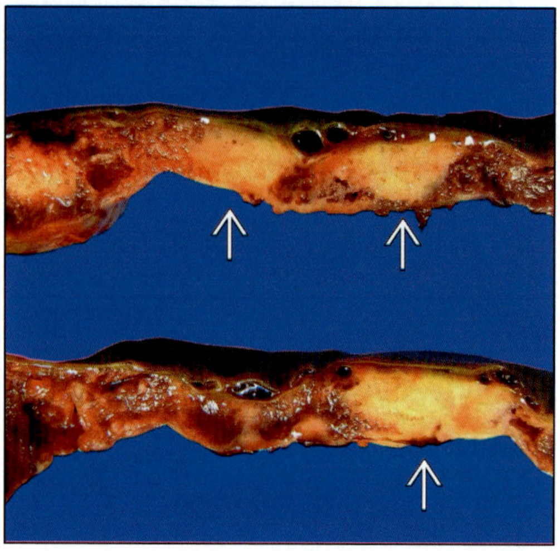

This placenta had multiple remote infarcts ➔ in association with maternal preeclampsia. The infarcts and other changes of maternal malperfusion led to placental insufficiency and asymmetric fetal growth restriction.

TERMINOLOGY

Abbreviations

- Fetal growth restriction (FGR)
- Intrauterine growth restriction (IUGR)

Definitions

- FGR = IUGR
  - Moderate: Weight < 10th percentile for gestational age (GA), a.k.a. small for gestational age (SGA)
  - Severe: Weight < 3rd percentile for GA
- Placental insufficiency: Critical reduction of placental exchange capacity
  - Although often used in conjunction with placental malperfusion, it is not specific for any particular placental disease

EPIDEMIOLOGY

Incidence

- Term infants with SGA: 10% in developed countries, up to 23% in developing countries
- Preterm infants with SGA: 9-22% of preterm births

Gender

- Female infants tend to weigh less than male infants; separate growth curves used

ETIOLOGY/PATHOGENESIS

General Overview

- Adequate fetal growth depends on adequate supply of oxygen and nutrients to fetus
- FGR is associated with
  - Maternal factors: Maternal medical disease, infection, hypoxemia, toxic exposure, medications
  - Fetal factors: Karyotypic abnormalities, genetic syndromes
  - Placental factors: Placental function is significantly compromised, may be secondary to maternal or fetal factors
    - Compromise of any placental component that affects maternal-fetal exchange over significant length of time can lead to poor fetal growth
    - FGR is more likely associated with lesions that are chronic, multiple, or single yet affect significant amount of parenchyma
  - Chronic placental pathologies include
    - Uteroplacental malperfusion
    - Fetal thrombotic vasculopathy, e.g., due to umbilical cord abnormalities
    - Extensive chronic villitis with fetal vasculopathy/ massive chronic intervillositis
    - Massive perivillous fibrin deposition
    - Chronic abruption

CLINICAL IMPLICATIONS

Imaging Findings

- Low estimated fetal weight
- Small abdominal circumference for age, abnormal head:abdominal circumference ratio (HC:AC), abnormal femur length:abdominal circumference ratio (FL:AC)
- Low amniotic fluid index/oligohydramnios
- Abnormal umbilical artery Doppler studies

Complications

- Term infants
  - Perinatal asphyxia, meconium aspiration, persistent pulmonary hypertension
- Preterm infants
  - Neonatal death, necrotizing enterocolitis, respiratory distress syndrome, bronchopulmonary dysplasia, pulmonary hemorrhage, pulmonary hypertension, postnatal growth failure, neurodevelopmental impairment

Embryonic Development

Crown-Rump Length (mm)	Days After Ovulation	Stage	Main External Feature	Placenta
	0-2	1	Fertilized egg	
	2-4	2	Morula	
	4-6	3	Blastocyst	
0.1		4	Bilaminar embryo	
0.2-0.4	6-15	5	Bilaminar embryo with yolk sac	
		6	Trilaminar embryo with primitive streak	Mesenchyme from primitive streak migrates to inner surface of trophoblast, early primary villous formation begins
0.4-1.0	15-17	7	Trilaminar embryo with notochordal process	
1.0-1.5	18-20	8	Primitive pit and notochordal canal formed	
1.5-2.0	20-22	9	Deep neural groove; 1st somites present; heart tubes begin to fuse	
2-3	22-24	10	Neural folds begin to fuse; heart begins to beat; embryo is straight; 4-12 pairs of somites	Yolk sac hematopoiesis established
3-4	24-26	11	Rostral neuropore closing; embryo slightly curved; 13-20 pairs of somites	
4-5	26-30	12	Upper limb buds appear; caudal neuropore closed; tail appearing	
5-6	28-32 (~ 6 weeks post LMP)	13	4 pairs of branchial arches; lower limb buds appear; tail present; 30 somites	Yolk sac-derived erythroblasts (large nucleated RBCs) arrive in placental vessels
6-7	31-35	14	Lens pits and nasal pits visible; optic cups present	
7-10	35-38	15	Hand plates formed; lens vesicles and nasal pits prominent	Erythropoiesis begins in liver
10-12	37-42	16	Foot plates formed; nasal pits face ventrally; pigment visible in retina	
12-14	42-44 (~ 8 weeks post LMP)	17	Finger rays appear; auricular hillocks developed; upper lip formed	Nonnucleated RBCs (liver origin) appear in placental fetal vessels
14-17	44-48	18	Toe rays and elbow region appear; eyelids are forming; ambiguous genital tubercle seen	Nonnucleated RBCs comprise 10% of placental fetal vessel RBCs at 9 weeks post LMP
16-20	48-51	19	Trunk elongating and straightening; midgut herniation into umbilical cord	Progressive replacement of yolk sac-derived erythroblasts (nucleated) with nonnucleated RBCs
20-22	51-53	20	Fingers distinct but webbed; scalp vascular plexus appears	
22-24	53-54	21	Fingers free and longer; toes still webbed	
24-28	54-56	22	Toes free and longer; eyelids and external ear more developed	
28-30	56-60 (~ 10-11 weeks post LMP)	23	Head more rounded; fusing eyelids	By 12 weeks post LMP, only 5% nucleated erythroblasts persist

LMP = last menstrual period; RBC = red blood cell. From Kalousek DK: Clinical significance of morphologic and genetic examination of spontaneously aborted embryos. Am J Reprod Immunol. 39(2):108-19, 1998; Szulman AE: Examination of the early conceptus. Arch Pathol Lab Med. 115(7):696-700, 1991.

1ST-TRIMESTER PREGNANCY LOSS

Gross Features

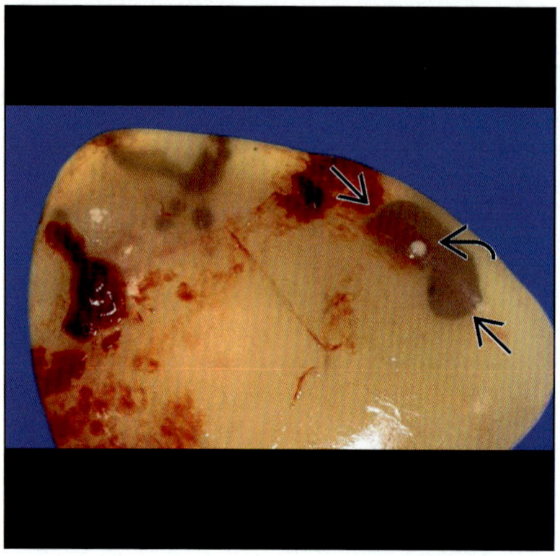
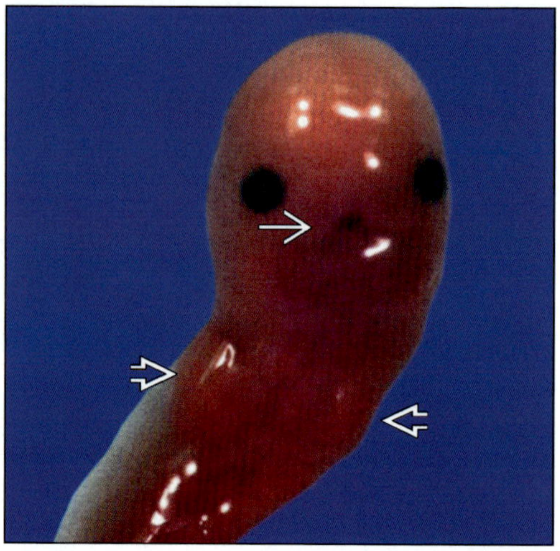

(Left) *This large gestational sac has a very small malformed embryo, which was found to have trisomy 13. The white structure overlying the fetus is the involuted yolk sac. (Courtesy B. Shehata, MD.)* ***(Right)*** *The embryo from the large gestational sac shows midline clefting and delayed limb development. Cytogenetics revealed trisomy 13. (Courtesy B. Shehata, MD.)*

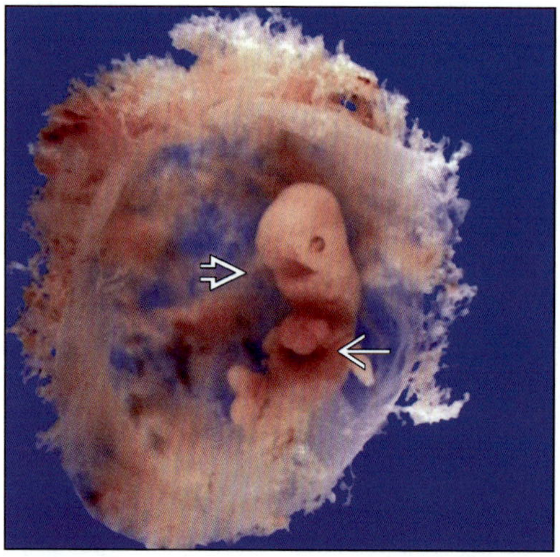
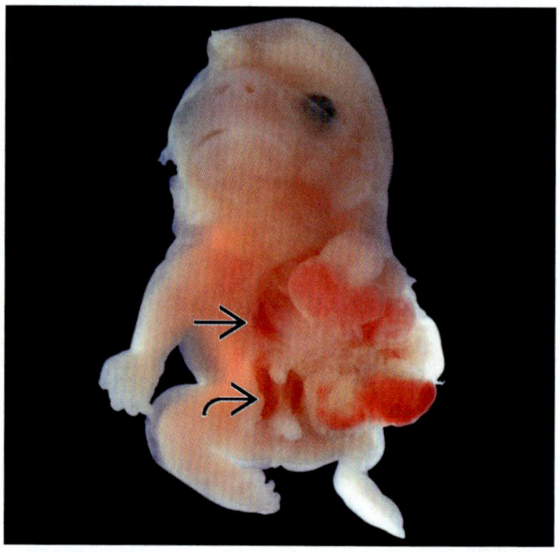

(Left) *This gestational sac from a 1st-trimester spontaneous abortion shows fetus with ectopia cordis. There is also a midline facial cleft.* ***(Right)*** *This embryo has a severe abdominal wall defect, allowing the entire abdominal contents to extrude into the amniotic sac, and also extrophy of the bladder. Asymmetry of the lower extremities indicates that this is likely a limb/body wall malformation.*

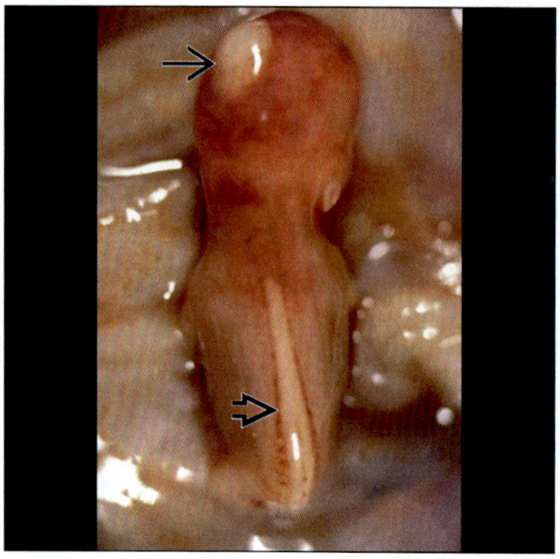
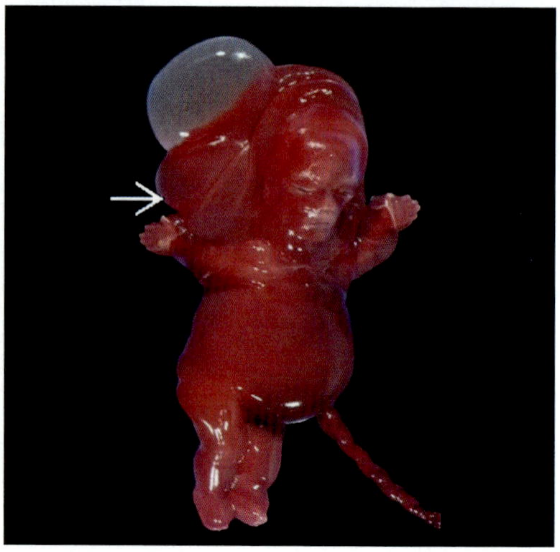

(Left) *An embryo (days 44-46) with an open neural tube defect and encephalocele is shown. The neural tube is completely closed at day 28 (Courtesy B. Shehata, MD.)* ***(Right)*** *This 11-week-gestation fetus has Turner syndrome (monosomy X). There is a large cystic hygroma of the neck and massive hydrops. (Courtesy B. Shehata, MD.)*

Microscopic Findings

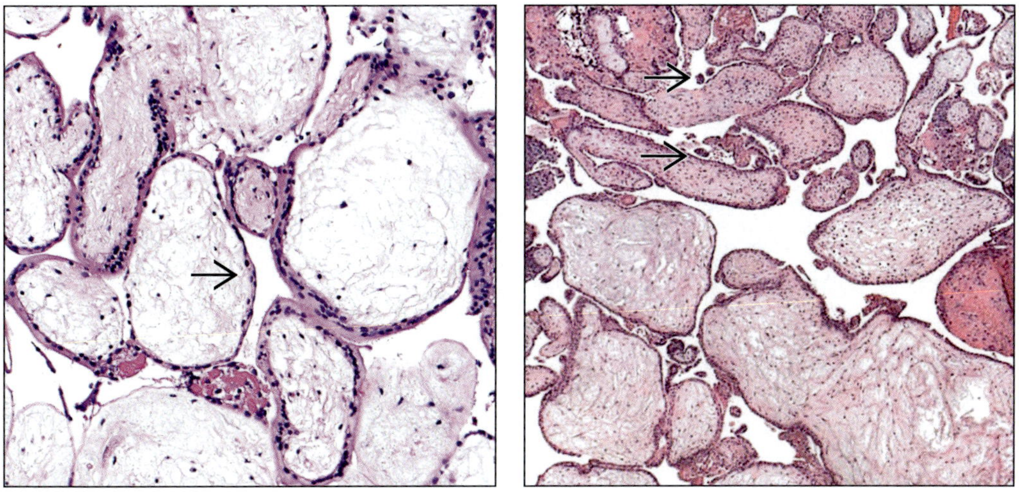

(Left) *Hydropic degeneration is a common finding with blighted ovum. The villi are nearly avascular with amphophilic stroma. The syncytiotrophoblast layer is thin and atrophic* →*, which accounts for the low hCG.* ***(Right)*** *The mixture of hydropic and fibrous-appearing villi is usually found later in 1st-trimester embryonic demise. Chromosomal abnormalities may have dysmorphic villi with marked variation in size and shape. Occasional syncytial knots* → *may be seen.*

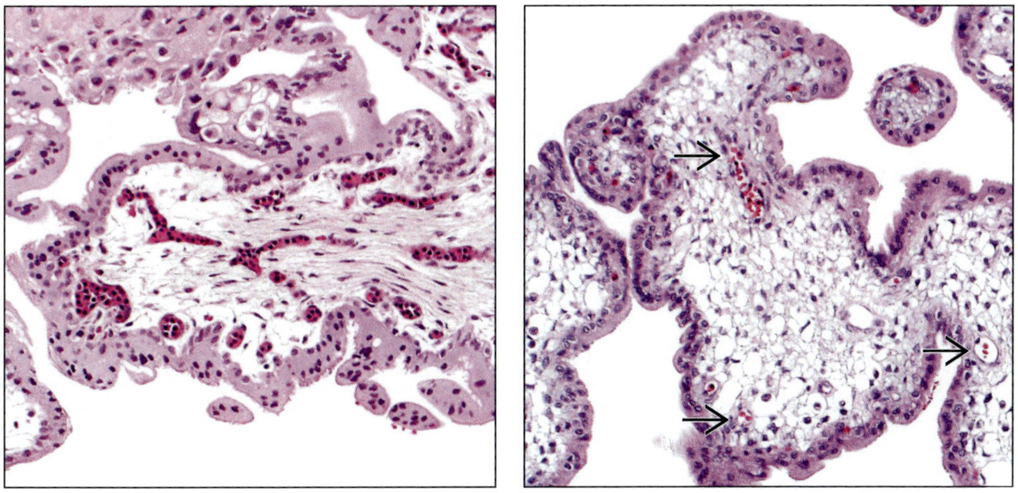

(Left) *The percentage of nucleated RBCs in the villous capillaries help date the embryonic age at demise. At 7 weeks (seen here), all of the erythrocytes are yolk sac-derived, enlarged nucleated forms. The villous RBCs persist even after capillaries degenerate.* ***(Right)*** *These villi from 11 weeks gestation (post LMP) show more admixed nonnucleated RBCs* →*. By this age, hepatic hematopoiesis replaces the nucleated, yolk sac-derived erythroblasts with erythrocytes.*

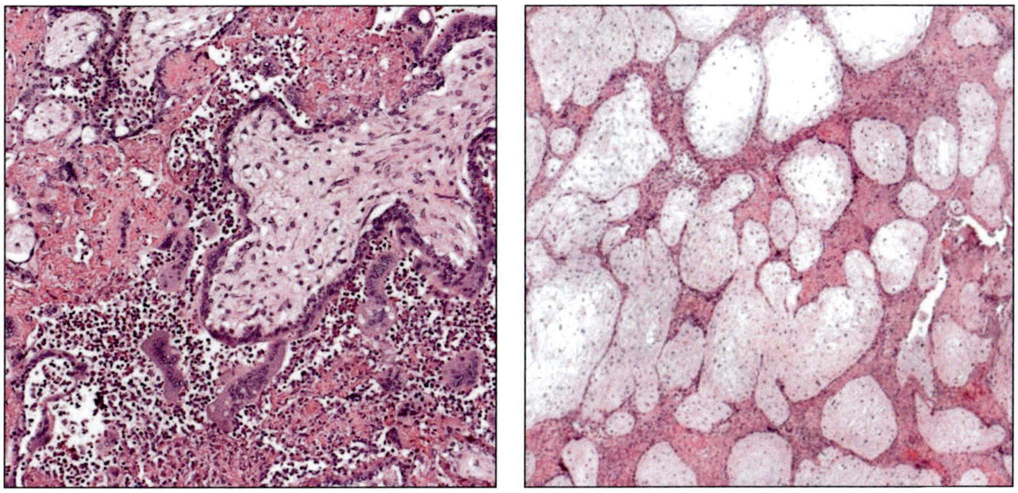

(Left) *This image shows chronic histiocytic intervillositis of unknown etiology in a 1st-trimester spontaneous abortion specimen. CD68 immunostaining confirms the presence of numerous intervillous histiocytes. This disorder is very likely to recur in future pregnancies.* ***(Right)*** *Massively increased perivillous fibrin is associated with recurrent pregnancy loss, especially in cases where extravillous cytotrophoblast are embedded in the fibrin.*

2ND-TRIMESTER FETAL DEMISE

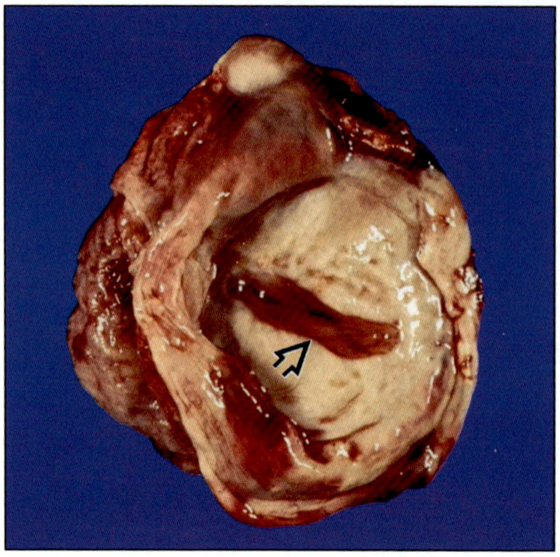

Late 2nd-trimester placenta shows purulent amniotic surface & membranes characteristic of subacute necrotizing chorioamnionitis. Umbilical cord is edematous & congested ➢. (Courtesy B. Shehata, MD.)

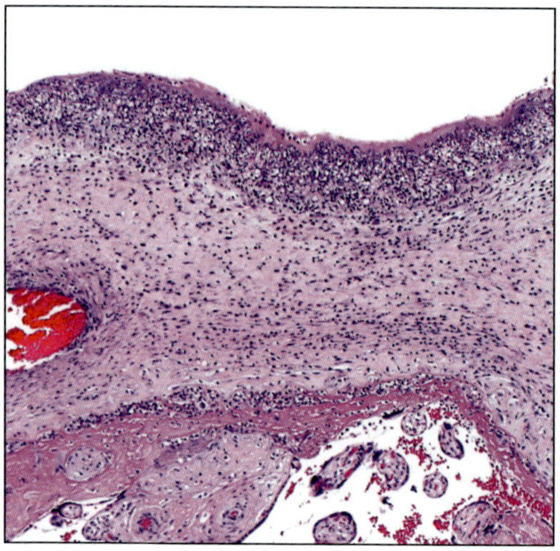

Subacute necrotizing chorioamnionitis, as seen in this case, is almost always seen in the 2nd trimester. Infection is usually present for up to 2 weeks. It may be associated with premature birth or fetal demise.

CONTENT

Scope of Discussion

- Placental and fetal findings of 2nd-trimester (gestation week 13 and 6 days through 27 weeks and 6 days) fetal demise
- Findings after termination of pregnancy for fetal anomalies

TERMINOLOGY

Definitions

- Stillbirth: Refers to in utero demise of potentially viable fetus (generally after 20 weeks gestation)
- Miscarriage: Lay term, usually refers to in utero demise of previable fetus (generally before 20 weeks gestation)

EPIDEMIOLOGY

Incidence

- Intrauterine fetal demise (IUFD) is relatively uncommon in 2nd trimester
  - 1-5% of pregnancies are lost at 13-19 weeks gestation
  - 0.3% of pregnancies are lost at 20-27 weeks gestation

ETIOLOGY/PATHOGENESIS

Fetal Chromosomal Abnormalities

- Comprise 24% of 2nd-trimester fetal deaths

Infection

- Ascending infection, chorioamnionitis (amniotic fluid infection sequence) comprises 40-60% of 2nd-trimester fetal death causes
  - Organisms, group B *Streptococcus*, *Neisseria gonorrhoeae*, *Gardnerella* spp., *Mycoplasma*/*Ureaplasma*, *Fusobacterium* spp.
- Hematogenous infection
  - TORCH infections: *Toxoplasma gondii*, other (syphilis, varicella-zoster virus, parvovirus B19), rubella, cytomegalovirus (CMV), herpes simplex virus (HSV)

Placental Insufficiency

- Placental function is unable to support further life of fetus due to loss of functional parenchyma
  - Uteroplacental malperfusion evidenced by small placenta, infarcts, distal villous hypoplasia, and maternal decidual vasculopathy
    - Usually occurs after 23 weeks gestation and is almost always associated with severe preeclampsia
  - Massively increased perivillous fibrin deposition
  - Extensive chronic inflammation
    - Chronic villitis in 2nd trimester is uncommon and more likely to be infectious
    - Chronic histiocytic intervillositis
  - Acute or chronic placental abruption

Impaired Fetal-Placental Perfusion

- Umbilical cord abnormalities
  - Nuchal or body entanglement, knots, amniotic bands, or excessively long and hypercoiled cord
- Fetal thrombotic vasculopathy (often in association with cord lesions above)
  - Differentiate from changes of fetal vascular involution after fetal demise

Fetal-Maternal Hemorrhage

- Fetal hydrops, edematous villi lacking fetal erythrocytes, nucleated red blood cells (NRBCs) in intervillous space ± intervillous thrombi

Maternal Conditions

- Cervical incompetence

- Uncontrolled chronic illness (e.g., diabetes, hypertension, autoimmune disease)
- Trauma (e.g., motor vehicle accident, physical abuse)
- Teratogen exposure and smoking/drug use
- Thrombophilia
- Müllerian duct and uterine anomalies, uterine septa or bicornuate uterus

Amniotic Band Syndrome

- Rupture of amniotic sac, usually before fusion with chorion in 1st trimester
  - Amniotic sheets may attach to skin of skull or face, resulting in malformations
  - Limb/body wall complex refers to contiguity of amnion with some portion of body wall, typically abdomen (early defect in morphogenesis)
  - Bands may constrict extremities &/or cord in otherwise normally developed fetus

CLINICAL IMPLICATIONS

Clinical Presentation

- Loss of fetal movement
- Vaginal bleeding
- Abdominal cramping
- Absence of fetal heartbeat

Imaging Findings

- Ultrasound may identify ≥ 1 fetal anomaly
- Placental and umbilical cord lesions are less commonly identified

Procedures

- Dilation and evacuation (D&E): Fetus and placenta are fragmented on receipt in surgical pathology
- Induction of labor: Less commonly performed; intact fetus is delivered

MACROSCOPIC FINDINGS

General Features

- Majority of 2nd-trimester intrauterine fetal demise or termination of pregnancy specimens are fragmented after D&E
  - D&E specimen: Surgical pathology specimen requiring pathologic examination
    - Autopsy may be requested
  - Use of standardized template improves ability to find causes of intrauterine fetal demise
  - Surgical pathology exam should confirm that all major fetal skeletal parts are present
    - Retention of fetal part in uterus is uncommon but may have associated maternal morbidity
  - Placenta and cord examination should be performed as thoroughly as possible
    - Especially useful in cases of unexplained intrauterine fetal demise
  - Anomalies identified on ultrasound are variably confirmed on pathologic examination
    - Central nervous system (CNS) malformations almost never confirmed due to disruption of brain tissues
    - Genitourinary anomalies frequently confirmed as intact kidneys and bladder are readily identified
    - Cardiac malformations are variably confirmed, expertise in dissection along lines of flow is useful: Intracardiac potassium chloride injection with fetal termination yields macerated heart tissue; difficult to assess
    - Abnormalities of extremities (e.g., polydactyly, heterodactyly) usually confirmed
    - Neural tube defects variably confirmed; sac is usually disrupted but bony defects are present
- Most institutions require consent for examination of intact fetus > 20 weeks gestation, some require consent for dissection of intact fetus at any gestational age
- Sections to be submitted
  - Sections of umbilical cord, membranes, chorionic plate, and placental parenchyma should be submitted as for intact placenta
  - Fetal lung and cross sections of fetal stomach aid in confirming amniotic fluid infection sequence as cause of fetal demise
  - Fetal heart, liver, and kidney are useful for dating in utero demise to delivery interval and confirming pathology such as renal cystic disease
- Ancillary studies
  - Skin or placental samples for cytogenetics (if not obtained in operating room)
  - In cases of fetal growth restriction with no identifiable cause, consider genomic evaluation of placenta for confined placental mosaicism
    - 4 samples from different regions of placenta sampled for karyotype (fresh tissue), array of comparative genomic hybridization (CGH), or single nucleotide polymorphism (SNP) array (fresh, formalin-fixed, or formalin-fixed, paraffin-embedded tissue)
  - Microbiology cultures may be performed on placental and fetal tissues if clinically desired
  - Specimen radiographs may be useful in suspected skeletal dysplasia

MICROSCOPIC FINDINGS

Placenta, Cord, and Membranes

- Look for evidence of amniotic fluid infection; special stains for organisms may be considered
- Look for fetal thrombi and changes of fetal thrombotic vasculopathy; correlate with gross umbilical cord findings
- Look for villous parenchymal processes, e.g., chronic villitis, chronic histiocytic intervillositis, massive previllous fibrin deposition
- Look for changes of uteroplacental malperfusion, e.g., distal villous hypoplasia, villous agglutination, infarcts
- Look for evidence of hematogenous infection

2ND-TRIMESTER FETAL DEMISE

Findings Compatible With Specific Chromosomal Abnormalities on D&E Examination

Chromosomal Abnormality	Gross Finding
Monosomy X (Turner syndrome)	Fetal hydrops, prominent dorsal edema of hands and feet, coarctation of aorta
Trisomy 18	Overlapping fingers, rocker-bottom feet, polydactyly
Trisomy 13	Severe craniofacial abnormalities, including holoprosencephaly, midline cleft lip, abnormal skull base, polydactyly, splenopancreatic fusion, and heart defects
Trisomy 21	Wide space between 1st and 2nd toes, clinodactyly, single palmar crease, heart defects, and duodenal atresia
Triploidy	Syndactyly of 3rd and 4th digits

From Ernst LM et al: Pathologic examination of fetal and placental tissue obtained by dilation and evacuation. Arch Pathol Lab Med 137:326-337; 2012.

- Plasmacytic chronic villitis, viral inclusions in CMV; correlate with fetal organ histology, confirm with immunohistochemistry or PCR
- Fetal erythroblastosis with intranuclear inclusions and hydrops in parvovirus B19

- Look for evidence of fetal-maternal hemorrhage
  - Extensive villous edema, erythroblastosis, intervillous NRBCs
  - Correlate with maternal Kleihauer-Betke or flow cytometry for fetal hemoglobin studies for fetal-maternal transfusion

Fetal Organs

- Evaluate lungs and stomach lumen for aspirated or swallowed neutrophils in amniotic fluid infection sequence
- Liver and adrenal glands useful for identification of viral inclusions of CMV and HSV
- Heart, lung, kidney, and liver autolysis useful for estimating in utero demise to delivery interval
- Kidney especially useful in estimating gestational age
- Specific anomalies such as cystic kidneys may be further classified

CHECKLIST FOR EVALUATION OF D&E SPECIMEN

Fetal Tissues

- Separate fetal tissues from placental and decidual tissues
- Measure foot length for assessment of growth
- Confirm skeletal parts are complete
- Note degree of maceration (dull, tan skin and dehydrated tissue in prolonged retention after fetal demise)
- Examine tissues for anatomic anomalies other than procedure-related disruption
  - Head (usually collapsed with fragments of cranium)
  - Face
    - Note presence and any abnormalities of eyes, ears, nose, mouth, and palate
    - Ear position is difficult to assess in young &/or fragmented fetus, but cleft palate is easily identified
  - 4 extremities
    - Fingers, palmar creases (develop in early 2nd trimester), toes, foot length
  - Fragments of rib and vertebral column
  - External genitalia
    - Urethral groove closes in male by 12 weeks, develops into labia in female
  - Internal genitalia (identified in 40% of D&E specimens)
  - Loose organs
    - Heart, lungs, GI tract, liver, and kidneys are nearly always identified
    - Adrenal glands are found in majority of specimens
    - Internal genitalia, pancreas, spleen, and thymus are found in < 50% of specimens

Placenta

- Placental tissues should be examined as completely as possible and standard tissue submitted for microscopic examination

Disposition of Specimen

- Determined by state law and hospital policy; hospital disposal often acceptable for < 20-week fetus
- Family may request burial or cremation of intact or disrupted fetal remains at any gestational age

SELECTED REFERENCES

1. Pinar H et al: Placental findings in singleton stillbirths. Obstet Gynecol. 123(2 Pt 1):325-36, 2014
2. Ernst LM et al: Pathologic examination of fetal and placental tissue obtained by dilation and evacuation. Arch Pathol Lab Med. 137(3):326-37, 2013
3. Gawron LM et al: Perinatal pathologic examination of nonintact, second-trimester fetal demise specimens: the value of standardization. Arch Pathol Lab Med. 137(8):1083-7, 2013
4. Gambhir PS et al: Chronic umbilical cord entanglements causing intrauterine fetal demise in the second trimester. Pediatr Dev Pathol. 14(3):252-4, 2011
5. Heller DS et al: Second-trimester pregnancy loss at an urban hospital. Infect Dis Obstet Gynecol. 11(2):117-22, 2003

Aneuploidy

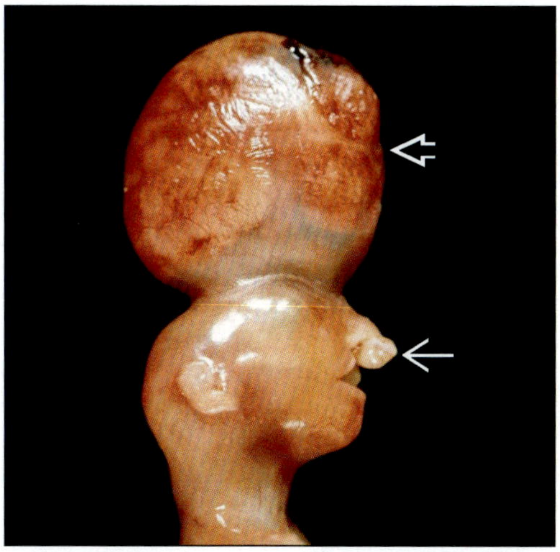

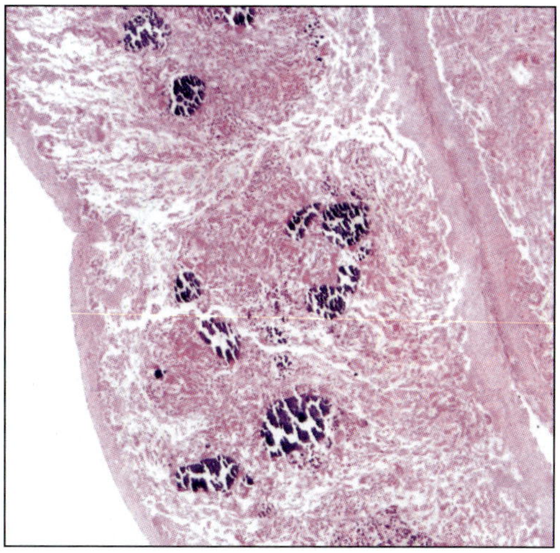

(Left) *This intact fetus with trisomy 13 has a cleft lip and palate ➔ and exencephaly ➔. In the fragmented fetus, facial clefting may still be identified, as well as fragments of skin overlying the exencephalic brain tissue. (Courtesy B. Shehata, MD.)* ***(Right)*** *Aneuploidy is associated with echogenic bowel on prenatal ultrasound, which is most likely the result of these block-like calcifications within the bowel contents. These are preserved even with severe maceration.*

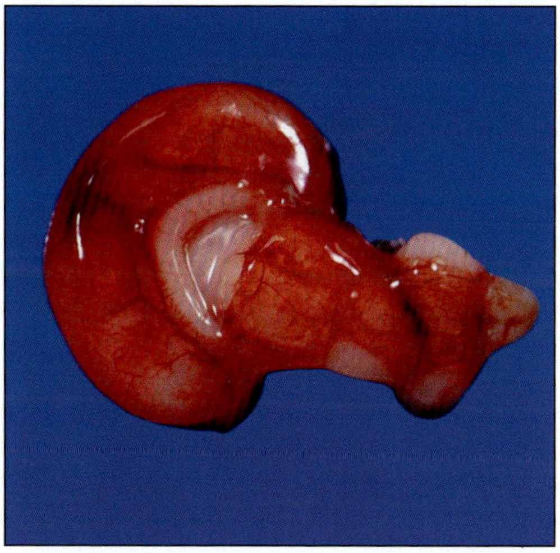

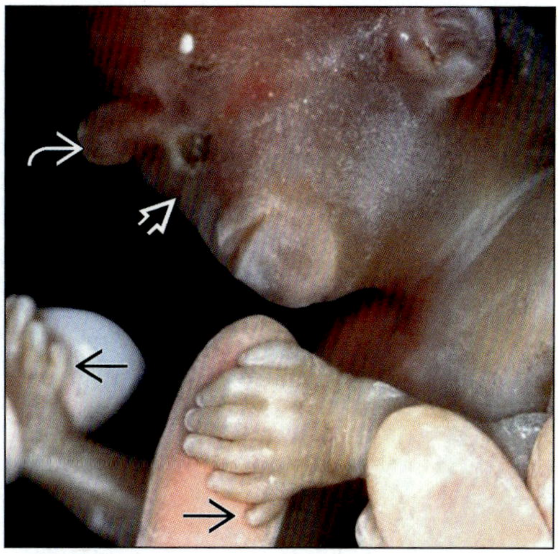

(Left) *Alobar holoprosencephaly, cup type is characteristic of trisomy 13 and triploidy. Malformations such as this, hydrocephalus, Dandy-Walker, lissencephaly, and polymicrogyria are rarely identified in D&E specimens.* ***(Right)*** *Gross photo shows trisomy 13 with post-axial polydactyly ➔. There is also cyclopia with incomplete fusion of the eyes ➔ and proboscis ➔ that is usually associated with alobar holoprosencephaly.*

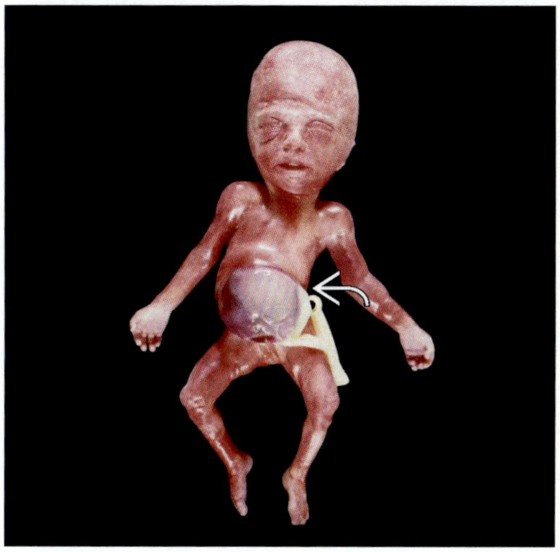

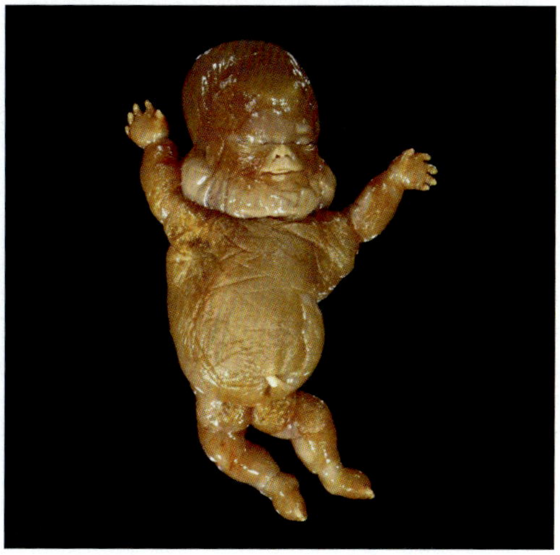

(Left) *This trisomy 18 fetus has a large omphalocele ➔. Omphalocele and gastroschisis are only variably identifiable in the fragmented fetus of a D&E procedure.* ***(Right)*** *Marked fetal edema may be associated with Turner syndrome (monosomy X), trisomy 21 (as in this case), or erythroblastosis fetalis and parvovirus B19 infection.*

Fetal Malformations

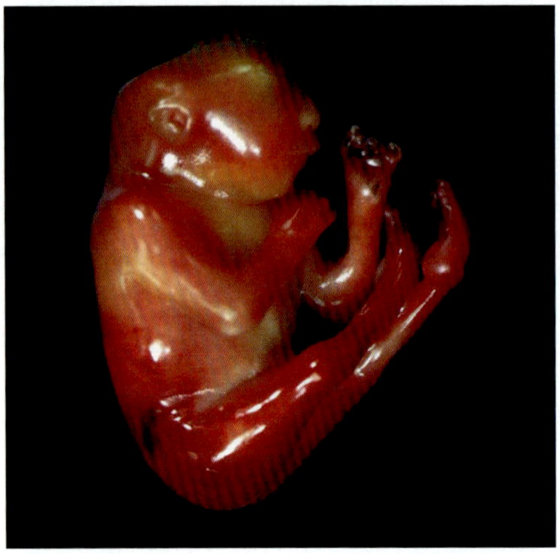

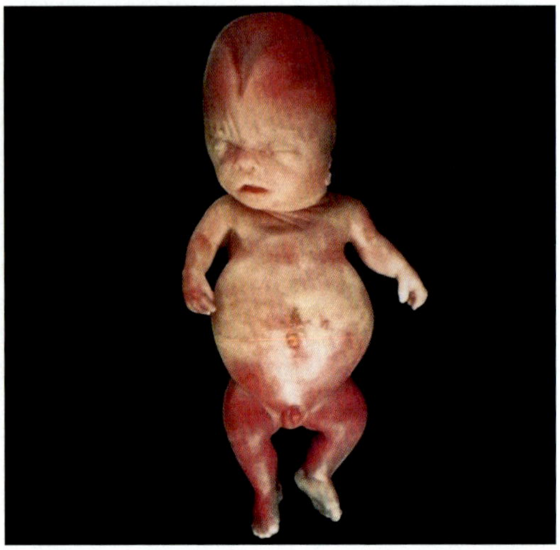

***(Left)** 2nd-trimester fetus shows anencephaly. Compared to other CNS malformations, anencephaly is usually confirmed in D&E specimen. Upper extremities show flexion contractures and the lower extremities fixed extension, consistent with arthrogryposis. (Courtesy B. Shehata, MD.) **(Right)** Thanatophoric dwarfism is the most common lethal chondrodysplasia. This type of fetus should always be x-rayed, and multiple bones should be decalcified for microscopic examination including calvarium, vertebra, and femurs.*

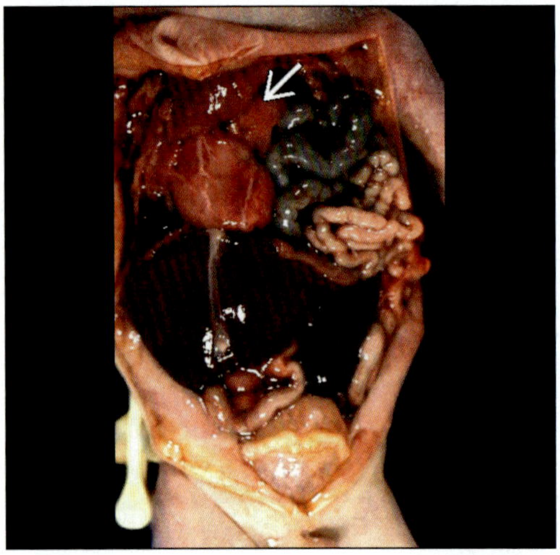

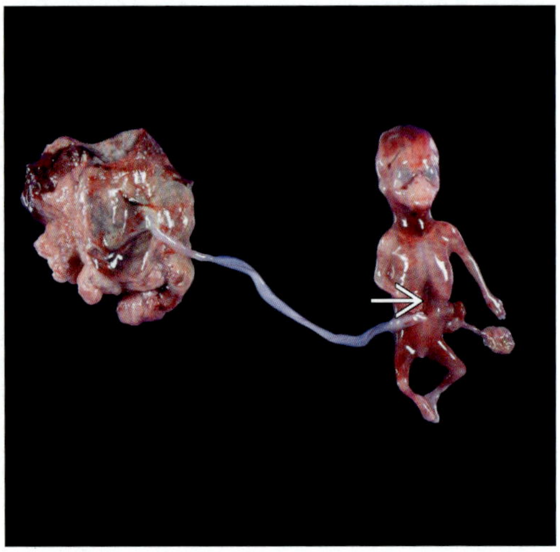

***(Left)** Diaphragmatic hernia is seen here with the majority of the intestines occupying the left chest, shifting the heart to the right. The hypoplastic left lung ➡ is pushed to the right. Liver, when present within the left chest, is associated with more severe pulmonary hypoplasia. (Courtesy B. Shehata, MD.) **(Right)** This fetus shows extrusion of bowel loops through a defect ➡ in the abdominal wall (gastroschisis). The defect is usually to the left of the umbilical cord.*

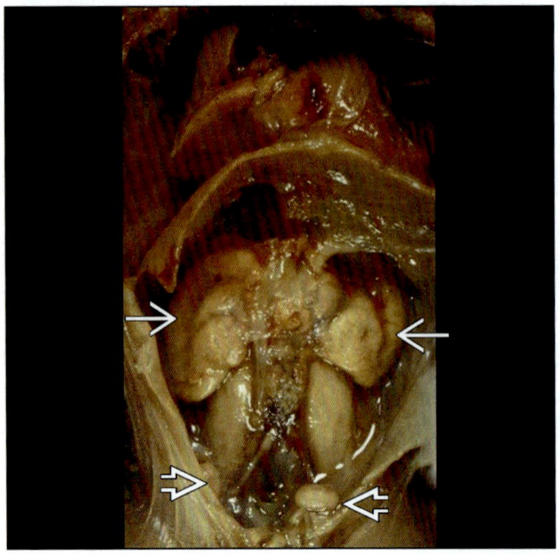

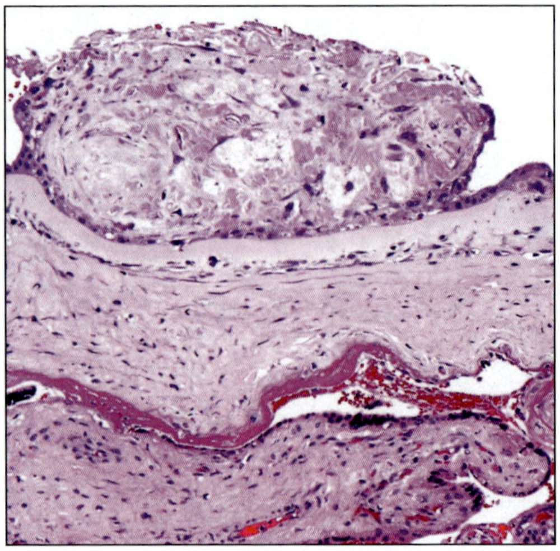

***(Left)** Bilateral renal agenesis is associated with severe pulmonary hypoplasia and oligohydramnios. In the absence of kidneys, the adrenal glands ➡ assume a flattened configuration in the retroperitoneum, which on ultrasound may be mistaken for kidneys. The testes ➡ are seen within the abdominal cavity. **(Right)** Amnion nodosum is seen in renal agenesis, due to accumulation of amniotic fluid debris with severe and prolonged oligohydramnios.*

Dilation and Evacuation

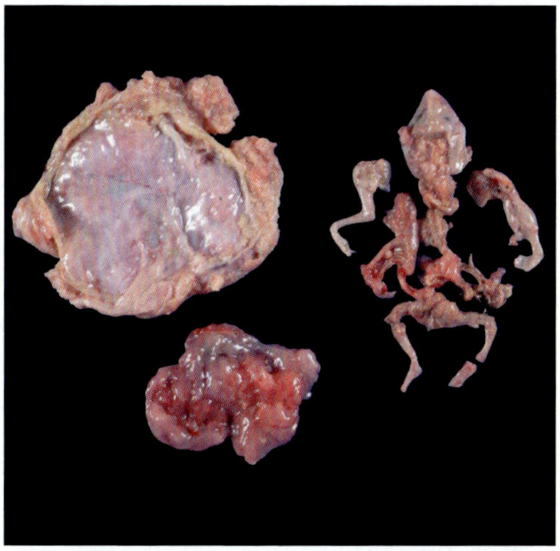

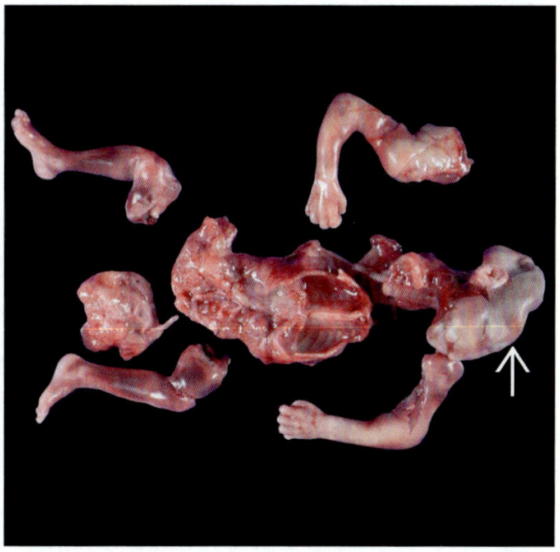

(Left) *Separation of D&E tissues into fetal, placental, and decidual parts is a necessary component of surgical pathology examination. Careful attention to fetus can confirm anomalies from ultrasound and find new abnormalities.* ***(Right)*** *Anencephaly ➡ is one of the few CNS abnormalities identifiable in fragmented fetus. Cranium is usually collapsed in D&E fetus to allow removal, with extensive disruption of brain tissues. In anencephaly, head may be delivered intact.*

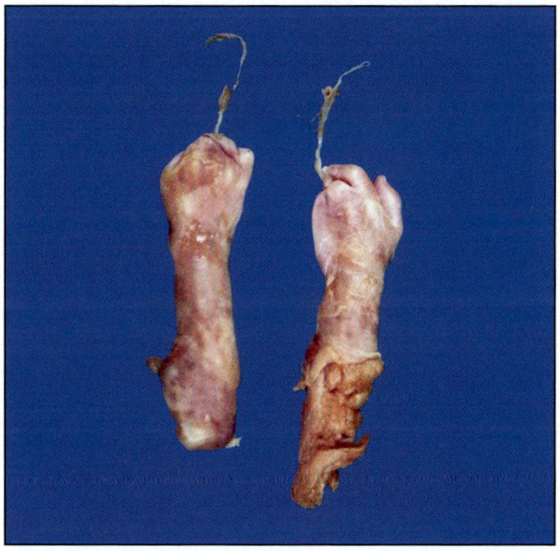

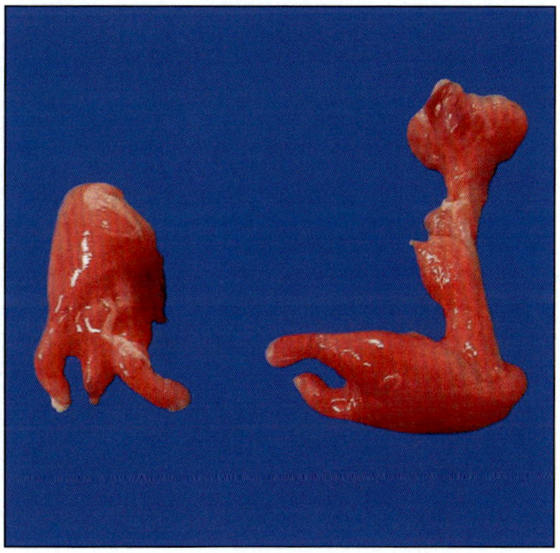

(Left) *These upper extremities show multiple amputations of the fingers with the attached bands, due to early amnion rupture.* ***(Right)*** *These upper extremities show severe abnormalities of the fingers, thumbs, and radii. The DDx would include numerous syndromes such as VATER, Holt-Oram, and Roberts-SC phocomelia. Careful documentation of anomalies allows the general surgical pathologist to work together with medical geneticists in establishing a diagnosis for the family.*

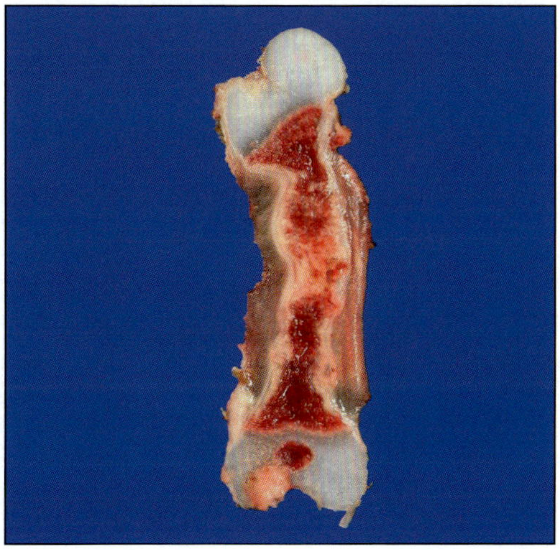

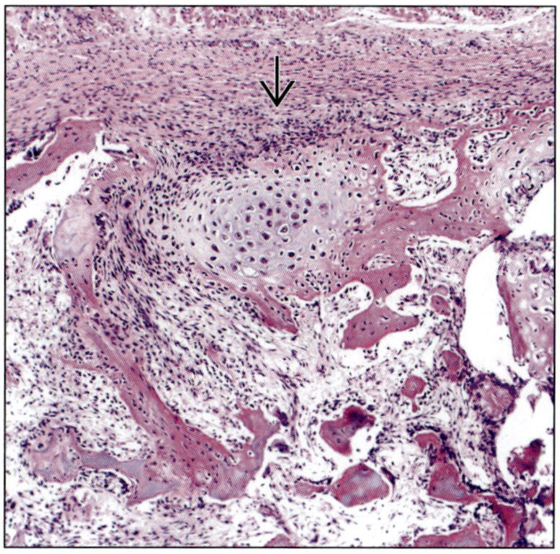

(Left) *This femur from a fetus with osteogenesis imperfecta shows the "crinkled" bone appearance of multiple cortical fractures.* ***(Right)*** *The histology of osteogenesis imperfecta type II shows disrupted cortical bone with a nodule of cartilage* ➡ *and irregularly oriented trabecular bone, consistent with a healing fracture.*

2ND-TRIMESTER FETAL DEMISE

Placental Pathology

*(**Left**) Amniotic bands → may also constrict the umbilical cord, causing fetal demise. Note the opacity of the chorionic plate → due to thickening of the denuded chorion. (**Right**) Chorion nodosum occurs after prolonged rupture of the amnion. There is thickening of the chorion, which has embedded amniotic fluid debris →.*

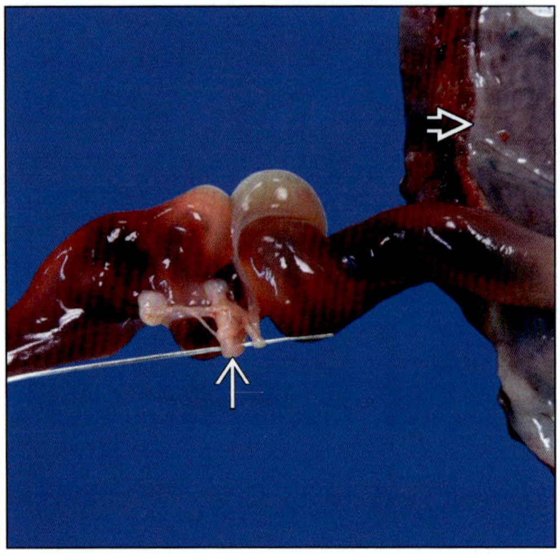

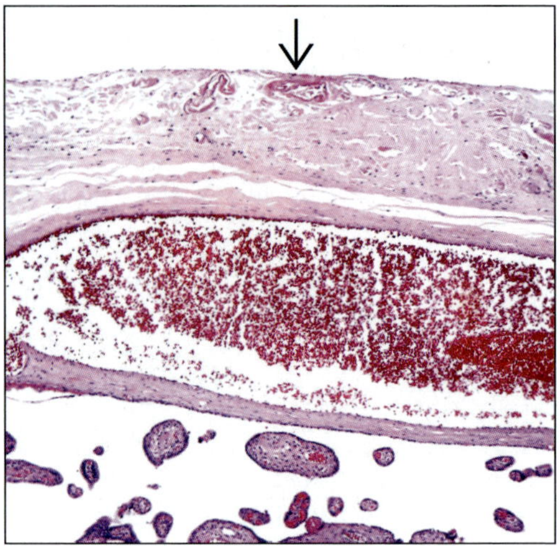

*(**Left**) This fetus was delivered intact after in utero demise due to umbilical cord pathology. The cord is long and hypercoiled with stricture → at the abdominal insertion. (**Right**) Fetal thrombotic vasculopathy is associated with umbilical cord compromise. This stem vessel has fibroblast proliferation and extravasation of red blood cells with avascular villi ↪. Focality of the changes helps distinguish them from involution after fetal demise.*

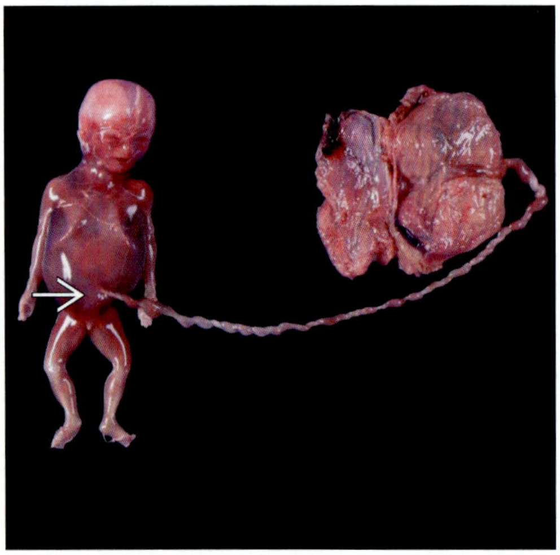

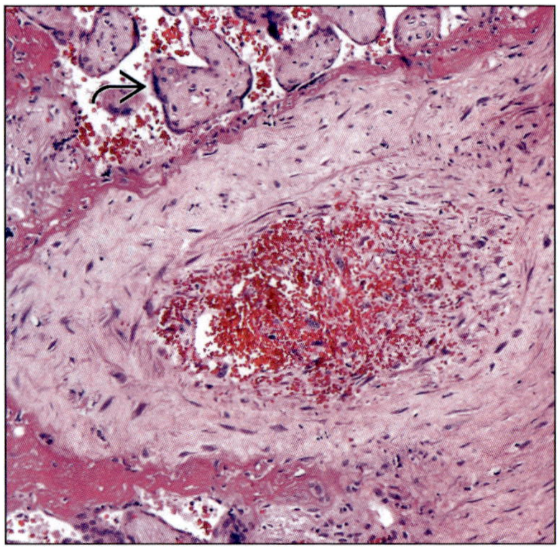

*(**Left**) Uteroplacental underperfusion may cause growth restriction, premature birth, or in utero death. This image shows distal villous hypoplasia with small, poorly vascularized villi and exaggerated syncytial knots. These changes are often associated with preterm preeclampsia. (**Right**) Retroplacental hemorrhage may cause fetal demise. This image shows residua of a subchorionic hematoma noted on early ultrasound. Longstanding hemorrhage may show hemosiderin-laden macrophages in the chorion.*

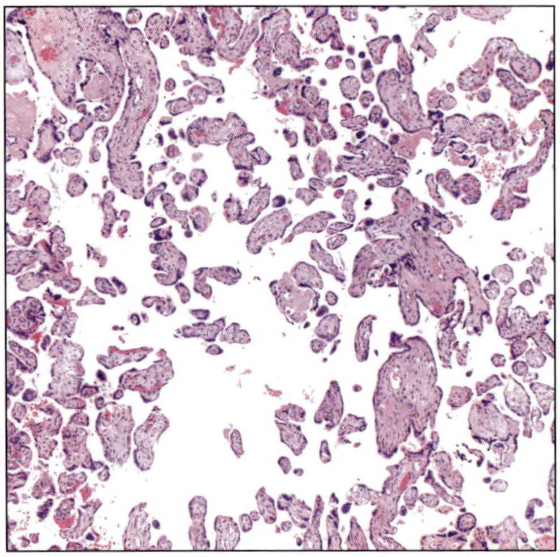

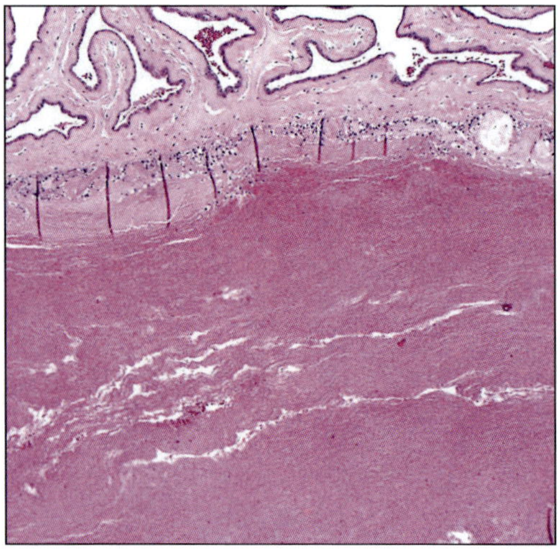

Placental Pathology

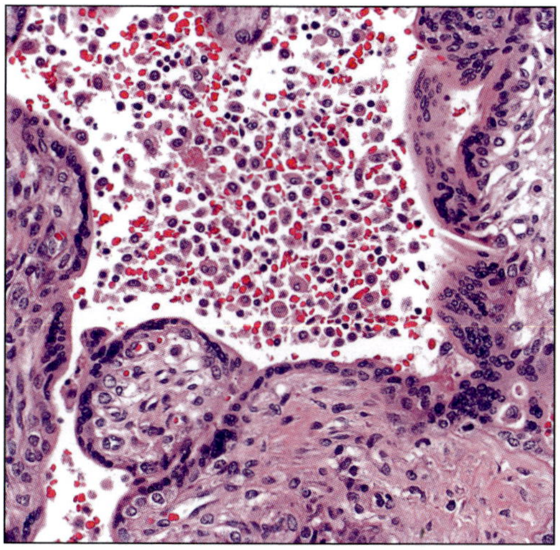
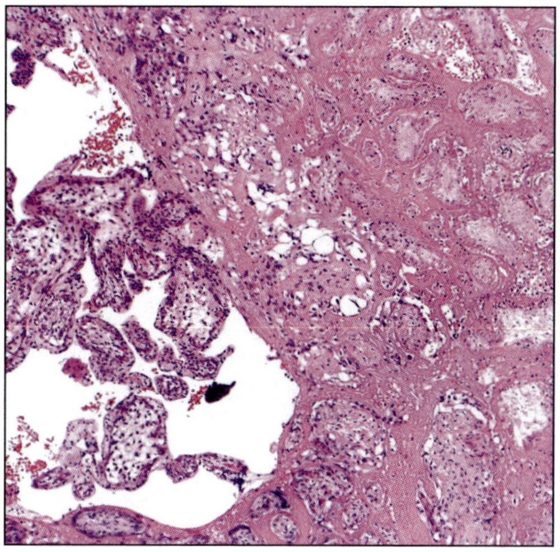

(Left) *Chronic histiocytic intervillositis is a rare cause of placental insufficiency and fetal loss, with frequent recurrence in subsequent pregnancies.* ***(Right)*** *Massive perivillous fibrin deposition (MPVFD) is associated with severe intrauterine growth restriction and fetal demise. It also has a significant risk for recurrence. Preserved villi are surrounded by placental matrix-type fibrin, with numerous extravillous trophoblast embedded in the fibrin.*

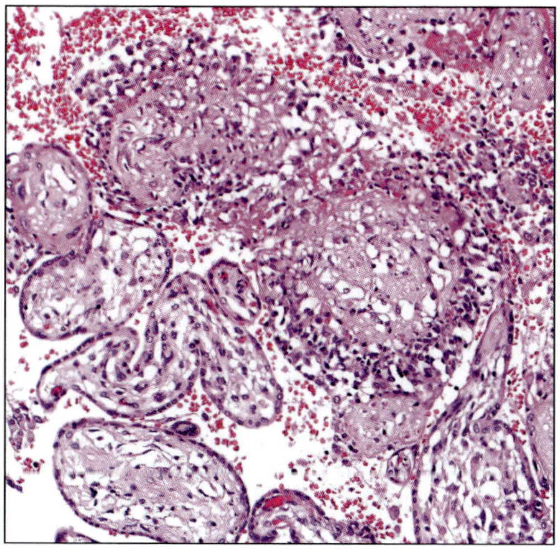
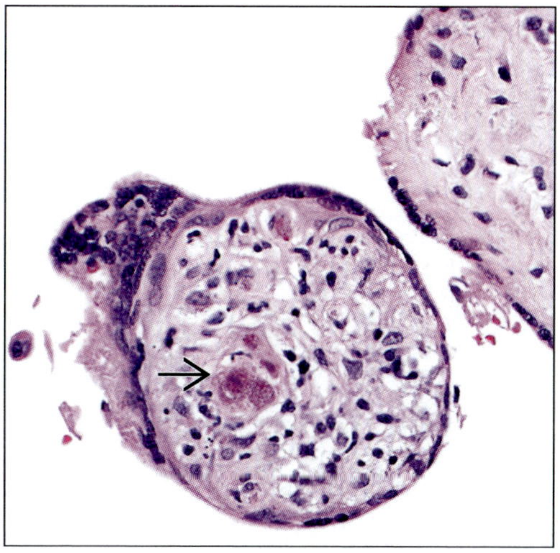

(Left) *Chronic villitis of unknown etiology (VUE) is less common in the 2nd trimester; infection should be strongly considered, especially with fetal demise.* ***(Right)*** *This case of chronic villitis is secondary to CMV infection, seen here with viral inclusions* →.

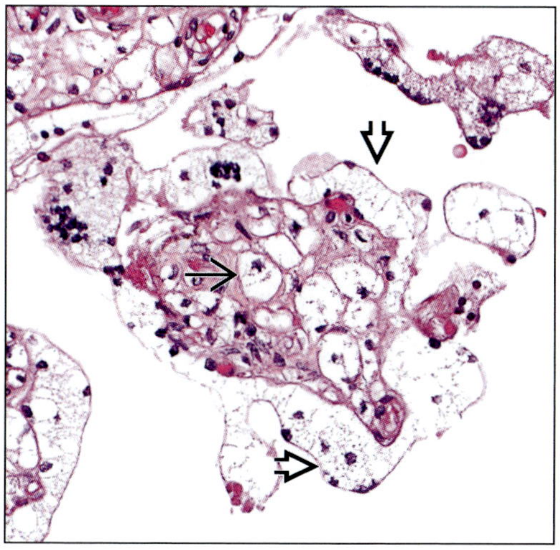
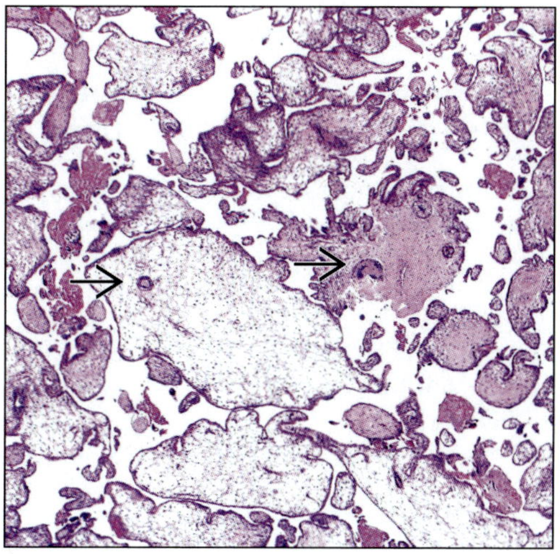

(Left) *The placenta also contains clues to genetic disorders of the fetus. Villi from this fetus with galactosidosis show massive vacuolization of the syncytiotrophoblast* ⇨ *and Hofbauer cells* →. ***(Right)*** *Dysmorphic villi are frequently associated with chromosomal abnormalities. The villi show marked variation in size and shape. There are large edematous villi and small fibrotic villi. Irregular contours result in formation of trophoblast pseudoinclusions* →.

3RD-TRIMESTER FETAL DEMISE

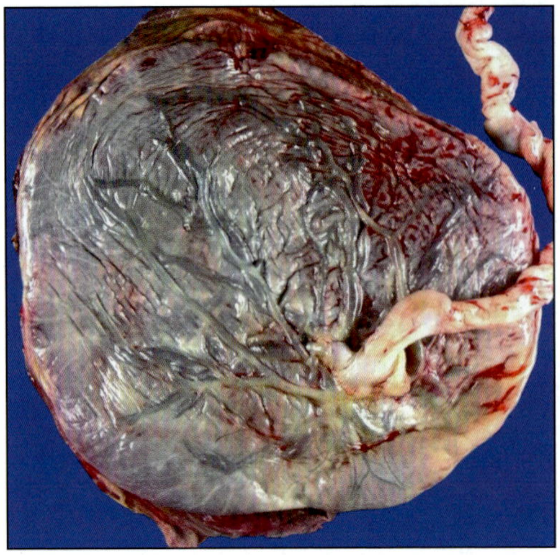

Severe acute chorioamnionitis, as seen in this case with purulent membranes, can be a cause of premature birth of a sick baby or 3rd-trimester fetal demise. The processes are on a continuum.

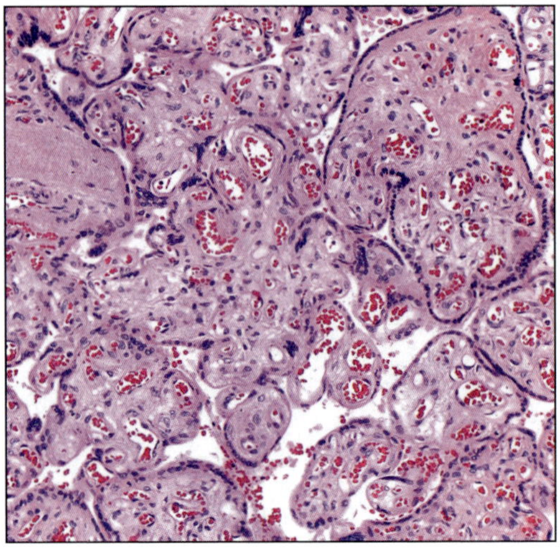

Placental maturation defect (a.k.a. distal villous immaturity) is associated with late fetal demise. The lack of sufficient vasculosynctial membranes in distal villi impairs gas and nutrient exchange.

TERMINOLOGY

Definitions

- Demise or stillbirth of fetus after 24 weeks of pregnancy

EPIDEMIOLOGY

Incidence

- 0.3% of pregnancies are lost at 24-40 weeks gestation

ETIOLOGY/PATHOGENESIS

Placental Causes of Fetal Demise

- No single acute, subacute, or chronic placental finding is specific for in utero demise
  - Conditions associated with fetal demise are similar to those causing intrauterine growth restriction, premature birth, and significant neonatal morbidity
    - These unfortunate outcomes are on same biologic continuum
  - Fetal demise may result from multiple additive maternal, fetal, and placental processes
- Subacute and chronic processes
  - Increased fetal growth in 3rd trimester imposes further demands on placental function
    - Compromised placenta may be unable to meet those demands
  - Subacute/chronic conditions
    - Uteroplacental malperfusion (characterized by small placenta, infarcts, distal villous hypoplasia, maternal decidual vasculopathy)
    - Extensive chronic villitis (usually villitis of unknown etiology)
    - Massively increased perivillous fibrin deposition
    - Impaired fetoplacental perfusion (single umbilical artery, marginal, velamentous or furcate cord insertion, hypercoiled cord, fetal thrombotic vasculopathy)
    - Complications of twin or higher order birth gestations (twin-twin transfusion, small placental share)
    - Prolonged amniotic fluid infection
    - Chronic fetal-maternal transfusion
    - Villous maturation defect/distal villous immaturity
- Acute processes
  - Placental abruption
  - Acute umbilical cord obstruction
    - May be caused by umbilical cord prolapse, cord rupture, kinking/compression, thrombosis
    - Also acute on chronic exacerbation of a nuchal/limb/body cord entanglement, due to increased fetal growth and physical changes in intrauterine environment with labor
  - Ruptured vasa previa
  - Massive fetal-maternal hemorrhage
  - Acute amniotic fluid infection (fetal morbidity may depend upon lethality of microorganism)

Maternal Conditions

- Uncontrolled chronic illness
  - Hypertension, preeclampsia, hemolysis, elevated liver enzymes, low platelets (HELLP) syndrome
    - May show changes of abruption &/or uteroplacental malperfusion in placenta
  - Diabetes, especially pregestational diabetes
    - May show distal villous immaturity in placenta
  - Systemic lupus erythematosus and other immunologic conditions
  - Post-term pregnancy
- Severe acute illness
  - Maternal sepsis, acute pneumonia, pyelonephritis, appendicitis, diabetic ketoacidosis
- Incompetent cervix
  - May show changes of amniotic fluid infection

- Uterine leiomyomata
- Alcohol, smoking, drug use, and teratogen exposure
- Trauma (e.g., motor vehicle accident, physical abuse, etc.), uterine rupture
- Thrombophilia
  - Factor V Leiden, protein S deficiency, and prothrombin G20210A mutation

Fetal Factors

- Syndromes and single malformations account for ~ 10% of stillbirths; these include aneuploidies
  - Chromosomal abnormalities
    - 4% of 3rd-trimester stillbirths are due to aneuploidy
    - Majority have characteristic dysmorphic features and malformations
  - Anatomic malformations
    - Congenital heart defects (CHDs) most common; recurrence risk in subsequent pregnancies is 2-3%
    - 25-33% of CHDs have syndromic features, 5-10% have chromosomal defects, 3% are attributed to single gene defects
    - Neural tube defects, renal abnormalities, congential diaphragmatic hernia are less common
- Developmental disruptions, dysplasias, and metabolic disorders comprise < 5% of stillbirth causes
  - Metabolic/storage diseases are very rare
  - Severe fetal anemia with hydrops
    - 30% die in utero
    - Hydrops occurs once critical level of anemia is reached (hematocrit of < 15%)
- Congenital tumors
  - Most commonly sacrococcygeal teratoma, usually associated with hydrops due to high-output failure
- Complications of twinning
  - Twin-to-twin transfusion, acardiac twinning, conjoined twins

MACROSCOPIC FINDINGS

General Features

- Placental examination is essential to determine cause of fetal demise
  - While fetal autopsy is ideal for thorough investigation, placental exam identifies cause of fetal demise more frequently than autopsy or cytogenetics
    - Placenta yields cause of death in up to 35% of stillbirths; may be only source for diagnosis in 16%
- Careful attention to umbilical cord pathology is warranted
  - Portions of umbilical cord may be submitted for cultures or other laboratory studies
    - If possible, these should be retrieved for pathologic examination after necessary samples are obtained

MICROSCOPIC FINDINGS

General Features

- Placental findings in stillbirth are similar to those associated with intrauterine growth restriction or premature birth

Infection

- Ascending infection
  - Amniotic fluid infection sequence
    - Maternal inflammatory response: Acute or subacute chorioamnionitis
    - Fetal inflammatory response: Umbilical vasculitis, chorionic plate vasculitis
    - Frequent cause of post-term in utero demise (after 41 weeks gestation)
- Hematogenous infection: Chronic villitis and intervillositis
  - Chronic villitis in 3rd trimester is usually due to idiopathic maternal immune response
  - ~ 5% of cases are due to infections (especially CMV)
    - Fetus may have hydrops

Uteroplacental Malperfusion

- Often associated with maternal hypertensive conditions, preeclampsia
- Acute retroplacental hemorrhage
- Chronic marginal abruption
- Small placenta with multiple infarcts, distal villous hypoplasia, accelerated villous maturation, increased syncytial knots
- Maternal decidual vasculopathy

Fetoplacental Malperfusion

- Umbilical cord pathology
  - Includes gross abnormalities, such as
    - Single umbilical artery
    - Abnormal insertion
    - Hypercoiling
    - Obstruction
    - Thrombi
  - Proposed criteria for diagnosis of umbilical cord compromise as cause of stillbirth
    - Dilated fetal vessels (vascular ectasia to ≥ 4x diameter of adjacent muscular vessel)
    - Thrombi of fetal muscular vessels (organized thrombi, organizing thrombi, and loss of endothelial integrity with bridging strands of fibrous connective tissue and extravasation of endothelial cells [fibromuscular sclerosis])
    - Focal or regional restriction of avascular villi or villous stromal karyorrhexis
    - Familiarity with vascular involutional changes after fetal demise is essential for proper utilization of proposed criteria, as similar changes are due to demise alone

Villous Maturation Defect

- Frequently associated with late in utero demise
  - After 37 weeks
- Associated with hypercoiled umbilical cords

Probable and Possible Causes of Stillbirth

Category	24-27 Weeks	28-31 Weeks	32-36 Weeks	≥ 37 Weeks	Entire 3rd Trimester
Placental disease (~ 50% due to uteroplacental malperfusion, maternal vasculopathy)	36%	25%	27%	25%	28%
Infection (fetus, placenta, or mother)	8%	6%	8%	12%	8%
Fetal/genetic structural abnormality	11%	14%	18%	13%	14%
Maternal medical complications (including gestational diabetes, antiphospholipid antibody syndrome)	10%	4%	8%	11%	8%
Hypertensive disorders (hypertension and preeclampsia)	16%	17%	10%	5%	12%
Umbilical cord abnormalities (cord prolapse, strictures, thrombi)	11%	6%	13%	14%	11%
Obstetric complications (abruption, multiple gestation, preterm labor/premature rupture of membranes, cervical insufficiency, chorioamnionitis)	19%	21%	17%	14%	18%
Other (hydrops, early amniotic rupture)	3%	6%	3%	2%	4%

All cases included complete placental examination, autopsy, and cytogenetics. From Stillbirth Collaborative Research Network Writing Group: Causes of death among stillbirths. JAMA. 306(22):2459-68, 2011.

Placental Findings More Frequent in Stillbirth Compared to Livebirth

Placental Finding	24-31 Weeks	32-36 Weeks	≥ 37 Weeks
Single umbilical artery	Yes	Yes	Yes
Distal villous immaturity (placental maturation defect)	No	No	Yes
Chorionic plate vascular degenerative changes*	Yes	Yes	Yes
Retroplacental hematoma	Yes	Yes	No
Focal infarction	No	Yes	No
Multifocal infarction	No	Yes	No
Diffuse infarction	Yes	Yes	Yes
Massive perivillous fibrin deposition	No	Yes	No
Intraparenchymal thrombus	No	No	Yes
Chorionic plate thrombi	No	Yes	Yes
Focal avascular villi	Yes	No	Yes
Multifocal avascular villi	No	No	Yes
Diffuse avascular villi*	Yes	Yes	Data unavailable
Diffuse villous edema	No	No	Yes

*The frequency of these findings in stillbirth was significantly increased compared to livebirths of comparable gestational ages. Many pathologies are present in both preterm birth and in utero demise. *Chorionic plate vascular degenerative changes and diffuse avascular villi may occur as pathologic processes or as secondary findings after fetal demise. From Pinar H et al: Placental findings in singleton stillbirths. Obstet Gynecol. 123(2 Pt 1):325-36, 2014.*

- Characterized by poor vasculosyncytial membrane (VSM) formation in mature distal villi
  - < 1 VSM per 4 distal villi
  - Present in > 10 high-power (400x) fields
- Histologic overlap with distal villous immaturity seen in gestational diabetes

Other Placental Pathologies

- Uncommon causes of fetal demise, but important to recognize as placental cause of death with recurrent potential
  - Massive perivillous fibrin deposition/maternal floor infarction
  - Chronic histiocytic intervillositis of unknown etiology
  - Extensive chronic villitis of unknown etiology

SELECTED REFERENCES

1. Pinar H et al: Placental findings in singleton stillbirths. Obstet Gynecol. 123(2 Pt 1):325-36, 2014
2. Stillbirth Collaborative Research Network Writing Group: Causes of death among stillbirths. JAMA. 306(22):2459-68, 2011
3. Pauli RM: Stillbirth: fetal disorders. Clin Obstet Gynecol. 53(3):646-55, 2010
4. Pinar H et al: Placenta and umbilical cord abnormalities seen with stillbirth. Clin Obstet Gynecol. 53(3):656-72, 2010
5. Parast MM et al: Placental histologic criteria for umbilical blood flow restriction in unexplained stillbirth. Hum Pathol. 39(6):948-53, 2008
6. de Laat MW et al: Hypercoiling of the umbilical cord and placental maturation defect: associated pathology? Pediatr Dev Pathol. 10(4):293-9, 2007

Uteroplacental Blood Flow Abnormalities

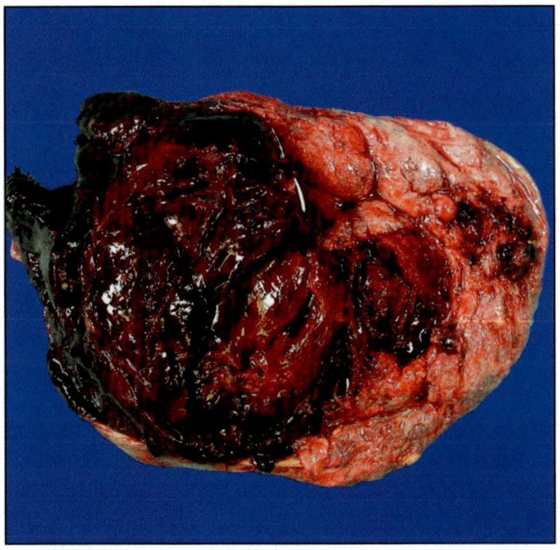

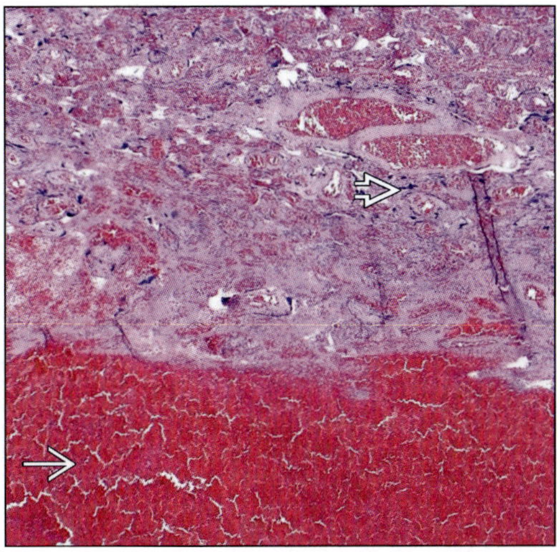

(Left) *Massive placental abruption is commonly associated with preeclampsia. Abruption of > 30-50% of the placental basal surface has a high fetal mortality rate.* ***(Right)*** *H&E shows acute retroplacental hemorrhage → with overlying acute infarct. Infarction is evinced by collapse of the intervillous space and the smudged appearance of syncytiotrophoblast nuclei ⇨.*

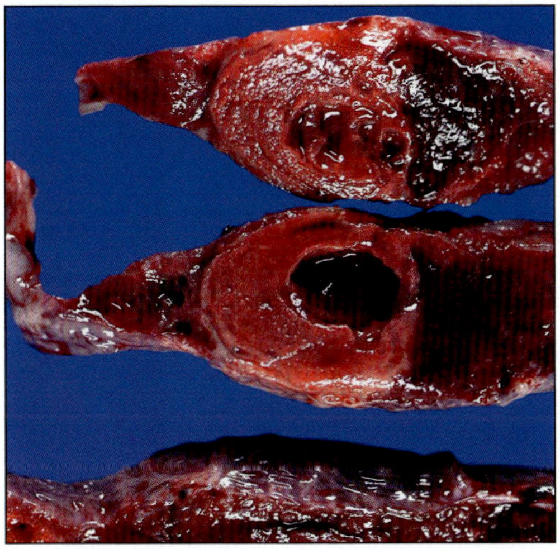

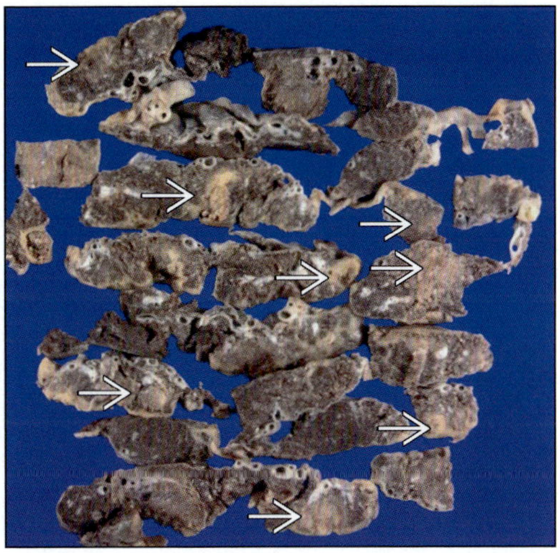

(Left) *This large subacute infarct with central hemorrhage (infarction hematoma) was associated with fetal demise. The hemorrhage may be a reperfusion injury.* ***(Right)*** *Multiple large or nonmarginal infarcts are seen in preeclampsia. They are associated with growth restriction, prematurity, and fetal demise. Gross photo shows numerous poorly circumscribed, tan foci → in this placenta due to multiple remote infarcts.*

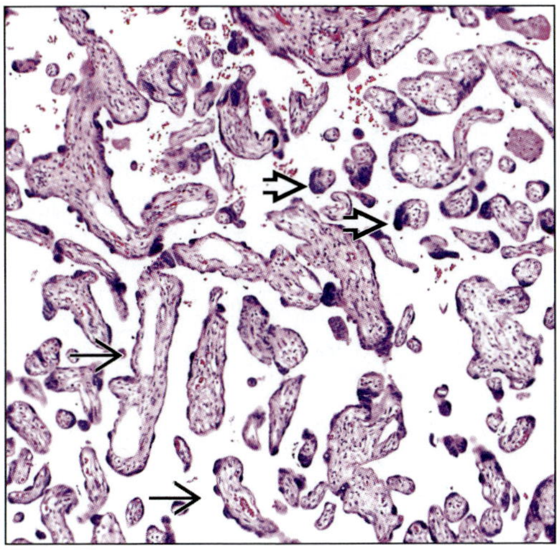

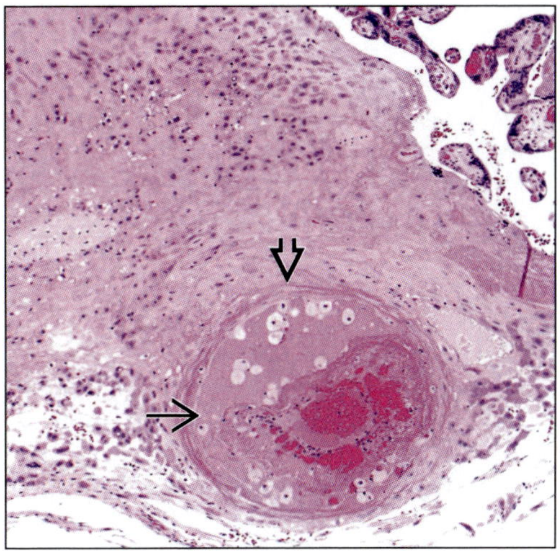

(Left) *Distal villous hypoplasia (accelerated villous maturation) is characterized by increased elongate slender villi → and exaggerated syncytial knots ⇨ (Tenney-Parker change). The findings reflect longstanding uteroplacental malperfusion and are characteristic of preterm preeclampsia.* ***(Right)*** *Uteroplacental malperfusion in preterm preeclampsia is associated with decidual vasculopathy. Note the fibrinoid necrosis → and foamy macrophages ⇨ in this spiral artery.*

Fetal-Placental Blood Flow Abnormalities

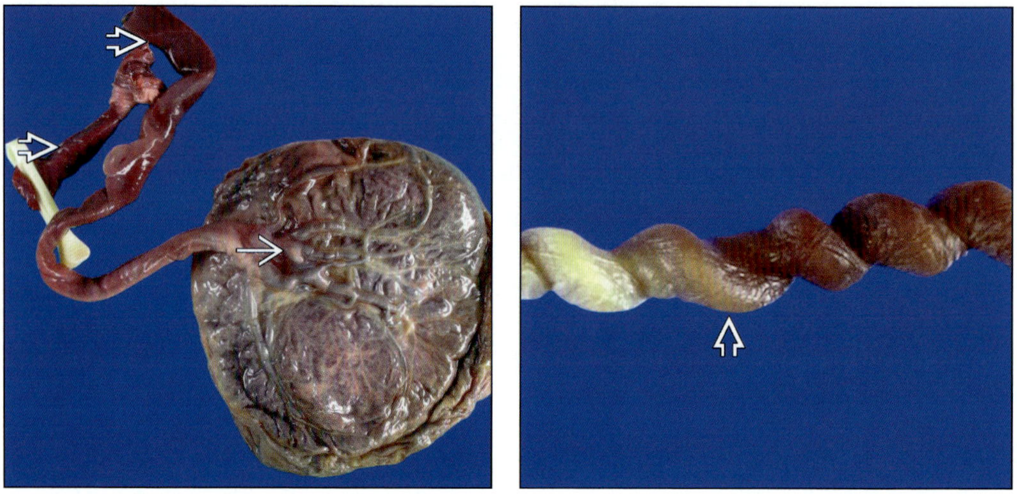

(Left) *Close attention to cord lesions is essential in 3rd-trimester fetal loss. In this case associated with a nuchal cord, the looped portion of the cord is flattened and appears macerated. A thrombus is visible in a proximal chorionic plate vein.* ***(Right)*** *Abrupt changes in cord color may suggest vascular pathology, as in this severely hypercoiled cord. Hypercoiled cords are associated with both chronic fetal-placental underperfusion and placental maturation defect.*

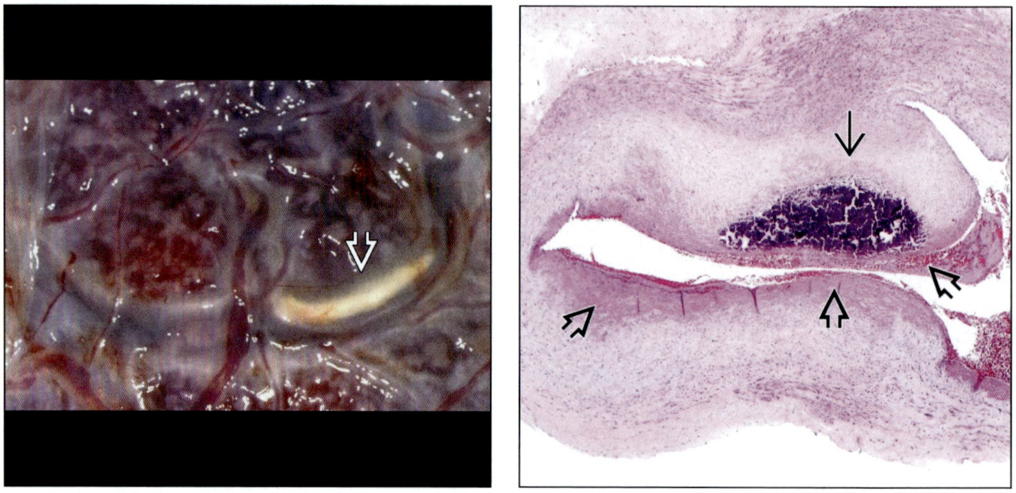

(Left) *Here, a remote thrombus is visible in a chorionic plate vein.* ***(Right)*** *This chorionic plate vessel displays an organizing thrombus. Within the endothelial cushion, there is mural calcification and subendothelial fibrin forming a fibrin cap. These changes are consistent with occlusion of flow in vivo and are usually associated with distal villous changes of fetal thrombotic vasculopathy.*

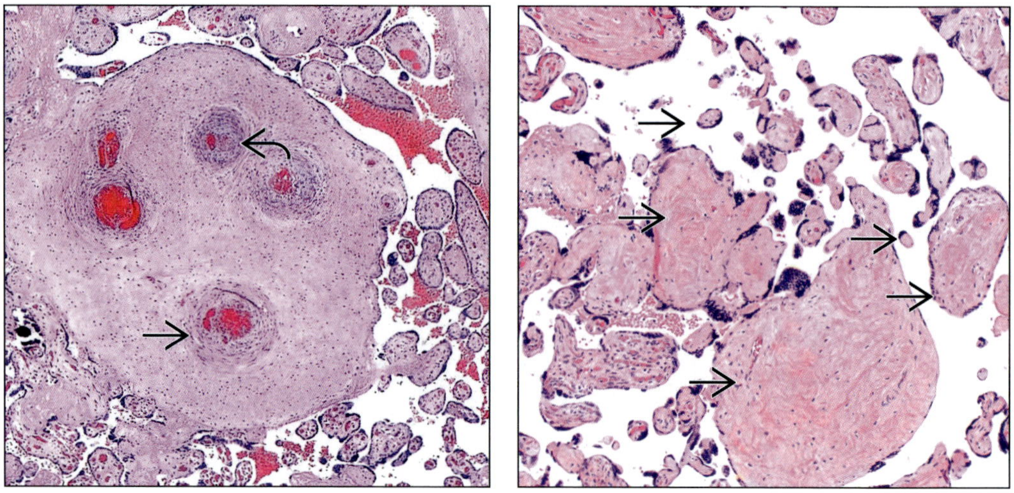

(Left) *Stem villous changes of fetal thrombotic vasculopathy include organizing thrombi as well as fibromuscular sclerosis with fibroblast proliferation and red blood cell extravasation.* ***(Right)*** *Distal villi become avascular with cessation of fetal perfusion. The syncytiotrophoblast layer remains intact and the intervillous space is preserved. This will occur throughout the placenta after prolonged in utero demise but regionally when due to focal thrombi.*

COMPLICATIONS OF MONOCHORIONIC MONOAMNIOTIC TWIN GESTATIONS

  - Single umbilical artery (SUA) (2-vessel cord) more common than MCDA twins or singletons, usually only affecting 1 twin
- Twin-twin transfusion syndrome
  - Much less common and much less morbid in MCMA twins than in MCDA twins
    - Anastomoses are usually large caliber, bidirectional, and resulting in compensatory parenchymal changes
    - No intraamniotic pressure differences that could differentially alter blood flow
- Asymmetric growth
  - Usually NOT due to twin-twin transfusion
  - Contributing factors can include cord anomalies and discrepant placental mass
  - Discordant twins have increased risk of death
- Intrauterine death
  - Monochorionic twins have highest mortality rates of all twinning types
  - Many early demises show genetic and phenotypic abnormalities
  - Late demises can occur suddenly and without observable warning signs
    - May be due to sudden cord compromise
    - May be due to acute exsanguination of viable twin to demised twin through large caliber anastomoses
- Acardiac twinning
  - Incidence
    - 1 in 35,000 deliveries, 1% of monozygotic pregnancies
  - 40-50% are MCMA
  - Increased incidence of 3% in monozygotic triplet pregnancies
  - Acardiac twin loses its vascular connection to placenta and receives all blood supply from pump twin
  - Direct artery-artery and vein-vein anastomoses between cords
  - Twin reversed arterial perfusion (TRAP)
    - Acardiac twin receives blood through artery-artery anastomosis
  - 33-42% of acardiac twins have single umbilical cord
    - Artery may enter directly into aorta of acardiac twin
    - Artery may be persistent vitelline artery rather than true umbilical artery
  - 33-50% of acardiac twins have chromosomal abnormalities
  - Acardiac twin has lethal malformation and pump twin has 50% mortality without treatment
  - Pump twin may have high-output failure, especially if acardiac twin is > 50% weight of pump twin
    - Fetoscopic laser coagulation of acardiac twin umbilical cord → 80% survival of pump twin
- Conjoined twins
  - Symmetric
    - Incidence: 1:30,000-100,000 births
    - F:M = 3:1
    - 28% die in utero death, 50% die in neonatal period
    - Ability to surgically separate twins is based on anatomical arrangement and shared organs
  - Asymmetric (parasitic twins)
    - Incidence: ~ 1 in 1,000,000 births
    - May have high-output cardiac failure or significant disability depending upon location
    - Generally can be resected
  - Fetus in fetu
    - May create a vascular steal or mass effect

MACROSCOPIC FINDINGS

General Features

- MCMA placental membranes form single sac without dividing membrane
  - Carefully examine placental surface for amnion
    - Amnion may become stripped off surface during delivery, giving false appearance of absent dividing membrane
  - Umbilical cords are usually inserted close to one another
  - Vascular anastomoses between placental territories of twins are always present
- Acardiac twin
  - Umbilical cords are close together or one may branch from the other
  - Acardiac twin umbilical cord is usually very short
  - Direct vascular connections between the 2 cords are present
  - Acardiac twin morphology varies
    - ~ 50% have some cardiac tissue, although nonfunctional
    - 68% acardius acephalus (no head development)
    - 15% acardius anceps (partial head development)
    - Less common: Acardius amorphus (least differentiated) and acardius acormus (only head development)
    - Lower extremities are typically much more developed than upper extremities or head (except in acardius amorphus and acardius acormus)
    - Multiple malformations include intestinal atresia, imperforate anus, renal agenesis (usually no lung parenchyma)
- Conjoined twins
  - Symmetric
    - Most common forms are thoracoomphalopagus, ischiopagus, and dicephalus
    - 87% are joined front to front, or side to side (ventral union)
    - 48% are joined rostral (dicephalus or cephalopagus, thoracopagus, omphalopagus)
    - 11% are joined caudal (ischiopagus)
    - 28% are joined lateral (parapagus, pelvis and variable trunk)
    - 13% are joined back to back (dorsal union)
    - 5% are joined craniopagus (joined at cranial vault)
    - 2% are joined rachipagus (joined at vertebral column)
    - 6% are joined pygopagus (joined at sacrum)
  - Asymmetric, parasitic twins

- Common sites are upper jaw, palate, basal skull, epigastrium, and back
- Varying external and internal differentiation
  - Fetus in fetu
    - Location: 75% upper retroperitoneum, 12.5% intracranial, 12.5% intrascrotal or testicular
    - Degree of differentiation that exceeds teratoma; axial skeleton
    - Some forms have umbilical cords and amniotic sac-like structures; rare chorionic villous tissue described

Specimen Handling

- Cords
  - Look for evidence of cord entanglement or communicating vessels between cord insertion sites
  - Note abnormal cord insertion patterns (marginal, velamentous, etc.)
  - Note number of umbilical arteries
  - Features suggestive of ongoing vascular compromise
    - Cord narrowing
    - Grooving (from knots or compression)
    - Thrombosis (from stasis and mural damage)
  - Cords from acardiac fetus will also vary
    - May be 2 cords, with acardiac generally having SUA
    - May be 1 cord that branches
  - Cords from conjoined twins will vary depending on area of fusion
    - Fusion of abdomen will have 1 cord with 4, 5, or 6 vessels
- Chorionic plate vasculature
  - Measure and estimate relative disc surface area supplying each twin based on vascular network from each cord
  - Look for superficial vascular anastomoses (usually artery-artery), noting number and caliber
  - Injection studies (air, milk, or dye) may help identify superficial anastomoses, but their presence may or may not be clinically relevant
- Membranes
  - Examine membranes to confirm monoamniotic placentation; ensure that amnion is present over fetal surface
    - Disruption of membranes with stripped amnion commonly occurs during delivery of twins
  - Amniotic surface should be continuous and smooth between cord insertion site, without disruption or excess membranes (could be site of separated dividing membrane)
  - Amnion itself may peel up from fetal surface of disc and mimic dividing membrane
- Parenchyma
  - Note any differences in congestion between the 2 sides (suggesting blood flow issues)
- Sections
  - Each vascular geographic zone should be treated as separate entity with submission of standard sections from each

MICROSCOPIC FINDINGS

General Features

- Twin gestations in general are frequently premature
- Changes of uteroplacental malperfusion are not uncommon
- Increased incidence of fetal thrombotic vasculopathy associated with abnormal cord insertions, cord compromise

DIFFERENTIAL DIAGNOSIS

MCDA

- Pseudomonoamniotic placentation occurs with rupture of dividing membrane of MCDA placenta
  - Disruption may occur intentionally with septostomy treatment of twin-twin transfusion syndrome
  - Disruption may occur unintentionally during laser therapy for twin-twin transfusion syndrome
  - Spontaneous rupture may occur
  - Loss of dividing membrane creates single amniotic cavity with risk for cord entanglement
- Amnion may be stripped off fetal surface during delivery and dividing membrane may be missed

SELECTED REFERENCES

1. Lewi L et al: The vascular anastomoses in monochorionic twin pregnancies and their clinical consequences. Am J Obstet Gynecol. 208(1):19-30, 2013
2. Aston KI et al: Monozygotic twinning associated with assisted reproductive technologies: a review. Reproduction. 136(4):377-86, 2008
3. Diehl W et al: Selective cord coagulation in acardiac twins. Semin Fetal Neonatal Med. 12(6):458-63, 2007
4. Dickinson JE: Monoamniotic twin pregnancy: a review of contemporary practice. Aust N Z J Obstet Gynaecol. 45(6):474-8, 2005
5. Giménez-Scherer JA et al: Malformations in acardiac twins are consistent with reversed blood flow: liver as a clue to their pathogenesis. Pediatr Dev Pathol. 6(6):520-30, 2003
6. Roqué H et al: Perinatal outcomes in monoamniotic gestations. J Matern Fetal Neonatal Med. 13(6):414-21, 2003
7. Spitz L et al: Conjoined twins. JAMA. 289(10):1307-10, 2003
8. De Paepe ME et al: Demonstration of placental vascular anatomy in monochorionic twin gestations. Pediatr Dev Pathol. 5(1):37-44, 2002
9. Pijnenborg JM et al: The monoamniotic twin: a riskful event. Eur J Obstet Gynecol Reprod Biol. 86(1):51-3, 1999
10. Bajoria R: Abundant vascular anastomoses in monoamniotic versus diamniotic monochorionic placentas. Am J Obstet Gynecol. 179(3 Pt 1):788-93, 1998
11. Feldman DM et al: Iatrogenic monoamniotic twins as a complication of therapeutic amniocentesis. Obstet Gynecol. 91(5 Pt 2):815-6, 1998
12. D'Alton ME et al: Syndromes in twins. Semin Perinatol. 19(5):375-86, 1995
13. Van Allen MI et al: Twin reversed arterial perfusion (TRAP) sequence: a study of 14 twin pregnancies with acardius. Semin Perinatol. 7(4):285-93, 1983

Monochorionic Monoamniotic Twins

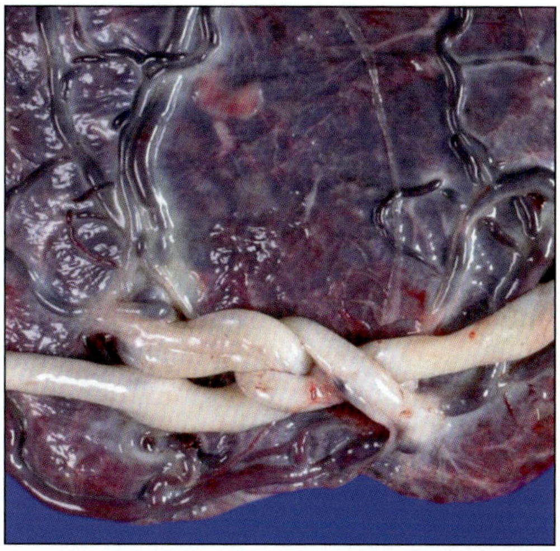

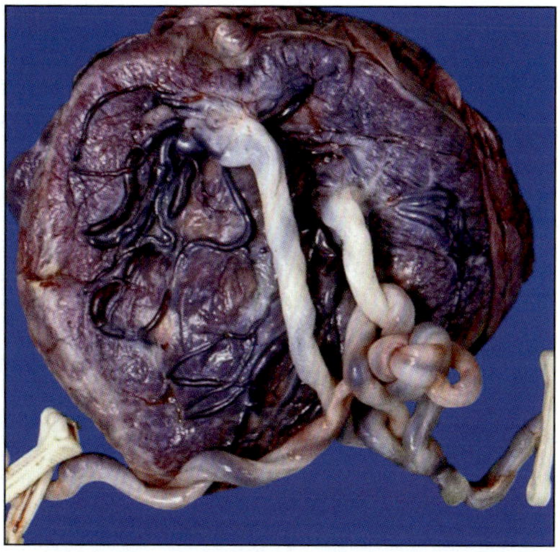

(Left) *Monochorionic monoamniotic (MCMA) twin placentas usually have cord insertions close to one another. The absence of a dividing membrane allows for cord entanglement.* ***(Right)*** *Severe cord entanglement in this MCMA placenta was fortunately associated with a good outcome for both twins.*

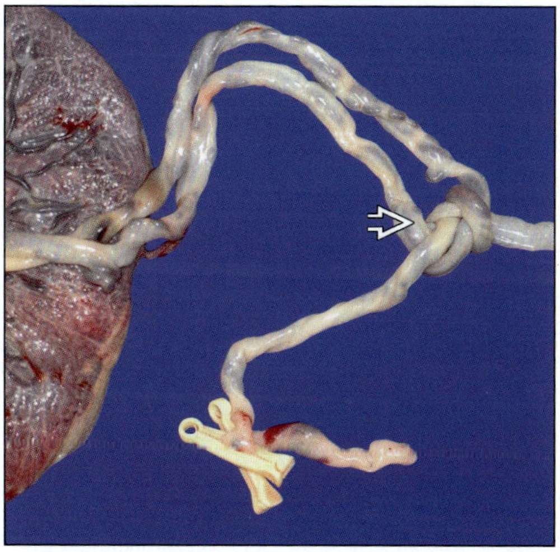

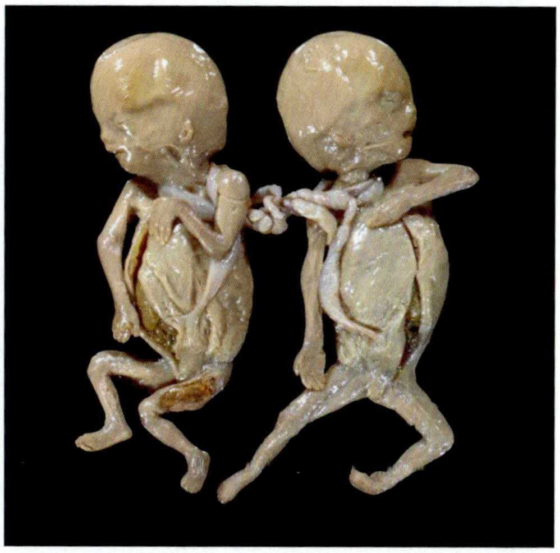

(Left) *A complex knot ⇨ has formed involving the midportions of both cords.* ***(Right)*** *Multiple cord loops around the neck of each fetus with additional entanglements between the 2 cords are the obvious cause of 2nd-trimester fetal loss in this case.*

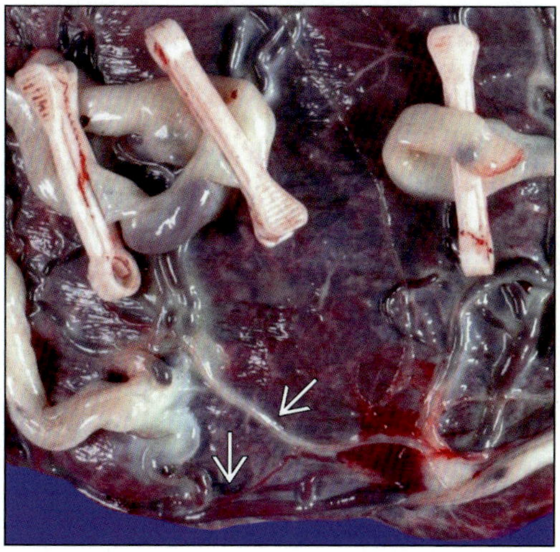

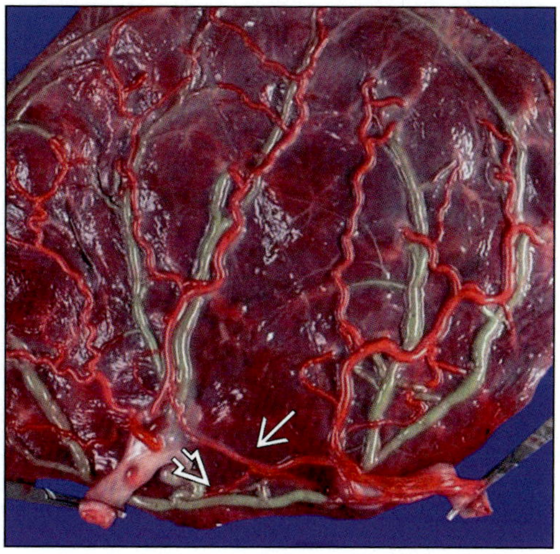

(Left) *Vascular anastomoses are always present in the MCMA placenta. Two superficial anastomoses → are seen in this placenta.* ***(Right)*** *Injection with dyes allows precise description of the various types of anastomoses in the same placenta. The 2 anastomoses are now more clearly identified as artery to artery →, and vein to vein ⇨.*

COMPLICATIONS OF MONOCHORIONIC MONOAMNIOTIC TWIN GESTATIONS

Acardiac Twin

*(**Left**) Gross photo shows a branched umbilical cord. The smaller 2-vessel cords ➔ of the acardiac twin anastomoses with the larger cord of the pump twin. (**Right**) The number of umbilical vessels may vary within the shared umbilical cord. This cord has 3 arteries and 2 veins ➔, consistent with 1 twin having a single umbilical artery.*

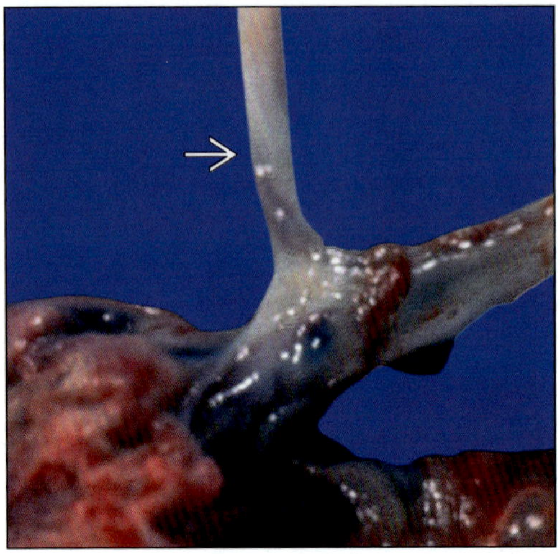

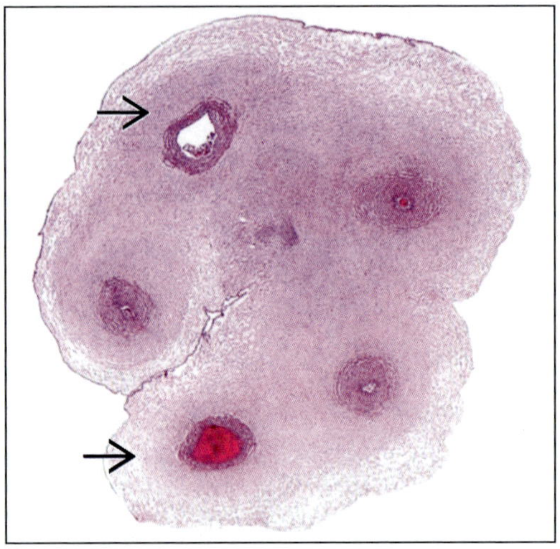

*(**Left**) Acardiac twinning is commonly associated with close approximation of the umbilical cords. There is a large artery to artery anastomosis ➔ noted between the 2 cords. (**Right**) This acardiac/acephalic twin was from a case of twin reversed arterial perfusion (TRAP). In TRAP, the acardiac twin shunts blood from the more normal pump twin. The pump twin dies in 50% of cases. (Courtesy S. Kostadinov, MD.)*

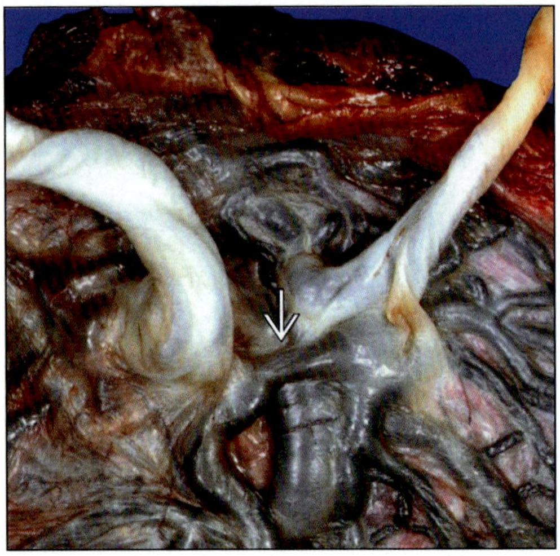

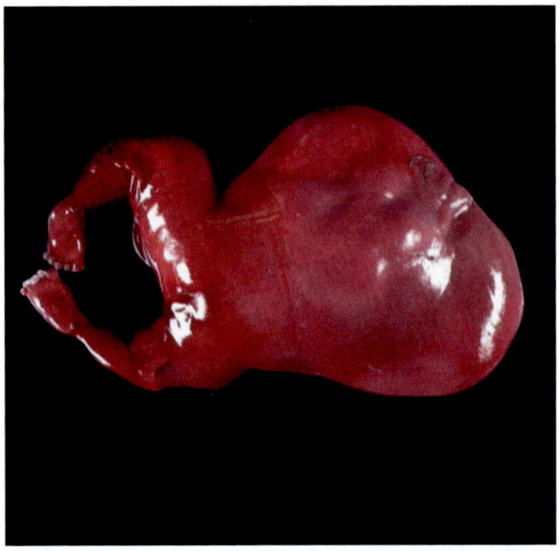

*(**Left**) This acardiac twin demonstrates well-formed lower extremities and relatively normal external male genitalia. There is only 1 rudimentary upper extremity ➔ and no cranial formation. (**Right**) Specimen radiographs help define anatomy of acardiac or conjoined twins to better guide dissection.*

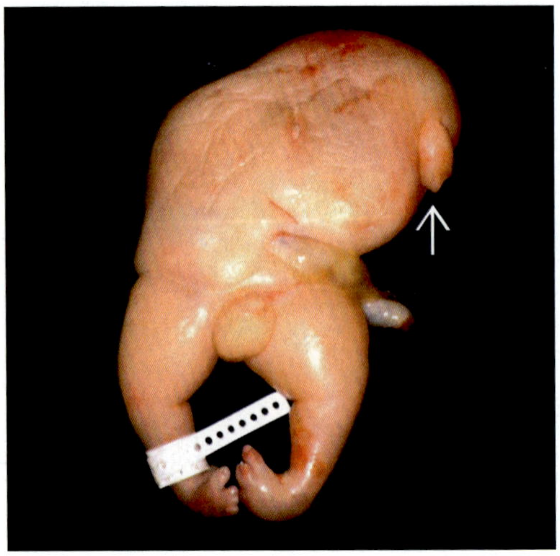

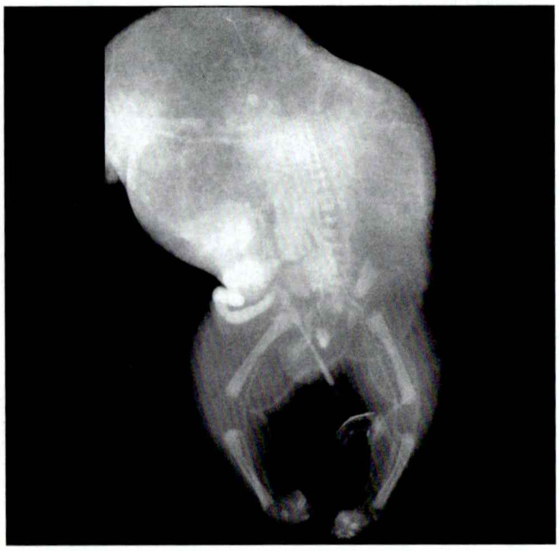

- Upregulation of atrial natriuretic peptide and endothelin-1
  - Cardiovascular anomalies

CLINICAL IMPLICATIONS

Clinical Presentation

- Most clinically relevant during 2nd trimester of pregnancy
- Usually incidental finding during routine ultrasound follow-up of monochorionic pregnancy
  - Oliguric oligohydramnios in 1 twin; polyuric polyhydramnios in other twin
- Less frequent presentations: Uterine distension, contractions, dyspnea

Imaging Findings

- Monochorionic pregnancy
- Oligohydramnios-polyhydramnios
  - Donor twin: Oligohydramnios (deepest vertical pool in amniotic sac ≤ 2 cm)
  - Recipient twin: Polyhydramnios (deepest vertical pool ≥ 8 cm); TTTS-related cardiomyopathy

Staging of TTTS

- Used to determine optimal management strategy
  - Based on ultrasound studies, including Doppler
  - Quintero staging system most widely used
  - Adaptations (e.g., Cincinnati system) include echocardiographic findings

MACROSCOPIC FINDINGS

General Features

- Monochorionic twin placenta: Single disc, thin 2-layered intertwin membrane (amnion only), intertwin vascular communications
- No pathognomonic TTTS features
- Overall: Increased frequency of uneven sharing, peripheral cord insertion, absence of AA anastomoses, and presence of VV anastomoses

Specimen Handling

- Routine examination of twin placenta
- Examination of choriovascular intertwin anastomoses
  - ± dye injection
  - Anatomic hallmarks of choriovasculature
    - Arteries superficial to accompanying veins
    - AA and VV anastomoses superficial and direct
    - AV anastomoses deep and indirect
  - Large AA and VV anastomoses identifiable without injection
- Injection of chorionic vasculature
  - Not routinely indicated for all monochorionic placentas
  - Potential indications
    - Examination of placenta following fetoscopic laser coagulation of TTTS
    - Monochorionic twin pregnancies with atypical course

MICROSCOPIC FINDINGS

General Features

- Poorly described; variable
  - Dependent on timing and degree of syndrome
  - Confounded by perinatal acute twin-twin transfusion
  - Influenced by associated placental anatomic features

DIFFERENTIAL DIAGNOSIS

Discordant Severe Intrauterine Growth Restriction

- Uneven placental sharing
- Peripheral cord insertion

Twin Reversed Arterial Perfusion (TRAP) Sequence

- Acardiac fetus
- Single large AA and VV shunts

Twin Anemia-Polycythemia Sequence (TAPS)

- Large intertwin difference in hemoglobin levels without TOPS
- Spontaneous or after laser coagulation
- AA anastomoses usually absent

Acute Perinatal TTTS

- Clinical presentation highly variable
- Occurs during birth
- Usually large AA &/or VV anastomoses present

DIAGNOSTIC CHECKLIST

Clinically Relevant Pathologic Features

- Relative distribution of placental territory
- Cord insertion types
- Presence/absence of AA and VV anastomoses
  - Description of AV imbalance potentially relevant in absence of AA anastomoses
- Confirmation of chorionicity
- Parenchymal lesions (type and extent)

SELECTED REFERENCES

1. De Paepe ME et al: What-and why-the pathologist should know about twin-to-twin transfusion syndrome. Pediatr Dev Pathol. 16(4):237-51, 2013
2. De Paepe ME et al: Placental markers of twin-to-twin transfusion syndrome in diamniotic-monochorionic twins: A morphometric analysis of deep artery-to-vein anastomoses. Placenta. 31(4):269-76, 2010
3. De Paepe ME et al: Demonstration of placental vascular anatomy in monochorionic twin gestations. Pediatr Dev Pathol. 5(1):37-44, 2002
4. Denbow ML et al: Placental angioarchitecture in monochorionic twin pregnancies: relationship to fetal growth, fetofetal transfusion syndrome, and pregnancy outcome. Am J Obstet Gynecol. 182(2):417-26, 2000
5. Machin G et al: Correlations of placental vascular anatomy and clinical outcomes in 69 monochorionic twin pregnancies. Am J Med Genet. 61(3):229-36, 1996

TWIN-TWIN TRANSFUSION SYNDROME

Gross Features

*(**Left**) In these diamniotic monochorionic twin-twin transfusion syndrome (TTTS) twins at 20 weeks gestation, the recipient twin is shown on the left and the smaller donor twin on the right. (**Right**) This organ overview highlights the striking difference in organ sizes between the twins, particularly affecting the heart and lungs. The organs of the recipient twin are shown on the left.*

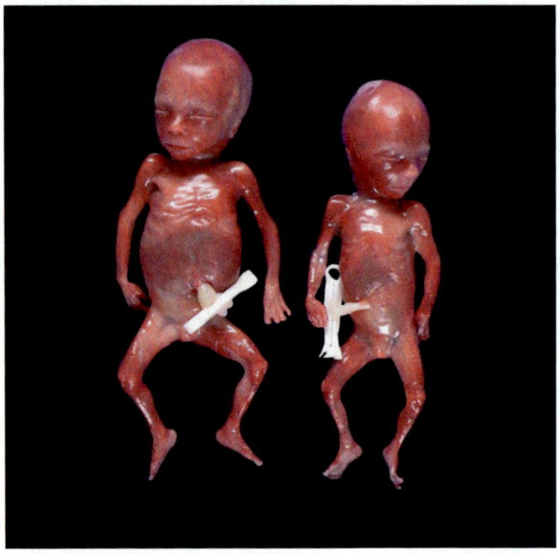

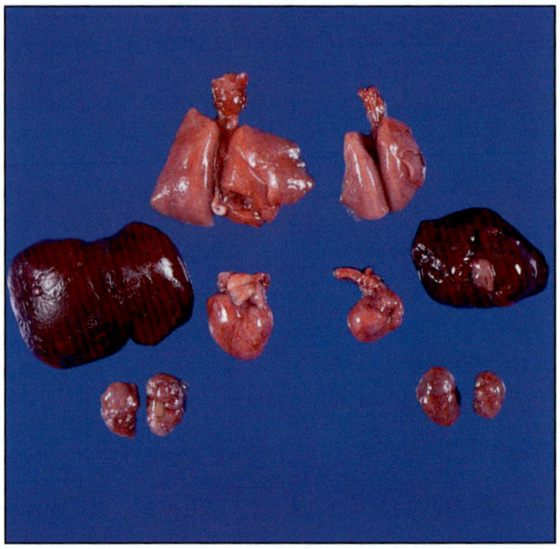

*(**Left**) This diamniotic monochorionic twin placenta from a pregnancy complicated by TTTS shows a thin and velamentously inserted cord of donor twin A, a larger and paracentrally inserted cord of recipient twin B, and uneven sharing of the placental mass. The dividing membrane is shown ⇨. (**Right**) This image shows the same placenta after vascular injection using the following color code: Twin A (donor): Artery is red and vein is yellow; twin B (recipient): Artery is red and vein is green. An artery-to-artery (AA) anastomosis is present ⇨.*

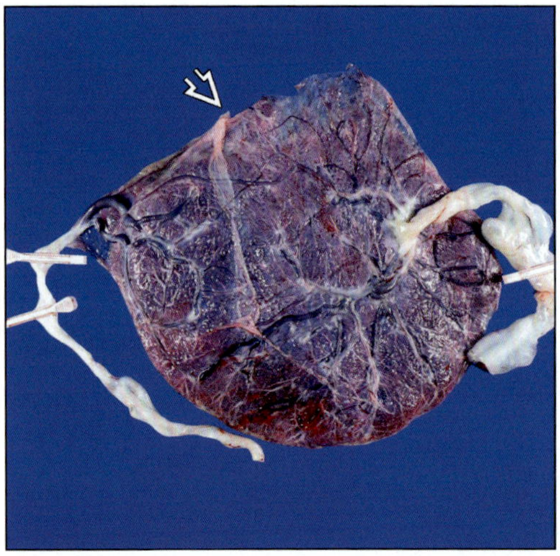

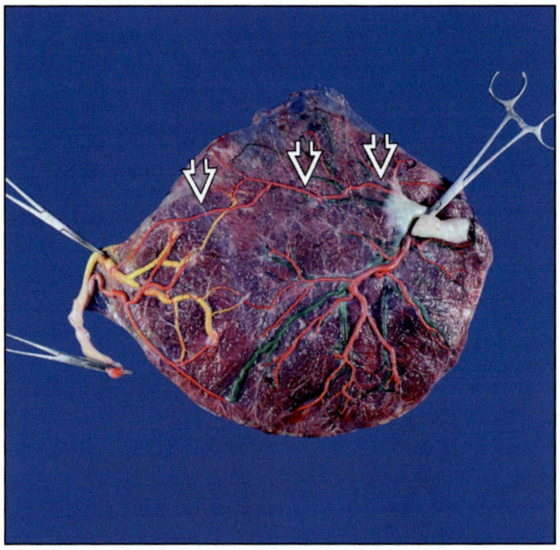

*(**Left**) A closer view of the upper portion of the placenta shows the superficial AA anastomosis ⇨, as well as a deep artery-to-vein (AV) anastomosis from recipient twin B to donor twin A ➡. (**Right**) The lower portion of the placenta displays deep AV anastomoses from twin B to twin A ➡ and a deep AV anastomosis from twin A to twin B ↪.*

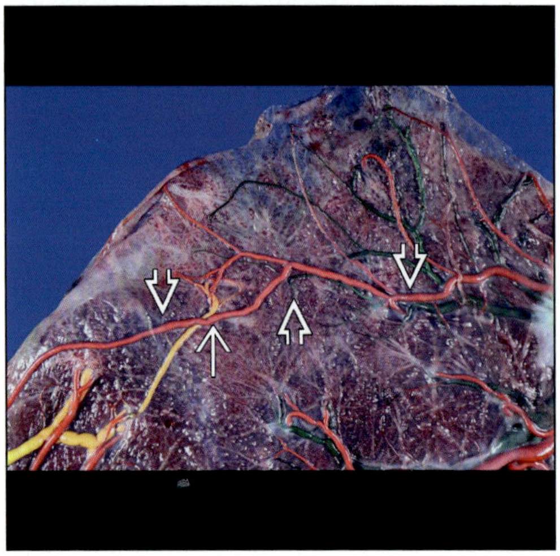

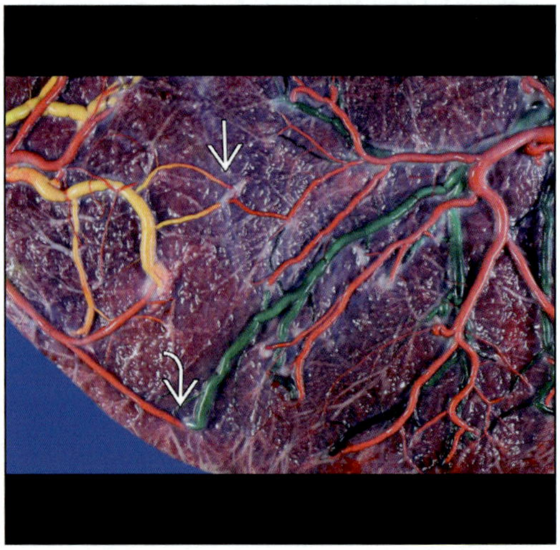

Suggested Microscopic Sections

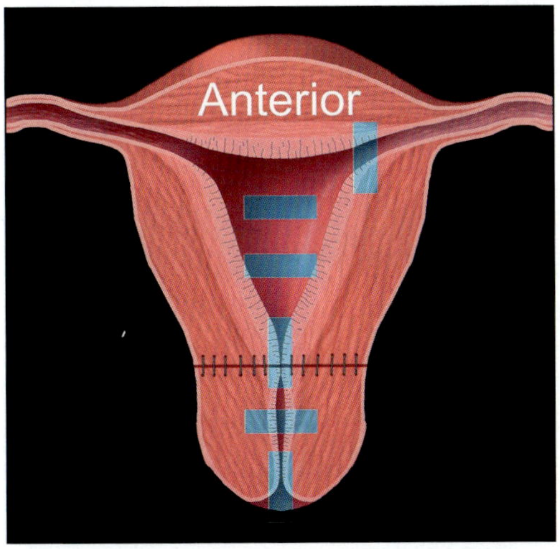

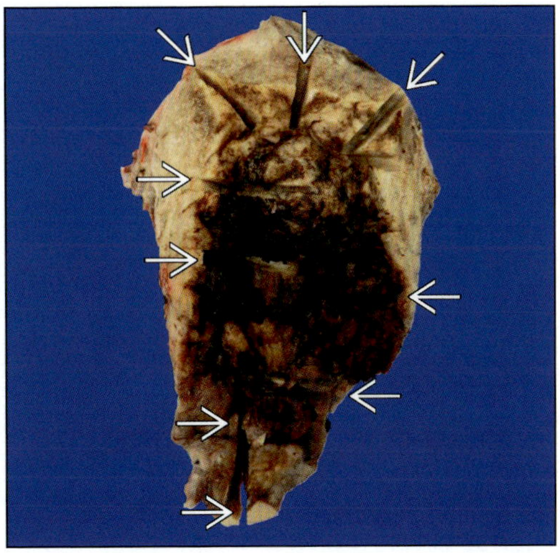

(Left) *This diagram shows suggested sections in blue to assure identification of the implantation site. Sections also include areas with known deficiency of decidualization: Lower uterine segment, current and prior cesarean section incision, and cornua of the fallopian tubes.* ***(Right)*** *This bivalved uterus shows a thick myometrium and adherent blood clot. Sections submitted for microscopic examination were taken at regular intervals to assure identification of the implantation site.*

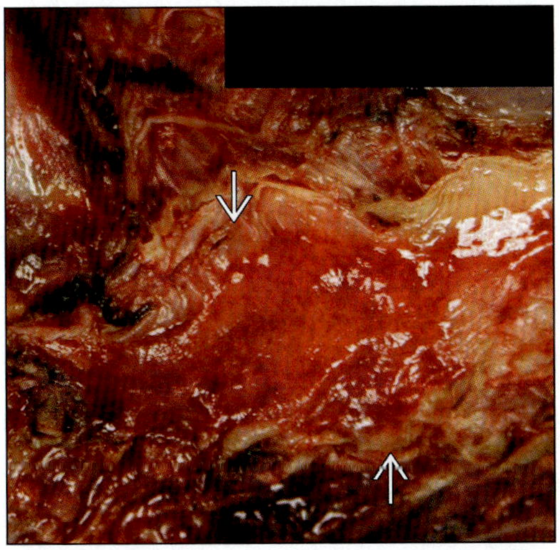

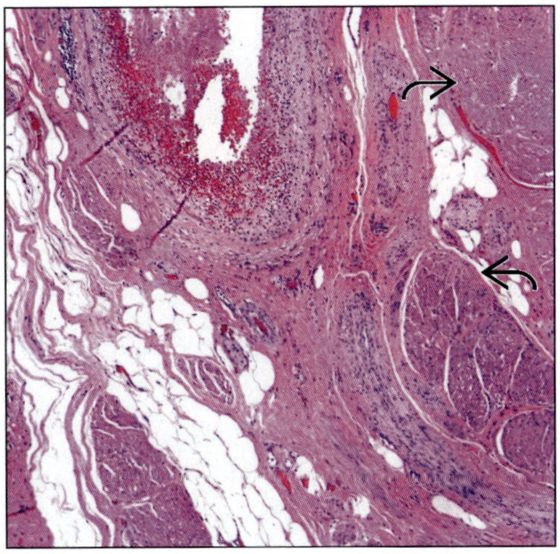

(Left) *The anterior surface of this uterus shows dense adhesions and red urinary bladder mucosa. A small portion of the bladder was removed at the time of hysterectomy due to inability to create a plane between the uterus and bladder.* ***(Right)*** *Dense adhesions on the anterior uterus is a common finding associated with history of previous C-section. This adhesion has a portion of urinary bladder smooth muscle. Bladder mucosa is usually not present.*

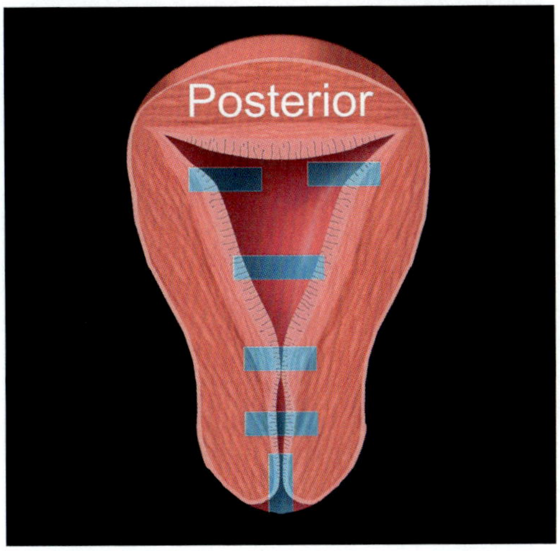

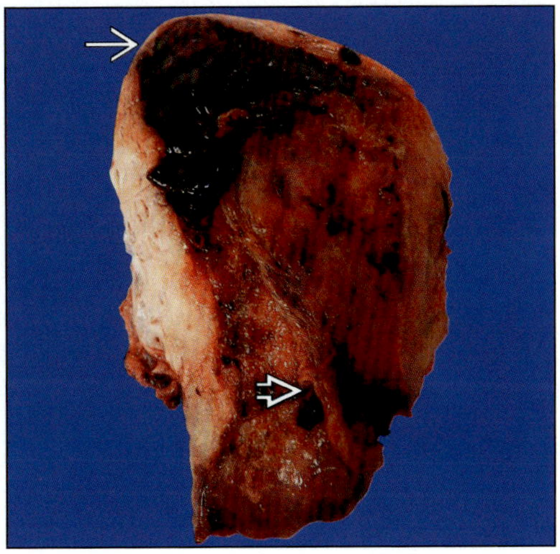

(Left) *The posterior uterus should also be systematically sectioned to identify the placental implantation site. The normal site of placental implantation is fundal and posterior.* ***(Right)*** *This specimen shows cornual placenta accreta with overlying blood clot. Villi are not readily visible. Placental membranes are noted in the mid body. Retained membranes are rarely associated with postpartum bleeding but may be a source of infection.*

Cervical Abnormalities

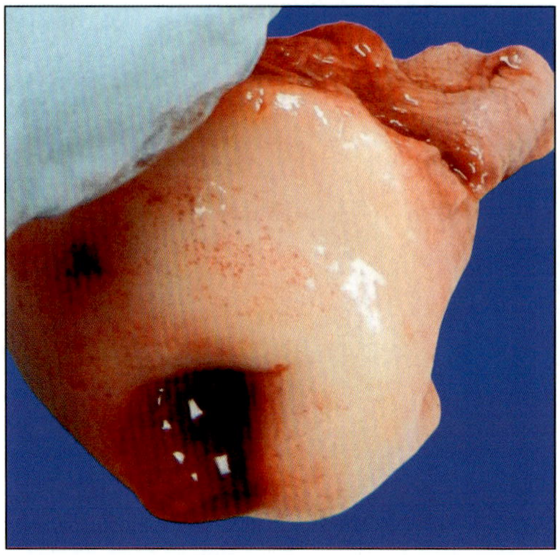
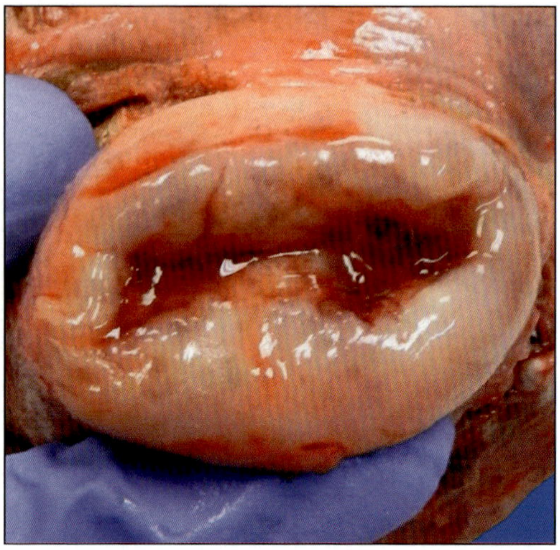

(Left) *This separately submitted cervix shows a round os, consistent with no prior vaginal delivery.* ***(Right)*** *This gaping os is consistent with a parous cervix, but this pregnancy was delivered via cesarean section with a nonlabored cervix.*

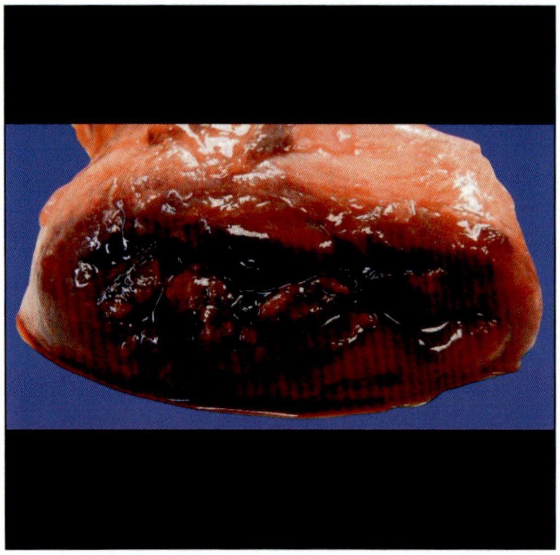
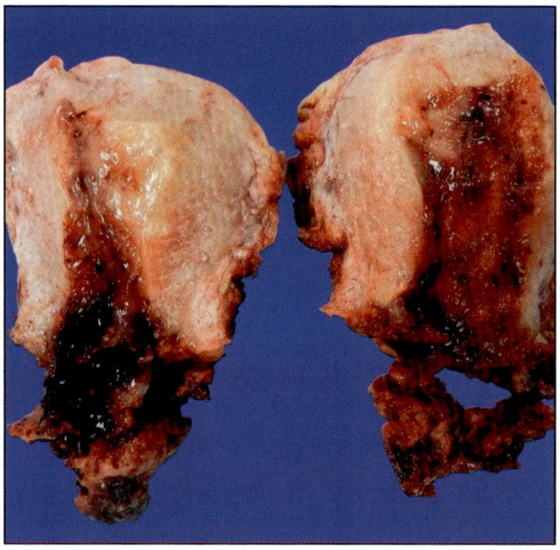

(Left) *This hemorrhagic edematous cervix is from a recent vaginal delivery. A small cervical laceration would be very difficult to identify in this type of specimen.* ***(Right)*** *Extensive disruption of the endocervix was associated with excessive hemorrhage due to a cervical pregnancy in this case.*

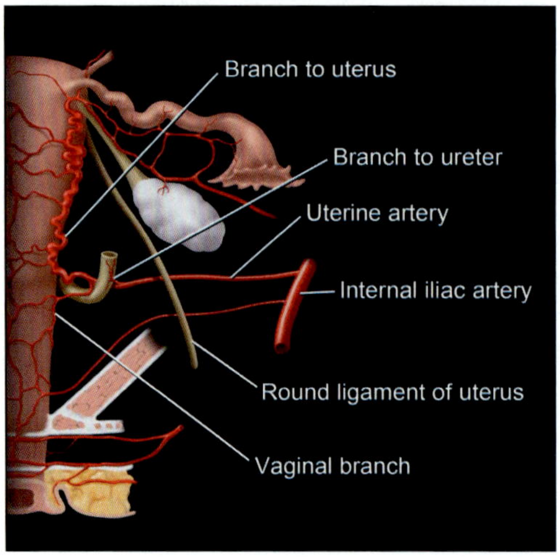

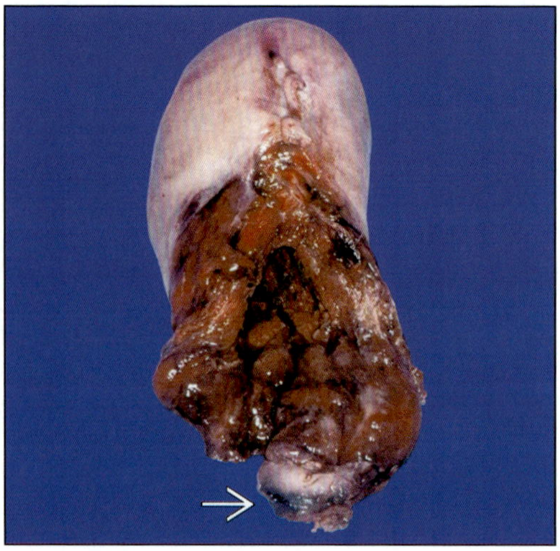

(Left) *This illustration of the cervical and uterine vasculature shows the vulnerability of the lateral lower uterine segment and cervical regions.* ***(Right)*** *This gross photograph shows massive uterine rupture involving the lateral aspect of the lower uterine segment and endocervix. The ectocervix ➔ is partially detached.*

Uterine Atony

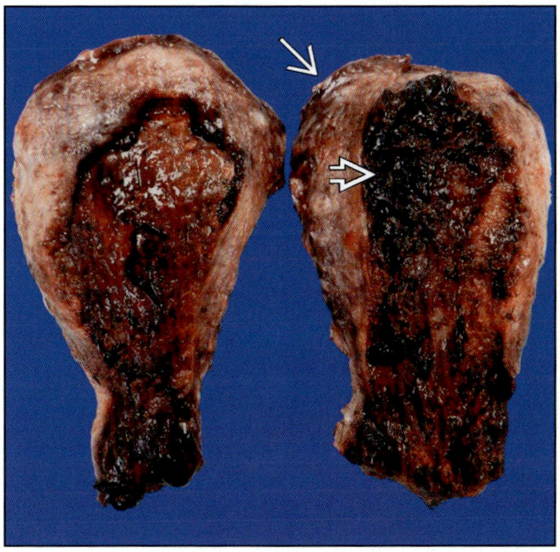

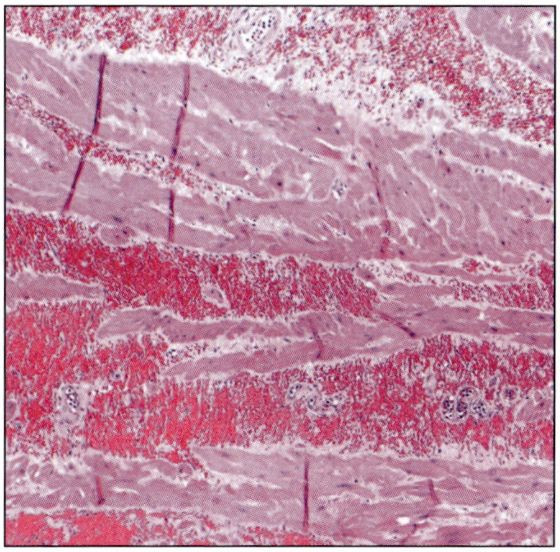

(Left) *This uterine cavity is enlarged with a thin, flabby myometrium, consistent with atony. Early postpartum hemorrhage occurred after acute abruption with fetal demise at 35 weeks and vaginal delivery. The dusky myometrium suggests a Couvelaire uterus (extension of placental abruption hemorrhage to the peritoneum). The implantation site was located beneath the adherent clot.* ***(Right)*** *Extensive acute hemorrhage dissects between myometrial fibers on microscopic exam.*

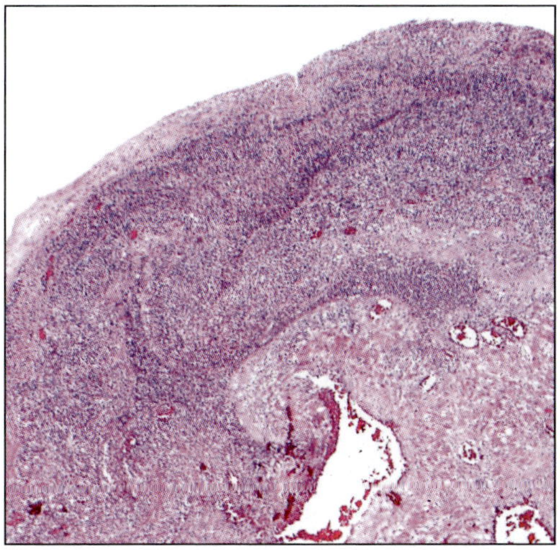

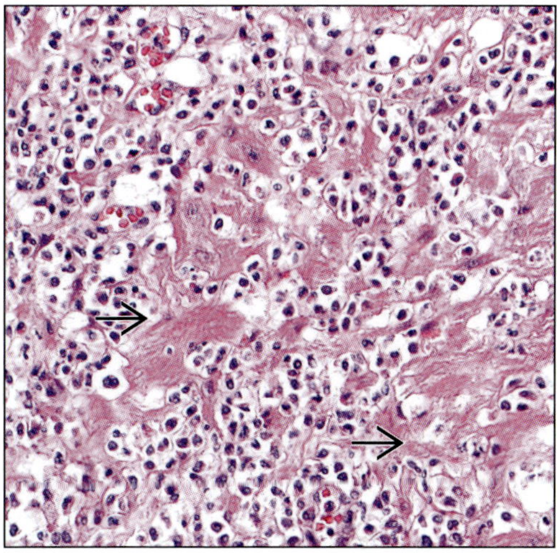

(Left) *This case of uterine atony was associated with severe acute endometritis. The placenta showed severe necrotizing chorioamnionitis.* ***(Right)*** *The same case also had severe acute myometritis. The neutrophils extend deeply into and between the myometrial smooth muscle fibers. Acute chorioamnionitis is associated with dysfunctional uterine contractions and uterine atony, even without such severe inflammation as seen here.*

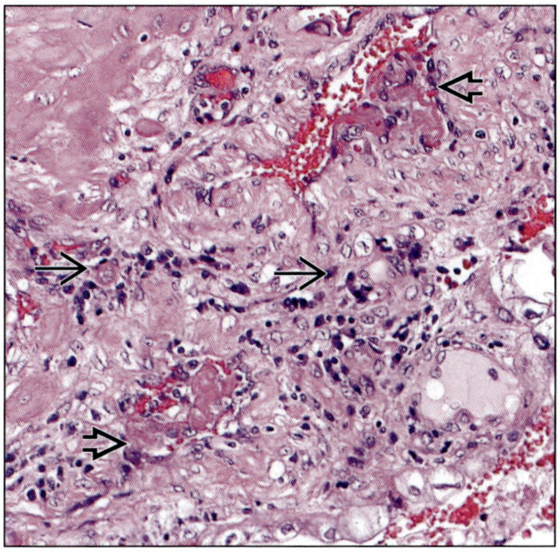

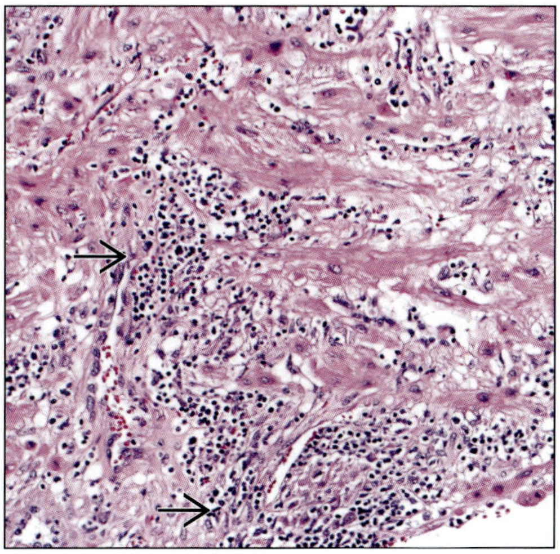

(Left) *Uterine atony may be associated with abnormal chronic inflammation. Within the deep endometrium, there are plasma cells. This is not from the implantation site, as the maternal vessels are not adapted for pregnancy. They contain small fibrin thrombi, suggestive of maternal coagulopathy.* ***(Right)*** *This section is from an atonic peripartum hysterectomy and shows a moderate lymphocytic infiltrate extending into the myometrium.*

POSTPARTUM HEMORRHAGE

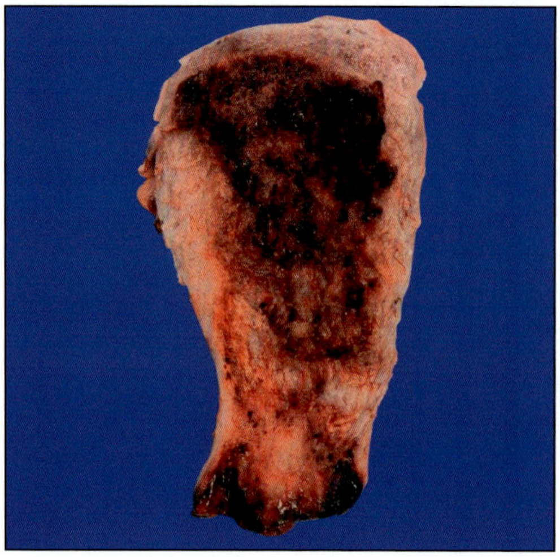

Features of uterine atony are present in this postpartum hysterectomy. The endometrial cavity is large and the myometrium is thin. The cervix shows features of a vaginal delivery.

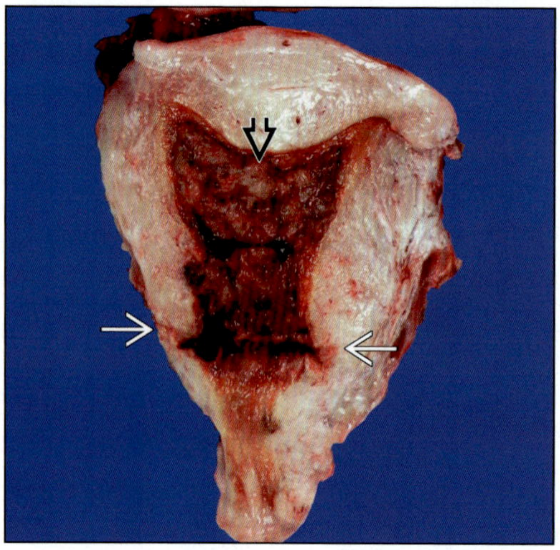

This uterus is a cesarean hysterectomy specimen. The hysterotomy incision ➔ is present in the lower uterine segment. The cervix is unlabored. Lush endometrium ⇨ is present in the fundus.

TERMINOLOGY

Abbreviations

- Postpartum hemorrhage (PPH)

Definitions

- Early PPH occurs in first 24 hours after delivery
  - > 500 mL after vaginal delivery
    - Incidence: 4-8% after vaginal deliveries
    - Bleeding may occur prior to, with, or after delivery of placenta
  - > 1,000 mL after C-section
    - Incidence: 2% after C-section
  - Because amount of bleeding is difficult to estimate, the following have been proposed to indicate PPH
    - Decrease in hematocrit of > 10%
    - Need for red blood cell transfusion
- Late PPH occurs 24 hours to 6 weeks after delivery
- Cesarean hysterectomy is performed at same time as C-section delivery of baby
- Postpartum hysterectomy is performed some time after baby is delivered either vaginally or by C-section

ETIOLOGY/PATHOGENESIS

Early Postpartum Hemorrhage

- Uterine atony accounts for 40-56% of early postpartum hemorrhage
  - Uterine overdistention
    - Multiple gestations, macrosomia, or polyhydramnios
  - Overworked uterus
    - Arrest of dilation or descent &/or prolonged 2nd stage of labor
    - Induction of labor or augmentation with oxytocin
    - Grand multiparity, parity > 7
    - Precipitous delivery
  - Infection
    - Chorioamnionitis results in dysfunctional uterine contractions
  - Relaxed uterus
    - Use of tocolytics, terbutaline, magnesium sulfate, or general anesthesia
  - Other risk factors
    - Prior postpartum hemorrhage
    - Advanced maternal age ≥ 35 years
    - Preeclampsia
    - Abruption
    - Placenta previa
    - Instrumented vaginal delivery
- Genital lacerations account for 20% of early PPH
  - Cervical lacerations often at 3-o'clock and 9-o'clock positions, may extend into cervix from lower uterine segment
  - Risk factors include uncontrolled vaginal delivery, traumatic vaginal delivery with shoulder dystocia, and operative vaginal delivery (vacuum or forceps)
- Uterine rupture, affects 1/1,000-3,000 deliveries
  - May occur prior to onset of labor or during labor and delivery
  - Occurs in scarred and unscarred uteri
    - Highest risk is with previous classical C-section
    - Most common location in scarred uterus is area of previous C-section incision
    - Incidence with trial of labor after C-section: 0.2-0.8%
  - Increased risk with high parity
  - Increased risk with overstimulation with oxytocin
- Uterine inversion, occurs in 1/2,000-2,500 deliveries
  - Accompanied by massive hemorrhage and hypovolemic shock
  - Predisposing factors include: Myometrial weakness, placenta accreta, short umbilical cord, fundal placental implantation, excessive traction on umbilical cord with delivery of placenta, manual removal of placenta
- Bleeding diathesis

POSTPARTUM HEMORRHAGE

Key Facts

Terminology
- Postpartum hemorrhage (PPH)
- Early PPH occurs in first 24 hours after delivery
  - > 500 mL after vaginal delivery
  - > 1,000 mL after C-section
- Late PPH occurs 24 hours to 6 weeks after delivery

Etiology
- Uterine atony
  - Uterine overdistention: Multiples, macrosomia, polyhydramnios
  - Overworked uterus: Prolonged labor, Pitocin, grand multiparity, precipitous delivery
  - Infection: Chorioamnionitis
  - Relaxed uterus: Tocolytics, general anesthesia
- Retained placenta
  - Accessory lobe, bilobate placenta or accreta
- Lacerations: Cervix, vagina, or inner myometrium
  - Instrumented or uncontrolled vaginal delivery
- Uterine rupture
  - Can occur in scarred and unscarred uterus
- Hemorrhagic disorders
  - Thrombocytopenia, disseminated intravascular coagulopathy for any reason
- Late PPH
  - Subinvolution of placental site
  - Placenta accreta
  - Infection
  - Gestational trophoblastic disease

- Thrombocytopenia: Pregnancy induced or idiopathic thrombocytopenia purpura
- Inherited coagulopathy such as hemophilia A, von Willebrand disease
- Coagulopathy associated with hypertensive disorders such as preeclampsia, HELLP syndrome
- Disseminated intravascular coagulopathy, associations include
  - Hypofibrinogenemia with retention of dead fetus (usually for > 4 weeks, does not occur with death of only 1 twin)
  - Amniotic fluid embolus syndrome, usually with rapid or tumultuous labor, sudden onset of shortness of breath
  - Abruption, especially with large retroplacental hematoma

Early or Late Postpartum Hemorrhage
- Retained placenta: Accounts for 10% of PPH
  - Accessory lobe or bilobate placenta with a portion left behind
  - Placenta adherens (failed contraction of myometrium behind a portion of placenta)
  - Trapped placenta (detached placenta trapped behind closed cervix)
  - May form polypoid endometrial mass (placental polyp)
- Placenta accreta: Accounts for 20-64% of hemorrhage
  - Increasing incidence in past few years as incidence of C-section has increased
    - 35% risk with prior C-section and placenta previa
    - 18-60% risk with prior uterine curettage
  - Increased risk with history of manual placental removal or prior retained placenta
  - Marked risk with pregnancy after endometrial ablation

Late Postpartum Hemorrhage
- Subinvolution of placental site
  - Most commonly occurs 2nd week post partum
  - May occur alone or be associated with retained placenta or infection
  - Implantation site vessels remain adapted for pregnancy without reversion to nonpregnant state
  - Placental site nodule is a related phenomenon with persistence of implantation site trophoblast, but usually presents with later dysfunctional uterine bleeding that occurs later than subinvolution
- Infectious endometritis
- Dehiscence of C-section scar
- Leiomyoma
- Gestational trophoblastic disease

CLINICAL ISSUES

Presentation
- Sudden massive hemorrhage
- Constant seepage
  - Postpartum uterus may hold up to 1,000 mL of blood
- Hemoperitoneum

Treatment
- Surgical approaches
  - Direct uterine massage or bimanual compression
  - Uterine or vaginal packing or use of balloon tamponade
  - Curettage to remove any placental fragments
  - B-Lynch compression sutures
  - Ligation of internal iliac arteries (hypogastric) and uterine arteries
  - Endovascular therapy, such as embolization or balloon occlusion
  - Hysterectomy
- Drugs
  - Uterotonics; oxytocics (Cytotec, Hemabate), Methergine

Prognosis
- Postpartum hemorrhage is 1 of top 5 causes of maternal mortality
  - Placenta accreta has 4-6% maternal mortality

- Uterine rupture is associated with maternal morbidity
  - High fetal morbidity and 50-70% fetal mortality
- Amniotic fluid embolus is associated with high maternal and fetal mortality
- Uterine inversion is associated with 13-41% maternal morbidity and mortality
  - Symptoms of shock far exceed amount of blood loss

MACROSCOPIC FEATURES

General Features

- Uterine atony
  - Boggy uterus, large endometrial cavity, may be isolated to lower uterine segment, generalized thin myometrium
- Placenta accreta
  - Uterus may be boggy or contracted
  - Accreta may be grossly visible, but is usually microscopic, with exception of planned hysterectomy for placenta accreta
- Abruption
  - Couvelaire uterus with extension of blood into myometrium, visible through serosa
  - Retroplacental hematoma
- Infection
  - Generally appears atonic; prior placenta may have shown chorioamnionitis
  - Late PPH due to infection may be associated with myometrial abscess or necrosis
- Uterine inversion
  - Endometrial surface extends out through cervix
- Subinvolution of maternal spiral arteries
  - Uterus is usually boggy with large thrombosed vessels visible on cut surface beneath endometrium

MICROSCOPIC PATHOLOGY

Histologic Features

- Uterine atony
  - Variable pathology
    - Acute endomyometritis, usually associated with chorioamnionitis
    - Microscopic placenta accreta
    - Focal smooth muscle injury that is not due to delayed fixation of specimen
    - Chronic endomyometritis
    - Fibrinoid necrosis of maternal vessels in implantation site with perivascular lymphocytes
- Placenta accreta
  - Villi adjacent to myometrium without intervening decidua
  - Must identify placental implantation site, which may need to be extensively sampled
  - Very difficult diagnosis to make on curettage samples
- Abruption
  - May have significant bleeding into myometrium, extending to serosal surface (Couvelaire uterus)
  - Retained retroplacental hematoma may result in hypofibrinogenemia
- Subinvolution of maternal spiral arteries
  - Normal involution occurs with a proliferation of fibroblast that initially obliterates vessel lumen; vessel then becomes reendothelialized with patent lumen and reformation of smooth muscle
  - Subinvolution is associated with large, patent vessels, and containing variably aged thrombi
    - Abnormal vessels may be adjacent to normally involuted vessels
  - Bcl-2, an oncoprotein that inhibits apoptosis, is increased in subinvoluting vessels
  - Retained placenta will also result in some degree of subinvolution of maternal vessels
- Amniotic fluid embolus
  - Amniotic fluid debris within small vessels and capillaries of lungs
  - Amniotic fluid debris in vessels in cervix and lower uterine segment

SELECTED REFERENCES

1. Mousa HA et al: Treatment for primary postpartum haemorrhage. Cochrane Database Syst Rev. 2:CD003249, 2014
2. Roux I et al: Pregnancy after endometrial ablation. A report of three cases. J Reprod Med. 58(3-4):173-6, 2013
3. Sellmyer MA et al: Physiologic, histologic, and imaging features of retained products of conception. Radiographics. 33(3):781-96, 2013
4. Bateman BT et al: The epidemiology of postpartum hemorrhage in a large, nationwide sample of deliveries. Anesth Analg. 110(5):1368-73, 2010
5. Weeks AD: The retained placenta. Best Pract Res Clin Obstet Gynaecol. 22(6):1103-17, 2008
6. Oyelese Y et al: Placenta previa, placenta accreta, and vasa previa. Obstet Gynecol. 107(4):927-41, 2006
7. Weydert JA et al: Subinvolution of the placental site as an anatomic cause of postpartum uterine bleeding: a review. Arch Pathol Lab Med. 130(10):1538-42, 2006
8. Keski-Nisula LT et al: Myometrial inflammation in human delivery and its association with labor and infection. Am J Clin Pathol. 120(2):217-24, 2003
9. Khong TY et al: Bcl-2 expression delays postpartum involution of pregnancy-induced vascular changes in the human placental bed. Int J Gynecol Pathol. 16(2):138-42, 1997
10. Khong TY et al: Delayed postpartum hemorrhage: a morphologic study of causes and their relation to other pregnancy disorders. Obstet Gynecol. 82(1):17-22, 1993

Placenta Previa and Abruption

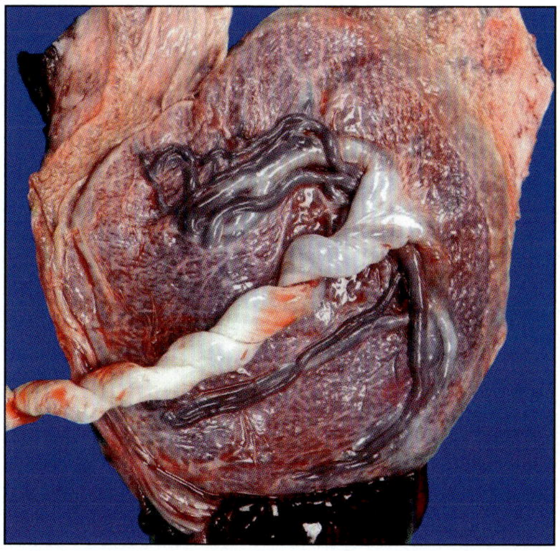
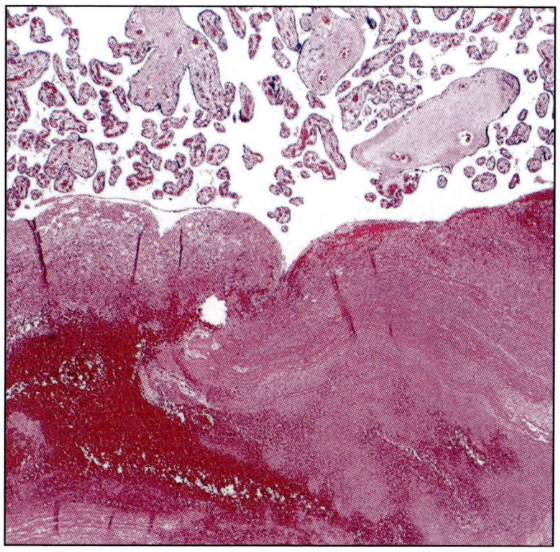

(Left) *Placenta previa may grossly be associated with a large, marginal hematoma that may be acute, as seen here. Usually, there will be a combination of recent and remote hemorrhage.* ***(Right)*** *Most often, the portion of placenta over the cervix in placenta previa is associated with microscopic evidence of remote marginal hemorrhage.*

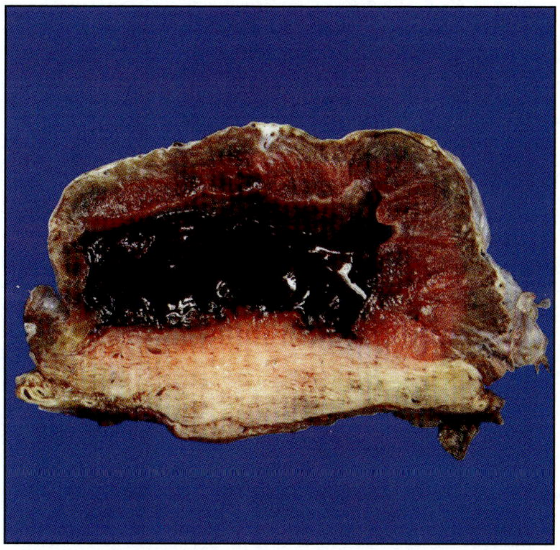
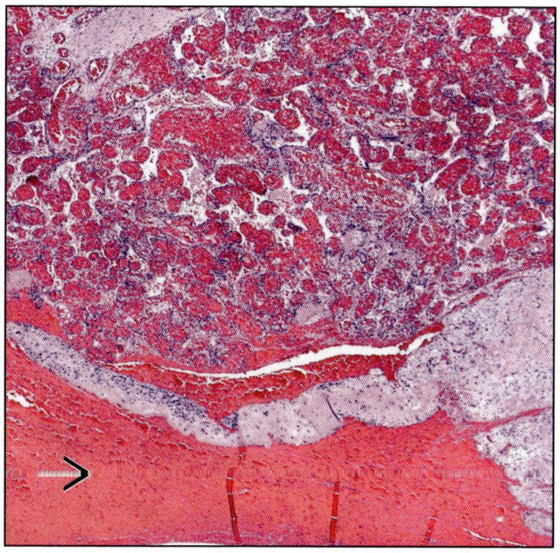

(Left) *In situ placental abruption is present in this cesarean hysterectomy. The patient presented with preterm labor and known placenta accreta.* ***(Right)*** *Acute placental abruption may be associated with a retroplacental hematoma* ⇒ *and villous stromal hemorrhage.*

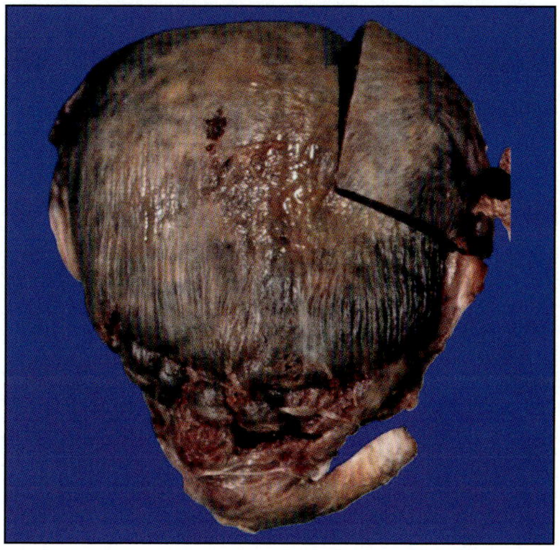
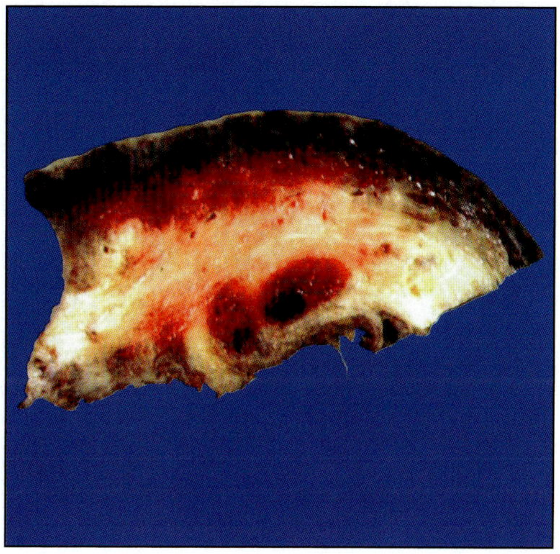

(Left) *This is a Couvelaire uterus with a large amount of blood evident beneath the serosal surface. "Couvelaire" refers to the extension of blood from placental abruption through the myometrium to the serosa.* ***(Right)*** *The cut surface of the Couvelaire uterus has extensive hemorrhage, mostly noted beneath the serosal surface.*

Early Postpartum Hemorrhage

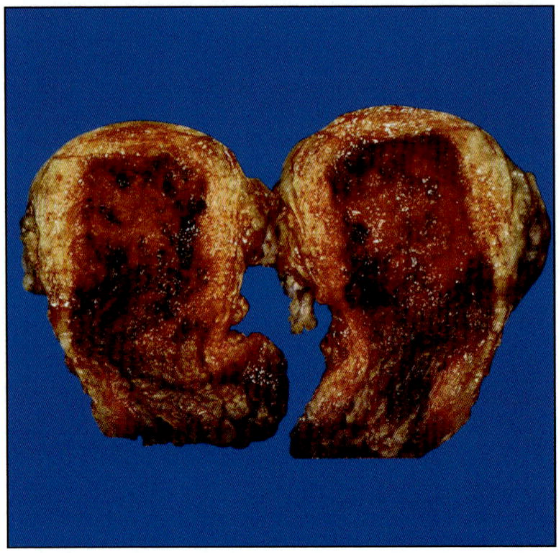

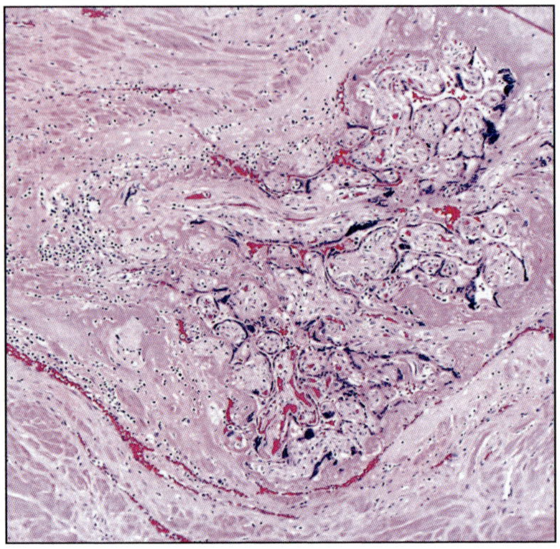

(Left) *Uterine atony after a term vaginal delivery typically shows a large endometrial cavity, thin myometrium, and no grossly evident residual placental tissue in the uterus.* ***(Right)*** *Placenta accreta associated with uterine atony may be microscopic, necessitating extensive sectioning of the placental implantation site.*

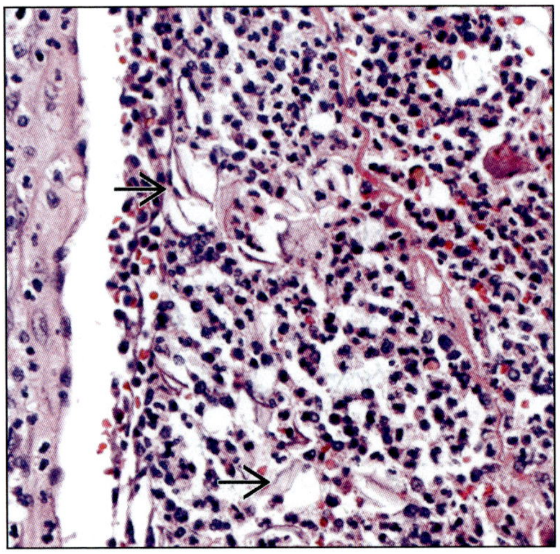

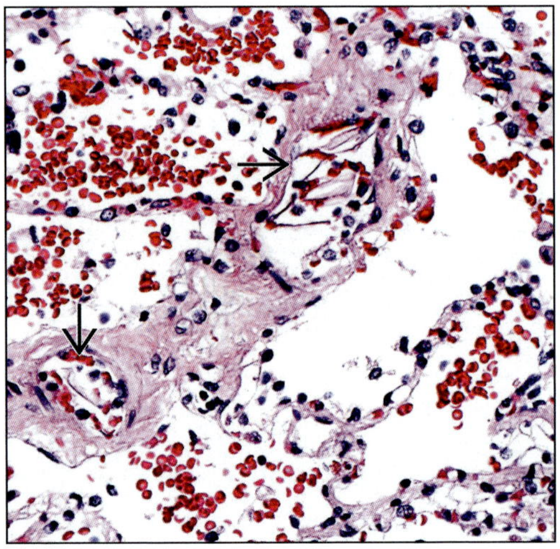

(Left) *This is a section of a uterine vessel from the cervical region of a postpartum hysterectomy specimen. The lumen contains abundant acute inflammation and squamous epithelial cells → that are presumed to be of fetal origin.* ***(Right)*** *This lung section shows fetal squamous cells → within small vessels, diagnostic of amniotic fluid embolus. Just as in the uterine cervix, there may be a large number of inflammatory cells, particularly eosinophils, associated with the emboli.*

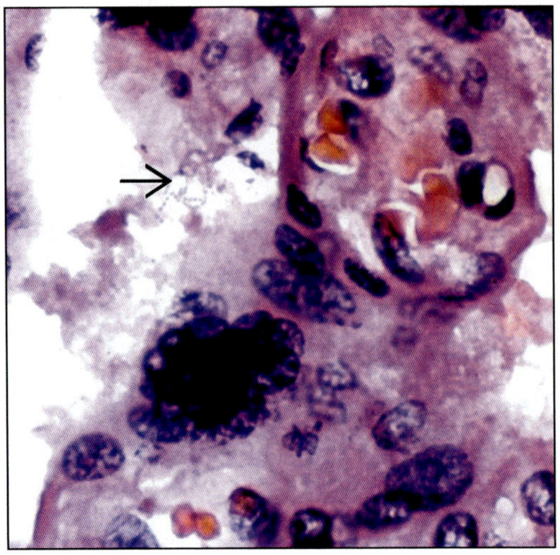

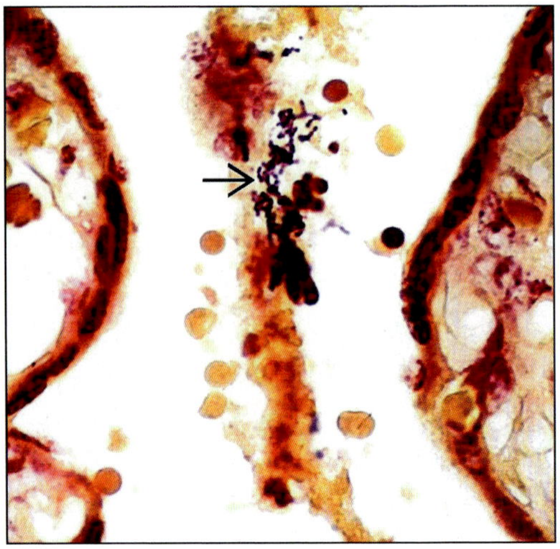

(Left) *Maternal shock and hemorrhage may rarely be associated with maternal sepsis. Rare cocci in chains → are present within the maternal intervillous space, without a significant inflammatory reaction.* ***(Right)*** *Gram stain highlights the large number of gram-positive cocci → within the maternal intervillous space. The organism identified by culture was group A Streptococcus.*

Late Postpartum Hemorrhage

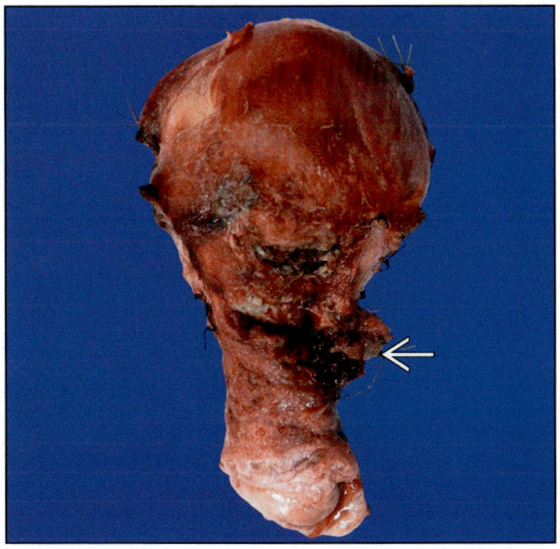

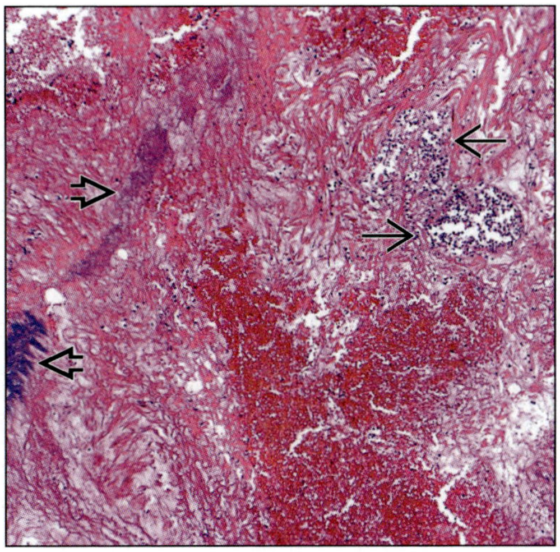

*(**Left**) Postpartum hysterectomy was performed several days after C-section. Large defect in anterior uterus is seen in the area of previous hysterectomy ➔. There was severe acute chorioamnionitis within the previously delivered placenta. (**Right**) This section shows acute endomyometritis with large aggregates of neutrophils ➔ and clouds of coccoid bacteria ⇨. The organism in this instance was group A Streptococcus, which is also associated with necrotizing fascitis.*

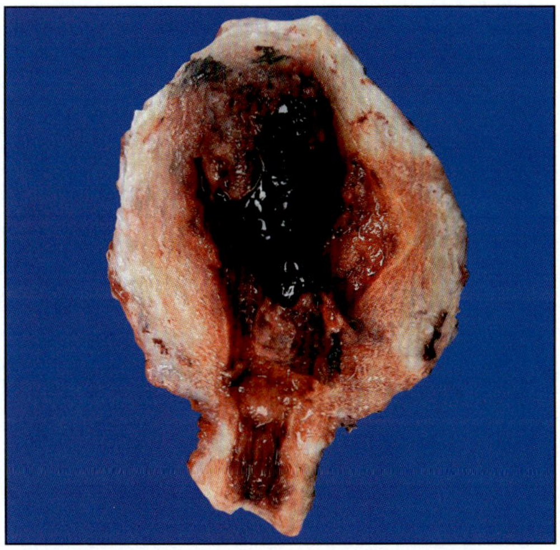

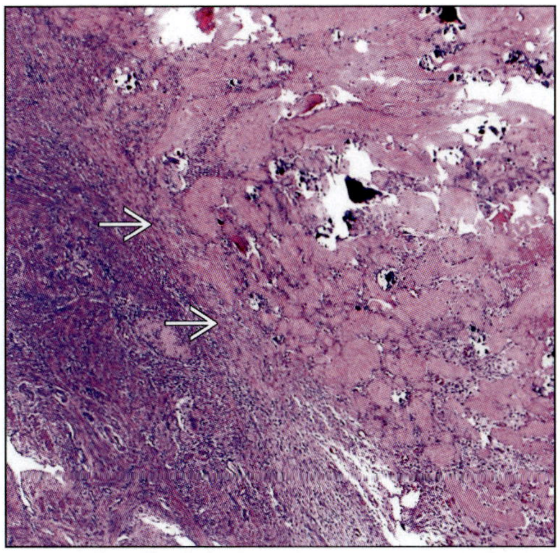

*(**Left**) This hysterectomy was performed for delayed postpartum hemorrhage. The specimen shows a large blood clot in the region of the uterine cornu. (**Right**) The cornua of the uterus and fallopian tubes is an area with deficient decidua and is prone to abnormal implantation. This image shows placenta accreta, with fibrotic villi ➔ adjacent to the myometrium.*

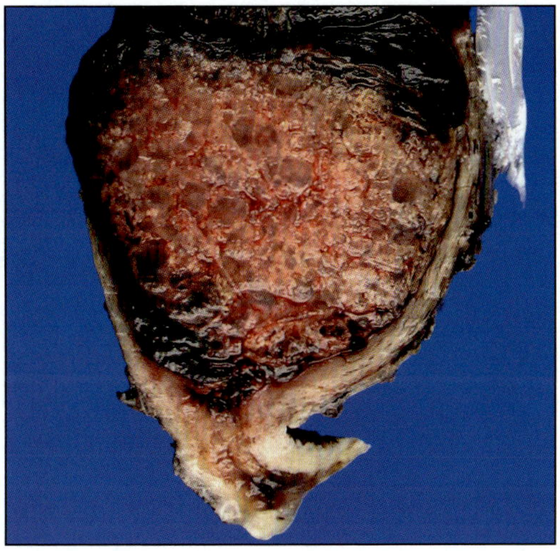

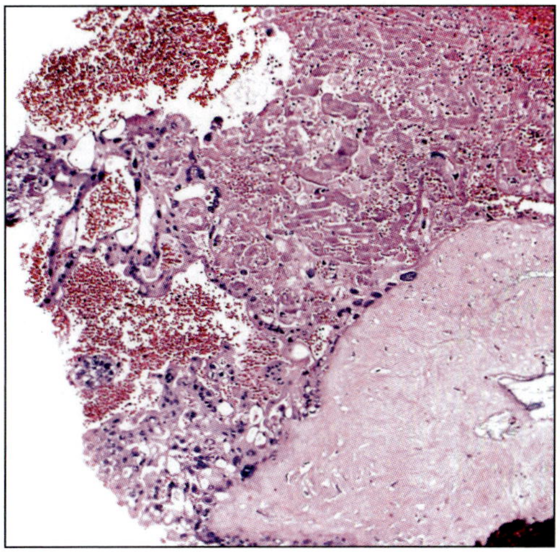

*(**Left**) Postpartum hemorrhage may rarely be due to complete mole, as seen here. The implantation site of the complete mole is prone to extensive hemorrhage. (**Right**) The rare residual villus with atypical trophoblast proliferation after evacuation of complete hydatidiform mole may also be associated with hemorrhage.*

POSTPARTUM HEMORRHAGE

Subinvolution of Maternal Arteries

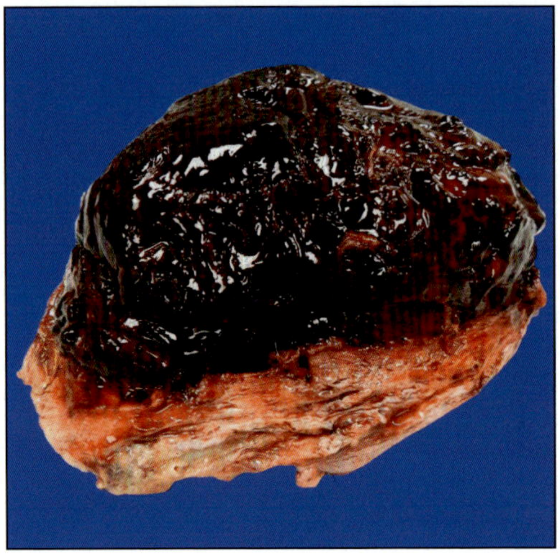

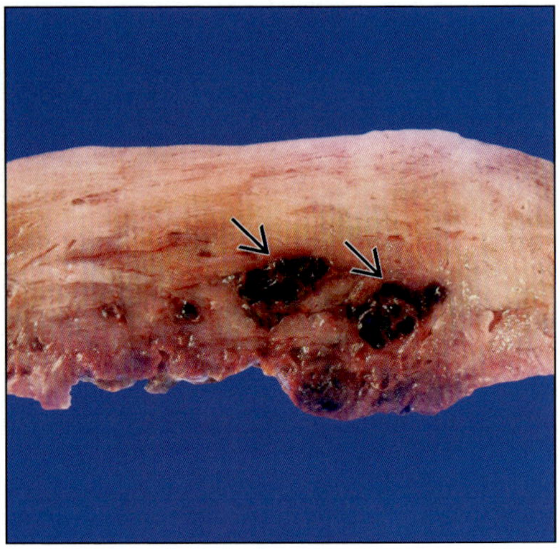

(Left) *This hysterectomy was done 5 weeks after a preterm vaginal delivery. The mother presented with sudden, massive uterine bleeding. The clot within the uterus was nearly 500 g.* ***(Right)*** *This section of the uterus shows large thrombosed myometrial vessels → in a case of delayed involution of the placental site. The maternal vasculature remains adapted for pregnancy with enlarged lumina and persistence of trophoblast-associated remodeling changes.*

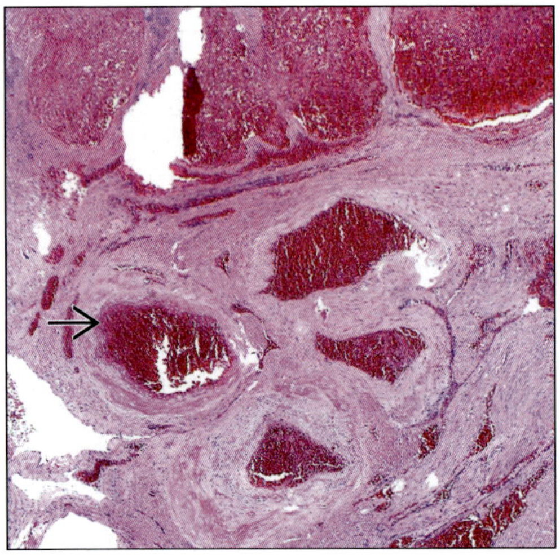

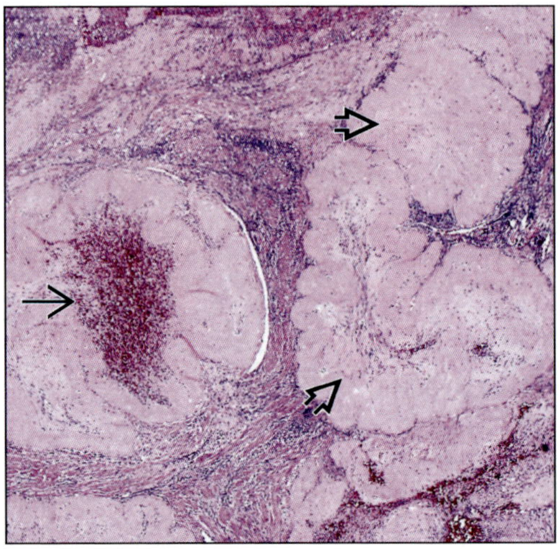

(Left) *The maternal spiral arteries → shown here have no involutional changes. They remain dilated with fibrin in the walls instead of vascular smooth muscle.* ***(Right)*** *This image shows delayed involution of 1 vessel →, immediately adjacent to involuted vessels with fibroblast proliferation ⇨. The vessels are surrounded by fibrinoid and a few invasive trophoblasts, consistent with the recent pregnancy.*

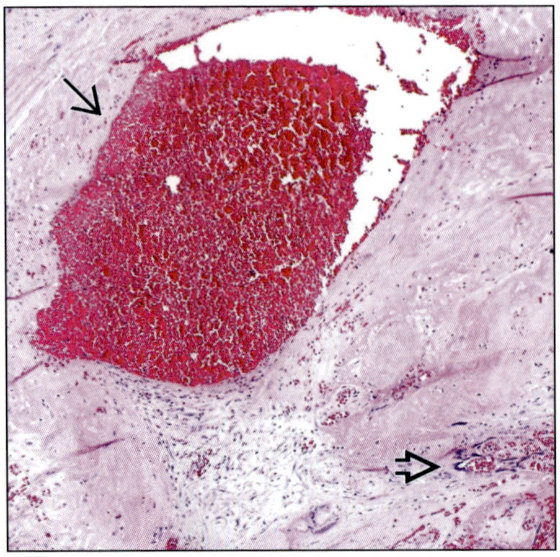

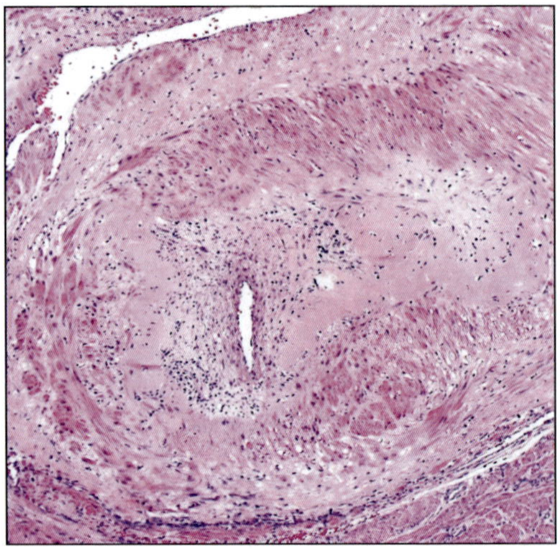

(Left) *This patient presented with uterine bleeding 5 weeks post partum. There is subinvolution of this maternal vessel →. Immediately adjacent, there are rare intravascular chorionic villi ⇨. The etiology of hemorrhage is more likely due to delayed involution rather than the very rare residual villus.* ***(Right)*** *This spiral artery shows near complete involution at 10 weeks post partum, with reformation of the vascular smooth muscle peripherally and centrally around a lumen.*

Postpartum Bleeding

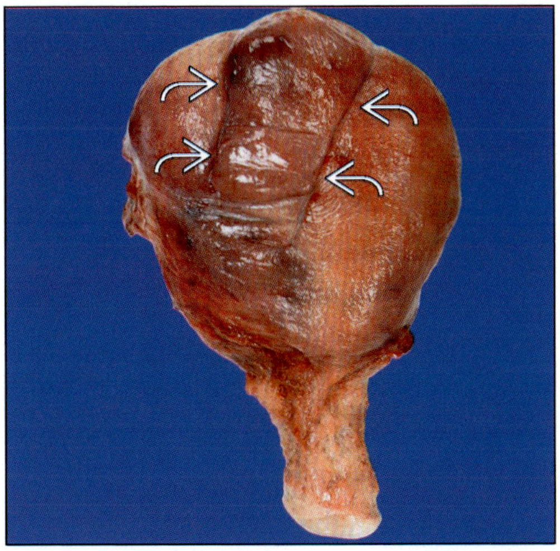

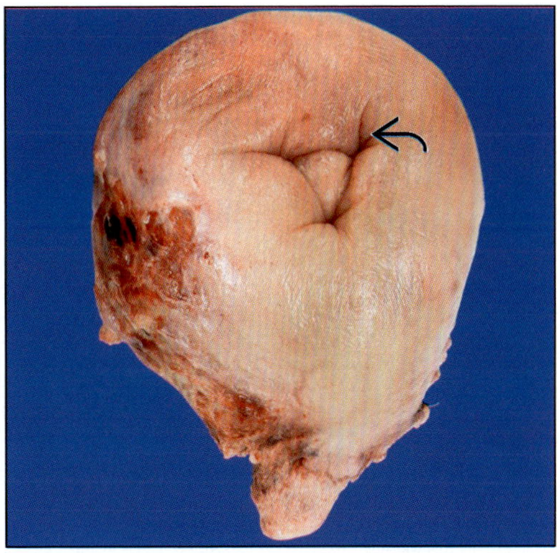

(Left) *Classic B-Lynch compression sutures ➩ are placed in the uterus in an attempt to reduce postpartum hemorrhage and prevent the need to perform a hysterectomy.* ***(Right)*** *Sutures ➩ were placed through the uterus in an alternative fashion in an attempt to stop postpartum hemorrhage.*

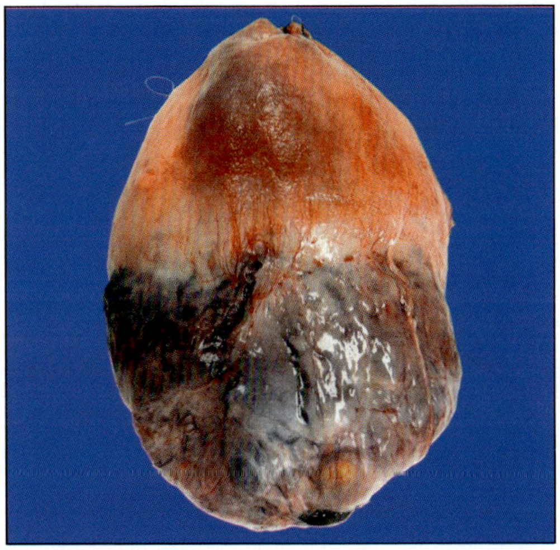

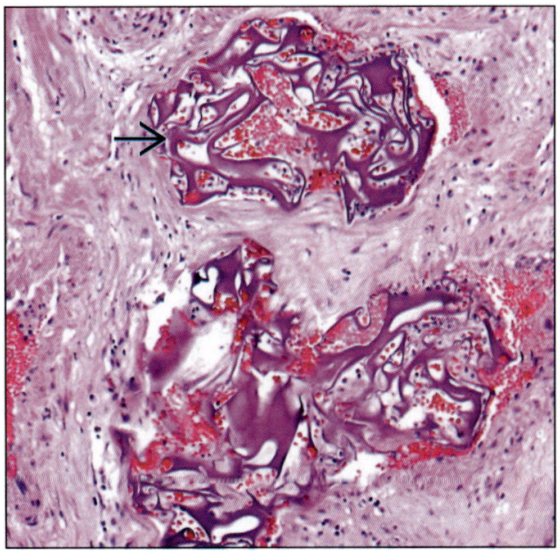

(Left) *The severity of placenta percreta in this case was evident at the time of delivery. In order to prevent excessive blood loss, Gelfoam embolization of maternal vessels was performed to reduce blood loss during the hysterectomy.* ***(Right)*** *This is the microscopic appearance of Gelfoam ➙ in uterine vessels.*

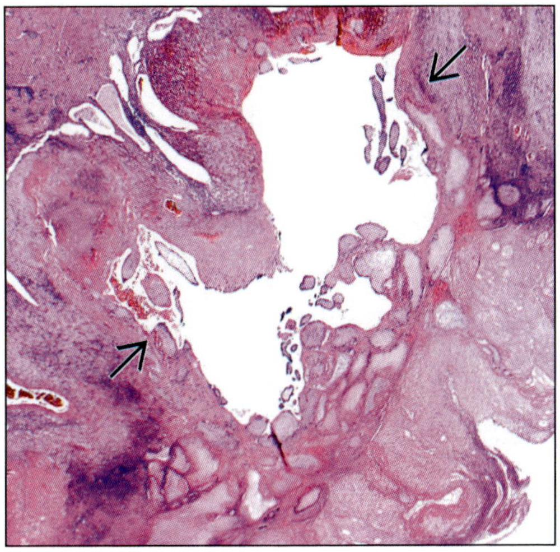

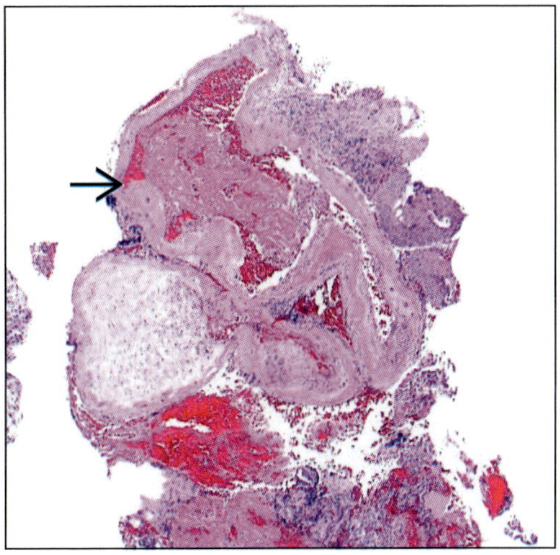

(Left) *The pathology of dysfunctional uterine bleeding can be similar to postpartum hemorrhage, with retention of products of conception, sometimes not clinically recognized. This case was found to be secondary to a retained empty gestational sac ➙.* ***(Right)*** *Dysfunctional bleeding was present 3 months post dilation and curettage for spontaneous abortion in this case. A repeat curettage shows enlarged residual maternal vessels ➙, which have failed to involute.*

Reference Charts for Placental Evaluation

WEIGHTS FOR SINGLETON PLACENTAS

Reference Weights for Trimmed Singleton Placentas

Gestational Age (Weeks)	10th Percentile	25th Percentile	Mean	75th Percentile	90th Percentile	Fetal:Placental Weight Ratio
21	114	128	143	158	172	2.54
22	122	138	157	175	191	2.78
23	120	152	181	220	260	2.96
24	129	153	197	228	280	3.11
25	142	169	200	242	270	3.28
26	160	184	212	260	300	3.47
27	154	186	225	280	330	3.72
28	210	238	270	302	331	3.97
29	229	259	293	327	357	4.19
30	249	281	316	352	384	4.38
31	269	303	340	377	411	4.58
32	290	325	364	403	438	4.78
33	311	347	387	428	464	4.97
34	331	369	411	453	493	5.28
35	352	391	434	477	516	5.56
36	372	412	457	501	542	5.81
37	391	432	478	524	566	6.04
38	409	452	499	547	589	6.37
39	426	470	519	567	611	6.65
40	442	487	537	587	632	7.23
41	456	502	553	605	651	

Formalin fixation may increase weight by 5-8% and prolonged refrigeration may decrease weight. Although large series provide untrimmed weights from delivery room, significant variation in amount of adherent blood, length of cord received, etc. make untrimmed weights a less reliable method for evaluation of placentas submitted to pathology. Weights are trimmed weights from fresh placentas. Placentas comprising the data for ages 23-27 weeks (Hecht et al) were selected from premature births with normal fetal growth (i.e., cases with fetal birth < 2 standard deviations below the mean were excluded). The placentas from the excluded cases in general showed features of uteroplacental malperfusion. Placentas comprising the data for gestational ages 21-22 weeks and 28-41 weeks were characterized as uncomplicated deliveries, excluding cases with intrauterine growth restriction, prolonged rupture of membranes, amniotic fluid infection sequence (chorioamnionitis), pregnancy-induced hypertension, infarcts, perivillous fibrin deposition, or thrombi. Data is derived from Hecht JL et al: Reference weights for placentas delivered before the 28th week of gestation. Placenta. 28(10):987-90, 2007 and Pinar H et al: Reference values for singleton and twin placental weights. Pediatr Pathol Lab Med. 16(6):901-7, 1996. Fetal:placental weight ratio is from Kalousek DK et al: Pathology of the human embryo and previable fetus: an atlas. New York: Springer, 1990.

WEIGHTS FOR TWIN PLACENTAS

Reference Weights for Trimmed Twin Placentas

Gestational Age (Weeks)	10th Percentile	25th Percentile	Mean	75th Percentile	90th Percentile
19	161	185	212	239	263
20	166	190	218	245	270
21	176	202	231	260	286
22	191	219	251	282	310
23	210	241	276	311	343
23 unfused	79	99	143	160	220
24	232	267	307	346	382
24 unfused	115	131	171	190	280
25	257	297	341	386	426
25 unfused	117	140	179	203	250
26	284	330	380	430	475
26 unfused	133	160	197	242	260
27	314	365	421	478	528
27 unfused	160	181	222	245	282
28	345	401	464	527	584
29	377	439	509	579	641
30	409	478	554	631	700
31	441	516	600	683	758
32	472	554	644	734	815
33	503	590	687	783	870
34	531	624	727	830	923
35	558	656	764	873	971
36	582	684	798	912	1014
37	602	708	827	945	1051
38	619	728	850	972	1082
39	631	743	868	993	1105
40	639	753	879	1005	1118
41	642	756	882	1009	1123

All data is from unfixed, trimmed placental discs (after cord and membranes have been trimmed away). Majority of data is from "normal" twin placentas, free of common placental pathologies (Pinar et al 1996). For each gestational age, these data encompass combined weight of dichorionic placentas with separate discs, weight of dichorionic fused placental discs, and monochorionic twin placentas. Data is supplemented with unfused placenta weights from Hecht et al (2007). "Unfused" weights refer to weights of individual dichorionic twin placental discs. Hecht data was normalized by inclusion of infants with birth weight Z scores between -2 and 2. From Hecht JL et al: Reference weights for placentas delivered before the 28th week of gestation. Placenta. 28(10):987-90, 2007 and Pinar H et al: Reference values for singleton and twin placental weights. Pediatr Pathol Lab Med. 16(6):901-7, 1996

WEIGHTS FOR TRIPLET PLACENTAS

Reference Weights for Trimmed Triplet Placentas

Gestational Age (Weeks)	90th Percentile	Mean	10th Percentile
20	285	253	226
21	320	284	257
22	345	319	289
23	400	361	331
24	445	406	371
25	498	456	408
26	558	509	444
27	630	564	480
28	697	621	516
29	772	673	553
30	849	738	591
31	925	797	631
32	1,000	855	674
33	1,072	911	719
34	1,139	965	768
35	1,200	1,017	821
36	1,297	1,108	940
37	1,330	1,147	1,007

The weights for each gestational age include trichorionic separate discs weighed in aggregate, trichorionic fused, as well as all combinations of dichorionic fusion or monochorionicity for the respective triplet placentas. From Pinar H et al: Triplet placentas: reference values for weights. Pediatr Dev Pathol. 5(5):495-8, 2002.

REFERENCE VALUES FOR FETAL AND PLACENTAL GROWTH IN EARLY PREGNANCY

Reference Values for Fetal and Placental Growth From 8-20 Weeks Gestation

Postmenstrual Gestational Age	Mean Placental Weight (g) (95% CI)	Mean Umbilical Cord Length (mm)	Fetal Crown Rump Length (mm)	Fetal Foot Length (mm) ± SD	Fetal:Placental Weight Ratio
8	1.6 (0.0-3.7)	20	14	4	0.18
9	15.2 (13.3-17)	33	20	5	0.25
10	28.8 (27.2-30.4)	55	26	6	0.38
11	42.4 (41.1-43.8)	92	33	7	0.58
12	56.1 (54.8-57.3)	126	40	9	0.65
13	69.7 (68.4-71)	158	48	12 +/- 2	0.72
14	83.3 (81.8-84.8)	188	56	17 +/- 3	0.73
15	96.9 (95.2-98.6)	215	65	19 +/- 1	0.80
16	110.5 (108.5-112.5)	240	75	22 +/- 2	1.0
17	124.2 (121.8-126.5)	264	88	25 +/- 3	1.29
18	137.8 (135.0-140.5)	287	99	28 +/- 2	1.63
19	101	309	112	29 +/- 4	1.78
20	112	330	125	33 +/- 2	2.23

CI = confidence interval; SD = standard deviation. Placental weight data for 19 and 20 weeks gestation are from a separate reference; note that mean placental weight is smaller than one would expect from weeks 8-18. Foot length can be used to assess fetal growth in disrupted fetuses. Data for umbilical cord length are derived from ultrasonographic studies (Weissman A et al: Sonographic measurements of the umbilical cord and vessels during normal pregnancies. J Ultrasound Med. 13(1):11-4, 1994). Other data is derived from Kalousek DK et al: Pathology of the human embryo and previable fetus: an atlas. New York: Springer, 1990; Boyd J et al: The Human Placenta. Cambridge: Heffer & Sons, 1970; Streeter CL: Weight, sitting height, head size, foot length and menstrual age of the human embryo. Carnegie Inst. Contrib. Embryol. 11:144, 1920.

D

INDEX

E

INDEX

INDEX

G

H

INDEX

I

INDEX

K

L

INDEX

M

INDEX

N

O

P

INDEX

INDEX

R

INDEX

INDEX

INDEX

INDEX

W

X

Z